Feline Emergency and Critical Care Medicine

Feline Emergency and Critical Care Medicine

Edited by

Kenneth J. Drobatz

Merilee F. Costello

Hillsborough Community
College LRC

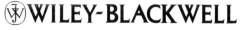 **WILEY-BLACKWELL**

A John Wiley & Sons, Inc., Publication

Edition first published 2010
© 2010 Blackwell Publishing Ltd.

Blackwell Publishing was acquired by John Wiley & Sons in February 2007. Blackwell's publishing program has been merged with Wiley's global Scientific, Technical, and Medical business to form Wiley-Blackwell.

Editorial Office
2121 State Avenue, Ames, Iowa 50014-8300, USA

For details of our global editorial offices, for customer services, and for information about how to apply for permission to reuse the copyright material in this book, please see our website at www.wiley.com/wiley-blackwell.

Library of Congress Cataloging-in-Publication Data

Feline emergency and critical care medicine / edited by Kenneth J. Drobatz, Merilee F. Costello.
    p. ; cm.
  Includes bibliographical references and index.
  ISBN 978-0-8138-2311-9 (pbk. : alk. paper)   1. Cats–Wounds and injuries–Treatment–Handbooks, manuals, etc.
2. Cats–Diseases–Treatment–Handbooks, manuals, etc.   3. Veterinary emergencies–Handbooks, manuals, etc.
4. Veterinary critical care–Handbooks, manuals, etc.   I. Drobatz, Kenneth J.   II. Costello, Merilee F.
  [DNLM: 1. Cat Diseases–therapy.   2. Critical Care–methods.   3. Emergencies–veterinary.   4. Emergency
Treatment–veterinary.   SF 985 F3142 2010]
  SF985.F415 2010
  636.8'0896025–dc22

                                                          2009049306

A catalog record for this book is available from the U.S. Library of Congress.

Set in 9 on 11.5 pt Sabon by Toppan Best-set Premedia Limited
Printed in Singapore by Markono Print Media Pte Ltd

2 2011

Dedications

To Lita, my wife, my best friend, and the best move I have EVER made!

Kenneth J. Drobatz

To Amy and Evie for all the love and joy you bring me every day
To my mother for always believing in me
To all the students, interns, residents, and nurses I have worked with—thank you for all you have taught me

Merilee F. Costello

Contents

Contributors

Jill L. Abraham, VMD, DACVD
Massachusetts Veterinary Referral Hospital
20 Cabot Road
Woburn, MA 01801

Amy J. Alwood, DVM, DACVECC
Critical Care Specialist
Monroeville, PA

Matthew W. Beal, DVM Diplomate ACVECC
Associate Professor, Emergency and Critical Care
  Medicine
Director of Interventional Radiology Services
College of Veterinary Medicine
Michigan State University
East Lansing, MI 48824-1314

Elise Mittleman Boller, DVM, DACVECC
Staff Veterinarian, Intensive Care Unit
Department of Clinical Studies
College of Veterinary Medicine
University of Pennsylvania
Philadelphia, PA 19104

Manuel Boller, Dr. Med. Vet., DACVECC
Senior Research Investigator, Critical Care
Department of Clinical Studies
School of Veterinary Medicine
3900 Delancey Street
Philadelphia, PA 19104

Benjamin M. Brainard, VMD, DACVA,
  DACVECC, Assistant Professor
Department of Small Animal Medicine and
  Surgery
College of Veterinary Medicine
University of Georgia
Athens, GA

Andrew J. Brown, MA, VetMB, DACVECC,
  MRCVS
Assistant Professor
Department of Small Animal Clinical Sciences
College of Veterinary Medicine
Michigan State University
East Lansing, MI

Jamie M. Burkitt, DVM, Dipl. ACVECC
Critical Consultations
Davis, CA 95616

Daniel L. Chan, DVM, DACVECC, DACVN,
  MRCVS
Lecturer in Emergency and Critical Care
Clinical Nutritionist, Nutrition Support Service
Department of Veterinary Clinical Sciences
Royal Veterinary College
University of London
North Mymms
Hertfordshire, AL9 7TA
United Kingdom

Anne Marie Corrigan, DVM, MS, DACVIM
Associate Professor
Small Animal Medicine and Surgery
St. George's University
Grenada, West Indies

Merilee F. Costello
Critical Care Specialist
Allegheny Veterinary Emergency Trauma and
  Specialty
Department of Critical Care
Monroeville, PA

Armelle deLaforcade, DVM, DACVECC
Assistant Professor
Department of Clinical Sciences
Cummings School of Veterinary Medicine
Tufts University
North Grafton, MA

Kenneth J. Drobatz , DVM, MSCE, DACVIIM,
    DACVECC
Professor and Chief, Section of Critical Care
Director, Emergency Service
Department of Clinical Studies—Philadelphia
University of Pennsylvania
School of Veterinary Medicine
Philadelphia, PA

Daniel J. Fletcher, PhD, DVM, DACVECC
Assistant Professor of Emergency and
    Critical Care
Cornell University Hospital for Animals

Susan G. Hackner, BVSc, MRCVS, DACVIM,
    DACVECC
Veterinary Specialty Consulting
New York, NY

Daniel Z. Hume
Staff Veterinarian, Emergency Services
Diplomate of American College of Veterinary
    Internal Medicine—Small Animal
Diplomate of American College of Veterinary
    Emergency and Critical Care
Matthew J. Ryan Veterinary Hospital at the
    University of Pennsylvania
3900 Delancey, Room #2018
Philadelphia, PA

L. Ari Jutkowitz, VMD, Dipl. ACVECC
Assistant Professor, Emergency and Critical Care
College of Veterinary Medicine
Michigan State University
East Lansing, MI 48824-1314

Lesley G. King, MVB, DACVECC, DACVIM
Professor, Section of Critical Care
Department of Clinical Studies
School of Veterinary Medicine
University of Pennsylvania
Philadelphia, PA

Lynne I. Kushner DVM, DACVA
1858 Huron Ave.
Roseville, MN 55113

Cathy Langston
Head of Nephrology, Urology, and Hemodialysis
    Unit
Animal Medical Center
510 E. 62nd Street
New York, NY

Douglass K. Macintire, DVM, MS
Professor
Department of Clinical Sciences
College of Veterinary Medicine
Auburn University
Auburn, AL 36849

Annie Malouin, DVM, DACVECC
Emergency and Critical Care Services
VCA Sacramento Veterinary Referral Center
Sacramento, California

Deborah C. Mandell, VMD, DACVECC
Staff Veterinarian, Emergency Medicine
Adjunct Assistant Professor
Section of Critical Care
Matthew J. Ryan Veterinary Hospital of the
    University of Pennsylvania
Philadelphia, PA

Linda G. Martin, DVM, MS, DACVECC
Assistant Professor, Small Animal Emergency and
    Critical Care
Department of Clinical Sciences
College of Veterinary Medicine
Auburn University
Auburn, AL

Maureen McMichael, DVM, DACVECC
Associate Professor
Section Chief SA Emergency and Critical Care
Director SA Medicine and Surgery Internship
    Program
Director Small Animal Blood Bank
Department of Veterinary Clinical Medicine
University of Illinois at Urbana-Champaign
1008 West Hazelwood Drive
Urbana, IL 61802

Mark A. Oyama, DVM, DACVIM-Cardiology
Associate Professor
Department of Clinical Studies—Philadelphia
School of Veterinary Medicine
University of Pennsylvania
3900 Delancey St.
Philadelphia, PA 19104

Garret Pachtinger, VMD
Veterinary Specialty and Emergency Center
1900 W. Old Lincoln Hwy.
Langhorne, PA

April Paul, DVM, DACVECC
Critical Care Specialist
Tufts VETS
Department of Emergency and Critical Care
Walpole, MA

Robert H. Poppenga, DVM, PhD, Dipl ABVT
Professor of Clinical and Diagnostic Toxicology
Head, Section of Toxicology
California Animal Health and Food Safety
   Laboratory
School of Veterinary Medicine
University of California–Davis
Davis, CA

Jennifer E. Prittie, DVM, ACVIM, ACVECC
Staff Criticalist
Department of Emergency and Critical Care
Animal Medical Center
New York, NY

Erica L. Reineke, VMD, DACVECC
Assistant Professor, Emergency and Critical Care
   Medicine
Department of Clinical Studies–Philadelphia
University of Pennsylvania
School of Veterinary Medicine
3900 Delancey Street
Philadelphia, PA 19104

Elizabeth Rozanski, DVM, DACVIM, DACVECC
Department of Clinical Sciences
Cummings School of Veterinary Medicine
Tufts University
North Grafton, MA

Deborah Silverstein, DVM, DACVECC
Assistant Professor of Critical Care
3850 Delancey Street
Matthew J. Ryan Veterinary Hospital at the
   University of Pennsylvania
Philadelphia, PA 19104-6010

Meg M. Sleeper, VMD
Associate Professor of Cardiology
Department of Clinical Studies
School of Veterinary Medicine
University of Pennsylvania
Philadelphia, PA

Sean D. Smarick, VMD, DACVECC
Director
Allegheny Veterinary Emergency Trauma and
   Specialty
Monroeville, PA

Sara Snow, DVM
D208 VMC
MSU
East Lansing, MI 48824-1314

Jessica M. Snyder, DVM, DACVIM (Neurology)
Staff Neurologist
VCA Veterinary Specialty Center of Seattle
20115 44th Avenue W
Lynnwood, WA 98036

Simon W. Tappin, MA, VetMB, DipECVIM-CA,
   MRCVS
Dick White Referrals
The Six Mile Bottom Veterinary Specialist Centre
London Road
Six Mile Bottom
Suffolk
CB8 0UH
ENGLAND

Tara K. Trotman, VMD, DACVIM
Staff Veterinarian, Internal Medicine
Department of Clinical Studies
Matthew J. Ryan Veterinary Hospital of the
   University of Pennsylvania
Philadelphia, PA

Amy Trow, DVM DACVECC
Ocean State Veterinary Specialists
East Greenwich, RI

Amanda E. Veatch, DVM
Small Animal Intern
Department of Veterinary Clinical Sciences
College of Veterinary Medicine
Washington State University
Pullman, WA 99164-6610

Lori S. Waddell, DVM, DACVECC
Adjunct Assistant Professor, Critical Care
Department of Clinical Studies
College of Veterinary Medicine
University of Pennsylvania
Philadelphia, PA

Cynthia R. Ward, VMD, PhD, DACVIM
Chief of Staff, Small Animal Medicine
Professor of Medicine
College of Veterinary Medicine
University of Georgia
501 DW Brooks Drive
Athens, GA 30602

Page E. Yaxley, DVM
Resident, Emergency and Critical Care Medicine
Department of Small Animal Clinical Sciences
D208 VMC
College of Veterinary Medicine
Michigan State University
East Lansing, MI 48824-1314

Acknowledgments

I would like to thank Dougie Macintire for all her support through my career and all the doors and opportunities she has opened for me.

Kenneth J. Drobatz

I would like to thank Dr. Ken Drobatz for always being an inspiring teacher and excellent mentor, and for giving me this wonderful opportunity.

Merilee F. Costello

Feline Emergency and Critical Care Medicine

1
APPROACH TO THE CRITICALLY ILL CAT

Kenneth J. Drobatz

Unique Features
The major point to emphasize regarding cats is that they are very subtle in their manifestation of critical illness/disease. What might appear to be subtle clinical signs may only be the tip of the iceberg regarding the severity of the condition. A full assessment of the vital parameters of a cat that "is not doing well" is essential to avoid missing serious underlying problems.

A. The general approach to the critically ill cat involves three phases: triage, primary survey, and secondary survey. The first two phases are for rapid assessment and recognition of the most life-threatening conditions.
   a. Triage is a process for sorting injured or sick animals based on their need for or likely benefit from immediate medical treatment.
   b. The primary survey is a more in-depth assessment utilizing the triage principles.
      i. Telephone triage (box 1.1)
         1. The initial contact between the client and the veterinary hospital is often via telephone. This conversation can allow for triage of the cat, help in the diagnosis, and provide information regarding first aid treatment.
            a. Immediate aims of telephone triage: Determine if the cat needs to be assessed by a veterinarian on an emergency basis, provide information for first aid for the cat, and calm the owner.
            b. Questions asked on the phone should determine the following:
               i.   The nature of the injury
               ii.   Respiratory status
               iii. Mucous membrane (mm) color
               iv.   Level of consciousness
               v.   Presence and severity of bleeding
                     1. Owners often overinterpret the severity of the bleeding.
               vi.   Heart rate
               vii. Presence/severity of wounds
               vii. Ability to ambulate
               ix.   Presence of fractures
               x.   Presence/severity of vomiting and diarrhea
               xi.   Ability to urinate (especially male cats)
               xii. Abdominal distention
               xiii. Ingestion of toxins (rare in cats)

Box 1.1. Telephone triage—symptoms to determine.
1. Nature of problem/injury
    a. Cardiovascular status (HR, mm color)
2. Neurologic status (mentation/seizures/ability to ambulate)
3. External hemorrhage
4. Vomiting/diarrhea severity
5. Ability to urinate
6. Toxin ingestion
7. Pain
8. Hiding/not eating/listless (warrants evaluation)

---

       xiv. Coughing (rare in cats)
       xv. Seizures/altered mentation
      xvi. Presence and severity of pain (difficult for owner to assess accurately)
  c. Conditions that demand immediate attention
      i. Respiratory distress (open-mouth breathing is generally a sign of severe respiratory distress in cats).
     ii. Severe bleeding
    iii. Straining to urinate without passing urine (often confused with constipation by owners)
    iv. Bleeding from body orifices
     v. Seizures/altered mentation/decreased level of consciousness.
    vi. Toxin ingestion.
   vii. Severe coughing (often confused by owners with retching or vomiting)
  viii. Protracted vomiting or diarrhea
    ix. Extreme pain
     x. Hiding/not eating/listless
       1. Owners often just state that their cat is hiding/not eating or listless. The range of severity of disease with this complaint can be wide, and therefore it should be recommended that the cat be evaluated by a veterinarian. Cats hide disease very well.
  d. Advising first aid
      i. Relying on the owner's interpretation of the cat's problem can be risky.
     ii. If the problem is clear (e.g., previous condition with same clinical signs, etc.), then advice over the phone is reasonable.
    iii. If in doubt at all about the cat's condition, the default recommendation is that the cat should be brought in for evaluation.
    iv. If trauma has occurred:
       1. The cat should be placed on a board or blanket/towel for support that will minimize movement of fractured bones.
       2. Although rolling newspapers into splints has been recommended for stabilization of fractures, we advise against this for both the cat's and the owner's sakes.
       3. Owners should be warned that handling a painful cat is dangerous as even the most docile cat may bite when it is painful.
2. Calming the owner
  a. The owner may be extremely upset about the pet while talking on the phone.
  b. If the owner is overly upset, it is advisable to ask if there is someone else present who can drive him or her and the pet to the clinic.

Box 1.2. Waiting room triage.
1. Obtain capsule history.
2. Assess respiratory (loudness, rate, rhythm, effort).
3. Cardiovascular (mm color, CRT, pulse rate and quality)
4. Neurologic (mentation, ability to ambulate)
5. Urinary tract (palpation of urinary bladder)
6. General
    a. Toxin exposure (ingestion, inhalation, topical)
    b. Potential for infection disease
    c. Limb fractures
    d. Severe pain
    e. Dystocia
    f. Prolapsed organs
    g. External bleeding
    h. Open wounds
    i. Owner's concerns

---

      c. Clear directions should be given on how to get to the clinic.
        i. It is best to have sets of directions for all areas around the clinic prewritten at the reception desk so the directions can be clear and consistent all the time.
        ii. Try to estimate the time of arrival and notify the rest of the medical staff about the potential condition the cat may be in and when it might arrive.
  ii. Waiting room triage (box 1.2)
    1. All cats presenting to an emergency clinic should be assessed immediately.
    2. Triage is the assessment and classification of patients to determine priority of need and proper placement of treatment.
    3. Steps of waiting room triage:
      a. Obtain a capsule history (ideally this should take <2–3 minutes):
        i.   The nature of the complaint and its progression
        ii. Previous major medical problems
        iii. Current medications and treatment
      b. Rapid physical evaluation. (Cats in carriers or wrapped in owner's arms or blankets should be removed from these coverings to be assessed. Be cautious with fractious cats or cats that might jump free. If in doubt, the cat should be assessed in a closed examination room if possible.)
      i. Four major body systems to assess:
        1. Respiratory
          a. Assess rate rhythm and effort
          b. Signs of respiratory compromise that require immediate transfer to the treatment room include the following (see chap. 2—Cardiopulmonary-Cerebral Resuscitation (CPCR):
            i.   Increased respiratory rate (many times the only sign in cats, even those with substantial respiratory compromise)
            ii. Increased respiratory effort
            iii. Loud upper airway sounds
            iv. Open-mouth breathing

        v.   Abducted elbows (rare in cats)
        vi. Extended head and neck (rare in cats)
        vii. Paradoxical respirations
        viii. Flaring of nares
        ix. Cats exhibiting signs iv–viii are generally in extreme respiratory distress.

2. Cardiovascular system (assessing for poor tissue perfusion)
   a. Assess mucous membrane color, capillary refill time, pulse quality, pulse rate, and rhythm (see chap. 3—Shock)
   b. Signs of cardiovascular system derangement that require immediate transfer to treatment room (see chap. 3—Shock)
      i.   Pale, gray, or hyperemic mucous membranes (normal feline mucous membranes tend to be less pink than in the canine, and cats' hyperemic mucous membranes don't tend to be as red as the dogs').
      ii. Very rapid or prolonged capillary refill time (<1 second and >2–3 seconds).
      iii. Weak or bounding pulses (cats' pulses don't tend to get as bounding as dogs')
      iv. Very rapid, slow, or irregular pulse/heart rhythm
3. Neurologic system
   a. Assess mentation and ability to ambulate (see chap. 25—General Approach and Overview of the Neurologic Cat)
   b. Signs of neurologic system abnormalities that require immediate transfer to the treatment area:
      i. Severe changes in mentation (stupor, coma, obtundation, extreme hyperexcitability, seizures)
      ii. Inability to walk or move legs
4. Urinary tract system
   a. Assess ability to urinate and palpate urinary bladder (especially sick male cats)
   b. Abnormalities in urinary tract system that require immediate transfer to the treatment area (see chap. 23—Urologic Emergencies: Ureter, Bladder, Urethra, GN, CRF):
      i. Inability to urinate
      ii. Large, firm, nonexpressable urinary bladder
5. Other assessments that require immediate transfer to the treatment area:
   a. Recent ingestion of toxin
   b. Topical exposure to toxin
   c. Severe vomiting and diarrhea (rare in cats compared to dogs)
   d. Owner is very concerned.
   e. Obvious limb fractures
   f. Severe pain
   g. Recent trauma
   h. Burns (fire, chemical, or hot water)
   i. Excessive bleeding
   j. Dystocia
   k. Prolapsed organs
   l. Open wounds
   m. Animals that have died
   n. Insect or snake bites
   o. If in doubt, transfer to treatment area for further assessment.

  c. Primary survey (see box 1.3)
    i. The primary survey is a more detailed and in-depth assessment of the four major body systems. The goal is to establish the relative stability of the cat and to further determine if immediate therapy is warranted.

Box 1.3. Primary survey.

1. Respiratory system
   a. Physical: mm color, respiratory rate/effort, upper airway sounds, thoracic auscultation
   b. Objective: Pulse oximetry, arterial blood gas analysis
2. Cardiovascular system
   a. Physical: mm color, CRT, pulse rate/quality, cardiac auscultation, rectal-to-toe temperature difference
   b. Objective: ECG, blood pressure, lactate concentration, CVP (central venous pressure)
3. Neurologic system
   a. Physical: mentation, cranial nerve function, ability to ambulate/motor movement, limb pain sensation, and spinal reflexes
   b. Objective: none on an emergency basis
4. Urinary tract:
   a. Physical: Palpate urinary bladder for distention; palpate kidneys for size, shape, pain, symmetry.
   b. Objective: Measure BUN, creatinine, blood gas analysis, potassium concentration.

---

    ii. Respiratory system

      1. Similar parameters should be assessed as in triage: mucous membrane color, upper airway sounds, respiratory rate, rhythm, and effort.

      2. Auscultation of all regions of the thorax and trachea

      3. Pulse oximetry and arterial blood gas give more objective and detailed information regarding lung function (the stress of obtaining an arterial blood gas may outweigh the benefit in a cat with respiratory compromise).

      4. Any animal showing signs of respiratory compromise should be given oxygen supplementation (see chap. 10—Respiratory Emergencies and Pleural Space Disease).

        a. Evaluation for the underlying cause should be immediately undertaken if the cat will tolerate this further assessment.

   iii. Cardiovascular system

      1. Similar parameters should be assessed as in triage: mucous membrane color, capillary refill time, pulse quality, rate, and rhythm. Cardiac auscultation and rectal-to-toe temperature difference can also provide assessment of tissue perfusion status.

      2. More objective assessments include ECG evaluation, blood pressure determination, blood lactate concentration, central venous pressure measurement, pulmonary artery catheterization and determination of pulmonary artery hemoglobin saturation with oxygen, measurement of cardiac output, tissue oxygen delivery, and consumption. (The pulmonary artery catheter is rarely used in cats for these determinations. See chap. 3—Shock.)

        a. Anecdotal impression is that cats with poor tissue perfusion often have low rectal temperature.

        b. Cats in shock often are bradycardic compared with dogs, which are usually tachycardic.

      3. Cardiovascular system derangements are life-threatening and should be addressed immediately (see chap. 3—Shock).

    iv. Neurologic system

      1. Assessment of the neurologic system is primarily through physical examination.

      2. Abnormalities of brain function may manifest as changes in mentation, gait, or cranial nerve function.

      3. Abnormalities of spinal cord or peripheral nerve function are manifested with normal mentation/cranial nerves, but abnormal limb findings such as loss of conscious proprioception, ataxia, changes in limb reflexes, altered sensation, and motor function.

4. Abnormalities in brain function require rapid assessment and treatment of the underlying cause before irreversible damage can occur (see chap. 25—General Approach and Overview of the Neurologic Cat).

5. Note: cats with severe altered perfusion may have abnormal neurologic function until perfusion abnormalities are corrected. Use caution when interpreting abnormal neurologic findings when perfusion is severely compromised.

  v. Urinary tract system

1. Initial primary survey physical evaluation of the urinary tract system is palpation of the urinary bladder, determination of urethral obstruction, and palpation of the kidneys for size, shape, symmetry, and pain.

2. More objective primary survey rapid assessment includes determination of blood urea nitrogen (BUN), serum creatinine and potassium concentrations, and blood gas analysis.

d. Secondary survey (box 1.4)

  i. The secondary survey occurs after assessment and stabilization of the immediate life-threatening conditions.

  ii. The secondary survey includes a full physical assessment ("head-to-tail" physical examination), a detailed medical history, imaging studies, and clinical pathology as indicated. Response to therapy may also be included as part of the secondary survey.

  iii. A comprehensive diagnostic and therapeutic plan can be developed; prognosis and costs can be estimated as well.

e. Emergency clinical pathology database (box 1.5)

  i. Rapid assessments of packed cell volume (PCV), total solids (TS), dipstick blood glucose, dipstick BUN, and a blood smear provide relatively immediate and essential information for evaluation of the critically ill patient.

1. The blood for these evaluations can be obtained by filling three heparinized capillary tubes from the hub of an intravenous catheter that is being placed or by filling them from the hub of a 25-gauge needle placed in a peripheral vein.

2. Detailed evaluation of the findings of the emergency database can be obtained from their respective following chapters.

Box 1.4. Secondary survey.
1. Head-to-tail physical examination
2. Detailed medical history
3. Imaging studies
4. Clinical pathology
5. Response to therapy

Box 1.5. Emergency database.
1. PCV
2. Total solids
3. Dipstick BUN
4. Dipstick glucose
5. Blood smear

3. General interpretation of abnormal emergency database findings
    a. PCV and TS should be interpreted together.
        i. Increased PCV and TS
            1. Dehydration (anecdotally TS is a more sensitive assessment of dehydration in the cat).
        ii. Increased PCV and normal TS
            1. Polycythemia
            2. Dehydration with protein loss
        iii. Normal PCV and increased TS
            1. Dehydration (common)
            2. Dehydration and anemia (common)
            3. Increased globulin production
            4. Lipemic serum or severely hemolyzed serum can give an increased TS reading on a refractometer.
        iv. Decreased PCV and decreased TS
            1. Blood loss (most common)
            2. Nonregenerative anemia with protein loss
            3. Nonregenerative anemia and liver dysfunction
            4. RBC destruction and protein loss
    b. Increased glucose
        i. Stress (most common)
        ii. Diabetes mellitus
        iii. Iatrogenic (intravenous glucose supplementation)
    c. Decreased glucose
        i. Insulin overdose
        ii. Liver failure
        iii. Sepsis
        iv. Neonatal/juvenile hypoglycemia
    d. Decreased BUN
        i. Diuresis
        ii. Liver dysfunction/failure
    e. Increased BUN
        i. Prerenal (most common)
            1. Dehydration (common)
            2. GI hemorrhage (uncommon)
        ii. Renal dysfunction/failure (common)
        iii. Postrenal (common in male cats)
    f. Blood smear evaluation
        i. Accurate evaluation of blood smear is highly dependent upon the quality of the smear that is made. A quality smear should:
            1. Have a feathered edge and a broad monolayer in which RBC are evenly distributed and have minimal overlap. This area is where WBCs are most easily identified and where RBC abnormalities can be most readily seen. Abnormal cell types, platelet clumps, and microfilariae may be found along the feathered edge.
        ii. For emergency purposes, gross evaluation of the three major cell lines is all that is needed.
            1. For rapid assessment of platelets and WBC count, first look at the feathered edge at low to medium power.
                a. Gross decreases in WBC (panleukopenia) can be recognized rapidly by the paucity of WBCs on the feathered edge (WBCs tend to accumulate at the

feathered edge; therefore, if the feathered edge lacks them, it is very likely that the WBC count is very low).

   b. Platelet clumps on the feathered edge suggest adequate platelets. These clumps can result in a falsely low estimate of platelet numbers when the estimate is based on the count from the monolayer.

2. After viewing the feathered edge, move to the monolayer just inside the feathered edge and evaluate the quality (see above) of the smear.

   a. Evaluate WBCs: Estimate the absolute number as low, normal, or high by using the high dry magnification.

      i. Estimate a differential WBC count using high dry magnification.

      ii. Evaluate leukocyte morphology using the oil immersion magnification.

   b. Evaluate platelets: Estimate the number. Adequate platelet number (enough to prevent bleeding) is indicated by observing 3–4 platelets/oil immersion field or noting several platelet clumps at lower magnification. In cats with a normal RBC count, one platelet per 20 RBCs suggests a normal platelet count as well.

   c. Evaluate RBCs: RBCs should be evaluated for size, shape, color, and parasites.

g. Evaluation of hematocrit tube supernatant

   i. A large buffy coat indicates a high WBC count.

   ii. Icteric serum could be due to prehepatic, hepatic, and posthepatic causes.

   iii. Hemolyzed serum can be due to poor blood collection technique or intravascular hemolysis (rare in cats).

   iv. Lipemic serum can be due to pancreatitis, immediately postseizure (anecdotal), or postprandial.

f. The emergency plan (box 1.6)

   i. After the initial assessment, a problem list should be generated with prioritization of most life-threatening to least life-threatening.

   ii. Plans (diagnostic, therapeutic, and monitoring) should then be made for each of those problems.

      1. The plan itself depends upon the problem, the stability of the cat, the nature of the cat (e.g., fractious), and the number and skill of the available nursing staff.

      2. After making a plan for each problem, they should be collated so that a comprehensive, cohesive, and clear order sheet can be written.

      3. Categories covered by emergency orders:

         a. Fluid therapy

         b. Medications to be given

         c. Diagnostics to be performed

         d. Parameters to be monitored

         e. Nursing care

Box 1.6. General emergency plan.

(Should be made for each problem separately and then consolidated for final order sheet)

1. Fluid therapy (type, route, rate)
2. Medication to be administered (type, dose, rate, frequency, compatibility)
3. Diagnostic plan (imaging, clinical pathology, etc.)
4. Monitoring (physical parameters, clinicopathology, electronic)
5. General nursing care orders

4. Fluid therapy orders should include (see chap. 8—Fluid Therapy) the following:
   a. Type of fluid to be administered
   b. Route of administration
   c. Rate of administration
5. Medication orders should include the following:
   a. Type of medication
   b. Dose of medication
   c. Rate of administration
   d. Frequency of administration
   e. Medications should be reviewed for compatibility with other administered therapies, as well as whether they are tolerated by cats, and potential untoward reactions that may occur.
      i. The orders should note monitoring for these reactions, and contingency orders should be available in case a reaction occurs.
6. Diagnostic plan
   a. Should be considered for all problems and then listed together in order of priority of completion.
      i. The stability of the cat, as well as the importance of the information in the emergency management of the cat, should determine the priority.
7. Monitoring plans
   a. Monitoring plans can be categorized into physical examination, clinicopathologic, and electronic parameters.
   b. Monitoring is extremely important in critical care to detect trends. This allows anticipation of problems before they occur.
   c. Common physical parameters that are monitored
      i.   Mucous membrane color
      ii.   Capillary refill time
      iii. Pulse rate and rhythm
      iv.   Pulse quality
      v.   Lung sounds
      vi.   Respiratory rate and effort
      vii. Neurologic function
          1. Mentation
          2. Cranial nerves
          3. Long tracts (especially voluntary motor capabilities and pain sensation for spinal cord injuries).
          4. Urination. Bladder size is easily palpable in cats and gives an estimate of urine production.
          5. Vomiting/bowel movements
          6. Rectal temperature
          7. Abdominal palpation
          8. Assessing skin and mucous membranes for petechiations/ecchymoses
      viii. Body weight
   d. Common clinicopathologic parameters
      i.   PCV, TS, dipstick BUN, and glucose
      ii. Electrolytes
      iii. Blood gas parameters
      iv. Blood smear
      v.   Coagulation parameters
   e. Electronic monitoring parameters
      i.   Central venous pressure

        ii. Electrocardiogram

        iii. Blood pressure

        iv. Pulse oximetry

        v. Pulmonary artery catheter placement (not commonly done in cats) to measure cardiac output, oxygen delivery, oxygen consumption, peripheral vascular resistance, and mixed venous oxygen saturation.

     f. Common nursing orders

        i. Keep patient clean and dry.

        ii. Check comfort (pain, etc.).

        iii. Turn patient as needed.

        iv. Other nursing orders will be for the specific patient needs.

  iii. General comments

     1. Emergency plans will need to be tailored to individual patient needs, the specific disease condition, the severity of the cat's condition, the physiologic stability of the cat, and the number and skill of the nursing staff. Additionally, the owner's personal needs and financial capability must also be considered.

     2. If the best emergency plan cannot be accommodated by your facility, then referral should be considered and discussed with the client.

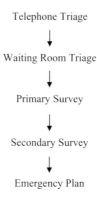

Telephone Triage

↓

Waiting Room Triage

↓

Primary Survey

↓

Secondary Survey

↓

Emergency Plan

Fig. 1.1. Algorithm for "Approach to the Critically Ill Cat."

2
CARDIOPULMONARY-CEREBRAL RESUSCITATION (CPCR)

Sean D. Smarick

Unique Features

Cats warrant some special consideration in CPCR:
- Fixed and dilated pupils are delayed in CPA.
- Airway management is more challenging due to laryngospasm.
- Size and conformation call for circumferential compressions.
- Faster compression rates
- Vasopressin use has not been reported in feline CPCR.
- Lidocaine dosage is decreased.
- IV and IT saline flushes are reduced in volume.

Offer technical challenges to invasive monitoring

A. Definitions
    a. Cardiopulmonary-cerebral resuscitation (CPCR) is the treatment for a cardiopulmonary arrest which incorporates basic, advanced, and brain-oriented prolonged life support.
    b. Cardiopulmonary arrest (CPA) is the lack of effective respiration and circulation that is the common pathway preceding death.
B. Precipitating factors
    a. Cardiopulmonary arrest can be caused by anything that can lead to death, so quickly identifying treatable underlying conditions is crucial for survival.
    b. The American Heart Association suggests ruling out "Hs and Ts" as potentially treatable factors leading to CPA. Adapted for cats, they include (see box 2.1) the following:
        i.   Hypoxia
        ii.   Hypovolemia
        iii. Hypoglycemia
        iv. Hyperkalemia
        v.   H+ (acidosis)
        vi. Hypothermia
        vii. Tablets (drugs/anesthesia)
        viii. Thromboembolism
        ix. Tension pneumothorax (extremely rare in cats)
        x.   Tamponade (cardiac, relatively rare in cats)
        xi. Trauma (head)

Box 2.1. Cardiopulmonary arrest.
A. Reversible precipitating factors
    a. Hypoxia
    b. Hypovolemia
    c. Hypoglycemia
    d. HyperK+
    e. H+ (acidosis)
    f. Hypothermia
    g. Tablets(drugs/anesthesia)
    h. Thromboembolism
    i. Tension pneumothorax
    j. Tamponade (cardiac)
    k. Trauma (head)

C. Clinical signs
    a. Observations and physical examination
        i. Unconsciousness and unresponsiveness
        ii. Lack of chest wall movement or agonal respirations
        iii. Auscultation will reveal no or agonal breath and no heart sounds.
        iv. Palpation will not yield an apex heart beat or peripheral pulse.
        v. Fixed and dilated pupils may take up to 90 seconds after a CPA in cats, whereas in primates it is almost immediate.
    b. Electrocardiogram (ECG)
        i. Asystole (flatline on ECG)
        ii. Pulseless electrical activity
            1. Previously called electromechanical dissociation
            2. Appears on the ECG as organized electrical activity that is not associated with any mechanical contraction of the heart
        iii. Ventricular fibrillation (VF)
        iv. Cats in respiratory arrest or early CPA also have had other arrhythmias reported, such as, sinus bradycardia, ventricular tachycardia, A-V block, and so on, that affect perfusion.
        v. Electrical activity on the ECG does not ensure mechanical activity; conversely, a lack of a discernable ECG rhythm may be due to poor electrode-patient coupling, machine malfunction, and so on, rather than CPA.
            1. Auscultation should always be done to fully evaluate cardiac activity in a patient with confirmed or suspected CPA.
    c. Other continuous patient monitors used during anesthesia or in critically ill patients can support, but are not specific for, a CPA.
        i. Doppler blood flow intensity drops precipitously or stops completely.
        ii. Capnometer alarms apnea or end-tidal carbon dioxide concentrations ($PetCO_2$) acutely trend downward toward 0 mmHg.
        iii. Pulse oximeter plethysmograph or LED pulse meter will indicate no pulsatile blood flow; saturation is not a reliable indicator as many dead patients will display a normal SpO_2.
D. Prognosis
    a. Return of spontaneous circulation (ROSC) in cats suffering a CPA has been reported in 15–61% of patients.
    b. Survival to discharge in cats with CPA has been reported as 2–22%, with the larger studies reporting <10% survival.

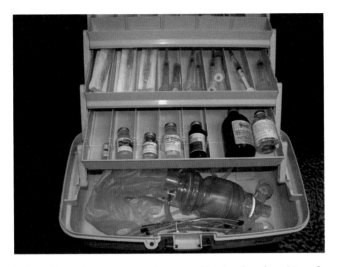

Fig. 2.1. Ideally, a dedicated cart for patients undergoing CPA is often found in referral centers; however, a converted fishing tackle box that is readily available to the treatment, surgical preparation, or surgical areas can save valuable time. See box 2.2 for a basic list of supplies. These supplies must be checked daily.

Box 2.2.   CPR box supplies.
3.0-mm to 5.5-mm cuffed endotracheal tubes with air syringe
Lidocaine 2% in an atomizer or 1-cc syringe to prevent laryngospasm
Muzzle gauze, umbilical tape, or other material to secure the endotracheal tube
Infant Ambu bag
Atropine injectable
Epinepherine injection 1:10,000 or 1:1,000
Sodium bicarbonate (8.4%)
0.9% saline for flushing IV catheters
1-cc and 3-cc syringes with 1-inch needles
Intraosseus needles/spinal needles
24-, 22-, and 20-ga IV catheters
Infusion caps or T-sets
Bag of LRS or saline
Infusion set

---

    c. In a study of cats with only respiratory arrest, 58% were discharged from the hospital.
    d. Factors associated with discharged feline survivors of CPA:
       i. CPA generally related to anesthesia and the perioperative period, although other causes have been successfully resuscitated.
      ii. Duration of CPCR less than 15 minutes
     iii. Do not rearrest.
E. General recommendations
    a. A dedicated area, cart, or tackle box for CPCR supplies should be maintained (fig. 2.1 and box 2.2).
    b. CPCR should be reviewed and practiced regularly by the staff.
    c. In the absence of a documented owner "do-not-resuscitate" order or signs of obvious death such as rigor, decapitation, and so on every CPA should be treated.

Treatment

A. Basic life support provides initial care in or out of the hospital and consists of the "ABCs" (box 2.3):
  a. Access airway
    i. Extend the neck (in a nontraumatized patient), pull the tongue forward, and if laryngospasm is observed or intubation imminent, instill 2% lidocaine by an atomizer or a drop or two via a 1-cc syringe onto the larynx.
      1. In a patient with a known or suspected traumatic injury, care should be taken to minimize manipulation of the neck until cervical injury has been ruled out.
    ii. Place and secure an appropriately sized endotracheal tube.
    iii. Confirm initial and continued placement with capnometry, visualization, or palpation.
    iv. If an airway obstruction is suspected, that is, the endotracheal tube cannot be passed or the patient cannot be ventilated, perform the following:

Box 2.3. Cardiopulmonary cerebral resuscitation BLS: "ABCs"

A. Assess unresponsiveness
B. Airway access
C. Breathing
  a. 20 bpm RA
  b. 8–10 bpm CPA
D. Circulation
  a. Circumferential compressions
  b. 120 compression/minute
  c. Open chest if chest, pleural space, or pericardial pathology

ACLS: "D–G"
A. Differential diagnosis
  a. Hs (see box 2.1)
  b. Ts (see box 2.1)
B. Drugs
  a. IV access
  b. Treatment for underlying cause
  c. Epinephrine
  d. Atropine
  e. $NaHCO_3$
C. Evaluate ECG
  a. Asystole/PEA/sinus bradycardia
  b. VF
D. Fibrillation treatment PRN
E. Gauge effectiveness

PLS (prolonged life support): "H and I"
A. Hypothermia
B. Intensive care
  a. Maximize cerebral perfusion (blood pressure) (see box 2.4)
  b. Avoid hypoxemia and hypercapnea
  c. Anticipate other organ dysfunction

> **Box 2.4.**   Quick reference CPCR drug volumes for the average-size (5-kg) cat.
>
> | Epineprhine | 0.1 mL of 1:1000 (low dose) |
> | | 1 mL of 1:10,000 (high dose) |
> | Atropine | 0.5 mL |
> | NaHCO$_3$ | 5 mL of 1 mEq/mL (8.4%) IV |

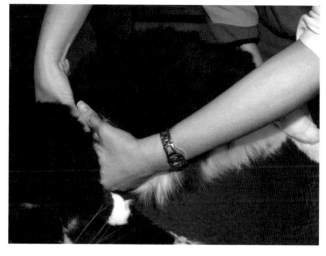

Fig. 2.2.   Proper hand positioning for circumferential compressions. Note that both hands are used and encompass the cranial thorax.

    1. Suction laryngeal/pharyngeal area of any vomitus or secretions.
    2. Physically remove any visible foreign body or use a polypropylene urinary catheter as a stylet to guide the endotracheal tube around the obstruction.
    3. Consider a foreign body obstruction and perform a Heimlich maneuver by making a sharp ventrocraniodorsal compression just cranial to the umbilicus.
    4. Perform a tracheostomy if an upper airway obstruction cannot be relieved.
  b. Breathing
    i. Provide positive pressure ventilation (PPV) via an ambu-bag, Baines or other nonbreathing circuits, or anesthesia machine, ideally with 100% oxygen supplementation.
    ii. PPV may also be provided by mouth-to-snout or a tight-fitting mask in the absence of endotracheal intubation but runs the risk of gastric distension resulting in poor circulation or aspiration of gastric contents.
      1. 20 breaths/minute in respiratory arrest
      2. 8–10 breaths/minute in CPA.
  c. Circulation
    i. External chest compressions
      1. Circumferentially place the hands around the cranial thorax of the cat in lateral recumbency (fig. 2.2).
      2. Decrease the chest diameter by about 30%.

    3. Maintain a 1:1 compression-to-relaxation ratio.

    4. Compress at a rate of 120 beats/minute and minimize interruptions.

    5. If unsatisfactory results are obtained, changing compressors or placement of hands and varying the rate and depth may offer some benefit.

    6. Interposed abdominal compressions may have benefit but have not been clinically evaluated in the cat; compress the mid-cranial abdomen with the palmar surface of the fingers or hand during the relaxation phase of the chest compressions.

    7. Simultaneous ventilation-compression CPCR and caudal binding/MAST trouser application are no longer recommended.

    8. Complications of external chest compressions include rib/sternum separations or fractures, hemothorax, pneumothorax, pulmonary contusions, and hepatic and splenic lacerations.

  ii. Internal cardiac compressions (ICC) is an advanced cardiac life support maneuver.

    1. Despite ongoing debate of the role of ICC, it is generally accepted that ICC must be employed within 2–5 minutes to realize the benefits of the intervention on survival.

    2. Indications include chest wall defect (e.g., rib fractures), penetrating trauma, cardiac tamponade, loss of chest wall compliance, and pleural space disease.

    3. A lateral thoracotomy is performed at the left 6th intercostal space by incising the skin with a scalpel blade, stabbing into the pleural space and extending the incision dorsally and ventrally stopping short of the vertebral arteries and internal thoracic with curved mayo scissors.

    4. Alternatively, excising the diaphragm during a ceilotomy offers an approach during an intraoperative CPA.

    5. Baby Balfour abdominal retractors or Finochetto rib spreaders are used for incision retraction.

    6. Deliver the heart from the pericardial sac (with the mayo scissors); and using the palmar surfaces of the fingers and thumb, compress the heart from the apex to the base at a rate of 150 beats/minute.

    7. Occlude the descending aorta by digital compression or by blunt dissection and occlusion with red rubber catheter, penrose drain, or Rumel tourniquet.

    8. With ROSC, release the aortic occlusion over 5–10 minutes and close the chest routinely after pleural lavage.

B. Advanced cardiac life support incorporates more sophisticated care usually available only in a hospitalized setting and continues the alphabet mnemonic letters D through G (box 2.3).

  a. D: Differential diagnoses are considered and identified reversible causes of CPA (see heading "Precipitating Factors") are addressed.

  b. D: Drugs

    i. Inhalant anesthetics are discontinued and 100% oxygen is given. Reverse any reversible injectable anesthetic drugs that were given.

    ii. Obtain vascular access if it is not already in place.

    1. Central intravenous catheters are ideal for administering drugs, but placement is technically difficult during CPCR, and the long length is not ideal for administering fluid boluses.

      a. A short (1–2 inch), large-bore catheter placed in the jugular vein facilitates rapid infusion of drugs and fluids but can be technically difficult in an arrest situation. A cutdown can be helpful in visualization and placement.

    2. Intraosseous access in the proximal cranial humerus or trocanteric fossa of the femur is especially useful in kittens and a good alternative in adult cats.

    3. Peripheral intravenous catheters are most common, but a cranial placement is preferred to shorten the time of drug delivery to the heart. After drug administration, flush the catheter with 2–5 mL of saline and elevate the extremity for 20 seconds but do not let this interfere with compressions and ventilations.

      4. If vascular access is delayed, the intratracheal route can be used to administer naloxone, atropine, vasopressin, epinephrine, and lidocaine (NAVEL). The drug amount should at least be double the IV dose and suspended in 3–5 mL sterile water for injection or 0.9% saline, injected via (i.e., red rubber) catheter to the level of the carina and followed by the administration by two breaths.

      5. Sublingual administration of medications has been only anecdotally recommended.

  iii. Narcotics and other anesthetic agents should be reversed with the appropriate antagonists during an anesthetic arrest.

  iv. Hyperkalemia and hypoglycemia are treated immediately.

      1. Hyperkalemia treatment

         a. Calcium gluconate

           i. 3–4 mL 10% calcium gluconate slow IV bolus over 1 minute during cardiac arrest.

         b. Dextrose bolus (0.25–0.5 g/kg) IV with insulin (1 unit regular insulin/cat) slow IV bolus over 1–2 minutes

         c. $NaHCO_3$ 1 mEq/kg slow IV bolus over 15–20 minutes.

      2. Hypoglycemia

         a. Dextrose 0.5 g/kg IV bolus

  v. If hypovolemia is the cause of or contributed to the CPA, appropriate boluses in 10–30-mL increments of 0.9% saline or LRS are indicated; however, in euvolemic CPA, minimize fluid administration as this may impede myocardial muscle perfusion by increasing right atrial pressure.

  vi. As the majority of CPA ECG rhythms in cats call for both a pressor and vagolytic therapy, it is reasonable to empirically administer them if an ECG interpretation is not readily available or the interpretation is delayed.

      1. If there has been no response, repeat epinephrine 0.01–0.02 mg/kg IV every 3–5 minutes. For endotracheal administration, use the 0.1–0.2 mg/kg dose.

      2. Vasopressin is used in people and dogs at 0.8 U/kg once as an alternative to epinephrine, but no feline studies have been performed.

      3. Atropine 0.004–0.04 mg/kg, repeated once in 5 minutes PRN. The low dose is used for suspected vagal-mediated (vomiting or urination followed by collapse) arrests.

      4. Sodium bicarbonate ($NaHCO_3$) is given for known metabolic acidosis, hyperkalemia, and after 10 minutes of CPCR at 1 meq/kg, then 0.5 meq/kg every 10 minutes. It is contraindicated in hypercarbia and requires adequate ventilation to avoid intracellular acidosis.

c. E: ECG Evaluation

  i. Asystole (flatline), pulseless electrical activity (wide, often bizarre bradyarrhythmia with no or ineffective mechanical cardiac activity), and severe sinus bradycardia are most often observed in cats with CPA.

      1. Administer epinephrine and atropine if not already given.

      2. Transthoracic electrical pacing (available on many defibrillators) may play a role in treatment of severe bradyarrhythmias. (Caution, as this can be quite painful to the cat if mistakenly applied when the cat still has brain function.)

  ii. Ventricular fibrillation (saw tooth waveform) is initially encountered in approximately 20% of feline CPA.

      1. It is possible VF may spontaneously terminate due to the small heart size.

      2. Immediate fibrillation therapy is indicated because the longer a heart fibrillates, the less likely is survival.

d. F: Fibrillation treatment

  i. Electrical defibrillation is the only effective therapy.

      1. A quick clip of the electrode area is ideal, but in short-haired cats, good paddle contact with appropriate conducting gel may suffice (avoid alcohol as it creates an explosion/fire hazard!).

2. The cat can be squeezed between the two standard "paddles" on opposite sides of chest with the paddle marked "sternum" over the patient's right thorax. Alternatively, the flat paddle marked "apex" is slid under the cat in left lateral recumbency, and the "sternum" paddle is pushed down on patient's right thorax; internal paddles are applied directly to either side of the heart if a thoracotomy has been employed.

3. Select 5–10 J/kg for monophasic (older) defibrillators or about 40% less with newer biphasic defibrillators. Internal defibrillation is approximately 10% of external settings.

4. Apply firm pressure to handheld paddles and use coupling gel or saline-soaked gauzes to decrease transthoracic impedance.

5. As contact with the patient or an item connected to the patient during defibrillation creates a shock hazard, the person using the defibrillator should announce while they insure
   a. "I am clear."
   b. "You (the resuscitation team) are clear."
   c. "All clear"

6. Administer one shock as above then perform compressions, ventilation, and drug therapy for 1 minute, repeating this cycle until VF is terminated.

ii. Pharmacologic attempts at defibrillation have been grossly disappointing, but pharmacologic intervention may be helpful in electroconversion with amiodarone 5 mg/kg (half the dose may be repeated once). Magnesium is only indicated in hypomagnesemic states or Torsades de pointes: 20 mg/kg diluted in D_5W over 5 minutes. The use of lidocaine has been questioned and is not recommended at this time.

iii. In the absence of a defibrillator, a precordial thump consisting of a closed fist hit over the middle sternum from 6 inches above can be attempted, but it is not recommended for routine use.

e. G: Gauge resuscitative efforts
   i. End tidal carbon dioxide values >15–20 mmHg, coronary perfusion pressure >15–20 mmHg or diastolic direct arterial pressure >30 mmHg support adequate circulation, but require monitoring equipment.
   ii. No other clinical indicators including pulse checks and pulse oximetry have proved reliable for real-time evaluation of CPCR effectiveness.
   iii. ROSC is proof of effective resuscitation; and, if it is not obtained:
      1. Confirm endotracheal tube placement.
      2. Augment compressions.
      3. Consider buffer therapy.
      4. Reevaluate ECG rhythm.
      5. Revisit differential diagnosis ("Hs and Ts") to address reversible cause.
      6. Consider discontinuing CPCR if there has been no ROSC after 15–30 minutes, sooner if the patient was presented in CPA or the underlying cause was a disease already receiving maximal support (i.e., septic shock on maximal pressors).

C. Prolonged life support PLS (see box 2.3) is postresuscitative care aimed at maximizing neurological recovery, represented by the letters H and I in the alphabet mnemonic. Invasive monitoring and PPV in cats are technically more challenging than in larger species.

a. H: Hypothermia
   i. Do not actively rewarm unless hypothermia was a precipitating factor.
   ii. Cooling hemodynamically stable patients by permissive means, cooling blankets, or ice packs down to approximately 93.5°F (34°C) for 12–24 hours may improve neurological recovery.

b. I: Intensive care to maximize cerebral perfusion and support the other organ systems is often needed for successful recovery.
   i. Supplemental oxygen or PPV is administered to maintain an arterial blood gas $PaO_2 > 80$ mmHg or pulse oximeter $SpO_2 > 95\%$.

Box 2.5. CRI setup.
- Dose of drug in µg/kg/dose × body weight in kg × 0.6 = # of mg placed into 50 mL at 5 mL/hr via syringe pump

Or
- Dose of drug in µg/kg/min × body weight in kg × 3 in 250 mL of saline @ 5 mL/hr via infusion pump

---

ii.   Maintain normocapnea with PPV assessed by arterial blood gas ($PaCO_2$ = 32 mmHg), venous blood gas ($PvCO_2$ = 35 mmHg) or end tidal ($PetCO_2$ = 30 mmHg).

iii. Constant rate infusions (CRI, Box 2.5) of norepinephrine (0.05–0.3 µg/kg/min), dopamine (10–20 µg/kg/min), and epinephrine (0.1–1 µg/kg/min), in order of decreasing preference, along with addressing acidemia are often needed to meet the goal of maintaining the MAP > 100 mmHg (or Doppler systolic >140 mmHg) for the first 12 hours and normotension thereafter.

iv.   Arrhythmias and rearrests are common and warrant continuous ECG monitoring. Arrhythmias that affect BP or are deteriorating warrant appropriate antiarrhythmic therapy.

v.   Acid-base balance is initially normalized to a pH of 7.35 using central venous pH by maximizing perfusion, maintaining normocapnea, and correcting pH with $NaHCO_3$ (0.3 meq/kg/meq of base deficit). Arterial samples do not accurately reflect the patient's acid-base status during CPCR but may be used after equilibration with the venous circulation.

vi.   Normoglycemia of 100–150 mg/dL is maintained by supplementing with dextrose (0.1 gm/kg bolus then 2.5%–10% CRI) or by administering insulin (0.5 u/cat regular insulin IM PRN).

vii. Due to global ischemic nature of CPA, monitoring for and treating other organ dysfunction is also needed.
  1. Coagulopathy
  2. Pneumonia
  3. Sepsis
  4. Renal failure
  5. Seizures

viii. Prognostic factors at 24 hours post-ROSC in people indicating poor neurological outcome or death include the absence of a corneal flex, a pupillary light response, a pain withdrawal response, or any motor responses.

Recommended Reading

American Heart Association guidelines for cardiopulmonary resuscitation and emergency cardiovascular care. Circulation 2005; 112(24 Suppl):1–203.

American Heart Association in collaboration with the International Liaison Committee on Resuscitation. Guidelines 2000 for cardiopulmonary resuscitation and emergency cardiovascular care. Circulation 2000; 102(8 Suppl).

Cole SG, Otto CM, Hughes D. Cardiopulmonary cerebral resuscitation in small animals: A clinical review. Part I. J Vet Emerg Crit Care 2003; 12(4):261–267.

Cole SG, Otto CM, Hughes D. Cardiopulmonary cerebral resuscitation in small animals: A clinical review. Part II. J Vet Emerg Crit Care 2003; 13(1):13–23.

Gilroy BA, Dunlop BJ, Shapiro HM. Outcome from cardiopulmonary resuscitation in cats: Laboratory and clinical experience. J Amer Anim Hosp Assoc 1987; 23:133–139.

Hofmeister EH, Brainard BM, Egger CM, Kang S. Prognostic indicators for dogs and cats with cardiopulmonary arrest treated by cardiopulmonary cerebral resuscitation at a university teaching hospital. J Am Vet Med Assoc. 2009 Jul 1; 235(1):50–57.

Kass PH, Haskins SC. Survival following cardiopulmonary resuscitation in dogs and cats. J Vet Emerg Crit Care 1992; 2(2):57–65.

Plunkett SJ, McMichael M. Cardiopulmonary resuscitation in small animal medicine: an update. J Vet Intern Med. 2008 Jan–Feb; 22(1):9–25.

Rush JE, Wingfield WE. Recognition and frequency of dysrhythmias during cardiopulmonary arrest. J Am Vet Med Assoc 1992; 200(12):1932–1937.

Waldrop JE, Rozanski EA, Swanke ED, et al. Causes of cardiopulmonary arrest, resuscitation management, and functional outcome in dogs and cats surviving cardiopulmonary arrest. Can Vet J 2005; 14(1):22–29.

Wingfield WE, Van Pelt DR. Respiratory and cardiopulmonary arrest in dogs and cats: 265 cases (1986–1991). J Am Vet Med Assoc 1992; 200(12):1993–1996.

3
SHOCK

Merilee F. Costello

Unique Features
- Cats in shock (particularly septic shock) may present with an inappropriately low heart rate (<160 bpm).
- Hypothermia is common in these patients and should be addressed once initial fluid therapy has been administered.
- Pain can be difficult to assess in cats, so analgesics should be administered if there is any question.
- Nutrition is important, as cats with poor perfusion rapidly develop a catabolic state which can lead to hepatic lipidosis.

A. Definition
  a. Decreased effective circulating volume and oxygen delivery to the tissue
    i. Oxygen delivery (DO_2) must equal oxygen consumption (VO_2).
      1. DO_2
        a. Oxygen delivery is determined by cardiac output multiplied by oxygen content ($CO \times CaO_2$).
          i. $CaO_2 = (Hb \times 1.34 \times SaO_2) + (PaO_2 \times 0.003)$
      2. VO_2
        a. Oxygen consumption is relatively constant in a normal animal.
        b. Causes of increased VO_2
          i. Status epilepticus (relatively rare)
          ii. Heatstroke (rare)
          iii. Tremorogenic mycotoxins (rare)
          iv. Malignant hyperthermia (rare)
      3. If DO_2 is less than VO_2, the result is cellular oxygen and energy debt leading to the following:
        a. Lactic acid production
        b. Intracellular acidosis
        c. Decreased intracellular enzyme function
        d. Decreased activity of the Na-K-ATPase pump, which leads to the following:
          i. Cell swelling
          ii. Loss of function
          iii. Cell death
          iv. Cytokine release

1. Further cellular damage
2. Cell death
3. Systemic inflammation
    a. Can lead to progressive failure of compensatory mechanisms and irreversible organ damage and failure
B. Clinical signs
    a. Clinical signs of poor perfusion are similar regardless of the category or underlying cause of the shock, and may include the following:
        i.   Poor pulses
        ii. Prolonged capillary refill time
        iii. Cold extremities
        iv. Hypothermia
        v.   Tachycardia or bradycardia
            1. Bradycardia is a unique pathophysiologic response to shock (particularly septic shock) in cats.
C. Categories of shock
    a. Cardiogenic shock
        i. Failure of the heart to maintain cardiac output
            1. Decreased cardiac output results in a decrease in oxygen delivery.
        ii. Etiology
            1. Low cardiac output heart failure (see chaps. 14—General Approach and Overview of Cardiac Emergencies and 15—Management of Specific Cardiac Diseases)
                a. Occurs when systolic dysfunction impairs the ability of the heart to effectively maintain cardiac output
                b. Most commonly seen in cats with dilated cardiomyopathy
                c. Can also occur in severe cases of restrictive or unclassified cardiomyopathy
            2. Arrhythmias (see chap. 17—Management of Life-Threatening Arrhythmias)
                a. Tachyarrhythmias
                    i. Significant increase in heart rate impairs ventricular filling and subsequent cardiac output.
                b. Bradyarrhythmias
                    i. Significant decrease in heart rate impairs ability of the heart to provide adequate cardiac output
                    ii. Cats may become bradycardic secondary to critical illness and shock, so differentiating primary bradyarrhythmia as a cause of shock versus bradycardia secondary to shock can be challenging.
            3. Pericardial effusion (see chap. 14—General Approach and Overview of Cardiac Emergencies)
                a. Clinically significant pericardial effusion leading to cardiac tamponade is rare in the cat.
                b. When cardiac tamponade occurs, increased pressure within the pericardial sac leads to impaired filling of the right side of the heart. This results in poor cardiac output and poor tissue perfusion.
        iii. Clinical signs
            1. Hypothermia common
            2. Cold extremities, poor to absent pulses
            3. Irregular heart rate, pulse deficits, tachycardia (HR >200–220) or bradycardia (HR <140–160)
            4. In cases of pericardial effusion, the heart sounds may be muffled and there may be jugular vein pulses or jugular vein distention (can be seen with just right-sided cardiac failure as well).
            5. A heart murmur is usually present, but the presence or absence of a heart murmur does not rule cardiogenic shock in or out.
            6. If congestive heart failure is present, increased lung sounds or pulmonary crackles may be ausculted.

       7. In cases with concurrent pleural effusion, lung sounds will be muffled (pleural effusion can occur in cats with left-sided heart failure).

b. Hypovolemic shock

  i. Hypovolemic shock is impaired perfusion secondary to a decrease in effective circulating volume.

  ii. Etiology

    1. Hemorrhage

      a. Hemoperitoneum

      b. Gastrointestinal hemorrhage

      c. Epistaxis

      d. Trauma resulting in significant tissue damage and hemorrhage

    2. Isotonic losses/severe dehydration

      a. Vomiting

      b. Diarrhea

      c. Severe polyuria without compensatory polydipsia (e.g., sick diabetic ketoacidotic cat)

    3. Third space loss

      a. Ascites

      b. Pleural effusion

  iii. Clinical signs

    1. Poor pulse quality

    2. Pale mucous membranes (especially if blood loss)

    3. Prolonged CRT

    4. Tachycardia

      a. Bradycardia possible in severely ill cats

    5. Abdominal fluid wave

      a. Hemoabdomen

      b. Ascites

c. Distributive shock

  i. This class is characterized by syndromes that result in inappropriate vascular tone, vasodilation, and impaired microcirculation.

  ii. The etiologies generally associated with this syndrome include septic shock and anaphylactic shock.

  iii. Anaphylactic shock

    1. This is the systemic sequelae of a Type I or immediate hypersensitivity.

      a. Mediated by IgE antibodies

    2. Can occur independent of IgE mediation; this is termed an anaphylactoid reaction.

    3. Occurs due to direct activation of the complement cascade

    4. Diagnosis

      a. Anaphylaxis can occur secondary to any stimulus of the immune system, including insect bites, snake envenomation, vaccines, drug reactions, transfusion reactions, and mast cell tumors.

      b. The signs of anaphylaxis in cats most commonly start in the gastrointestinal tract (often severe vomiting) and then progress to clinical signs of hypoperfusion.

    5. Treatment

      a. Removal of the underlying cause, if known

      b. Benadryl 1–2 mg/kg IM

      c. Epinephrine 0.1 mL/cat IV or IM (1 : 1,000 solution)

      d. Fluid therapy and supportive care (see "Septic shock" below)

  iv. Septic shock

    1. Sepsis is defined as a systemic inflammatory response syndrome (SIRS) secondary to an infectious process.

Table 3.1. SIRS criteria in the cat.

Temperature	>103.5°F, <100°F
Heart rate	>225, <140 beats/minute
Respiratory rate	>40 breaths/minute
White blood cell count	>19,500, <5,000, or >5% bands

2. Septic shock is a progression of this inflammatory response resulting in cardiovascular dysfunction and compromise.
3. SIRS can result from a number of different disease processes.
   a. The criteria for the diagnoses of SIRS are different in cats (see table 3.1).
4. Potential sources of infection include the following:
   a. Pulmonary
      i. Pyothorax
      ii. Pneumonia
         1. It is important to note that in a study of histopathologically diagnosed pneumonia in cats, significant pneumonia was associated with minimal or no changes on thoracic radiographs or CBC in some cats.
      iii. Endocarditis (extremely rare in the cat)
   b. Abdominal
      i.   Septic peritonitis
      ii. Septic pancreatitis
      iii. Pyelonephritis
      iv. Bacteremia secondary to severe gastrointestinal disease
      v.   Pyometra
      vi. Hepatic abscesses
   c. Neurologic
      i. Meningitis
   d. Severe bite wounds and subsequent tissue infection
5. Clinical signs
   a. Bradycardia common in septic cats (HR <140 bpm)
   b. Tachycardia (HR >225 bpm)
   c. Hypothermia
   d. Poor to absent pulses
   e. Prolonged CRT
   f. Pale, icteric mucous membranes
      i. The classic hyperemic, red mucous membranes with a rapid CRT is generally not appreciated in cats.
   g. Abdominal pain
      i. This was reported independent of intra-abdominal pathology in a study of severe sepsis in cats.
D. Treatment of shock
   a. Goals of therapy are to maximize oxygen delivery to the tissues
      i. Oxygen delivery (DO_2) = cardiac output × oxygen content
         1. Oxygen content = $(1.34 \, Hb \times SpO_2) + (0.003 \times PaO_2)$
      ii. Addressing each of these components (hemoglobin, oxygen saturation and PaO_2) will maximize your oxygen delivery.
   b. Fluid therapy (see chap. 8—Fluid Therapy for more details)
      i. Cardiac output = heart rate × stroke volume

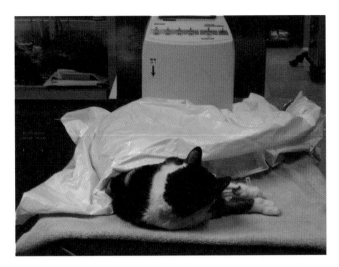

Fig. 3.1. Cat being externally rewarmed using a Bair Hugger circulating air blanket.

    1. Fluid therapy will improve preload and subsequently improve stroke volume.

    2. Although cats in shock may be bradycardic, atropine should not be administered to increase heart rate as this will increase myocardial oxygen consumption.

        a. Fluid resuscitation and rewarming generally will result in a normalization of the heart rate.

  ii. Fluid therapy is an integral part of the therapy in all categories of shock except cardiogenic shock resulting from low cardiac output heart failure.

  iii. The lung is the shock organ in the cat, so care must be taken with fluid therapy to avoid pulmonary edema or fluid overload.

  iv. The shock bolus in cats is 60 mL/kg of isotonic fluids or 3–5 mL colloid intravenously.

    1. This bolus should be given in smaller increments to affect.

    2. Initial bolus of 15–30 mL/kg of isotonic crystalloids over 15–20 minutes and repeat as needed to the full 60 mL/kg to improve perfusion parameters.

    3. Initial therapy should be isotonic fluids, but if patient is hypoproteinemic or perfusion parameters (pulse quality, heart rate, CRT) fail to improve with crystalloids, then colloids should be administered. The dose of colloidal solutions (e.g. Hetastarch) should be 2–3 ml/kg over 15–20 minutes.

    4. The initial treatment should be with a warmed isotonic fluid if the cat is hypothermic.

 c. Rewarming

  i. Rewarming is initially done by administering warm intravenous fluids.

  ii. After an initial bolus, external warming should be instituted.

    1. Forced-air heating (Bair Hugger, Arizant Healthcare Inc., Eden Prairie, MN; fig. 3.1)

    2. Circulating water blankets

    3. Incubator

  iii. A continuous rectal temperature probe can be invaluable in these patients to monitor response to warming as well as to watch for any evidence of hyperthermia or relapse of hypothermia.

  iv. Cats generally require improvement in their body temperature before improvement in perfusion parameters are appreciated.

    1. After initial fluid bolus of 15–30 mL/kg, rewarming should be initiated.

 d. Catecholamines

  i. In cats that remain hypotensive (Doppler <100 mmHg, mean arterial pressure <70) despite adequate fluid therapy and normothermia, exogenous catecholamine therapy may be indicated.

1. Dopamine
   a. Vasopressor with dose-dependent effects of the following:
      i. 5–10 μg/kg/min (affects B1 adrenergic receptors)
         1. Positive inotropic and chronotropic effects
      ii. >10 μg/kg/min (affects alpha-1 adrenergic receptors resulting in vasoconstriction)
2. Dobutamine
   a. Dose 5–20 μg/kg/min
   b. Positive inotropic and chronotropic effects
   c. Cats treated with dobutamine should be observed closely, as there are reports of seizures in cats treated with dobutamine CRIs for greater than 24 hours.
      i. If a patient has seizures on dobutamine, administer 0.5 mg/kg of diazepam and discontinue the dobutamine immediately.
3. Norepinephrine or epinephrine
   a. Can be used in cats that are not responding to dopamine or dobutamine
   b. Norepinephrine 0.1–3 μg/kg/min
   c. Epinephrine 0.1–2 μg/kg/min
4. Vasopressin
   a. Potent pressure agent
   b. No officially reported doses, although anecdotally it has been used as a last-ditch effort in cats that have not responded to all the other measures listed above (dose 0.5–2 mU/kg/min as a CRI). Should never be used as a first-line agent.
e. Antibiotic therapy
   i. Antibiotics should only be administered in cases of documented or suspected infectious components to the clinical presentation.
   ii. In cats with septic shock, appropriate antibiotic therapy is an integral part of the therapy.
   iii. Culture and sensitivity should be used to identify effective antibiotics. Broad spectrum antibiotics should be instituted pending sensitivity results. Combination choices include the following:
      1. Ampicillin 22 mg/kg IV every 8 hours and Baytril 5 mg/kg IV every 24 hours
      2. Clindamycin 10 mg/kg IV every 12 hours and Baytril 5 mg/kg IV every 24 hours
      3. Timentin (Ticarcillin and Clavulanate Potassium) 40–50 mg/kg IV every 6–8 hours
f. Glucocorticoids
   i. High-dose corticosteroids are no longer recommended for the treatment of shock.
      1. Potential risks of high-dose corticosteroid use for shock include increased risk of infection, delayed wound healing, and gastric irritation/ulceration (although cats are relatively more resistant to these effects compared to dogs).
   ii. Recent studies, however, have suggested that septic human patients may benefit from physiologic doses of steroids.
      1. In humans the current recommendation is the use of replacement doses of glucocorticoids in patients with refractory septic shock.
      2. A recent study in septic cats documented a decreased adrenal response, but no study has documented an improved outcome in cats treated with physiologic steroids as compared to conventional therapy.
         a. However, in cats with refractory septic shock that remain hypotensive despite adequate volume replacement, normothermia, vasopressor therapy, and treatment with physiologic steroids may be indicated.
            i. Dexamethasone sodium phosphate 0.08 mg/kg IV every 12–24 hours
               1. Equivalent to 0.5 mg/kg prednisone
g. Blood products
   i. Administration of red blood cells to an anemic patient will improve the oxygen carrying capacity of the blood and therefore improve oxygen delivery.

    1. Red blood cell transfusions should be considered in any poorly perfused cat with a PCV <20
       a. Initial dose of 1 unit (~ 20–30 mL) per cat
   ii. In cats with a coagulopathy, replacement of coagulation factors with plasma therapy minimizes
       further blood loss.
    1. Plasma should be administered in cats with prolonged coagulation times.
       a. Dose 5–10 mL/kg
 h. Nutritional support
    i. Cats in shock can rapidly develop a catabolic state.
       1. This can rapidly result in a significant nutritional deficiency, and nutritional needs should be
          addressed early.
   ii. Nutrition can be provided enterally by a naso-esophageal, esophagostomy, or PEG tube if the
       patient is not vomiting and is normothermic (see chap. 9—Nutritional Support for the Critically
       Ill Feline Patient).
  iii. In cats that cannot tolerate enteral feeding, total parenteral nutrition may be necessary (see chap.
       9—Nutritional Support for the Critically Ill Feline Patient).
 i. Glycemic control
    i. In humans, maintaining normoglycemia significantly improves outcome in critically ill patients.
   ii. Cats that are stressed frequently become hyperglycemic.
       1. If this is persistent throughout hospitalization and despite improving perfusion, judicious
          regular insulin therapy may be indicated to try and maintain a blood glucose of less than 250.
          a. This is particularly important in patients receiving TPN.
 j. Pain management (see chap. 7—Pain Management in Critically Ill Feline Patients)
    i. Pain can be difficult to recognize in veterinary patients, particularly in critically ill cats.
       1. The severity of illness may result in reluctance to treat with analgesic agents.
   ii. Untreated pain in these cats will lead to depression, inappetance/anorexia, decreased mobility,
       and an increase in stress hormones furthering the negative nitrogen balance.

4
TRAUMA
Erica L. Reineke

Unique Features	
Clinical signs of shock	Bradycardia (HR <160 bpm) in addition to other commonly cited signs of shock
Treatment of shock	Crystalloid shock bolus: 40–60 mL/kg
	Colloid shock bolus: 3–5 mL/kg
	Note: In cats, caution must be exercised, with administration of fluid therapy, as pleural effusion and pulmonary edema can occur as a result of fluid overload.
Response to hemorrhage	Limited ability of the spleen to contract and release additional red blood cells during blood loss
Clinical signs of respiratory distress	wsevere respiratory distress. Open-mouth breathing is a sign of severe respiratory distress.

I. Overview of trauma
   A. Definition of trauma: tissue injury that occurs more or less suddenly and includes any physical damage to the body caused by violence or accident
   B. Trauma is one of the most common emergencies seen in the hospital. Severe trauma is generally associated with significant blood loss or extensive soft tissue and orthopedic injury, and often involves vital organs. The unique physiology of the feline patient makes the treatment of trauma difficult and different from that of canine patients.
   C. Feline patients may suffer from unique traumatic injuries such as high-rise syndrome, dryer and fan belt injuries, and common traumatic injuries such as vehicular injury and bite wounds.
II. Physiologic response to trauma
   A. Trauma elicits complicated physiologic responses designed to prevent further tissue injury and promote adequate cellular oxygen delivery.
      1. Sympathetic nervous system stimulation will lead to release of catecholamines and cortisol.
         a. Increasing heart rate, contractility, and blood pressure through vasoconstriction
         b. This initially results in increases in skeletal muscle blood flow and decreases in splanchnic blood flow.
         c. Ongoing increases in circulating catecholamines will lead to activation of the renin-angiotensin system and secretion of vasopressin, ultimately intensifying vasoconstriction.

       d. Blood flow is redistributed to the lungs, heart, and brain, and away from the skin, skeletal muscle, kidneys, and other abdominal organs.

     2. Activation of intrinsic and extrinsic coagulation cascades occurs.

     3. Immune system up-regulation leads to the production of acute phase proteins and cytokine release.

  B. Exuberant physiologic responses to trauma can initiate a cascade of inflammatory and metabolic responses that predispose to the development of systemic inflammatory response and multiple organ dysfunction syndrome.

III. Approach to the feline trauma patient

  A. Assessment of the respiratory system

     1. Observation

       a. Evaluate respiratory rate and effort and pattern of breathing.

          i. Signs of respiratory distress include tachypnea, open-mouth breathing, cyanotic mucous membranes, stridor or stertor, restlessness, extended head and neck, nasal flare, and paradoxical respiration.

          ii. Keep in mind that cats develop more subtle signs of respiratory distress compared with dogs, and tachypnea alone may be indicative of severe respiratory compromise. Open-mouth breathing is generally considered to be a sign of severe respiratory compromise.

       b. Evaluate for thoracic injuries such as penetrating chest wounds or flail chest.

       c. Evaluate for injuries that could impair the upper airways, including jaw fractures, skull fractures, tracheal avulsion, or direct injury to the laryngeal and pharyngeal area.

       d. Hypoventilation may occur due to severe pain, trauma to the thorax, or neurologic disease.

     2. Auscultation

       a. Pulmonary crackles or harsh lung sounds may indicate the presence of contusions.

       b. Dull lung sounds may be heard with pleural space disease (pneumothorax, hemothorax, diaphragmatic hernia).

     3. Diagnostics

       a. Thoracic radiography is useful in identifying rib fractures (relatively rare in cats due to very compliant ribs compared to dogs), pulmonary contusions, diaphragmatic hernia, and pleural space disease. Chest radiographs should be performed with caution as they can be life-threatening due to both the manual restraint and positioning required.

       b. Thoracic ultrasound may be useful in identifying the presence of pleural fluid or diaphragmatic hernia (recently, its use for identifying pneumothorax and thoracic injury has been reported in dogs with traumatic injury).

       c. Pulse oximetry can be used to evaluate for hypoxemia, although results may be affected by poor perfusion and pigmented mucous membranes.

       d. Arterial blood gas analysis may be used to assess for hypoxemia and hypoventilation. Arterial blood gas sampling is generally difficult to perform in a cat and requires restraint, which may further compromise the patient. Therefore, venous CO_2 may be used with caution as an indicator of hypoventilation as long a perfusion is good. Poor perfusion may cause an increase in venous CO_2 despite normal or low arterial $PaCO_2$.

     4. Treatment

       a. Provide supplemental oxygen either with flow-by, mask, or oxygen cage.

       b. Thoracocentesis should be immediately performed if respiratory compromise is suspected to be secondary to pleural space disease. Tension pneumothorax (extremely rare in the cat) will not only cause severe respiratory compromise due to lung collapse but will also decrease venous return and impair cardiac output.

       c. Consider intubation and positive pressure ventilation if respiratory distress does not improve with oxygen support or thoracocentesis. This is rarely needed, and most cats will significantly improve following oxygen supplementation and minimizing handling, which may exacerbate stress.

      d. Emergency tracheostomy may need to be performed if there is an upper airway obstruction from traumatic injuries. This procedure is rarely necessary in the feline trauma patient.

B. Assessment of the cardiovascular system

  1. Physical examination

    a. Evaluate for shock: hypovolemia and anemia can occur in the feline trauma patient following external hemorrhage from wounds or hemorrhage into a body cavity (abdomen, thorax, or retroperitoneal space) or fracture site. Significant and life-threatening internal hemorrhage can occur even without obvious evidence of external injuries or wounds.

      i. Mucous membrane color and capillary refill time: pale or white mucous membranes may indicate vasoconstriction from hypoperfusion and/or anemia.

      ii. Heart rate and rhythm

        1. Tachycardia (heart rate >200 bpm) or bradycardia (heart rate <160 bpm) may be supportive of shock.

        2. Bradycardia has been reported in cats in response to severe systemic illness. The mechanism by which this occurs in unknown but may be secondary to cytokine release or increased vagal tone.

        3. Arrhythmias can occur secondary to blunt myocardial trauma or electrolyte abnormalities.

      iii. Pulse rate and quality: poor pulse quality or absent femoral or dorsal metatarsal pulses are indicative of shock. Extremities may also feel cool to the touch.

      iv. Measure rectal temperature. Hypothermia can occur commonly in the feline trauma patient and is another indicator of shock.

  2. Diagnostics

    a. Measurement of indirect arterial blood pressure:

      i. A systolic blood pressure ≤90 mmHg is supportive of hypotension.

      ii. Blood pressure measurements should be interpreted in light of the physical exam findings.

    b. ECG

    c. Packed cell volume (PCV) and total solid concentration:

      i. Unlike the dog, the feline spleen has a limited ability to contract and release additional red blood cells during acute blood loss.

    d. Blood lactate concentration: elevations in venous blood lactate are supportive of hypovolemia.

      i. In contrast to the dog, cats may only develop very high blood lactate concentrations in response to severe life-threatening hemorrhage. Therefore, even mild elevations in blood lactate concentration should prompt the clinician to evaluate for hypovolemic shock.

    e. Central venous pressure monitoring: this is generally not performed immediately due to the need for central catheter placement. However, a decreased central venous pressure (<0–5 mmHg) with concurrent physical examination findings of shock is supportive of hypovolemia.

  3. Treatment

    a. Evidence of poor tissue perfusion (pale mucous membranes, slow capillary refill time, bradycardia or tachycardia, weak or absent pulses, depressed mentation) should be immediately treated.

      i. 40–60 mL/kg is the shock bolus a of a balanced crystalloid solution, whereas 3–5 mL/kg is the bolus for a colloid solution.

      ii. Typically, one-third to one-half of the shock bolus is initially administered over 15–20 minutes and additional fluids are given depending on the patient's response to fluid therapy.

      iii. Transfusions of packed red blood cells (10 mL/kg) or fresh whole blood (20 mL/kg) should only be administered to patients who develop severe anemia (PCV ≤15%–20%) from hemorrhage. Hemoglobin-based fluids, such as Oxyglobin (2.5–10 mL/kg given at a rate of ≤5 mL/kg/hr), should be used cautiously in cats as they may lead to pulmonary edema and pleural effusion due to the potent oncotic effect of these solutions. In addition, these solutions have not been approved for use in cats at this time.

    iv. The goal of fluid therapy in a patient should be to alleviate peripheral vasoconstriction, increase systolic blood pressure to at least 90 mmHg, and restore urine output through restoration of an adequate intravascular volume.

    v. Caution must be exercised when administering fluid therapy to feline patients, especially if a heart murmur or arrhythmia is ausculted, as fluid overload resulting in pleural effusion and pulmonary edema is common. This may occur secondary to increased vascular permeability, myocardial dysfunction, or decreased oncotic pressure due to hypoalbuminemia.

  b. Major external hemorrhage (extremely rare in traumatized cats) should be managed by use of direct and indirect pressure and compressive bandaging.

  c. Hypothermia should be initially treated through the administration of warm intravenous fluids. Once the intravascular volume has been restored, circulating warm water blankets or forced air blankets can be used.

  d. Institute pain management:

    i. Some studies have shown that pain may worsen traumatic conditions and increase mortality from shock.

    ii. Opiods are this author's drug choice for controlling pain from trauma as they cause minimal cardiovascular and respiratory depression. Nonsteroidal anti-inflammatory medications should be avoided initially until renal and gastrointestinal perfusion is adequate and there is no evidence of kidney injury.

  e. Emergency surgery should be performed in patients with uncontrolled internal or external hemorrhage. This is rarely indicated, and most patients can be stabilized through fluid therapy, blood products, and pain management.

C. Assessment of the neurologic system

  1. Physical examination

    a. A complete examination of the neurologic system should be completed after evaluation of the respiratory and cardiovascular systems and after fluid resuscitation and respiratory support have been initiated.

    b. Evaluate for trauma to the skull: scleral hemorrhage, skull fractures, ocular injuries.

    c. Evaluate mentation

      i. Depressed or dull mentation may be secondary to pain or hypoperfusion but may also indicate elevations in intracranial pressure (ICP).

        1. These patients should be continually reassessed during fluid resuscitation as the patient may become more responsive when fluid therapy or pain management is initiated.

      ii. Obtunded, stuporous, or comatose patients should alert the clinician to likely increases in ICP secondary to brain edema or hemorrhage.

    d. Evaluate cranial nerves: assess pupil size and shape as well as presence of nystagmus or other cranial nerve abnormalities.

    e. Evaluate motor ability (and ability to ambulate once stable) and spinal reflexes.

    f. Seizures should alert the clinician to elevations in ICP.

  2. Diagnostics

    a. Monitor heart rate and blood pressure: hypertension with associated bradycardia (Cushing's reflex) indicates elevations in ICP.

    b. Blood glucose: hyperglycemia is often seen in patients with head trauma and may have an association with worse brain injury.

  c. Radiography to assess for skull and spinal fractures (only once the patient has been stabilized).

  d. Monitor for hypoventilation with serial arterial CO_2 measurements or end-tidal CO_2 monitoring. CO_2 should be maintained within the normal range (30–40 mmHg). Hypoventilation can lead to cerebral vasodilation and worsening of elevations in ICP. Too low of a $PaCO_2$ (<20 mmHg) can result in excessive brain blood-vessel vasoconstriction.

  e. We are currently limited in our ability to directly measure intracranial pressure in patients with head trauma.

 3. Treatment

  a. Suspected elevations in ICP (see chap. 25—General Approach and Overview of the Neurologic Cat and chap. 26—Neurologic Emergencies: Brain)

   i. Elevate head 15–30 degrees to encourage venous drainage, being careful to keep both the head and neck straight.

   ii. Provide oxygen support.

   iii. Consider administration of mannitol (0.5 g/kg–1 g/kg intravenously over 20–30 minutes) or hypertonic saline (3–5 mL/kg) intravenously to reduce cerebral edema.

   iv. Maintain adequate mean arterial blood pressure (>90 mmHg) to ensure cerebral perfusion.

   v. Jugular venous blood sampling should be avoided.

   vi. If patient's neurologic status is deteriorating, consider intubation and positive pressure ventilation. Patients may be temporarily hyperventilated to decrease ICP as this will cause cerebral vasoconstriction.

  b. Suspected spinal trauma: avoid moving patient and consider imaging and stabilization of spinal fractures.

D. Assessment of the renal system

 1. Physical examination

  a. Evaluate for the presence of a urinary bladder. The absence of a palpable urinary bladder should alert the clinician to the possibility of a ruptured bladder. Serial evaluations for the presence of a bladder should be performed following fluid resuscitation.

   i. Damage to the urinary system may not be evident for several hours following the initial trauma.

   ii. In addition to a ruptured bladder, urine may leak into the retroperitoneal space from trauma to the kidneys or ureters. Therefore, monitoring for adequate urine output in addition to serial monitoring of blood urea nitrogen and creatinine is essential.

 2. Diagnostics

  a. Monitor urine output. Normal urine output is 1–2 mL/kg/hour in an adequately hydrated and perfused patient.

  b. Monitor renal values at least once daily. Elevations in blood urea nitrogen, creatinine, and potassium with a decreased urine output should alert the clinician to the possibility of urinary tract rupture.

  c. Abdominal radiography: evaluate for the presence of a urinary bladder or loss of serosal detail in the abdominal or retroperitoneal space, which may indicate effusion.

  d. Renal ultrasonography: evaluate for the presence of a urinary bladder. In addition, trauma to the kidneys, ureters, and presence of abdominal or retroperitoneal effusion can be assessed.

  e. Retrograde urethrocystogram and/or intravenous pyelography to assess for leakage of urine along the urinary tract.

  f. A uroabdomen may be diagnosed by comparing abdominal effusion creatinine to serum creatinine and abdominal effusion potassium to serum potassium.

   i. An abdominal effusion creatinine to serum creatinine ratio of 2.0 : 1 or abdominal effusion potassium to serum potassium of 1.9 : 1 is diagnostic of a uroabdomen.

   3. Treatment
       a. Until surgery, placement of a urinary catheter for bladder rupture can decrease leakage of
          urine into the abdominal cavity.
       b. A pigtail catheter can be placed into the abdominal cavity to facilitate removal of urine from
          the peritoneal space until surgery.
       c. Exploratory laparotomy can be used to identify and repair damage to the urinary system.
   E. Additional evaluation
       1. Once the patient is stabilized, a thorough evaluation for orthopedic and soft-tissue injuries should
          be performed.
          a. Radiography should be utilized to diagnose fractures, luxations, and penetrating wounds. If
             a fracture is suspected, a soft padded bandage should be applied to immobilize the fracture
             fragments, preventing further injury and alleviating pain.
          b. All wounds should be clipped and cleaned. If wounds are extensive or degloving wounds are
             present, surgical debridement and placement of wet-to-dry bandages may be indicated. Broad-
             spectrum antibiotic therapy should be instituted.
IV. Specific types of trauma
   A. High-rise syndrome
       1. Overview
          a. High-rise syndrome is defined as traumatic injuries sustained by cats falling at least two
             stories.
          b. It occurs more commonly in younger cats and may be more frequent in warmer weather.
          c. Extent of injuries depends both on the length of fall and landing surface.
          d. After falling five stories, the cat reaches terminal velocity (60 mph) and may relax, positioning
             its legs horizontally (splay-legged or spread-eagled). In this position, the cat distributes forces
             evenly throughout its body during landing.
       2. Common injuries
          a. Shock: either from internal or external hemorrhage
          b. Thoracic injuries: pulmonary contusions, pneumothorax, trauma to the chest wall. In one
             study, up to 90% of cats that fell from the seventh story or higher had associated thoracic
             injuries.
          c. Abdominal trauma: hemoperitoneum, urinary tract rupture, and diaphragmatic hernia
          d. Facial injuries: facial trauma, hard palate fractures, mandibular fractures, dental injuries
          e. Skeletal injuries: limb, spinal fractures, and luxations. These injuries should be addressed once
             the patient is stabilized.
       3. Prognosis
          a. Dependent on the severity of the injury. Reported survival rates are between 90% and
             96.5%.
          b. In one study, only one-third of the cats required emergency treatment. Surviving cats fell a
             range of 2 to 32 stories.
   B. Dryer injury
       1. Overview
          a. The natural curiosity of the cat in addition to its heat-seeking behavior may lead to dryer
             injury.
          b. The severity of injury will depend both on the length of time the cat is in the dryer and the
             temperature setting of the dryer.
          c. Compared with dogs, cats are naturally heat resistant.
       2. Common injuries
          a. Heatstroke: once the body temperature rises above 106°F, the cat is at risk for developing
             thermal injury to tissues.
             i. Thermal injury can occur to all tissues of the body, including the central nervous system,
                liver, kidneys, and gastrointestinal and coagulation systems.

        ii. Sepsis can result from heatstroke secondary to bacterial translocation from the gastrointestinal tract.

    b. Head trauma

    c. Burns

    d. Thoracic injuries such as rib fractures, hemothorax, pneumothorax, and diaphragmatic hernia

    e. Skeletal and spinal injuries

3. Approach to the patient with dryer injury

    a. Evaluate the cardiovascular system. Shock should be treated as recommended previously with the administration of either intravenous crystalloids and/or colloids.

    b. Evaluate the respiratory system and institute therapy as above.

    c. Evaluate for hyperthermia: if the rectal temperature is >105°F, the cat should be actively cooled.

        i. Cooling methods that could be considered include saturating the hair coat with room-temperature water, using fans, and/or placing the cat on a cool surface such as an examination table.

        ii. Cold water or immersion in ice baths should be avoided as this may lead to peripheral vasoconstriction which will inhibit heat dissipation.

    d. Evaluate for evidence of head trauma.

    e. Evaluate for burns and orthopedic injury. Burns should be cleaned. Silver silvadene can be applied, and broad spectrum antibiotic therapy should be initiated.

4. Diagnostics

    a. Complete blood count, chemistry screen, and urinalysis to evaluate for thermal injury to organs

    b. Coagulation profile: if DIC is suspected, treatment with fresh frozen plasma may be considered (dose = 10 mL/kg).

    c. Radiography to assess for thoracic and skeletal injuries

    d. Serial blood pressure and ECG monitoring

    e. Abdominal ultrasonography

5. Prognosis

    a. Depends on severity of injuries sustained, in addition to thermal injury.

    b. Prognosis is guarded in cats that develop sepsis and multiple organ failure as a result of thermal injury.

C. Fan-belt injuries

1. Overview

    a. Fan-belt injuries most commonly occur in cold weather as cats seek a warm place to sleep. The cooling engine block of a car can be very enticing for both the warmth radiating from the block and the shelter provided by the hood and fenders.

    b. Trauma to the cat occurs when the owner of the car starts the engine, causing the fan blades to spin and placing the cat at risk for contact with either the belt or blades.

2. Common injuries

    a. Head trauma

    b. Abrasions and lacerations: most wounds may be managed medically, but if a puncture into a body cavity is suspected or uncontrolled hemorrhage is present, surgical intervention is warranted.

    c. Burns: ear tips, face, and foot pads

    d. Degloving injuries

    e. Limb/spinal fractures

        i. Closed fractures should be bandaged to immobilize fracture movement once the patient is stabilized.

        ii. Open fractures should be thoroughly lavaged followed by bandaging. In addition, antibiotic therapy should be initiated.

D. Predator injury and bite wounds
   1. Overview
      a. There are a number of animals that may prey on domestic and feral felines; however, the majority of wounds will be sustained following interactions with dogs. Cats may also develop bite-wound abscesses following fights with other cats. Generally, these are rarely life-threatening and are easily treatable.
      b. Bite wounds from dogs or other predators range in severity from simple lacerations to life-threatening injuries to the head, chest, and abdominal cavities.
      c. These injuries may lead to internal organ damage, a systemic inflammatory response, and sepsis.
   2. Approach to the feline with bite wounds
      a. Puncture wounds should be surgically explored as extensive injury can occur to the underlying tissues despite the relatively benign appearance of the overlying skin area.
      b. Radiography should be considered if wounds are suspected to penetrate the thoracic or abdominal cavity.
         i. Radiographic evidence of penetrating wounds includes the presence of free gas or effusion.
         ii. Wounds that are found to penetrate a body cavity warrant an exploratory laparotomy or thoracotomy to evaluate for injury to internal organs and to lavage the body cavity.
         iii. In addition, body wall defects or herniation warrant surgical evaluation and repair.
      c. Additional radiography should be considered if skeletal or spinal injuries are suspected.
      d. Wounds that are found to have extensive dead space should have drains placed.
      e. Broad spectrum antibiotic therapy and pain management (see chap. 7—Pain Management in Critically Ill Feline Patients) should be started.
      f. Complete blood count, chemistry screen, and urinalysis should be monitored to assess for organ injury or failure.
      g. Noninvasive blood pressure monitoring and pulse oximetry monitoring if indicated.
   3. Prognosis: dependent on severity of injuries and whether there is progression to a systemic inflammatory response and sepsis. Progression of the latter warrants a more guarded progression.

Recommended Reading

Aldrich J. Global assessment of the emergency patient. Vet Clin Small Anim, 2005; 35(2):281–305.

Driessen B, Brainard B. Fluid therapy for the traumatized patient. J Vet Emerg Crit Care, 2006; 16(4):276–299.

Muir W. Trauma: Physiology, pathophysiology and clinical implications. J Vet Emerg Crit Care, 2006; 16(4):253–263.

Syring RS. Assessment and treatment of central nervous system abnormalities in the emergency patient. Vet Clin Small Anim, 2005; 35(2):343–358.

Vnuk D, Pirkic B, Maticic D, et al. Feline high-rise syndrome: 119 cases (1998–2001). J Fel Med Surg, 2004; 6:305–312.

Whitney WO, Mehlhaff CJ. High-rise syndrome in cats. J Am Vet Med Assoc, 1987; 191(11):1399–1403.

5
GUIDELINES FOR ANESTHESIA IN CRITICALLY ILL FELINE PATIENTS

Lynne I. Kushner

A. Preanesthetic assessment
  a. The need to anesthetize a critically ill cat must outweigh the risks of postponing the surgery or procedure until the animal is stable. In some cases surgery to correct a life-threatening condition, for example, septic abdomen, cannot be postponed. However, stabilization of cardiovascular status must be initiated prior to anesthesia.
      i. Cats with heart failure, intracranial hypertension, pneumothorax, or pulmonary edema should be stabilized whenever feasible. Cats in acute respiratory distress may require sedation/anesthesia for diagnostic or therapeutic interventions (thoracocentesis, etc.).
  b. Preoperative assessment of history, HR and rhythm, blood pressure, hydration, respiratory rate and character, mental status, and temperament should be routine.
      i. A current, complete blood count and chemistry and acid-base status should be evaluated if time will allow. Tests of coagulation and blood typing may be indicated, depending on disease and needs of the patient.
      ii. All pertinent diagnostic modalities (chest radiographs, echocardiogram, ECG, etc.) should be available and reviewed by the anesthetist prior to anesthesia.
  c. Chronic diseases such as diabetes mellitus, renal and heart disease, poor body condition, or advanced age may often coexist with the acute disease.
      i. With cachexia, IV drugs remain in well-perfused tissues longer, resulting in more profound or prolonged effects; hypothermia can be severe.
      ii. With obesity, relative overdose of IV-administered drugs may occur if dosage is not modified for ideal weight; ventilation is compromised due to smaller functional residual capacity compounded by respiratory depressant drugs.
      iii. Aged cats have decreased functional physiologic reserves with decreased capacity for adaptation to physiologic changes.
  d. Classification of the patient's physical status (PS), although somewhat subjective, can be helpful in providing the anesthetist means of a consistent approach to case management (table 5.1).
      i. Critically ill cats (cats whose health status is life-threatening) and those who are moribund are generally classified as PS 4 and 5, respectively.
  e. Assessment of risk, anticipation of potential anesthetic complications, and management strategies to prevent or address them should be planned prior to anesthesia.
B. Pharmacologic considerations
  a. Drugs chosen for premedication and induction should depend on the disease(s) present as well as the temperament and condition of the cat (see anesthesia for specific diseases below).
  b. Cats who are critical (PS 4) typically do not require premedication, and agents can be titrated IV to effect for induction.

Table 5.1. Physical status (PS) classifications, modified from the American Society of Anesthesiologists.

PS 1	Normal healthy patient; usually elective procedure (OHE; minor laceration)
PS 2	Slight systemic disease, no obvious incapacity (early, simple urethral obstruction; healthy dystocia)
PS 3	Moderate systemic disease, but well compensated (diabetes M; significant cardiac disease, but not in failure; obstructed bowel with no perforation)
PS 4	Severe systemic disease that is a constant threat to life (perforated bowel; diaphragmatic hernia with pulmonary compromise; brain tumor with deteriorating mentation)
PS 5	Moribund; not expected to live
E	Emergency procedure applied to classification

   c. Mask induction may be appropriate if stress or hemodynamic instability is avoided.

      i. High inhalant concentrations ($\geq$1.5 MAC) typically result in unacceptable low blood pressures; critically ill cats may not tolerate low concentrations.

      ii. Mask induction is not appropriate if the need for rapid intubation is required (vomiting; airway or respiratory distress).

      iii. In general, drugs with significant cardiovascular depressive effects (acepromazine, alpha-2 agonists, propofol) should be avoided in PS 4 animals.

C. Intraoperative monitoring and management

   a. Although monitoring by a dedicated and competent individual is important during any anesthetic, it is imperative in critical patients (see "Anesthesia for Healthy Cats," monitoring).

      i. Monitoring with continuous ECG, blood pressure should be routine and end-tidal CO_2 is highly recommended.

      ii. Pulse oximetry should be monitored during thoracotomy, diaphragmatic hernia, thoracocentesis, or any case where oxygenation may be impaired. If in doubt, pulse oximetry monitoring should be performed.

      iii. Monitoring of body temperature and vital signs should continue at least every 30 minutes during the recovery period until the cat is normothermic and conscious. Critical patients may require hematologic and acid base monitoring along with continuous monitoring of vital signs with interventions (blood products, colloids, vasopressors) to achieve stable hemodynamics. Comfort level (signs of pain or anxiety) should always be monitored as a vital sign.

   b. Additional venous catheters should be secured in case administration of blood products or other infusions are needed.

      i. 5–15 mL/kg/hr balanced crystalloid volume solutions are recommended during anesthesia; rate will depend on the severity of surgical trauma and concurrent diseases.

      ii. Cats with low colloidal osmotic pressure (i.e., hypoalbuminemia) will benefit from colloids (Hetastarch 1–2 mL/kg /hr), which can maintain normovolemia while sparing excessive crystalloid rates. Hypotension due to hypovolemia may necessitate administration of a colloid bolus (3–5 mL/kg). Colloids maintain intravascular volume longer (2–5 hrs) than crystalloids, and initially may increase plasma volume by 2–4 mL per mL of colloid. In cats, the total dose of colloid should not exceed 12–15 mL/kg/24 hr.

      iii. Crystalloids replace estimated blood loss over 15–20 minutes 3 : 1; colloids, 1 : 1.

      iv. Packed RBCs or whole blood when PCV <15–18%. Factors to consider when making the decision to transfuse:

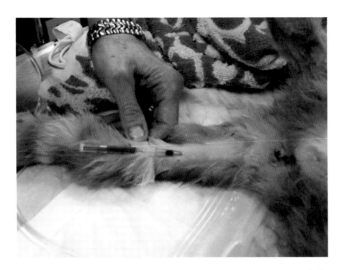

Fig. 5.1. The hair of the ventral aspect of the proximal third of the tail is clipped and cleaned with surgical scrub prior to placement of a 22-gauge venous catheter in the coccygeal artery. From the arterial catheter, direct blood pressure can be monitored and arterial blood may be sampled if needed.

  1. Acute vs. chronic blood loss
  2. Duration of anesthetic procedure and resulting fluid needs
  3. Ongoing blood loss
  4. Hemodynamic instability of patient
 v. Fresh frozen plasma if coagulation factors are needed at a rate of approximately 5 mL/kg.
c. Cats pose particular challenges to the anesthetist.
 i. Indirect blood pressure monitors (oscillometric, plethysmographic and ultrasound Doppler techniques) have been evaluated in anesthetized cats for reliability and accuracy. Many studies find that most indirect techniques, particularly Doppler, underestimate systolic but are good predictors of MAP; therefore, Doppler BP is subject to some interpretation.
  1. Indirect techniques may fail during periods of severe hypotension, hypothermia, and poor perfusion.
  2. Arterial catheterization for direct BP monitoring can be difficult, especially in hypotensive cats; but with skill, dorsal pedal, or coccygeal arteries can be catheterized (fig. 5.1).
  3. Limited accessibility under drapes during surgery
   a. Jugular catheters are most accessible and reliable for blood sampling and can be used to measure CVP (central venous pressure; fig. 5.2). Jugular catheters should be avoided in cats that are coagulopathic (hyper- or hypocoagulopathic).
   b. All peripheral catheter ports should be made accessible.
  4. Arterial or central venous blood should be sampled intraoperatively to assess changes in PCV and plasma proteins, electrolyte, acid-base, or blood gas abnormalities if significant blood loss, hemodilution, or acid-base imbalance is suspected.
  5. Small size can lead to severe hypothermia (<34°C), which can lead to bradycardia, hypotension, decreased enzyme and cell function, increased infection rate, prolonged recovery, and reduced anesthetic requirements.
   a. Forced warm air blankets or warm water circulating pads should be applied to the patient at induction of anesthesia (Bair Hugger, Arizant Healthcare Inc., Eden Prairie, MN; fig. 5.2).
d. Balanced anesthetic techniques reduce inhalant concentrations and allow for better cardiovascular stability, analgesia, and muscle relaxation (table 5.2).

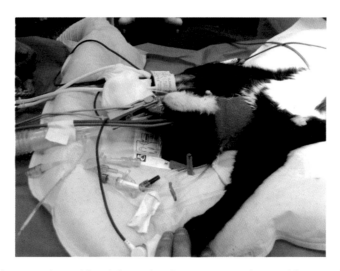

Fig. 5.2. A cat has been anesthetized for abdominal exploratory surgery for possible septic abdomen. In addition to a cephalic catheter, a double lumen catheter was placed in the jugular vein providing addition IV access if needed for administration of blood products, inotropes, or continuous infusions such as fentanyl. Blood samples such as PCV, TP, glucose, or electrolyes may be collected from the jugular catheter if needed during surgery. In addition, if necessary, central venous pressure (CVP) may be monitored from the jugular catheter. Note forced warm air blanket under cat.

Table 5.2. Anesthesia maintenance adjuncts.

Drug	Dosage	Comments
Fentanyl	2.5–5.0 µg/kg IV repeat as needed 0.5–1.0 µg/kg/min	Duration of effect ~15–20 min Significant bradycardia, respiratory depression, support ventilation; excellent analgesia, poor muscle relaxation; infusion may require partial reversal at recovery.
Morphine	IV bolus not recommended 1.7–6.7 µg/kg/min	Histamine release is dose, rate dependent and usually produces no clinical signs of histamine release in healthy animals.
Butorphanol	0.1–0.2 mg/kg IV	Duration ~45–60 min
Hydromorphone or Oxymorphone	0.05–0.1 mg/kg IV 0.025–0.05 mg/kg IV	Duration 45–90 min Bradycardia and respiratory depression are possible; support ventilation.
Etomidate	0.2–0.0.5 mg/kg IV	Cortisol depression, supplement with steroids if necessary; intravascular hemolysis possible. Duration 10–20 min
Diazepam or Midazolam	0.05–0.1 mg/kg 0.025–0.1 mg/kg	For improved muscle relaxation; duration 15–30 min; repetitive dosing may result in prolonged recovery.
Atracurium	0.05–0.1 mg/kg	For neuromuscular blockade; duration 15–20 min; institute IPPV; provide adequate anesthesia.
Ketamine	0.5–1.0 mg/kg IV 8–25 µg/kg/min	Can improve postoperative analgesia (low dose); can provide balanced anesthesia
Propofol	0.1–0.4 mg/kg/min	Will reduce or replace inhalant; avoid if significantly hypotensive.
Lidocaine	25–50 µg/kg/min	May reduce inhalant MAC; avoid prolonged infusions; can produce cardiovascular depression.

    i.   All inhalants produce dose-dependent decreases in BP, and the anesthetic concentration should be reduced or terminated if blood pressure falls to unacceptable levels (MAP <60 mmHg or Doppler <80 mmHg).

    ii.   Intraoperative opioid administration reduces isoflurane MAC requirements in cats by up to 35%, depending on opioid and patient responses.

        1. Opioids, however, do not provide good muscle relaxation and are not anesthetics (not hypnotics).

    iii.   Studies have determined that at equipotent doses, blood pressure is better maintained with propofol than with isoflurane.

        1. In a clinical study, cats undergoing orthopedic surgery due to trauma received either isoflurane (inspired 1.2%) and fentanyl (0.33 μg/kg/min) or propofol (0.2 mg/kg/min) and similar fentanyl. In that study, cats receiving isoflurane-fentanyl had significantly lower arterial blood pressures compared with the cats receiving propofol-fentanyl.

        2. However, both drugs can produce bradycardia and are potent respiratory depressants. Heart rate and $ETCO_2$ should be carefully monitored, and controlled ventilation should be instituted if necessary.

        3. In a different study, the minimal infusion rate of propofol to prevent response to various stimuli in 50% of cats breathing room air was 0.1–0.28 mg/kg/min, and cardiovascular and respiratory indices were well maintained.

            a. The addition of low- (23 μg/kg/min) or high- (46 μg/kg/min) dose ketamine significantly reduced the dose of propofol (~50%), even though there was no difference between the two doses.

            b. Although the addition of ketamine with the reduction of propofol did not alter most cardiovascular and blood gas values, it did significantly increase pulmonary arterial pressure and venous admixture and did significantly reduce PaO_2.

    iv.   Small doses of benzodiazepines (BZ) (0.05–0.1 mg/kg) can improve muscle relaxation.

    v.   Etomidate in small boluses (0.3–0.5 mg/kg) produces minimal C/V depression, but cortisol supplement (0.05 mg/kg Dexamethasone IV) may be warranted.

  e. Hypotension should be treated once volume depletion is corrected and anesthetic concentrations have been reduced.

    i.   Without complex hemodynamic monitoring, the vasopressor/inotrope chosen is based on clinical judgment and patient response.

        1. Dopamine 5–10 μg/kg/min; positive inotropic and chrontropic effects; will increase MAP; vasoconstriction at high doses

        2. Dobutamine 5–10 μg/kg/min; positive inotropic and chrontropic effects; less likely to increase MAP unless high dosage rates used

        3. Phenylephrine 0.1–4 μg/kg/min ; vasoconstriction; minimal change in HR

        4. Norepinephrine 0.05–0.2 μg/kg/min vasoconstriction

        5. Epinephrine 0.05–2 μg/kg/min positive inotropic and chrontropic effects; vasoconstriction

D. Anesthesia for cats with cardiovascular dysfunction

  a. Cardiovascular dysfunction may refer to a primary disorder of the heart, such as hypertrophic cardiomyopathy (HCM), or the vascular system (vasculogenic shock).

  b. Preanesthetic assessment

    i.   Cats who are hypovolemic from hemorrhage, third space losses, or vasculogenic disorders such as sepsis should be aggressively treated as appropriate prior to anesthesia (see chap. 3—Shock). Cats with a life-threatening surgical disease (e.g., perforated bowel) may require surgery before complete stabilization can be accomplished (PS 4, 5) and pose the most challenges to the anesthetist.

    ii.   Cats with preexisting cardiac disease without evidence of failure may require anesthesia and surgery for a variety of noncardiac causes.

Table 5.3. Suggested sedation and anesthesia protocols for cats with cardiac disease or hemodynamic instability.

Disorder	PS	Sedation/Premed	Induction IV	Comments
Mild-moderate hypertrophy	2, 3	AcP/Op; Op/BZ, Op/BZ/Ket ±AcP	Prop, Thio,	Caution AcP in PS 3; low dose Ket if necessary (2–5 mg/kg IM). Avoid thio if extrasystoles.
HCM severe; enlarged LA; dynamic LVOT obstruction	3, 4	Op/BZ	Op/BZ + Etom, Prop, Thio, mask	Minimize thio, prop but avoid with systolic dysfunction; avoid thio if arrhythmias; avoid Ket. Extreme caution with fluids.
Hemodynamic instability (sepsis, etc.); no primary cardiac disease	4	Not needed	Op/BZ, Etom Ket/BZ, mask	Avoid morphine for induction; caution with Ket; caution with inhalant concentrations; ensure adequate volume replacement.

Note: AcP (acepromazine 0.01–0.04 mg/kg IM), Op (hydromorphone 0.05–0.2 mg/kg; oxymorphone 0.025–0.1 mg/kg; butorphanol 0.1–0.4 mg/kg IM, IV; morphine 0.2–0.5 mg/kg IM), BZ (diazepam 0.2–0.4 mg/kg IV; midazolam 0.1–0.3 mg/kg IM, IV, Ket (ketamine 2–5 mg/kg IM, IV), Thio (thiopental 2–8 mg/kg IV), Prop (propofol 1–4 mg/kg), Etom (etomidate 0.3–1.5 mg/kg IV, use physiologic dose of dexamathasone sodium phosphate 0.05 mg/kg IV), mask (isoflurane, sevoflurane induction).

1. Murmurs and gallop rhythms auscultated preoperatively should be investigated to determine significance.
    a. Thoracic radiographs to evaluate heart size, evidence of edema, or effusions
    b. Echocardiography necessary to determine functional abnormalities
2. Cats with physiologic murmurs generally pose no additional concerns for anesthesia.
3. Cats with mild cardiac enlargement or thickening of ventricular walls but no evidence of obstructive or myocardial dysfunction pose some concern for possible fluid overload.
4. Cats with severe HCM and atrial enlargement; dynamic LV outflow tract obstruction (LVOT) present greater anesthetic concerns; caution with fluid rates; avoid tachycardia, hypotension

c. Pharmacologic considerations (table 5.3)
    i. Premedication may not be indicated in cats with hemodynamic instability (PS 4).
        1. Opioids, BZ are relatively devoid of significant cardiovascular depressive effects and are good choices as IV adjuncts for induction.
        2. Unlike the depressed dog, cats typically require small amounts of anesthetics with the above to accomplish intubation.
            a. Etomidate (0.3–1.0 mg/kg IV) provides the best hemodynamic stability.
            b. Ketamine (2–5 mg/kg IV) may be a good choice in most situations, but not in severe HCM. However, the direct depressive effects of ketamine may predominate in unstable patients with little sympathetic tone.
            c. Inhalant induction but may cause hypotension
    ii. Premedication may be warranted in stable cats (PS 2, 3) with heart disease, but drugs should be chosen according to the degree of dysfunction.
    iii. In general, ketamine and tiletamine/zolazapam are not recommended in cats with moderate/severe HCM because of their indirect sympathomimetic effects.

    iv.   Alpha-2 agonists in general should be avoided in cats with heart disease because of the profound cardiovascular effects they produce.

    v.   However, aggressive, fractious cats often become a real challenge to handle without sedation and require good chemical restraint.

       1. Opioid + BZ + small amounts (<5 mg/kg) of ketamine IM is usually well tolerated in cats with mild-moderate HCM.

       2. In an echocardiographic study of cats with significant HCM, disappearance of systolic anterior motion of the mitral valve and normalization of the gradient across the LVOT occurred after administration of 20 µg/kg medetomidine IM.

       3. Mask or tank induction can be an option if extreme excitement can be avoided.

       4. Therefore, risks and benefits of these techniques should be weighed against potential consequences of increasing heart rate and oxygen demands from excessive manual restraint and resulting increases in sympathetic tone.

    vi.   Anticholinergics should be administered only if needed to treat a clinically significant bradycardia.

    vii.   Propofol, thiopental should be avoided in cats with hemodynamic instability (PS 4, 5), but small amounts may be appropriate for cats with HCM.

    viii.   Cats receiving ACE inhibitors or calcium channel blockers may be at increased risk for intra-operative hypotension or bradycardia.

d. Anesthesia management and monitoring

    i.   Cats classified as PS 4, 5 or cats with functional abnormalities on echocardiogram undergoing prolonged anesthesia (PS 3, 4) ideally should have a central venous catheter for easy IV access and possible CVP monitoring as well as additional peripheral catheters depending on severity and duration of surgery.

    ii.   Cats with significant heart disease may not tolerate fluid volumes typically administered during anesthesia; fluid rates should be decreased during prolonged procedures.

       1. However, hypotension during anesthesia may occur secondary to hypovolemia if fluid losses are not adequately addressed.

       2. CVP monitoring may be helpful to assess volume overload or hypovolemia. Because of much intercat variation in CVP measurements, trends in CVP and the response to fluid challenges are more important than absolute values. Modest increases to fluid challanges (~2.0 mmHg after 6 mL/kg crystalloid in healthy cats) may be expected if heart failure is not present.

    iii.   Supplemental opioids or local anesthetic techniques to reduce inhalant concentrations should be routine.

       1. Opioid infusions (see table 5.2)

       2. Morphine epidural; lidocaine line block (see chap. 7—Pain Management in Critically Ill Feline Patients)

    iv.   Arterial or central venous blood may be sampled intraoperatively to assess changes in PCV and plasma proteins, as well as electrolyte, acid-base, or blood gas abnormalities.

    v.   Monitoring urine output during anesthesisa may be helpful to assess adequate CO and renal perfusion, although little information is available describing normal urine production in anesthetized cats.

    vi.   Hypotension (MAP <60–65 mmHg; Doppler <75 mmHg) should be treated with vasopressors or positive inotropes as needed after volume needs are addressed.

       1. Positive inotropes and chronotropes (dopamine, dobutamine) may be contraindicated in cats with HCM; modest amounts of vasoconstrictors (phenylephrine) may be better choices.

       2. Cats without HCM may benefit from a positive inotrope.

       3. Septic cats may require vasoconstrictors and positive inotropes and can be the most challenging to treat.

E. Anesthesia for the hyperthyroid cat
  a. Hyperthyroid cats are often aged, thin, and exhibit multisystemic abnormalities, including the following:
      i. High output cardiac state with murmurs, gallops, tachycardia
      ii. Renal insufficiency that may coexist
      iii. Behavior changes and hyperexcitability
  b. A euthyroid state should be attained prior to anesthesia but is not always possible.
      i. Thyroidectomy should be performed after medical management is instituted.
      ii. Hyperthyroid cats may require anesthesia for emergency procedures unrelated to thyroid disease.
          1. Significant tachycardia (>200 bpm) may require preoperative treatment with beta blockers (propranalol 0.5–2.0 mg/kg PO; esmolol 10–100 μg/kg /min) or calcium channel blockers (Diltiazem 7.5 mg/kg PO).
  c. Pharmacologic considerations
      i. Avoid agents that can potentiate catecholamine release or activity.
          1. Avoid ketamine.
          2. Thiopental (4–12 mg/kg) (if no dysrhythmia) or propofol (2–6 mg/kg) can be a good choice in most cats.
          3. Acepromazine (0.03–0.05 mg/kg IM) may blunt sympathetic activity and can minimize stress (avoid in PS 4).
          4. Opioids, ± BZ
          5. Avoid routine use of anticholinergics, but use if needed to correct a clinically significant bradycardia.
  d. Anesthetic management and monitoring
      i. Cardiac rate and rhythm must be closely monitored.
      ii. If significant tachycardia develops (HR >220 bpm) despite adequate depth of anesthesia, esmolol (0.01–0.1 mg/kg /min) may be indicated.
      iii. As some cats may be hypertensive with some degree of renal insufficiency, renal perfusion should be maintained by keeping BP in the range of high normal.
      iv. Caution with indirect-acting catecholamines (dopamine, ephedrine) as this may precipitate an exaggerated catecholamine response.
      v. Monitor body temperature, keep normothermic with external warming devices.
F. Anesthesia for cats with airway or respiratory diseases
  a. Cats presented in acute respiratory distress may require anesthesia for diagnostic or therapeutic purposes (chest tubes, thoracocentesis), or for repair of traumatic injuries suffered with concurrent thoracic trauma (stabilized pneumothorax, diaphragmatic hernia, or pulmonary hemorrhage)
  b. Preanesthetic assessment
      i. IV access should be secured with minimal stress; if not possible, sedation may be warranted. In all circumstances, close observation is necessary.
          1. The cat with moderate/severe respiratory disease may breathe well when conscious but can be severely compromised when sedated.
      ii. Cats with obstructive disease (nasopharyngeal polyps or masses) may be difficult to intubate necessitating small diameter tubes or tracheostomy, and this should be anticipated prior to induction.
      iii. Avoid drugs that may cause vomiting, such as α_2 agonists or pure opioid agonists; opioids can be administered if necessary once the airway is secured.
  c. Pharmacologic consideration (table 5.4)
      i. Acepromazine (0.01–0.05 mg/kg IM) provides mild/moderate sedation with little or no respiratory depression.
      ii. If good chemical restraint is necessary, ketamine 2–4 mg/kg IM with AcP or BZ produces minimal respiratory depression.
          1. Ketamine decreases bronchomotor tone and is a good choice for asthmatic cats.

Table 5.4. Examples of some sedation/anesthesia protocols for various diseases and procedures.

Disease/Condition	Procedure	Sedation/Anesthesia	Comments
Urinary obstruction With hyperkalemia	Catheterization	Ket/BZ IV*/IM But/BZ IV ± Ket; Prop IV	Brief restraint Ket (≤2 mg/kg) Prop (≤1 mg/kg) only if nec Intubation may be necessary; O₂.
Respiratory distress (mild) Severe respiratory distress	Radiographs Chest tube	AcP; Ket /Mid IM, IV Thio, Prop IV; Ket/Diaz	Ket (≤5 mg/kg) administer flow-by O₂ intubate if necessary Rapid intubation necessary; O₂.
Liver disease	Aspirate, biopsy	But ± BZ ± Prop IV	Midazolam (<0.2 mg/kg) preferable to diazepam— caution without flumazenil; be prepared to intubate when using Prop; provide O₂.
Neurologic disease	CSF collection	BZ + Thio or prop IV	Intubate; avoid hypoventilation; avoid high concentrations of inhalant or use propofol.

Note: Ket (ketamine 2–6 mg/kg), BZ (diazepam 0.2–0.3 mg/kg; midazolam 0.1–0.2 mg/kg), But (butorphanol 0.1–0.2 mg/kg), Prop (propofol 0.5–2 mg/kg increments), Thio (2–4 mg/kg increments), AcP (Acepromazine 0.025–0.05 mg/kg).
*Use lower dosages IV.

    iii. Thiopental (2–8 mg/kg IV), propofol (2–6 mg/kg IV), or KetBZ (5–8 mg/kg, 0.3–0.4 mg/kg) for rapid induction and intubation

    iv. Etomidate may cause wretching or vomiting and should be reserved for patients with hemodynamic instability.

    v. Volatile anesthetics also decrease bronchomotor tone.

  d. Anesthetic management and monitoring

    i. Avoid stress or excitement that can exacerbate respiratory distress.

      1. Premedication may be warranted.

    ii. Preoxygenation with 100% oxygen for 3–5 minutes should precede administration of a rapid sequence IV induction and intubation.

    iii. Controlled ventilation should be applied as necessary with attention to airway pressures and pulmonary compliance.

      1. Increased airway pressures >15 cm H_2O to achieve tidal volumes of 15 mL/kg or less may indicate poor pulmonary compliance and suggest airway obstruction, pneumothorax, or pleural effusion.

        a. Suction endotracheal tube to remove obstructive airway secretions.

        b. Thoracocentesis to remove air or fluid

          i. Discontinue positive pressure ventilation briefly during thoracocentesis to avoid iatrogenic pneumothorax.

        c. Bronchodilators (terbutaline 0.01 mg/kg IM IV) if bronchoconstriction is suspected. Hypotension can occur with rapid IV administration.

      2. Decreased SpO_2 <94% with 100% inspired oxygen (FiO_2 of 1.0) suggests that a large alveolar arterial oxygen gradient (P[A-a] O_2 gradient) in addition to the above can be caused by parenchyma diseases resulting in disruption of V/Q ratios.

      3. Positive pressure ventilation rather than spontaneous breathing may improve oxygenation.

        a. Positive end expired pressure (PEEP) can be applied by the anesthetist by maintaining up to 5 cm H_2O positive pressure within the rebreathing bag if a PEEP valve is not available.

        b. PEEP may result in lower blood pressure due to a decrease in venous return; if so, adequate volume replacement and inotropic or vasoactive agents may be indicated (see notes on hypotension above).

   iv. Pulse oximetry and $ETCO_2$ should be monitored.

   v. Prior to extubation, SpO_2 should be monitored.

        1. Placing the cat in sternal recumbency and careful reversal of opioids or BZ may be necessary to restore spontaneous respiration and adequate $PaCO_2$.

        2. Once spontaneous respiration is restored, SpO_2 should be monitored as the FiO_2 is reduced to determine the animal's O_2 requirements prior to extubation.

   vi. O_2 supplementation should be provided in recovery and the cat should be continuously monitored.

G. Anesthesia for cats with urinary tract diseases

  a. Cats with obstructive uropathy may require brief anesthesia or sedation for urinary catheterization; cats in renal failure that require general anesthesia for surgery (PU, ruptured bladder, or unrelated surgical diseases) should be stabilized as well as possible to correct electrolyte abnormalities and restore vascular volume.

  b. Preanesthetic assessment

   i. Cats who are severely hyperkalemic, demonstrating ECG abnormalities or idioventricular rhythms, are at great risk for mortality because of cardiac instability (PS 4).

        1. Treatment to stabilize cardiac conduction with calcium gluconate (50–100 mg/kg IV slowly) should be instituted before sedative or anesthetic agents are administered.

        2. Efforts to reduce serum K and the existing acidemia (fluids, Na, bicarbonate, glucose ± insulin) should be instituted (see chap. 23—Urologic Emergencies: Ureter, Bladder, Urethra, GN, and CRF).

   ii. Cats with advanced renal failure may have secondary cardiac disease, which should be identified prior to anesthesia, as this will greatly complicate anesthetic management (fluid administration).

   iii. Inhalant anesthesia generally depresses renal function transiently in healthy animals by altering autoregulation, renal blood flow, and glomerular filtration rate (GFR) via changes in cardiovascular function and neuroendocrine activity; therefore, cats with preexisting renal disease are at risk for further damage.

        1. BP should be maintained in the upper range of normal.

  c. Pharmacologic considerations (table 5.4)

   i. Ketamine in low/moderate dosages (<5 mg/kg with 0.25 mg/kg BZ IV) may be used in cats with mild or moderate renal disease.

        1. Ketamine is metabolized rapidly in the liver, and metabolism and redistribution are the major factors in reducing blood levels.

        2. Although renal excretion is responsible for elimination, only 10% of the administered ketamine and its metabolite were eliminated in the urine during recovery in healthy cats.

        3. Ketamine may increase RBF with little to no change in GFR.

   ii. Cats with obstructed uropathy can tolerate low dosages of Ket with BZ (as above) if needed for urinary catheterization; however, if severely hyperkalemic, Op/BZ would be a better choice.

        1. Ketamine should be avoided in cats with hyperkalemic cardiac conduction abnormalities, due to its indirect sympathomimetic effects.

   iii. Acepromazine may potentiate hypotension and should be avoided in PS 4 patients.

        1. However, in isoflurane-anesthetized dogs administered 0.1 mg/kg acepromazine or saline, RBF and GRF were similar between the two groups despite significantly lower MAP in the acepromazine group. However, this has not been specifically investigated in cats.

iv.   Thiopental and propofol produce little change in RBF and GFR providing CO and BP are well maintained.

1. Thiopental is a highly protein-bound weak acid that may reach receptor sites in higher concentrations in the presence of hypoalbuminemia and acidosis, as may occur with uremia.

v.   Etomidate may produce hemolysis and hemoglobinuria due to the high osmolality of its formulation (propylene glycol).

vi.   Sevoflurane presents some issues relevant to the renal system.

1. Although highly fluorinated, sevoflurane requires little intrarenal metabolism, which may result in lower inorganic Fl- concentrations as occurred with methoxyflurane.

a. Little work has been done in cats determining F- concentrations with sevoflurane.

b. Sevoflurane in the presence of CO_2 absorbents is degraded to compound A, a potential renal toxin. Although no further renal damage from sevoflurane has been documented in human patients with renal failure, it probably should be avoided unless non-rebreathing circuits are used.

2. Deep planes of inhalant anesthesia disrupt autoregulation and decrease RBF; balanced techniques will minimize inhalant concentrations.

3. Inhalants have weak Ca channel blocking effects, which can potentiate the cardiac effects of moderate hyperkalemia if not treated.

vii.   Cats with renal failure may be receiving Ca channel blockers, which may put them at risk for hypotension during anesthesia.

d. Anesthetic management and monitoring

i.   It is most important to maintain adequate perfusion to kidneys by maintaining CO, BP.

1. Hypotension should be managed by lowering inhalant anesthetic concentration, maintaining adequate vascular volume and administering inotropes such as dopamine or dobutamine at $\geq 5\,\mu g/kg$ /min to improve CO and consequently, RBF.

2. The practice of administering low-dose dopamine (1–$4\,\mu g/kg/min$) for providing protective renal effects has been questioned. Studies in humans have not confirmed intrinsic protective effects of dopamine on the kidney. Some studies failed to demonstrate dopamine receptors in the renal circulation of cats, although dopamine receptors have been identified in feline renal cortices.

ii.   Fluid rates should be administered at 10–$15\,mL/kg$, but care must be used to avoid fluid overload, especially if heart disease is present.

1. CVP should be monitored and fluids carefully administered, especially if heart disease is present.

H. Anesthesia for cats with hepatic disease

a. Cats with hepatic lipidosis, porto-systemic shunts, or biliary obstruction may be chronically debilitated, hypoproteinemic, icteric, exhibit various stages of liver dysfunction, and require anesthesia for liver biopsy, feeding tubes, or surgical exploration.

b. Pre-anesthetic assessment

i.   Blood count and chemistry with albumin should be current, and coagulation function (prothrombin time, partial thromboplastin time, activated clotting time) should be evaluated prior to surgery.

ii.   Cats with signs of hepatic encephalopathy (HE) demonstrate increased sensitivity to GABA-nergic neurotransmission and will have an increased sensitivity to CNS depressant drugs, in particular, the BZ.

c. Pharmacologic considerations (table 5.4)

i.   Acepromazine requires extensive metabolism, can transiently decrease platelet function and PCV and should be avoided in cats with severe liver disease.

ii.   Unless flumazenil is available, benzodiazepines should be used with extreme caution or not at all in cats with severe liver disease.

    1. Glucuronidation is required for elimination of BZ.

    2. HE may be potentiated by BZ administration.

     a. Evidence of improved mentation exists in people and animals with HE after receiving the BZ antagonist flumazenil (0.01–0.02 mg/kg).

  iii. Small doses of thiopental (<5 mg/kg) are not necessarily contraindicated in mild-moderate liver disease.

    1. It requires extensive hepatic metabolism and is highly protein bound; caution in severe liver disease.

  iv. Propofol is rapidly metabolized and eliminated in part due to extra hepatic mechanisms of removal and is a good induction agent for patients with liver disease, providing there is good cardiovascular stability.

  v. Opioids maintain C/V stability well, reduce induction and inhalant requirements, and can be reversed if necessary.

  vi. Ketamine is rapidly biotransformed in the cat via microsomal N–demethylation; use low dosages if necessary in cats with mild-moderate liver disease.

  vii. Hepatic metabolism of desflurane, isoflurane, and sevoflurane are negligible and none are associated with hepatic injury.

 d. Anesthetic management and monitoring

  i. In general, reduction of hepatic blood flow is proportional to decreases in arterial BP and cardiac output.

    1. Maintenance of good BP and CO is most important.

  ii. Cats who are severely hypoproteinemic are at risk for hypotension due to low oncotic pressure and relative hypovolemia.

    1. Colloids such as hetastarch (1–2 mL/kg/hr) as well as fresh frozen plasma if coagulation factors are needed, should be included as part of the fluid plan to maintain vascular volume, minimize crystalloid volumes, and prevent further dilution of existing plasma proteins.

I. Anesthesia in cats with neurologic disease

 a. Cats with neurologic disease (brain tumor or inflammatory DZ) may require anesthesia for cerebral spinal fluid collection or imaging. Cats suffering major trauma with evidence of head trauma (anisocoria; scleral hemorrhage; skull or jaw fractures) may require anesthesia for diagnostic purposes (radiography) or surgery for lacerations or fracture repairs.

 b. Preoperative assessment

  i. Cats with signs of increased ICP such as depression, abnormal mentation, irregular pupils, or seizure should be treated appropriately with furosemide or mannitol before anesthesia (see chap. 25—General Approach and Overview of the Neurologic Cat and 26—Neurologic Emergencies: Brain).

  ii. Hypertension (MAP >100 mmHg) may be the response to maintain cerebral perfusion pressure in the presence of increased ICP; treatment to decrease ICP should be instituted prior to anesthesia.

    1. Although bradycardia with hypertension is the classic Cushing's response to intracranial hypertension, tachycardia, arrhythmia, and marked T wave changes can be signs of intracranial pathology.

  iii. Cerebral blood flow (CBF) is dependent on cerebral perfusion pressure, $PaCO_2$, and PaO_2, and is autoregulated in the normal brain; this may be disrupted in disease.

 c. Pharmacologic considerations (table 5.4)

  i. Thiopental, propofol reduces cerebral metabolic rate ($CMRO_2$) and CBF by directly increasing cerebral vascular resistance.

  ii. BZ and opioids may decrease or not change CBF directly as long as hypoventilation is avoided.

  iii. Dissociatives should be avoided because they increase $CMRO_2$ and CBF by decreasing cerebral vascular resistance, although hyperventilation will minimize the increase in CBF.

    iv.   Isoflurane, sevoflurane, and desflurane (halothane should be avoided) decrease $CMRO_2$ but increase CBF and cerebral blood volume to varying degrees despite normal ventilation at ≥ 1 MAC.
        1.   Dose-dependent disruption of autoregulation of CBF occurs with inhalants but may be less altered by SEVO.
        2.   CBF and cerebral blood volume increase at <1 MAC in presence of poor intracranial compliance, and injectables such as propofol may be preferable.

  d. Anesthetic management and monitoring
    i.   The benefit of premedication must be weighed against the potential risks in the patient with poor intracranial compliance.
        1.   Avoid drugs that may induce vomiting or hypoventilation (increased pCO_2) before the airway is secured.
        2.   Avoid increases in MAP and occlusion of jugular veins as can occur with excessive restraint in uncooperative patients.
        3.   Rapid sequence induction is ideal to quickly secure the airway.
        4.   Lidocaine 2 mg/kg IV included at induction/extubation may minimize coughing, which can increase intracranial pressure.
    ii. $ETCO_2$ should be included as routine monitoring in animals with possible or confirmed intracranial pathology.
        1.   Ideally, the $paCO_2$–$ETCO_2$ gradient should be determined in order to maintain $ETCO_2$ at appropriate levels.
        2. $paCO_2$ should be kept in low-normal range (30–40 mmHg), and $paCO_2$ <25 mmHg or >50 should be avoided.
    iii.   Hypotension should be avoided to maintain adequate cerebral perfusion pressure.
    iv.   Avoid excessive fluid administration, but normovolemia must be maintained.
        1.   Hypertonic saline (2–4 mL/kg) may be the optimal fluid when ICP is of concern and hypovolemia is present.
        2.   Avoid glucose-containing solutions unless hypoglycemia is documented. Normoglycemia should be maintained.
    v.   Elevate head 30 degrees when possible to facilitate venous and CSF drainage.

Recommended Reading

Bostrom I, Nyman G, Kampa N, et al. Effects of acepromazine on renal function in anesthetized dogs. Amer J Vet Res 2003; 64:590–598.

Caulkett NA, Cantwell SL, Houston DM. A comparison of indirect blood pressure monitoring techniques in the anesthetized cat. Vet Surg 1987; 287:370–377.

Green SA. Renal disease; hepatic disease. In Thurmon JC, Tranquilli WJ, Benson GJ, eds, Lumb and Jones' Veterinary Anesthesia, 3d ed, pp 785–797. Baltimore: Williams and Wilkins, 1996.

Ilkiw JE. Anaesthesia and disease. In Hall LW, Taylor PM, eds, Anaesthesia in the Cat, pp 224–248. London: Bailliere Tindall, 1994.

Ilkiw JE, Pascoe PJ. Effect of variable-dose propofol alone and in combination with two fixed doses of ketamine for total intravenous anesthesia in cats. Am J Vet Res 2003; 64:907–912.

Ilkiw JE, Pascoe PJ, Fisher LD. Effect of alfentanil on the minimum alveolar concentration of isoflurane in cats. Am J Vet Res 1997; 58:1274–1279.

Ilkiw JE, Pascoe PJ, Tripp LD. Effects of morphine, butorphanol, buprenorphine and U50488H on the minimum alveolar concentration of isoflurane in cats. Am J Vet Res 2002; 63:1198–1202.

Lamont LA, Bulmer BJ, Sisson DD, et al. Doppler echocardiographic effects of medetomidine on dynamic left ventricular outflow tract obstruction in cats. J Am Vet Med Assoc 2002; 221:1276–1281.

Liehmann L, Mosing M, et al. A comparison of cardiorespiratory variables during isoflurand-fentanyl and propofol-fentanyl aneaesthesia for surgery in injured cats. Vet Anaesth Analg 2006; 33:158–168.

Pascoe PJ, Ilkiw JE, Pypendop BH. Effects of increasing infusion rates of dopamine, dobutamine, epinephrine, and phenylephrine in healthy anesthetized cats. Am J Vet Res 2006; 67:1491–1499.

Patel PM, Drummond JC. Cerebral physiology and effects of anesthetics and techniques. In Miller RD, ed, Miller's Anesthesia, 6th ed. Philadelphia: Churchill Livingston, 2005.

Pypendop BH, Ilkiw JE. The effects of intravenous lidocaine administration on the minimum alveolar concentration of isoflurane in cats. Anesth Analg 2005; 100:97–101.

Pypendop BH, Ilkiw JE. Hemodynamic effects of sevoflurane in cats. Am J Vet Res 2004; 65:20–25.

Steffey EP, Branson KR, Gross ME, et al. Drugs acting on the central nervous system. In Veterinary pharmacology and therapeutics, 8th ed, Adams HR ed, pp 153–360. Ames, Iowa: Iowa State Press, 2001.

6
ANESTHETIC PROTOCOLS FOR SYSTEMICALLY HEALTHY CATS

Lynne I. Kushner

Unique Features
- Feline patients may present challenges to the clinician with respect to their temperament, behavior, and response to sedative and analgesic agents.
- The cat's limited ability to eliminate drugs via glucoronidation, and the susceptibility of feline RBC to oxidative injury, can influence their response to some drugs such as benzodiazepines and propofol, respectively.
- Unlike dogs, profound chemical restraint is less likely to occur in cats after opioid tranquilizer administration unless alpha-2 agonists or dissociatives are included.
- Opioids can produce mild or moderate sedation and euphoria in calm cats that can make them more manageable for minor procedures.
- Opioids may produce hyperthermia that can be profound in some cats, although the mechanism and consequences are unclear.
- Securing accurate blood pressure readings may be more challenging in cats due to inconsistencies of some indirect methods and greater difficulty in performing arterial catheterization.

I. General Comments
   A. Systemically healthy cats may present with conditions of an acute nature where sedation or anesthesia is required to accomplish diagnostic or therapeutic interventions. The fractious or aggressive cat always poses a challenge to accomplish noninvasive tasks without good chemical restraint.
      1. Mild to moderate sedation may be needed to facilitate radiographic or ultrasound examinations, or to accomplish bandage or splint application.
      2. Heavy sedation and immobilization may be required to perform procedures such as urinary catheterization for urethral obstruction, needle/bone marrow aspirates/biopsies, thoracocentesis, or chest tube placement.
      3. Sedation prior to induction of general anesthesia is always recommended, with some exceptions, to facilitate IV catheterization, minimize stress related catecholamine release, and reduce IV induction dosage and inhalant requirements.
      4. Emergencies requiring anesthesia and surgery include cats with dystocia, intestinal foreign bodies, severe bite wounds, lacerations, and abscesses.
   B. Sedation implies a state of depressed consciousness that is qualitative.
      1. Mild: tranquilization or euphoria; where animal maintains mobility but is responsive to stimuli

2. Moderate: depression of consciousness, recumbent, easily aroused; small risk for respiratory depression and hypoxia

3. Heavy: depression of consciousness, not easily aroused but responsive to noxious stimuli; moderate risk for respiratory depression and hypoxia

4. Unconscious sedation = anesthesia; unable to be aroused; significant risk for respiratory depression and hypoxia

5. The degree of sedation required depends on the type and duration of procedure, the requirement for immobility, and physical status and temperament of animal.

C. Anesthesia implies loss of consciousness and perception to noxious stimuli and can be accomplished with injectable agents or inhalants. In either situation, with some exceptions (very brief, noninvasive procedures), endotracheal intubation should always be accomplished and oxygen provided.

D. Although we can never guarantee anesthesia or heavy sedation free from complications, it can be minimized by consideration of the following:

1. Evaluation of physical status of patient and recognition of any preexisting conditions

2. Basic hematological/biochemical screening should include PCV, TS, BUN, Creat, ALT

3. Continuous monitoring of vital signs during anesthesia through recovery by qualified individuals

   a. Type of monitoring may depend on duration and type of procedure being performed, and condition of patient

      i. Intermittent monitoring, at least every 10 minutes, of heart and respiratory rates, pulse quality, mucous membrane color, and CRT by auscultation and observation should be the minimum required for every patient under heavy sedation or brief anesthesia.

      ii. For patients not intubated, SpO_2 monitoring is most important. However, oxygen supplementation should always be provided.

      iii. For most patients during anesthesia in addition to the above, continuous ECG, blood pressure monitoring, and temperature should be routine.

      iv. End-tidal CO_2, SpO_2 monitoring is most important in patients with neurological or pulmonary diseases, respectively (see chap. 7—Pain Management in Critically Ill Feline Patients).

   b. Guidelines for intraoperative monitoring (ideal)

      i. HR should be at least >100 but <180 bpm.

      ii. Mean arterial BP should be at least ≥60 mmHg or a Doppler pressure of at least 80 mmHg.

      iii. Respiratory rate and tidal volume should maintain $ETCO_2$ between 30 and 45 mmHg, and controlled ventilation should be instituted when necessary.

      iv. Degree of CNS depression (depth of anesthesia) should be assessed continually and interpreted with respect to degree of muscle relaxation and autonomic responses.

4. Venous access should be secured on every patient heavily sedated or anesthetized.

   a. Fluids during surgery are administered to maintain vascular volume and oxygen delivery to tissues, replace acute fluid losses, counteract vasodilating effects of anesthetics, and normalize acid-base and electrolyte abnormalities.

      i. Crystalloids at 5–15 mL/kg/hr depending on severity of surgical trauma and concurrent diseases

      ii. Blood redistribution, net fluid reabsorption typically decrease PCV, plasma proteins during routine anesthesia.

   b. A healthy anesthetized animal can safely lose up to 40% of its blood volume if volume replacement is adequate.

   c. Crystalloid solutions should replace estimated blood loss by volume 3:1; colloids, 1:1.

5. Body temperature should be monitored and forced–warm-air blanket or circulating warm water pads should be applied at the time of induction.

6. Knowledge of the pharmacologic effects of sedative and anesthetic agents used

Table 6.1. Examples of sedation protocols for healthy cats (all doses are in mg/kg).

Drugs/combinations	mg/kg IM	mg/kg IV	Comments
Acepromazine Hydromorphone[a]	0.025–0.1 0.05–0.1	0.01–0.04 0.05–0.1	Mild-mod sedation, euphoria in calm cat; less effective in fractious cats; duration 0.5–2 hr Hyperthermia possible at recovery
Midazolam[b] Hydromorphone	0.1–0.25 0.05–0.1	0.1–0.25 0.05–0.1	Mild-mod sedation in calm or older cat; dysphoria possible; duration 0.5–2 hrs; hyperthermia possible
Acepromazine Buprenorphine	0.025–0.05–0.1 0.01–0.02	0.02–0.05 0.005–0.01	Mild sedation; dysphoria less likely than with hydromorphone; hyperthermia may be less likely
Dexmedetomidine	0.0025–0.020		Moderate sedation; duration 0.5–1.0 hr; severity of bradycardia variable
Xylazine Ketamine	0.5–1.0 4–8		Moderate-heavy sedation/immobilization duration 0.5–0.75 hrs; may vomit
Medetomidine Ketamine	0.005–0.02 2–6		Immobilization/anesthesia at the higher dosages; duration 0.5–1.5 hrs; severity of bradycardia variable
Ketamine Midazolam ± Hydromorphone	2–10 0.1–0.25 0.05–0.1	2–5 0.1–0.25 0.05–0.1	Heavy sedation /immobilization; duration 0.5–1 hr Hyperthermia possible
Telazol®	3–4	1–2	Heavy sedation/immobilization; duration 0.5–1.0 hr; larger doses may result in prolonged recoveries
Telazol® Hydromorphone[a]	2–3 0.05–0.1		Heavy sedation/immobilization; duration 0.5–1.0 hr
Diazepam Ketamine	0.2–0.5 5–10	0.2–0.4 2–5	Heavy sedation/immobilization/anesthesia; duration 0.5 hr

a. Hydromorphone can be substituted with oxymorphone 0.025–0.05 mg/kg, butorphanol 0.1–0.4 mg/kg.
b. Midazolam can be substituted with diazepam 0.1–0.5 mg/kg.

II. Sedatives (table 6.1)
    A. Phenothiazines (acepromazine; AcP)
        1. Blocks central postsynaptic transmission of dopamine in several areas of the brain, including basal ganglia, limbic, chemoreceptor trigger zone, hypothalamus, thermoregulatory centers; peripheral blockade of vascular adrenergic and H1 receptors
        2. Mild to moderate sedation depending on dosage and individual response
        3. Variable vasodilation, hypotension depending on dosage and individual response
          a. Splenic sequestration of blood results in drop in PCV, platelets
        4. Antihistaminic and antiemetic
        5. May decrease seizure threshold (controversial)
        6. Little change in HR but could decrease from decreased sympathetic tone
          a. Raises threshold to catecholamine-induced arrhythmia
        7. Little respiratory depression except in high doses
        8. Metabolized in liver

B. Benzodiazepines (BZ; diazepam, midazolam)
   1. Binds to specific BZ receptors, which facilitates inhibitory action of GABA and glycine on central and peripheral neuronal transmission; reduces polysynaptic reflex activity
   2. Anticonvulsant, sedation, muscle relaxation
   3. Significantly reduces induction doses of hypnotics via synergism at GABA sites
   4. BZ are not good sedatives in cats unless used in combination with other sedatives but may produce excitatement at high dosages.
   5. Diazepam formulated in propylene glycol may be irritating when administered IM (but not ineffective), unlike water-soluble midazolam.
      a. Midazolam is reported to be 1.5–3 times more potent than diazepam.
      b. Midazolam has shorter t ½s, but pharmacokinetics in cats have not been reported.
   6. In general, BZ are associated with minimal C/V and pulmonary depression; however, large doses IV can produce transient respiratory depression and apnea, decreased HR and BP.
   7. Metabolism of BZ require hydroxylation by microsomal enzymes and elimination by glucoronide reduction
      a. Cats have limited ability for glucoronidation, important for final elimination of BZ.
      b. Cats may have prolonged recoveries with BZ, and they should be used with caution in cats with significant liver disease if flumazenil (BZ antagonist) is not readily available (see chap. 14).
C. Alpha-2 agonists (medetomidine, xylazine)
   1. $\alpha_2 : \alpha_1$ ratio: medetomidine 1,600:1 vs. 160:1 xylazine
   2. Activation of central and peripheral presynaptic α_{2A} receptors mediate decreases in NE release; decreases sympathetic outflow from cardiovascular centers; increases vagal outflow; reduces polysynaptic reflex; activation of postsynaptic peripheral vascular α_{2B} receptors
   3. Sedation; analgesia; muscle relaxation
   4. Profound cardiovascular changes: bradycardia; initial vasoconstriction and increased BP followed by decreased BP to baseline or below; decreased CO
   5. Decreased sensitivity to increases in CO_2 when large dosages are administered
   6. Cardiovascular effects of alpha-2 agonists are qualitatively similar and specific effects will depend on species, dosage, route administered, and drug's affinity for and ability to activate central and peripheral α_2 receptor subtypes. Medetomidine has potency and efficacy greater than xylazine.
      a. It is the relative predominance of affinity at either α_{2A} or α_{2B} receptors that may determine overall hemodynamic effects of medetomidine.
      b. Duration and degree of sedation is dose-dependent, but C/V effects are similar over most dosage rates.
      c. Concomitant use of anticholinergics is controversial. Evidence demonstrates that increased HR along with increased afterload increases cardiac work, O_2 consumption, but some clinicians find it clinically useful.
   7. May cause vomiting: xylazine >> medetomidine
   8. Specific α_2 antagonism: atipamazole >> yohimbine
      a. May produce hypotension; caution if administered IV
D. Opioids (see chap. 7—Pain Management in Critically Ill Feline Patients for specifics on antinociception)
   1. Opioids are analgesics but are frequently used for its sedative effects.
   2. Opioids bind to a family of opioid receptors (μ, κ, δ) located in brain, spinal cord, and peripheral sites. The specific opioid receptor(s) they bind to, the concentration and sites of location, and clinical effects of the drug and its binding affinity to the receptor vary among drugs, species, and studies, making opioid pharmacology complex and often confusing.
   3. Bradycardia; reduced CNS sensitivity to CO_2, but usually is not a clinical problem in cats
   4. Causes little/no change in cardiac contractility or blood pressure although blood pressure may drop transiently in some patients after IV administration

5. Behavioral effects from opioids in cats have determined the following:
   a. Euphoria or dysphoria from most opioids and depends upon opioid, dosage, and condition of the cat
      i. Euphoria after hydromorphone; dysphoria after butorphanol; dysphoria rare after buprenorphine
   b. Vomiting after hydromorphone and morphine; no vomiting after butorphanol and buprenorphine
   c. Hyperthermia (>104°F) after hydromorphone and ± BZ in healthy cats. The mechanism and significance of these findings are uncertain at this time.
6. Opioids should be administered with tranquilizers to minimize potential dysphoria; can produce mild to moderate sedation in calm cats but unlikely to produce immobilization
   a. Greater sedative effects in aged cats
7. Morphine and meperidine associated with histamine release
   a. Morphine may be administered slowly IV in low dosage (<0.5 mg/kg) or as an infusion without adverse hemodynamic effects. IV administration of meperidine is not recommended because it can cause significant histamine release, vasodilation, and myocardial depression.
III. Drugs and drug combinations producing immobilization (see table 6.1)
   A. The addition of low dosages of an α₂ agonist or a dissociative such as ketamine or tiletamine-zolazapam to an opioid or tranquilizer is likely to produce immobilization or anesthesia
   B. Although mixing drugs may be complicated, it allows for lower dosages of any one drug with the advantage of additive or synergistic effects.
IV. Injectable anesthetics (table 6.2)
   A. Dissociatives (ketamine; tiletamine-zolazapam [Telazol])
      1. Ketamine binds to N-methyl-D-aspartate (NMDA) and non-NMDA glutamate receptors as well as to muscarinic and nicotinic cholinergic sites, monoadrenergic and opioid receptors. In addition, ketamine interacts with voltage-dependent ion channels of Na and Ca.
      2. NMDA receptor binding appears to be the primary site of anesthetic and analgesic action.
      3. Dose-dependent central nervous system depression leading to a state of dissociation between thalamo-neocortical and limbic systems.
      4. Subanesthetic dosages produce inhibition of central sensitization of spinal neurons (wind-up); anesthetic doses produce good somatic, weak visceral analgesia.

Table 6.2.   Injectable anesthetics and dosages typically required for endotracheal intubation.

Drug	Nonsedated	Sedated	Comments
Thiopental (2.0%) mg/kg IV	12–15	2–8	Administered to effect; may cause apnea with rapid administration; can potentiate catecholamine induced dysrhythmia
Propofol mg/kg IV	6–8	2–6	Administered to effect; apnea likely with rapid administration; vasodilation, hypotension; muscle twitching possible
Ketamine/Diazepam mg/kg/mg/kg IV	5–8/0.25–0.5	2–5/0.25–0.5	Ketamine should be administered with BZ; sympathomimetic effects may be blunted with increased dosage of BZ; respiratory depression possible
Etomidate mg/kg IV	2–3	0.25–1	Can produce myoclonic activity; can result in pigmenturia and hemolysis; minimal cardio/pulmonary effects
Telazol® mg/kg IV	2–3	1–2	Similar to ket/diazepam; larger doses may result in prolonged recoveries

    5. Good evidence that ketamine can reduce or reverse opioid tolerance

    6. Ketamine has direct cardio-depressive effects that are offset by the indirect sympathomimetic effects in normal patients.

       a. Inhibition of CNS-mediated intraneuronal and extraneuronal uptake of catecholamines, and inhibition of the vagal component of the baroreceptor reflex result in the increases in HR, CO, BP seen clinically.

       b. Sympathomimetic effects are minimized but may not be abolished by concurrently administered opioids, BZ and α_2 agonists.

       c. Animals with little/no sympathetic reserve or under general anesthesia may not benefit from the sympathomimetic effects.

    7. Minimal effects on central respiratory drive; produces the typical apneustic pattern of breathing. When used with other CNS depressants, may result in significant respiratory depression.

       a. Increases pulmonary arterial pressure; anecdotal reports, though rare, of cats with pulmonary edema after ketamine may be due to a direct increased pulmonary arterial pressure (cardiogenic) or central sympathetic stimulation (neurogenic)

       b. Ketamine is a bronchial smooth muscle relaxant and directly antagonizes the spasmogenic effects of carbachol and histamine.

    8. Ketamine is rapidly biotransformed in the cat via microsomal N-demethylation, but unlike other species, forms primarily only 1 metabolite (norketamine) which exerts little pharmacologic activity. Although ketamine and norketamine are excreted by the kidneys, in one study very little (10%) was recovered in the urine at recovery.

B. Tiletamine/zolazapam (T/Z) (1 : 1 ratio)

    1. T/Z produces dose dependent sedation/anesthesia with excellent muscle relaxation

    2. Cardiovascular/pulmonary effects similar to ketamine/diazepam

    3. Recovery may be prolonged with high dosages (>4 mg/kg) because of the relatively high concentration of BZ.

C. Hypnotics (propofol, thiopental, etomidate)

    1. Similarities (propofol and thiopental)

       a. Interacts with the CNS GABA$_A$ receptor, resulting in dose-dependent depression of cortical and postsynaptic cortical reflexes

       b. Produces dose-dependent sedation to unconsciousness (anesthesia) and provides no analgesia at subanesthetic concentrations

          i. Rapid redistribution; short acting

       c. Potent respiratory depressant

       d. Myocardial depressant

       e. Metabolized by microsomal oxidative enzymes

       f. Cerebral vasoconstrictor which reduces cerebral blood flow and volume (CBF) and intracranial pressure, and cerebral metabolic rate (CMR)

    2. Differences (propofol vs. thiopental)

       a. Propofol (phenolic compound) metabolism exceeds liver blood flow, suggesting extra hepatic sites (in cats, 60% first pass extraction found in the lung) and lack of pharmacokinetic alterations found in patients with liver disease

       b. Relatively nonaccumulative; however, in cats, prolonged recoveries are seen after continuous infusions.

          i. Full recovery in cats administered propofol at infusion rates for 2.5 hours were almost twice as long as those who received 30-minute infusions

       c. Because feline RBCs are susceptible to oxidative injury, Heinz body anemia and malaise have been documented in cats after consecutive day administration.

       d. Propofol has greater veno and vasodilatory actions; hypotension more likely.

       e. Propofol lacks the vagolytic effects of thiopental, and HR may decrease or not change.

      f. Although propofol lowers the threshold to catecholamine-induced dysrhythmia, probably less dysrhythmogenic

      g. Propofol may be inhibitory or excitatory at CNS sites and twitching or seizurelike motor activity is not uncommon.

   3. Etomidate (imidazole derivative)

      a. Probable mechanism for hypnosis is via GABA-ergic sites.

      b. Rapid hepatic hydrolysis

      c. Formulated in propylene glycol, etomidate in moderate amounts can cause hemolysis, hemoglobinuria because of high osmolality (>4,000 mOsm/L).

      d. Maintains cardiovascular stability with minimal respiratory depression

        i. Does not potentiate catecholamine-induced dysrythmia

      e. Etomidate transiently decreases cortisol production (see chap. 7—Pain Management in Critically Ill Feline Patients).

D. Local anesthetics (lidocaine 2%; bupivacaine 0.5%)

   1. Many toxicity studies using healthy cats have determined that seizure and cardiovascular collapse occur with dosages in excess of 11 mg/kg and 4 mg/kg of lidocaine and bupivaine, respectively.

   2. Infiltration of local anesthetics for line or nerve blocks may allow surgical procedures with only heavy sedation (small mass removals) or reduce the amounts of injectable or inhalant anesthetics (C-section)

      a. Lidocaine <4 mg/kg; bupivicaine <2 mg/kg

      b. Diluting lidocaine or bupivicaine with saline to 1% and 0.25%, respectively, will increase volume but not dose

   3. IV lidocaine (bupivacaine should NOT be administered IV) can be administered to cats in IV infusions for minimum alveolar concentration (MAC) reduction or analgesia, although documented efficacy is variable and questionable.

      a. One study documented a linear reduction of MAC over a large range of plasma concentrations.

        i. Cardiac index decreased significantly despite increases in MAP when plasma concentrations >5 µg/mL.

      b. Clinical experience suggests that up to 50 µg/kg/min can be administered without cardiovascular depression.

        i. Dosage should be reduced after 1–2 hours to avoid cardiovascular depression that may occur from accumulation of lidocaine.

   4. Lidocaine 2 mg/kg IV administered immediately prior to induction can produce mild sedation and may reduce dosage of hypnotics.

   5. Methemoglobinemia in cats has been documented with benzocaine but not lidocaine.

V. Volatile anesthetics (table 6.3)

A. Isoflurane (ISO) and sevoflurane (SEVO) are the most commonly used inhalants in veterinary medicine. Desflurane (DES) may be less commonly used because of its unique properties and atypical vaporizer design. Nitrous oxide (N_2O), commonly used in human medicine, is less useful in veterinary medicine because of its low potency. Halothane will soon follow methoxyflurane as being of historical significance.

B. Low blood-gas solubility coefficients of the volatile agents mean that alveolar concentrations change quickly with changes in inspired concentrations; thus induction and recovery times are rapid.

   1. Blood-gas solubilities: desflurane < sevoflurane < isoflurane < halothane

   2. This property may be most relevant during mask or tank induction.

C. Minimum alveolar concentration of inhalants, a measure of potency, is generally higher (less potent) in cats than in dogs.

Table 6.3. Some properties of the common inhalant anesthetics.

Inhalant	Blood/gas solubility coefficients at 37°C	Mean MAC_{50} values reported in cats (%)
Isoflurane	1.46	1.6–2.2
Sevoflurane	0.68	2.6; 3.4
Desflurane	0.42	9.8; 10.2
Halothane	2.54	0.8–1.2

MAC_{50} %: minimum alveolar concentration in 50% of animals.

D. Studies in cats comparing the C/V and pulmonary effects of SEVO, DES, and ISO found similar effects with minor differences.
   1. SEVO produced less vasodilation but greater decrease in CO compared to ISO.
   2. SEVO produced less CV depression with controlled ventilation compared to ISO.
E. Neither ISO, SEVO, or DES sensitizes the myocardium to catecholamines.
F. All have similar effects on the CNS and will produce decreases in CMR but increases in CBF at ≥1 MAC.
G. ISO, SEVO, and DES do not produce direct hepatic or renal toxicity, and hepatic and renal blood flow are well preserved in clinically relevant concentration as long as CO and BP are preserved.
   1. Sevoflurane reacts with CO_2 absorbents to produce a potentially renal toxic vinyl ether, "Compound A", a substance that produces dose-dependent nephrotoxicity at high concentrations in rats.
      a. There are no studies in cats specifically evaluating the toxic effects of SEVO, although studies in humans, horses, and dogs failed to document clinical toxicity.
   2. DES, ISO, and especially SEV produce carbon monoxide (CO) and extreme temperatures during reactions with dessicated CO_2 absorbents, and although rare, explosions/fire in canister with sevoflurane have been reported.
   3. The use of nonrebreathing circuits, which obviates the need for CO_2 absorbents, negates the concern of CO or Compound A (see VI. Breathing circuits).
VI. Breathing circuits
   A. Circle or rebreathing systems utilize CO_2 absorbents for removal of CO_2 and imply rebreathing (minus CO_2) some portion of exhaled gases, the amount of which depends on the fresh gas flow rate.
      1. Pediatric circles utilizing smaller volumes and diameters can be used for healthy cats as small as 2.5–3.0 kg.
      2. Maintenance O_2 flow rates are based on the recommendation of three times the patient's O_2 consumption, approximately 22–44 mL/kg.
      3. Advantages of a semiclosed rebreathing circuit are conservation of heat and moisture, and economy in usage of inhalant and O_2.
      4. Disadvantages are increased resistance to breathing across one-way valves and CO_2 canister, and potential concern for breakdown products of compound A and CO in the circuit.
   B. A nonrebreathing circuit is a common term describing circuits that do not utilize CO_2 absorbents and rely on high O_2 flow rates to avoid rebreathing.
      1. Recommended flow rates depend on type of nonrebreathing circuit, spontaneous vs. controlled breathing, and patient characteristics and are in ranges of two to three times patient's minute volume = 450–600 mL/kg/min.
      2. Advantages are minimal resistance, less work of breathing; no break down products of inhalants (compound A) in circuit
      3. Disadvantages are loss of heat and moisture, wasteful in oxygen and inhalant usage.

Recommended Reading

Andress JL, Day TK, Day DG. The effects of consecutive day propofol anesthesia on feline red blood cells. Vet Surg, 1995; 24:277–282.

Duncan B, Lascelles X, Robertson SA. Antinociceptive effects of hydromorphone, butorphanol, or the combination in cats. J Vet Intern Med, 2004; 18:190–195.

Euro J Drug Metab and Pharm, 1987; 12:219–224.

Ilkiw JE, Suter C, McNeal D, et al. The optimal intravenous dose of midazolam after intravenous ketamine in healthy awake cats. J Vet Pharmacol Therap, 1998; 21:54–61.

Lamont LA, Bulmer BJ, Grimm KA; Cardiopulmonary evaluation of the use of medetomidine hydrochloride in cats. Am J Vet Res, 2001; 62:1745–1762.

Paddleford, RR. Anesthetic equipment. In Manual of small animal anesthesia, 2nd ed, pp 89–109. Philadelphia: W.B. Saunders, 1999.

Pascoe PJ, Ilkiw JE, Frischmeyer KJ. The effect of the duration of propofol administration on recovery from anesthesia in cats. Vet Anaes Analg, 2006; 33:2–7.

Pypendop BH, Ilkiw JE. Hemodynamic effects of sevoflurane in cats. Am J Vet Res, 2004; 65:20–25.

Pypendop BH, Ilkiw JE. Assessment of the hemodynamic effects of lidocaine administered IV in isoflurane anesthetized cats. Am J Vet Res 2005; 66:661–668.

Pypendop BH, Ilkiw JE. The effects of intravenous lidocaine administration on the minimum alveolar concentration of isoflurane in cats. Anesth Analg 2005; 100:97–101.

Steffey EP, Branson KR, Gross ME, et al. Drugs acting on the central nervous system. In Adams HR, ed, Veterinary pharmacology and therapeutics, 8th ed, pp 153–360. Ames: Iowa State Press, 2001.

Thurmon JC, Tranquilli WJ, Benson GJ. Preanesthetics and anesthetic adjuncts. In Lumb and Jones' Veterinary Anesthesia, 3rd ed, pp 183–209. Baltimore: Williams and Wilkins, 1996.

7
PAIN MANAGEMENT IN CRITICALLY ILL FELINE PATIENTS

Lynne I. Kushner

I. Nociceptive transmission—and associated vocabulary
    A. Pain is a conscious unpleasant sensation caused by a noxious stimulus that produces some degree of tissue injury.
    B. *Transduction* occurs when nociceptors on peripheral, afferent Aδ and C nerve fibers respond to chemical, thermal, or mechanical stimuli and transform these signals into action potentials. If minimal/no damage to tissues occurs, physiologic pain results.
        i.   *Physiologic* pain is a normal innocuous response to a noxious stimulus that is transient and protective in nature (fig. 7.1).
        ii. *Clinical* pain is an exaggerated, prolonged physiologic pain associated with some degree of tissue damage and inflammation; it is typically acute and secondary to surgery or trauma.
        iii. When significant tissue damage occurs, prostaglandins, histamine, serotonin, and brandykinins are but a few of the compounds released from damaged tissues that sensitize nociceptors, reduce thresholds, and augment the response to further nociceptive stimulation leading to peripheral sensitization.
        iv. *Peripheral sensitization* may lead to hyperalgesia (see below) and allodynia (see below) at the site of injury.
    C. Action potentials are transmitted via afferent Aδ and C peripheral nerve fiber to the dorsal root ganglion and dorsal horn of the spinal cord.
    D. *Modulation* occurs throughout the peripheral and CNS when the interaction of neurotransmitters with receptors lead to activation of intracellular signaling cascades on the neuronal membrane, which can amplify, or inhibit, further intracellular signaling.
        i.   Excitatory amino acids and peptides (glutamate, substance P) released from afferent synaptic terminals on dorsal horn neurons bind to glutaminergic receptors a-amino-3-hydroxy-5-methyl-4-isoxazlepropionic acid (AMPA), kainite, and N-methyl-D-aspartate (NMDA), resulting in opening and phosphorylation of ion channels and regulatory proteins.
        ii. AMPA receptors respond more to acute and brief noxious impulses, but repetitive activation leads to the removal of the magnesium block in the NMDA channel.
        iii. NMDA receptor activation enhances further AMPA activity, which in turn activates more NMDA receptors, leads to amplification of responses of impulses, and increases its receptive field size in the spinal cord resulting in synaptic plasticity and central sensitization.
            a. *Central sensitization* thus is an increased responsiveness of sensory input into the spinal cord (also called *windup*).
            b. *Hyperalgesia* often results, which is pathologic pain that is an exaggerated response to a noxious stimuli at the site of injury (primary) but also may extend to areas outside the site of injury (secondary).

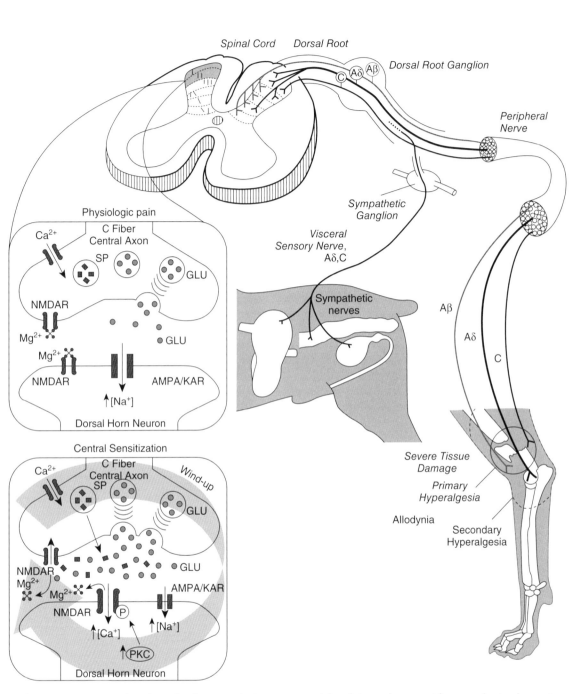

Fig. 7.1. Diagram describes what happens during severe peripheral tissue damage. After transduction by nociceptors on afferent Aβ, C and Aδ fibers, action potentials are transmitted to the dorsal horn of the spinal cord for further processing and modulation. During physiologic pain, most NMDARs are blocked by Mg^{2+}; consequently, there is no postsynaptic cumulative depolarization of the CNS. During somatic or visceral pathologic pain conditions, C fibers become sensitized by inflammatory mediators (peripheral sensitization), lowering the threshold to firing and producing spontaneous discharges resulting in a persistent release of glutamate and substance P on the C fibers of the dorsal horn. These substances produce a cascade of intracellular signaling leading to activation of phosphokinase C (PKC), phosphorylates, and NMDARs leading to the removal of the Mg block, central sensitization, and windup. From Pozzi, Muir, and Traverso 2006.

      c. *Allodynia* is pain perceived from a stimulus that would normally not be perceived as painful.

      d. *Neuropathic* pain is associated with damage to peripheral and central components of the nervous system and can be characterized by hyperalgesia and allodynia.

  E. *Projection* of nociceptive information is transmitted via ascending tracts to areas of the cortex where *perception* occurs. Further transmission and modulation occur via descending tracts.

    i.   The periaqueductal gray and ventromedial medulla are rich in serotonin, opioid, adrenergic receptors and are important centers for relaying descending information to the spinal cord where nociceptive input is further modulated (facilitated or inhibited).

II. Types of pain categorized by severity, duration, anatomic location, or neurobiological mechanisms

  A. *Somatic* pain arises from bone, skin, or muscle, and is generally transmitted via Aδ fibers, some C fibers.

    i.   Somatic pain is typically characterized as sharp and well localized.

  B. *Visceral* pain arises from stretching, distension, or inflammation of viscera, is transmitted along C fibers and Aδ fibers, and is associated with sympathetic and parasympathetic pathways.

    i.   Visceral pain is characterized as dull, aching, and poorly localized

  C. *Acute* pain typically is associated with trauma, surgery, or disease; it is physiologic pain that may evolve to clinical and inflammatory pain. Acute pain often responds favorably to opioids, NSAIDs.

    i.   Mild-moderate

      a. Lacerations, abscesses

      b. Surgical (pyometra; C-section)

    ii. Moderate-severe

      a. Fractures, blunt trauma; degloving injuries; burns

      b. Surgical (orthopedic, amputation, thoracotomy, extensive abdominal), radical mastectomy, enucleation

    iii. Clinical, inflammatory pain may result in pathologic or neuropathic pain if not treated aggressively.

  D. *Chronic* pain persists weeks or months beyond the time acute pain is expected to resolve and is associated with chronic disease processes.

    i.   Chronic pain is less responsive to conventional analgesics and is more difficult to treat; NMDA antagonists, systemically administered local anesthetics, antidepressants may be effective.

    ii. Mild to severe

      a. Dental, periodontal disease; glaucoma

      b. Osteoarthritis, interstitial cystitis

      c. Musculoskeletal pain

      d. Bone pain (neoplasia)

  E. Targeting the mechanism rather than the symptom and applying a multimodal approach is the best rationale for pain management.

III. Pain and the stress response

  A. Although pain can play a protective role in minimizing tissue damage, unrelieved pain induces stress and suffering, and pain and suffering are associated with maladaptive physiologic responses.

    i.   Increases in neuroendocrine activity can induce cardiovascular changes (tachycardia, hypertension) and metabolic consequences such as protein catabolism and modulation of the immune response.

    ii. Stress increases energy requirements, which may lead to weight loss and negative nitrogen balance if caloric intake is decreased.

IV. Assessing pain in the cat

  A. Any surgery or a trauma that would be painful to humans should be assumed to be painful to a cat; when in doubt, analgesics should be administered.

  B. Recognizing pain in the cat is a subjective assessment based on changes in the cat's behavior or appearance (table 7.1).

Table 7.1. Behavior or appearance that suggests a cat in pain.

Attitude	Aggression in an otherwise friendly cat; quite decreased responsiveness in an otherwise active cat; does not engage in otherwise normal interactions
Mobility	Unwillingness or slow to move; inability to jump; change in gait; hiding
Posture	Lying with tense muscle tone, less likely to sleep curled up; hunched appearance when standing
Reaction to touch	Flinching or increased muscle tension when stroked; hissing, growling when touched; aversive reaction to touch peripheral to site of surgery or injury
Other physiologic changes	Loss of appetite; change in elimination habits

Table 7.2. An example of an interactive simple descriptive score for assessment of pain in cats (modified from Cambridge, et al. 2000).

Stimulus by Observer	Cat's Response	Score
Approaches cat	Seeks interaction (rubbing, purring)	0
	Does not approach but raises head	1
	Does not move	2
	Withdraws head and body	3
	Avoids, moves away	4
Strokes cat	Responds favorably	0
	Does not move	1
	Withdraws from observer	2
	Moves away	3
Palpates wound	Does not respond	0
	Moves away	1
	Growls	2
	Reacts violently and moves away	3

      i.   Signs of pain in cats can be subtle, chronic pain particularly.

     ii.   It can be difficult to distinguish between attitude, malaise, and pain.

    iii.   Subject to observer variability

  C. Physiologic parameters such as cardiovascular, respiratory indices, and neuroendocrine concentrations, such as cortisol and catecholamines, have not been reliable indicators of pain or pain relief after analgesic administrations in various clinical studies.

  D. Using pain scales with specific descriptors that can be qualified and scored decreases observer variability, maintains a record of assessment or change of behaviors, and aids in evaluating response to analgesia. Few scoring methods in cats have been published or validated, however (table 7.2).

V.   Choosing the appropriate analgesic depends on many factors

  A. Type of pain—categorized by severity, duration, anatomic location, or neurobiological mechanisms

  B. Physical status and concurrent disease(s)

      i.   Critically ill or aged cats may not tolerate the cardiovascular effects of alpha-2 agonists; NSAIDS would be contraindicated in cats with renal disease.

  C. Routes available for administration

      i.   Oral administration of buprenorphine, tramadol, or transdermal application of fentanyl or lidocaine allows for better owner compliance.

Table 7.3.   Recommended dosages of opioids for cats.

Drug	Dose	Route	Interval	Side Effects/Comments
Morphine	0.1–0.5 mg/kg 0.1–0.2 mg/kg/hr 0.1 mg/kg	IM, SC IV Epidural	4–6 hours 8–12+ hours	Histamine release Urinary retention
Methadone	0.1–0.5 mg/kg 0.1–0.2 mg/kg	IM, SC, IV Epidural	2–4 hours 4 hours	Weak mu agonist NMDA antagonist Side effects rare
Hydromorphone	0.05–0.1 mg/kg	IM, SC, IV	4–6 hours	Hyperthermia common
Oxymorphone	0.05–0.2 mg/kg	IM, SC, IV	4–6 hours	Similar to hydromorphone
Meperidine	3–10 mg/kg	IM, SC	1–3 hours	Histamine release
Fentanyl	3–5 µg/kg 2–10 µg/kg/hr 5 µg/kg/hr 25 µg/hr/cat	IV IV Transdermal patch	5–90 minutes 1–3 days (6–12 hour onset)	Bradycardia marked Variable absorption
Butorphanol	0.1–0.8 mg/kg 0.1 mg/kg/min	IM, SC, IV	2–4 hours	Marked individual variability in response
Buprenorphine	0.01–0.02 mg/kg	IM, SC, IV, OTM	6–8 hours (onset 30 minutes)	Excellent buccal absorption

VI.   Opioids (table 7.3)
  A. Most effective systemically administered analgesics used to treat acute, severe pain.
  B. Opioid receptors are G protein–coupled receptors located in spinal and supraspinal sites.
     i.   Ultimately leads to decreased cAMP formation, membrane hyperpolarization, inhibits voltage sensitive Ca channels, and depresses terminal release of neurotransmitters from the cell.
  C. In humans, considerable genetic polymorphism exists in opiate receptor genes, as well as the isoenzymes responsible for opioid metabolism.
     i.   May account for individual variability in responses.
     ii. The cat is no exception in this regard.
  D. Potency depends on the affinity of the drug to the receptor and the intensity of the effect it produces for a given dosage.
     i.   Two drugs can be equi-effective (produce same effects), but the one that produces the maximal effect by occupying fewer receptors with a lower dose is more potent.
        a. Fentanyl >>> hydromorphone > morphine
     ii. The intensity of the pain will dictate the efficacy of the drug in that it may decrease its potency; that is, more receptors must be occupied to produce the effect.
     iii. Clinical impression suggests pure agonists (hydromorphone) are more effective for severe, acute pain than partial agonists (buprenorphine), which do not achieve maximum effect despite large dosage.
  E. Recent studies in cats have employed methods that apply a measured and repeatable noxious stimulus (thermal or pressure) for which a response can be determined objectively (flinching, vocalization). After baseline responses are measured, the response to various opioids and dosages can be compared. (table 7.4).
     i.   Thermal, mechanical stimuli assess somatic analgesia; other methods (e.g., colonic balloon model) may be more appropriate for visceral pain.
        a. Therefore, extrapolating results of experimental studies to clinical cases should be done cautiously.

Table 7.4. Summary of studies that have determined the effects of opioids on thermal thresholds in cats. The higher the temperature, the greater the analgesic effect.

Opioid	Dose mg/kg	Time (min) to significant analgesia	Duration (min)	Peak temp (°C)	Baseline (°C)	Observations
Morph Bupren Butorph IM n = 6	0.2 0.01 0.2	240 240 5	360 >480 30	49 51 50	<47 <48 <46	Similar peak responses despite different onset and duration; mild sedation, euphoria Vomited with morphine; mydriasis Robertson, et al. 2005a, b
Bupren OT Bupren IV n = 6	0.02 0.02	30 30	360 360	57 51	41.2 40.8	No vomiting; euphoria; no correlation between plasma concentration and effect Robertson, et al. 2005a, b
Fentanyl IV n = 6	0.02	5	110	55	41.8	No vomiting; euphoria; mydriasis Analgesia >1.07 ng/ml Robertson, et al. 2005a, b
Hydro IV n = 6	0.1	15	450	54	40.9	No vomiting but salivation; significant increase in skin and rectal temp; mydriasis; no concentration and effect relationship Wegner, et al. 2004
Meper IM n = 6	5	30	60	50	45	Normal behavior Dixon, et al. 2002
Butorph IV n = 6	0.1–0.8	15	90	48	<42	No difference between doses, results pooled; no vomiting; dysphoria associated with all doses; marked variation in response among cats Lascelles and Robertson 2004
Metha Morph Bupren SQ n = 8	0.2 0.2 0.02	60 45 45	180 60 45	3.4 3.4 2.9	0 0 0	Reported as increase from baseline; also tested pressure thresholds with similar results Steagall, et al. 2006
Hydro IV n = 7	0.025 0.05 0.1	— 5 20	— 80 200	No change 47 55	40.7 41.0 41.5	No excitatory behavior; hyperthermia only with high dose Wegner and Robertson 2007
Hydro Butorph Hydro+ Butorph n = 6	0.1 0.4 0.1 + 0.4	15 15 15	345 180 540	49 48 46	40	50% vomited with hydro only Dysphoria with butorph only Combo increased duration, decreased quality Lascelles and Robertson 2004

Note: morph = morphine; bupren = buprenorphine; butorph = butorphanol; meth = methadone; hydro = hydromorphone; meper = meperidine.

F. Morphine, a pure agonist, is the prototype to which other opioids are compared.
   i. May have delayed or unpredictable effects in cats due to a relative deficiency in metabolizing morphine to its more potent active metabolite, morphine 6 glucorinide (M6G). However, efficacy has been demonstrated in cats.
   ii. Avoid large or rapidly administered IV dosages due to histamine release.
   iii. Vomiting is commonly reported after morphine administration.
   iv. Dose: 0.1–0.5 mg/kg IM, SQ

G. Meperidine is an opiate agonist with anticholinergic, antispasmotic actions with a potency less than morphine.
   i. IV admininistration is contraindicated due to histamine release and significant vasodilatory and cardiac depressive effects.
   ii. Mild sedative effects
   iii. Vomiting uncommon
   iv. Short duration of analgesia (<2 hrs)
   v. The active metabolite normeperidine produces neuroexcitatory effects when in high concentrations.
      a. Seizures have occurred in humans with renal failure.
      b. Normeperidine has been recovered in the serum of cats.
   vi. Meperidine has intrinsic serotonergic properties and should not be used concurrently with MAO inhibitors, which could lead to serotonin syndrome: signs of tremors, hyperthermia, coma.
      a. Selegiline is a MAO B inhibitor which may minimize the likelihood of this interaction.
   vii. Dose: 3–10 mg/kg SQ, IM

H. Oxymorphone is a pure opiate agonist with a potency ten times that of morphine in humans. Little objective information concerning oxymorphone's effect on nociceptive thresholds in cats is known, although clinical studies and experience demonstrate positive responses.
   i. Dose: 0.05–0.4 SQ, IM, IV

I. Hydromorphone is reported as having five to seven times the potency of morphine in humans.
   i. May have supplanted oxymorphone in popularity because of its reliable availability and lower cost than oxymorphone.
   ii. Very effective analgesia and long duration of action (4–6 hrs)
   iii. Increases in skin and rectal temperatures were recorded in research cats.
      a. Retrospective evaluation of postanesthetic hyperthermia in feline hospitalized patients revealed a positive correlation to the use of hydromorphone.
   iv. Euphoria typically observed
   v. Dose: 0.05–0.2 mg/kg SQ, IM, IV

J. Methadone is a pure agonist with similar potency and duration to morphine.
   i. Demonstrates a relative potency of antagonism at the NMDA receptor
      a. ketamine ≥ dextromethorphan > methadone
   ii. Vomiting less common than with morphine
   iii. Dose: 0.1–0.5 mg/kg SQ, IM, IV

K. The phenylpiperidine derivatives, which include alfentanil, fentanyl, sufentanil, and remifentanil are potent synthetic opioids with relatively short durations of action.
   i. Commonly administered as continuous rate infusions to minimize inhalant and injectable anesthetic concentrations in order to preserve cardiovascular stability
   ii. Relative potencies: sufentanil ≫ fentanyl ≥ remifentanil > alfentanil
   iii. A ceiling effect in isoflurane MAC reduction (35%) with alfentanil
      a. Some cats demonstrated increase in rectal temperatures, $paCO_2$, and muscle rigidity during alfentanil–isoflurane anesthesia.
   iv. Infusions of fentanyl (0.1 µg/kg/min), alfentanil (0.5 µg/kg/min), and sufentanil (0.01 µg/kg/min) to cats significantly reduced the minimal propofol infusion dose to prevent purposeful movement.

  v. Remifentanil (0.2–0.3 µg/kg/min) prevented purposeful movement and cardiovascular responses in propofol-anesthetized cats undergoing ovariohysterectomy.
    a. Remifentanil is noncumulative and rapidly cleared due to metabolism by hydrolysis via nonspecific plasma esterases.
  vi. Although hemodynamic stability is associated with the use of these opioids, significant bradycardia and respiratory depression can occur.
L. Fentanyl transdermal patch
  i. Intended use in humans is for chronic pain rather than acute surgical pain.
  ii. Time to achieve steady state plasma concentrations in cats is reported to be from 12 to 72 hours and persist to up 18 hours after patch removal.
  iii. Partial removal of adhesive backing of a 25 µg/hr patch resulted in minimizing the plasma concentration of fentanyl and may be desirable in small or debilitated cats.
  iv. Hypothermic cats during isoflurane had significantly lower fentanyl plasma concentrations than normothermic anesthetized cats.
  v. Some clinical studies demonstrated improved pain scores in cats after ovariohysterectomy and onychectomy.
M. Butorphanol is primarily an agonist at kappa and antagonist at mu receptors.
  i. Some studies in cats found significant analgesia, but somewhat unpredictable and of short duration.
    a. Low dosages (0.1 mg/kg) effective in a colonic balloon model, representative of visceral pain
    b. Analgesic responses to electrical stimulation (somatic pain model) were significant and dose dependent (0.4, 0.8 mg/kg)
    c. Recent studies (thermal threshold, somatic pain) found significant analgesia that was not dose dependent but with a marked intercat variability in regard to efficacy.
  ii. Dysphoria has been reported as frequent in recent studies but not seen in other studies
  iii. Not associated with vomiting
  iv. Dosage 0.1–0.8 mg/kg IV, IM
N. Buprenorphine is a partial mu agonist and kappa antagonist that is reported to be 25–50 times more potent than morphine in humans.
  i. Binds avidly to the mu receptors, but long onset; slow dissociation resulting in long duration of action (≥6 hrs)
  ii. Produces a partial or "ceiling" effect in analgesia; efficacy best with mild-moderate pain
  iii. Purported to be difficult to reverse with antagonists
  iv. Bioavailability by the oral transmucosal route in cats was found to reach 100% and duration and efficacy were equal to similar IV dosage.
  v. Not associated with vomiting
  vi. Euphoria common
  vii. Dose: 0.01–0.02 mg/kg buccal mucosal, SQ, IM, IV
O. Tramadol (atypical opioid)
  i. Centrally acting analgesic whose actions are mediated through opioid, serotonergic, and adrenergic pathways; NMDA receptor inhibition reported
  ii. Pharmacokinetics of IV and oral tramadol and its main metabolite, O-desmethyl-tramadol, have been studied in cats.
    a. At 5 mg/kg PO good bioavailability with elimination t ½ of 3.4 hours (twice as long as reported in dogs)
    b. Pharmacokinetic profiles between metabolite and parent are very similar, and metabolite is thought to bind to mu receptors avidly.
    c. Euphoria observed in most cats
  iii. Few controlled analgesic studies available in cats

       a. One recent study demonstrated minimal effect on thermal or mechanical thresholds after 1 mg/kg dosage SQ.

       b. Euphoria and occasional dysphoria observed

    iv. Tramadol may be a good postoperative analgesic for home administration.

    v. Tramadol may lower the seizure threshold; serotonin syndrome (signs of sympathetic over-stimulation, seizure, coma) reported in humans with concurrent administration of antidepressants (SSRI, MAOI, tricyclics)

    vi. Published dosage for cats is 2–4 mg/kg PO/12 hrs.

VII. NMDA antagonists (ketamine, amantadine)

  A. Ketamine, in addition to providing chemical restraint and dissociative anesthesia, produces moderate somatic analgesia and weak visceral analgesia in dosage ranges of 2–8 mg/kg in cats.

    i. After 2 mg/kg, a delayed onset of hyperalgesia was demonstrated in one study.

  B. Recent advances in the study of nociception and its pathways have determined ketamine to be a potent noncompetitive inhibitor of the NMDA receptor at subanesthetic dosages, thus inhibiting central sensitization, hyperalgesia, and opioid tolerance.

    i. Acts centrally and peripherally at opioid, AMPA, NMDA, GABA-A receptors

       a. Blocks open ion channels and inhibits Ca entry in NMDA receptor

    ii. Experimental and clinical studies in experimental animals and humans have demonstrated higher nociceptive thresholds, lower pain scores, and opioid requirements when subanesthetic dosages of ketamine are administered prior to and during the noxious stimulus (surgery).

       a. Dosages used clinically in cats are extrapolations from other species; no dose response studies have been done in cats evaluating ketamine for the purpose of preventing or treating central sensitization.

    iii. Doses 0.1–0.6 mg/kg/hr after a loading dose of 0.5–1 mg/kg

  C. Amantadine has low affinity for NMDA receptors.

    i. Has been used in humans to treat neuropathic pain and adjunct to reduce opioid requirements and tolerance

    ii. Little documentation about efficacy in cats, but clinical experience supports use for chronic pain

    iii. Reported dosage for cat, 2–5 mg/kg PO/24 hrs

VIII. Anticonvulsants (Gabapentin)

  A. Gabapentin is a GABA analog, does not appear to interact directly with GABA but appears to bind to voltage gated calcium channels on a GABA subunit.

    i. Other actions include interactions with NMDA receptors and inhibition of release of a variety excitatory peptides and amino acids in the spinal cord.

    ii. Does not appear to alter nociceptive thresholds; rather, potentiates the effects of other analgesics.

    iii. In humans, good efficacy noted for neuropathic pain

    iv. Objective data in cats are lacking, but clinical impressions have determined good results in cats with chronic pain, with minimal side effects (sedation with high dosage).

    v. Published dosages 1.5–4 mg/kg SID; clinical experiences suggest up to 5–10 mg/kg/8–12 hrs

IX. Nonsteroidal anti-inflammatory drugs (NSAIDs; meloxicam, carprofen; table 7.5)

  A. NSAIDs inhibit production of prostaglandins by noncompetitive inhibition of cyclooxygenase (COX) enzymes, thus reducing fever, inflammation, and pain.

  B. COX-1 is important in physiological processes such as regulation of gastrointestinal and renal blood flow, while COX-2 is induced by inflammatory mediators, although there is some overlap of function.

  C. Choosing an NSAID with COX-2 specificity is best to minimize the potential for GI or kidney toxicities.

Table 7.5. Nonopioid drugs used to treat pain.

Drug	Dosage mg/kg	Route/Interval	Side Effects/Comments
Ketamine	0.3–0.6 mg/kg loading 0.1–0.6 mg/kg /hr	CRI	Dosages extrapolated from humans, rats
Tramadol	2–4	PO/12 hr	NMDA antagonist Avoid with SSRI and MAO inhibitors
Amantadine	2–5	PO/24 hr	NMDA antagonist Efficacy anecdotal in cats
Gabapentin	1.5–4 5–10	PO/24 hr PO/12	GABA analog; dosage; effects anecdotal in cats
Lidocaine	1–2 mg/kg loading 1.5–3 mg/kg/hr	CRI	Potential for cardiovascular depression
Meloxicam	0.1–0.2 mg/kg (acute) 0.05 mg/kg (chronic)	SQ or PO once SQ, PO 1–4 days	For chronic use monitor closely for side effects; avoid in hypovolemic /hypotensive cats
Carprofen	1–2 mg/kg	SQ; IV once	Avoid in hypovolemic/hypotensive cats

    i.   However, specificity of NSAIDs to COX receptors determined from in-vitro testing and susceptibility to toxicities are unique between species, and in-vitro data may not represent in-vivo conditions.

    ii.   NSAIDs may also interact with enzymes other than COX, such as 5-lipoxenase, which may be responsible for additional detrimental or beneficial effects.

  D. Many NSAIDs rely primarily on hepatic gluronidation for metabolism, which may reduce their margin of safety in cats.

  E. NSAIDs are contraindicated in cats with liver or renal disease and those that are hypovolemic or hypotensive.

  F. Meloxicam is the only NSAID registered for cats in the United States; it is also registered for use in cats in Europe, Australia, and New Zealand.

    i.   In-vitro study found that any meloxicam concentration producing COX- 2 inhibition always inhibited at least 20% of COX-1.

    ii.   One clinical study in cats undergoing onychectomy found better analgesia with meloxicam than butorphanol.

    iii. A short-term toxicity study following single dose in cats found no elevations in BUN, creatinine, or buccal mucosal bleeding time after 24 hours.

    iv. 0.1–0.2 mg/kg PO or SC has been recommended for perioperative pain followed by 0.05 mg/kg for 4 days. For chronic pain, 0.1 mg/kg followed by 0.05 mg/kg for 4 days then to the lowest effective dose every 24–48 hours.

    v.   0.2–0.3 mg/kg SC once prior to or after surgery is recommended.

  G. Carprofen

    i.   At the labeled dose, in-vitro testing found COX-2 inhibition at 100% with COX-1 inhibition 44%.

    ii.   Several clinical studies in cats report very effective analgesia after ovariohysterectomy, providing better analgesia than meperidine or buprenorphine, and no difference from meloxicam or ketoprofen.

      a. Only recommended for single dosing at 1–2 mg/kg SQ

X.   Alpha-2 agonists (medetomidine; dexmedetomidine)

  A. Like opioids, alpha-2 agonists bind to G protein–coupled receptors, leading to a variety of intracellular messenger signaling cascades, which ultimately results in diminished neurotransmitter release and inhibition of nociceptive transmission.

    i.   Alpha-2 receptors, like opioid receptors, are found in similar sites throughout the brain and spinal cord.

    ii.   Dexmedetomidine, the d-isomer of the racemate medetomidine, is twice the potency of medetomidine at equivalent dosage, but comparison at equipotent dosages finds little difference in quality of effects.

    iii. One study found that only 40 and not 2, 5, 10, or 20 μg/kg of dexmedetomidine IM significantly increased thermal thresholds in cats, and this response was less than that from a dosage of 20 μg/kg of buporenorphine; however, sedation increased in a dose-dependent manner.

B. Not typically a first-line analgesic because of marked sedative effects; however, relatively low dosage can potentiate the effects of other analgesics and sedatives; therefore, a multimodal pharmacologic approach to analgesia is most effective.

C. Low dosage of continuous rate infusions (1–2 μg/kg medetomidine; 0.05–1.0 μg/kg dexmedetomidine) can be beneficial in cats requiring analgesia with anxiolysis.

XI. Local anesthetics (lidocaine; systemic analgesia)

A. There is experimental and clinical evidence that lidocaine administered as an IV infusion is effective against acute and postoperative pain, hyperalgesia, and neuropathic pain in humans and experimental animals. Therefore, lidocaine continuous-rate infusions may be effective adjuvants for preventing and/or treating central sensitization and hyperalgesia in cats.

B. Possible mechanisms include decreased neuronal discharge secondary to blockade of selective sodium channel subtypes that are up-regulated after sensory nerve injury and neuronal hyperpolarization by enhancing inward potassium currents.

    i.   Lidocaine concentrations in the range of 0.6–5.7 μg/mL are reported to provide analgesia in a variety of species.

C. In toxicity studies, convulsive dosages of lidocaine administered IV to cats have ranged from 11.7 ± 4.6 mg/kg to 22.0 ± 4.4 mg/kg, and lidocaine plasma concentrations during seizures varied from 19.6 ± 5.5 to >100 μg/mL.

    i.   Subjective signs of toxicity such as dizziness occur in people at concentrations >5 μg/mL, although plasma levels and clinical signs are not always well correlated.

D. Few studies determining efficacy and safety of lidocaine as an analgesic/anesthetic in cats have been published.

    i.   No effect on thermal thresholds were determined when moderate lidocaine plasma concentrations (up to 4.3 μg/mL) were achieved; no adverse effects were noted in that study.

    ii.   In an IV-regional anesthesia study in isoflurane-anesthetized cats, cumulative dosage of 6 mg/kg 1% lidocaine over a 40-minute duration resulted in no significant decreases in blood pressure or adverse effects with concentrations in ranges of 1.5–6.4 μg/mL.

    iii. Lidocaine infusions administered to achieve target plasma concentrations decreased isoflurane requirements up to 52% at a maximum concentration of 11 μg/mL (estimated dosage, 3.4 mg/kg). However, cardiovascular depression was dose dependent and became severe when concentrations exceeded 5 μg/mL; investigators did not recommend lidocaine infusions for isoflurane MAC reduction in cats.

E. The safety and efficacy of transdermal lidocaine creams have been studied in cats.

    i.   One gram of EMLA (lidocaine/prilocaine) and 15 mg/kg of ELA-Max (liposome-encapsulated lidocaine) applied locally to intact skin were evaluated for determination of plasma concentrations, possible adverse effects, and efficacy in minimizing discomfort for jugular catheter placement in healthy and clinically ill cats.

        a. Although some cats objected to catheter placement, minimal plasma concentrations were measured in both studies, methemoglobin levels were negligible, and no adverse effects were noted in any cat.

        b. Lidocaine creams may be useful for minor surgical procedures such as mass removals.

        c. Lidoderm patch placed along incision lines is effective and appears to be safe in cats.

Table 7.6. Some common regional techniques and their indications. Parentheses denote alternative choice.

Procedure	Indications	Drug(s)	Dose mg/kg	Comments
Epidural	Femoral, pelvic, perineal traumas/ surgery	M (bupren) (bupiv) (lido)	0.1–0.15 (0.01–0.02) (0.5–1.0) (3)	Total volume 0.2 mL/kg Significant MAC reduction with local anesthetic
Epidural (fig. 7.3)	Sternotomy; cranial-abdominal analgesia	M (bupren) 0.7 saline	As above 0.25 mL/kg	No local anesthetic to avoid Potential blockade of autonomic or respiratory function
Brachial plexus block (fig. 7.2)	Traumas to forelimb, distal to mid-humerus, elbow	Bupiv	1.5	Add equal volume of saline for greater spread; with nerve locator less volume necessary
Line blocks (along incision lines)	C-section	Lido	4	Saline can be added to increase volume
Interpleural analgesia	Postthoracotomy; chest trauma; upper abdominal pain	Bupiv	1.5 with equal volume saline	Evacuate chest tube first; instill with affected side down

Note: M = morphine 1 mg/mL; bupren = buprenorphine 0.3 mg/mL; lido = lidocaine 20 mg/mL; bupiv = bupivicaine 5 mg/mL.

XII. Regional analgesic techniques (table 7.6)
  A. Local anesthetics applied via infiltration whenever possible can minimize intraoperative anesthetic concentrations and minimize post–operative pain and opioid requirements. Peripheral nerve blocks with local anesthetics can interrupt the impulse flow from the painful area to the CNS.
  B. Recommended dosages for local anesthetic infiltration techniques
    i. Lidocaine 1%; 2%: up to 4 mg/kg
    ii. Bupivacaine 0.25%; 0.5%: up to 2 mg/kg
  C. Epidural and spinal (subarachnoid l) administration of opioids, alpha-2 agonists, local anesthetics
    i. Generally applied at the lumbosacral space (fig. 7.3)
      a. In cats, the spinal cord ends at the cranial sacrum; therefore, subarachnoid penetration is not uncommon.
      b. Generally less volume (~½ epidural) should be administered.
    ii. Local anesthetics block all sensory input to the dorsal horn.
    iii. Opioids, alpha-2 agonists are applied in close proximity to its target (receptors); lower doses are required.
    iv. Less systemic effects (opioids), longer duration of action (morphine) than when administered systemically
    v. Contraindications include local infection, sepsis, bleeding disorders
    vi. Drugs used should be preservative free; may preclude the use of drugs not easily obtained in this form (alpha-2 agonists, some opioids)
    vii. Strict attention must be paid to sterile technique.
  D. Detailed descriptions of regional techniques in cats can be found in Tranquilli et al. 2007.

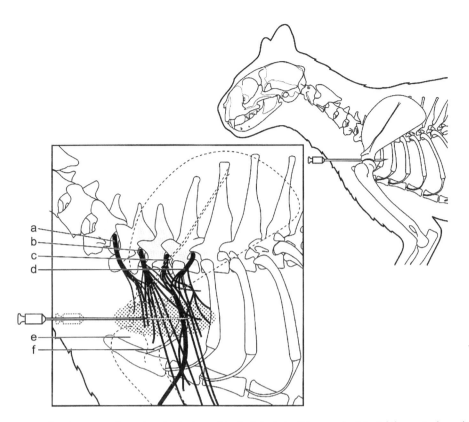

Fig. 7.2. Needle placement for a brachial plexus block. (a) sixth, (b) seventh, (c) eighth cervical, and (d) first thoracic spinal nerves; (e) tuberosity of humerus; (f) first rib. A 22-gauge 1.5-inch needle is placed in the axillary space proximal to the shoulder. The needle is advanced in a plane parallel to the scapula. The syringe should be aspirated for blood prior to injection. Equal volume of saline can be added to Bupivacaine 1.5 mg/kg or lidocaine 2 mg/kg and can be injected at the brachial plexus and as the needle is withdrawn. From Tranquilli, Thurmaon, and Grimm 2007.

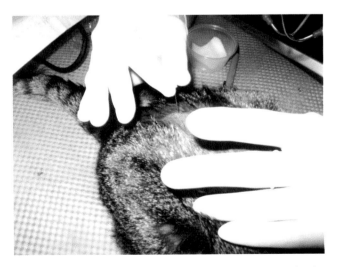

Fig. 7.3. The lumbosacral space has been palpated along the dorsal midline at a level immediately caudal to the wings of the ilia. A 22-gauge, 1.5 spinal needle is being introduced perpendicular to the dorsum and is advanced until a loss of resistance is appreciated, indicating that the ligamentum flavum has been punctured and the tip of the needle is in the epidural space. After the stylet is removed, a test injection of a small amount of air is made. When no resistance is encountered, the syringe with morphine and bupivacaine is injected.

Recommended Reading

Cambridge AJ, Tobias KM, Newberry RC, et al. Subjective and objective measurements of postoperative pain in cats. J Am Vet Med Assoc, 2000; 217:685–690.

Gaynor JS, Muir WW. Pain behaviors. In Gaynor JS, Muir WW, eds, Handbook of Veterinary Pain Management. St Louis: Mosby, 2002.

Kushner LI. Intravenous regional anesthesia in isoflurane anesthetized cats: Lidocaine plasma concentrations and cardiovascular effects. Vet Anaesth Analg, 2002; 29:140–149.

Lascelles BD, Court MH, Hardie EM, et al. Nonsteroidal anti-inflammatory drugs in cats: A review. Vet Anaes Analg, 2007; 34:228–250.

Lascelles BD, Robertson SA. Use of thermal threshold response to evaluate the antinociceptive effects of butorphanol. Am J Vet Res, 2004; 65:1085–1089.

Muir WW, Woolf CJ. Mechanisms of pain and their therapeutic implications. J Am Vet Med Assoc, 2001; 219:1346–1356.

Pozzi A, Muir WW, Traverso F. Prevention of central sensitization and pain by N-methyl-D-aspartate receptor antagonists. J Am Vet Med Assoc, 2006; 228:53–60.

Robertson SA, Lascelles BD, Taylor PM. PK-PD modeling of buprenorphine in cats: Intravenous and oral transmucosal administration. J Vet Pharm Therap, 2005a; 28:453–460.

Robertson SA, Taylor PM, Sear JW et al. Relationship between plasma concentrations and analgesia after intravenous fentanyl and disposition after other routes of administration in cats. J Vet Pharmacol Therap, 2005b; 28:87–93.

Skarda RT, Tranquilli WJ. Local and regional anesthetic and analgesic techniques: Cats. In Tranquilli WJ, Thurmon JC, Grimm KA, eds, Lumb and Jones' Veterinary Anesthesia and Analgesia, 4th ed. Ames, Iowa: Blackwell Publishing, 2007.

Steagall PVM, Carnicelli P, Taylor PM, et al. The effects of subcutaneous methadone, morphine, buprenorphine or saline on thermal and pressure thresholds in cats. J Vet Pharmacol Therap, 2006; 29:531–537.

Tranquilli WJ, Thurmon JC, Grimm KA, eds. Lumb and Jones' Veterinary Anesthesia and Analgesia, 4th ed. Ames, Iowa: Blackwell, 2007.

Wagner AE. Opioids. In Gaynor JS, Muir WW, eds, Handbook of Veterinary Pain Management. St Louis: Mosby, 2002.

Wegner K, Robertson SA. Dose-related thermal antinociceptive effects of intravenous hydromorphone in cats. Vet Anaes Analg, 2007; 34:132–138.

Wegner K, Robertson SA, Kollias-Baker C, et al. Pharmacokinetic and pharmacodynamic evaluation of intravenous hydromorphone in cats. J Vet Pharmacol Therap, 2004; 27:329–336.Recommended Reading

Woolf CJ, Max MB. Mechanism-based pain diagnosis, issues for analgesic drug development. Anesthesiology, 2001; 95:241–249.

8
FLUID THERAPY

Garret Pachtinger

> **Unique Features**
> - Compared to dogs, cats are more susceptible to fluid overload resulting in respiratory distress. Therefore, the patient should be monitored closely when using crystalloids, colloids, or hemoglobin-based solutions such as oxyglobin.
> - Feline vascular volume (40–60 mL/kg) differs from canine vascular volume (90 mL/kg). As a result, fluid resuscitation needs will differ between cats and dogs.
> - Physiologic responses in shock may be variable in the cat (i.e., while the physiologic response to decreased cardiac output in most species is tachycardia, cats can have a normal or bradycardic response to shock.)

The goal of fluid therapy is to expand intravascular volume, restore circulatory function, and ultimately deliver oxygen to tissues. Although in most situations the importance of fluid therapy is quite clear, there are many different opinions regarding the type of fluid, volume of fluid, and rate of fluid to be administered. Fortunately, as long as the heart and kidneys are working appropriately, normal homeostatic mechanisms allow a reasonable margin of error in the estimation of the fluid deficit and therapy required.

I. Crystalloid solutions (table 8.1)
   a. Electrolyte solutions are considered the mainstay of fluid therapy in veterinary medicine.
   b. Consist primarily of water with a sodium or glucose base, plus the addition of other electrolytes and/or buffers
   c. Can be used as maintenance or replacement solutions
   d. May be isotonic, hypotonic, or hypertonic based on the sodium concentration and osmolality of the fluid:
      i. Isotonic crystalloids contain a sodium concentration or osmolality similar to that of the cells in the body. This is the most common fluid type used in veterinary medicine. Examples include Normosol-R, 0.9% NaCl, Plasma-Lyte 148, and lactated Ringer's.
      ii. Hypotonic solutions contain a lower sodium concentration or osmolality than the cells of the body (0.45% NaCl, D_5W).
      iii. Hypertonic solutions contain a higher concentration of sodium or osmolality than cells of the body (i.e., 7.2%–23% NaCl).
   e. Using Isotonic crystalloids, only one-third of the volume administered remains within the intravascular space 1 hour after administration; therefore, larger volumes need to be used as compared to other types of fluid (Griffel, Elgart).

Table 8.1. Fluid categories.

Type of Solution	Examples
Crystalloid	
Isotonic	Normosol-R®, 0.9% NaCl, Plasma-Lyte 148®, lactated Ringer's
Hypertonic	7.2%–23% NaCl
Hypotonic	0.45% NaCl, D$_5$W
Colloid	
Natural	Albumin
Synthetic	Hetastarch, dextrans, gelatins
Other	Packed red blood cells, plasma, Oxyglobin®, PPN

Table 8.2. Shock doses of intravenous fluids.[a]

Fluid Type	Dose
Crystalloid	40–60 mL/kg; ¼ to ⅓ given over 20–30 minutes. Reassess patient to determine need for additional bolus or placement of fluid rate.
Colloid	2–4 mL/kg given over 20–30 minutes. Reassess patient to determine need for additional bolus or placement of fluid rate.
Hypertonic saline (7.2%)	2–3 mL/kg given over 20–30 minutes. Reassess patient to determine need for additional bolus or placement of fluid rate.

[a] Doses are patient dependent and may need to be altered based on underlying conditions such as cardiac disease.

   f. Examples of situations when crystalloid fluid therapy is indicated include volume depletion secondary to the losses associated with vomiting, diarrhea, third spacing, or diuresis (polyuria), as well as for replacement of intravascular volume seen with losses in shock and hemorrhage.

   g. Shock dose: 40–60 mL/kg in the cat. Most patients do not require the entire shock dose, and it is advisable to divide the total shock volume into two to four aliquots, giving each over 20 to 30 minutes and reassessing the patient between each increment to determine its effectiveness.

      i. An example would be to give a 5-kg cat in shock 75–100 mL over approximately 30 minutes and then reassess to determine effectiveness and future plan.

II. Colloid solutions

   a. When compared to crystalloids, colloids contain larger molecular weight substances, remain in the intravascular space longer, increase oncotic pressure, and increase vascular volume by retaining fluid within the vascular space (Rizoli, Concannon).

   b. Colloid therapy is often used in conjunction with crystalloid fluid therapy because colloids provide intravascular volume while crystalloids correct both intravascular and extravascular deficits (table 8.2).

   c. Use of colloids is generally considered when there is a low colloid osmotic pressure (<15 mmHg), or a low total protein (<3.5–4), or when edema develops following administration of isotonic crystalloids.

    d. Colloids can be divided into two categories: natural and synthetic.
       i. Natural—albumin is the only naturally occurring colloid.
          1. At this time, no species-specific albumin is available for cats.
          2. Plasma contains approximately 25 to 30 g/L of albumin. If a 5-kg cat has a serum albumin of 1.5 g/dL, the cat would require approximately 0.5 liters of FFP to increase the albumin to 2.5 g/dL (calculated using the following formula: albumin deficit = 10 × [Desired Alb – Patient Alb] × body weight (kg) × 0.3)
          3. Although administration of plasma is the optimal choice for albumin replacement, the cost of plasma, its limited supply, and the amount necessary to increase colloid osmotic pressure make plasma an unrealistic choice for colloid fluid therapy.
      ii. Synthetic—there are three types of synthetic colloids (gelatins, hydroxyethyl starches, and dextrans)
          1. Initial boluses of hydroxyethyl starch (Hetastarch) or Dextran 70 (not readily available anymore) given at a dosage of 2–4 mL/kg given over 15–20 minutes can be used in the cat.
          2. Maintenance therapy at 0.5–1 mL/kg/hr can be used for oncotic support.
    e. The main adverse effects of synthetic colloid administration are coagulopathy and decreased coagulability. When dosages >20 mL/kg/24 h are used, coagulopathic effects become apparent.

III. Hypertonic solutions (i.e., hypertonic saline)
    a. Provide rapid volume expansion with lesser volume administration.
    b. Cause an increase in the osmotic gradient, which "pulls water" from the interstitial space and intracellular space into the intravascular space, expanding intravascular volume.
    c. May be most efficacious in patients with acute hypovolemic shock (and therefore normal interstitial hydration) and may also be useful in resuscitation of patients with head trauma
    d. Since the initial volume expansion is followed by redistribution, hypertonic saline should not be used alone but followed with crystalloid fluid therapy.
    e. Due to the large sodium concentration and osmotic pull of fluid from the interstitial and intracellular spaces, hypertonic solutions are contraindicated in dehydrated or hypernatremic patients.
    f. A bolus of 2–3 mL/kg over 15 to 20 minutes is recommended in cats.
    g. A recipe for administration of hypertonic saline with a colloid is to dilute 23.4% NaCl with 6% hetastarch or dextran 70 (volume NaCl and volume colloid) to make a 7.5% solution of NaCl.

IV. Hemoglobin-based solutions
    a. Oxyglobin (Biopure Corporation, Cambridge MA) is a purified, polymerized bovine hemoglobin diluted in a modified lactated Ringer's solution.
    b. This fluid can carry and release oxygen in a manner similar to red blood cells.
    c. Advantages of Oxyglobin include the following:
       i. Long shelf life (approx. 3 years)
      ii. Immediate oxygen carrying capability because there is no requirement for 2,3-diphosphoglycerate.
      iii. No need for blood typing/crossmatching
      iv. Minimal risk of infectious disease transmission
      v. Contributes to osmotic pressure, offering an additional advantage in hypotensive patients
      vi. No known allergic reactions following repeat doses
      vii. Plasma half-life of approximately 24 hours
    d. Disadvantages of Oxyglobin
       i. Rapid fluid overload and development of pulmonary edema due to the high oncotic pressure.
      ii. Administration may cause a transient yellow-brown discoloration to mucous membranes, skin, sclera, and urine.
      iii. Fever
      iv. Diarrhea
      v. May cause an inability to measure certain normal bloodwork parameters:

Table 8.3. Shock categories and causes.

Category	Cause
Hypovolemic shock	Loss of intravascular volume from hemorrhage, vomiting, diarrhea, and severe polyuria without adequate polydypsia
Cardiogenic shock	Cardiac disease leading to a reduced cardiac output
Distributive shock	SIRS, sepsis, or anaphylaxis triggered by a dysfunction of the microcirculation that leads to inappropriate, widespread vasodilatation and results in relative hypovolemia
Obstructive Shock	A mechanical interference with ventricular filling from pericardial effusion leading to tamponade, caval syndrome of heartworm disease, aortic thromboembolism, and intracardiac neoplasia

1. While the PCV may decrease due to dilution, oxygen carrying capacity, and ultimately hemoglobin, can be measured with a hemoglobinometer. The hemoglobin concentration can be multiplied by 3 to estimate the PCV (i.e., a blood hemoglobin concentration of 10 correlates to a PCV of 30).
2. Oxyglobin may cause a transient red discoloration of the plasma resulting in the inability to detect hemolysis. Furthermore, due to this red discoloration, certain chemistry analyzers that use colorimetry may not give accurate values.

   e. Dose: 5 mL/kg is recommended. Due to the high oncotic pressure, smaller doses should be considered in patients with underlying cardiac disease.

V. Specific conditions requiring fluid therapy
   a. Shock (table 8.3): A complex group of conditions that result from inadequate oxygen delivery to tissues. While numerous classification schemes have been developed, clinically useful categories in feline emergency medicine include hypovolemic shock, cardiogenic shock, obstructive shock, and distributive shock (sepsis/SIRS; see chap. 3—Shock).
      i. Hypovolemic shock: can be either absolute or relative in nature
         1. Causes of absolute hypovolemic shock: hemorrhage, vomiting, diarrhea, and severe polyuria without adequate polydypsia
         2. Causes for relative hypovolemic shock: anaphylaxis or the use of vasodilatory drugs and an increased microvascular permeability
      ii. Cardiogenic shock: caused by a reduced cardiac output and often associated with cardiac disease. The end result of cardiogenic shock is global hypoperfusion.
      iii. Distributive shock: most commonly associated with SIRS, sepsis, or anaphylaxis triggered by a dysfunction of the microcirculation that leads to inappropriate, widespread vasodilatation and results in relative hypovolemia
      iv. Obstructive shock: results from a mechanical interference with ventricular filling. Examples include pericardial effusion leading to pericardial tamponade, caval syndrome of heartworm disease, aortic thromboembolism, and intracardiac neoplasia.
         1. From clinical experience, both hypovolemic and distributive shock syndromes respond to aggressive fluid therapy. Obstructive shock responds to fluid therapy, but identification and correction of the underlying cause will more rapidly improve patient outcome. Due to the underlying cardiac disease, fluid therapy is contraindicated in cardiogenic shock.
   b. Dehydration (table 8.4)
      i. Treatment involves administration of crystalloid fluids to both correct the fluid deficit as well as calculate and replace ongoing loss.

Table 8.4.   Physical assessment of dehydration.

Estimated % Dehydration	Clinical Signs
<4	Not detectable
4–5	Subtle loss of skin elasticity, "tacky" mucous membranes
6–8	Decreased skin turgor (when the skin is tented there is a slight delay in return to normal position), dry mucous membranes, slight prolongation of capillary refill time, eyes may be dull
10–12	Prolonged capillary refill time (>2 seconds), dry mucous membranes, sunken eyes, tented skin does not return to normal position, possible tachycardia, and weak pulses
12–15	Pale mucous membranes, capillary refill time >3 seconds, signs of shock, dementia, death imminent

Table 8.5.   Potassium supplementation chart.

Serum Potassium Concentration (mEq/L)	mEq KCl to Add to 500 mL Fluid	Maximum Infusion Rate (0.5 mEq/kg/h)
<2.0	40	6 mL/kg/h
2.1–2.5	30	8 mL/kg/h
2.6–3.0	20	12 mL/kg/h
3.1–3.5	14	18 mL/kg/h
>3.5–<5	5	25 mL/kg/h

Note: Potassium doses should not exceed K-Max (0.5 mEq/kg/h) unless clinically required and only when extremely close monitoring is implemented.

    ii. The fluid deficit is calculated based on the patient's body weight (kg) and the percentage of dehydration (see box 8.2).

    iii. Ongoing losses may be caused by diarrhea, vomiting, polyuria (without sufficient polydypsia), or other conditions that lead to an abnormal fluid loss.

       1. Losses such as these can be estimated by weighing diapers. This can be performed by subtracting the normal diaper weight from the diaper with the fluid loss (10 g = 0.01 kg = 10 mL).

c. Potassium supplementation (table 8.5)

    i. Potassium is vital in the function of tissues such as muscles and nerves.

    ii. Causes for hypokalemia include (but are not limited to) the following:

       1. Anorexia

       2. Diabetes mellitus

       3. Administration of potassium-free or low-potassium fluids

       4. Gastrointestinal fluid loss (vomiting or diarrhea)

       5. Renal disease/failure

       6. Hyperaldosteronism (Conns Syndrome)—a rare disease that leads to loss of potassium via the kidneys due to the activity of aldosterone (see chap. 32—Management of Specific Endocrine and Metabolic Diseases: Other and chap. 34—Electrolyte Disorders).

       7. Iatrogenic causes such as the administration of diuretics (e.g., furosemide).

    iii. Signs of hypokalemia include weakness, ventroflexion of the neck, lethargy, mental depression, arrhythmias, and death from respiratory muscle paralysis.

    iv. Potassium can be supplemented orally or added to intravenous fluids.

       1. Oral supplementation can be done by administering potassium gluconate (Tumil-K, Daniels Pharmaceuticals) at a dose of 2 mEq/4.5 kg PO q12 h.

       2. If oral supplementation is not possible or severe hypokalemia is present, intravenous potassium administration should be considered.

       3. The amount of potassium to add to maintenance fluids should be based on measured serum potassium. (When giving boluses of intravenous fluids, potassium should NOT be supplemented due to the risk of rapid hyperkalemia and cardiotoxicity. See table 8.5.)

       4. If oral or intravenous potassium administration is not possible, subcutaneous administration with solutions containing up to 30 mEq/L of KCL can be administered safely.

       5. Potassium doses should not exceed K-Max (0.5 mEq/kg/hour) unless clinically required. If required, strict monitoring should include heart rate, respiratory rate and effort, ECG, blood pressure, and mentation. Frequent evaluation of electrolytes (hourly to no less than every 6 hours) should be performed as well.

  d. Bicarbonate supplementation

    i. Usually reserved for a severe metabolic acidosis and pH disturbance (pH <7.1–7.2; base deficit >10; bicarbonate <14 mEq/L).

    ii. Bicarbonate deficit equation (mEq of bicarbonate to administer):

       1. $0.3 \times Bw(Kg) \times (24 - \text{patient bicarbonate})$

       2. One-fourth to one-third of this deficit should be given slowly over 2 to 4 hours.

       3. Alternatively, 1–3 mEq/kg can be administered with 1 mEq/kg for mild acidosis and 3 mEq/kg for severe acidosis.

       4. Blood gases should be taken after completion of this aliquot to determine if additional bicarbonate administration is necessary (i.e., if the patient pH is still less than 7.2 or clinical signs related to acidemia such as decreased response to pressor therapy, etc.)

       5. Bicarbonate administration is not recommended if blood gases are not available.

       6. Bicarbonate is not recommended if there is a respiratory dysfunction leading to an already elevated CO_2 as bicarbonate will be broken down into H_2O and CO_2, further exacerbating the existing respiratory compromise and hypercapnea.

       7. Complications of bicarbonate administration include hypernatremia, hyperosmolality, and additional electrolyte disturbances (decrease in ionized calcium and potassium) due to its alkalinizing effects.

  e. Maintenance fluid therapy (box 8.1)

    i. Defined as the volume needed per day for fluid balance (i.e., the intake of fluids should be equal to the loss of fluids).

    ii. Daily fluid requirements (mL/kg/day) parallel daily energy requirements (kcal/kg/day).

    iii. Normal feline energy requirements are 50–60 kcal/kg/day. Therefore, a rough estimate for fluid balance would be 50–60 mL/kg/day for the maintenance fluid requirement (see box 8.2).

    iv. Alternatively, an approximate dose for fluid maintenance is 2–3 mL/kg/h.

  f. Ongoing loss therapy

    i. The amount lost through vomiting, diarrhea, polyuria, and so on that should be measured/estimated and then added to the maintenance and dehydration fluid calculations

       1. Example: A 5-kg patient is estimated to be vomiting approximately 10 mL every 4 hours.

$$24 \text{ hours}/4 \text{ hours} = 6 \text{ episodes in } 24 \text{ hours}$$

$$6 \text{ vomiting episodes} \times 10 \text{ mL} = 60 \text{ mL}$$

Therefore, the patient's ongoing loss is estimated to be 60 mL over 24 hours.

> **Box 8.1.**   Fluid calculations.
> Feline maintenance fluid administration: 50–60 mL/kg/24 hours
> Fluid deficit from dehydration (in mL) =   % Dehydration × body weight (kg) × 1,000 mL
> Ongoing losses per hour in mL: Estimation of loss/24 hours

g. Fluid diuresis
  1. The goals are to increase the glomerular filtration rate, increase renal perfusion, and enhance the renal excretory function.
  2. Specific disease states where fluid diuresis may be considered include renal disease to eliminate renal toxins and improve azotemia as well as in cases of toxin ingestion to hasten the elimination of toxins that are excreted by the kidneys.
  3. In these situations, crystalloid fluids are the fluids of choice.
  4. Fluid rates required to induce a sufficient diuresis can be as high as 2–4 times a patient's maintenance requirements. Expected urine output for adequate fluid diuresis is 2–6 mL/kg/h.
  5. "Ins" and "outs" should be measured every 2–4 hours. A urinary catheter with a closed collection system is recommended to allow accurate monitoring and calculation of "outs."
  6. During fluid diuresis, careful monitoring should be made for signs of fluid overload such as abnormal lung sounds (crackles), generalized edema, hypertension, or jugular venous distension.

VI. Constant rate infusion (CRI) formulas

Formula 1:

[CRI dose (mg/kg/hr) × body weight (kg) × bag volume (mL)] ÷ fluid rate (mL/hr) = dose of drug (mg) to add to bag

Example: Morphine CRI at 0.1 mg/kg/hr for 10-kg cat with IV fluid rate of 20 mL/hr:

(0.1 mg/kg/hr × 10 kg × 1,000 mL) ÷ 20 mL/hr = 50 mg added to a 1-L bag

Formula 2 (for use if multiple CRI medications will be needed at the same time):

Fluids will run at 1 mL/kg/hr

CRI dose (mg/kg/hr) × bag volume (mL) = dose (mg) to add to bag

Additional maintenance fluids will need to be piggy-backed or placed through another catheter if additional fluids are required, as the CRI rate for this formula will only be 1 ml/kg/hr.

Formula 3:

Dosage (μg/kg/min) × W (kg) = mg to add to 250 mL base solution at a rate of 15 mL/h

Formula 4:

$$M = D \times W \times V/R \times 16.67$$

Abbreviation key:

M = milligrams of drug to add to the base solution
D = dosage of drug in micrograms per kilogram per minute
W = body weight in kilograms
V = volume in milliliters of base solution
R = fluid rate in milliliters per hour
16.67 = conversion factor

To determine the appropriate R if dosage is adjusted, the formula would be:

$$R = D \times W \times V / M \times 16.67$$

Box 8.2. Sample feline fluid therapy case.

Example: A 5-kg cat with a 1-day history of vomiting and diarrhea. On physical examination, the cat is 5% dehydrated (tacky mucous membranes, CRT 1.5 seconds, very slight decrease in skin turgor). The cat is vomiting 10 mL every 4 hours. PCV 45, TS 7.4, Na 153, K 3.2, BUN 41, Creat 1.8, Glucose 140.

Solution: Use a balanced electrolyte solution and replace the deficit over 12 hours.

Dehydration	= % dehydration × BW (kg) × 1,000 = mL of fluid needed
	= 0.05 × 5 × 1,000 = **250 mL**
Maintenance (×12 hours)	= 50–60 kcal/kg/day = 50–60 mL/kg/day
	= 300 mL/day
	= 300 mL/24 h
	= **150 mL in 12 hours**
	= 150 mL for 12 hours
Ongoing losses	= 10 mL in 4 hours
	= **30 mL in 12 hours**
Total	= 250 mL + 150 mL + 30 mL
	= 430 mL/12 hours
	= 35.8 mL/hour × 12 hours

Additives to the fluids:

Potassium is added to the fluid bag (14 mEq/500 mL) based on the KCL replacement chart.

During the fluid therapy and continued hospitalization, monitoring will include physical examination parameters (heart rate, pulse quality, respiratory rate, respiratory effort, mentation), electrolytes, blood pressure, mentation, and continued losses.

References and Recommended Reading

Brady CA, Otto CM. Systemic inflammatory response syndrome, sepsis, and multiple organ dysfunction. Vet Clin North Am Small Anim Pract, 2001; 31:1147.

Brown R. Potassium homeostasis and clinical implications. Am J Med, 1984; 77:3–10.

Concannon KT, Haskins SC, Feldman BF. Hemostatic defects associated with two infusion rates of dextran 70 in dogs. Am J Vet Res, 1992; 53(8):1369–1375.

Cote E. Cardiogenic shock and cardiac arrest. Vet Clin North Am Small Anim Pract, 2001; 31:1129.

Crystal MA, Cotter SM. Acute hemorrhage: a hematologic emergency in dogs. Compend Cont Educ Prac Vet, 1992; 14:1.

Day TK. Current development and use of hemoglobin-based oxygen-carrying (HBOC) solutions. J Vet Emerg Crit Care, 2003; 13(2):77–93.

DiBartola SP. Fluid, Electrolyte and Acid Base Disorders, 3rd ed. WB Saunders, 2005.

Elgart HN. Assessment of fluids and electrolytes. AACN Clin Issues, 2004; 15(4):607–621.

Gibson GR, Callan MB, Hoffman V, et al. Use of a hemoglobin-based oxygen-carrying solution in cats: 72 cases (1998–2002). J Am Vet Assoc, 2002; 221(1):96–102.

Glowaski MM, Moon-Massat PF, Erb HN, et al. Effects of oxypolygelatin and dextran 70 on hemostatic variables in dogs. Vet Anaesth Analg, 2003; 30(4):202–210.

Griffel MI, Kaufman BS. Pharmacology of colloids and crystalloids. Crit Care Clin, 1992; 8:235.

Gutierrez G, Reines HD, Wulf-Gutierrez ME. Clinical review: hemorrhagic shock. Crit Care, 2004; 8(5):373–381. Epub 2004 Apr 2.

Haldane S, Graves TK, Bateman S, Lichtensteiger CA. Profound hypokalemia causing respiratory failure in a cat with hyperaldosteronism. J Vet Emerg Crit Care, 2007; 17(2):202–207.

Johnson AL, Criddle LM. Pass the salt: indications for and implications of using hypertonic saline. Crit Care Nurse, 2004; 24(5):36–8, 40–4, 46 passim.

Kelly N, Rentko VT. Comparative cardiovascular response by Oxyglobin versus packed red blood cells in acute anemia. J Vet Emerg Crit Care, 1998; 8(3):252.

Kirby R. Septic shock. In Bonagura JD, ed, Current Veterinary Therapy XII. Philadelphia: W.B. Saunders, 1995.

Kumar A, Parillo JE. Shock classification, pathophysiology, and approach to management. In Parillo JE, Dellinger RP, eds, Critical Care Medicine: Principles of Diagnosis and Management in the Adult, 2nd ed. Philadelphia: Mosby, 2001.

Mendez CM, McClain CJ, Marsano LS. Albumin in clinical practice. Nutr Clin Pract, 2005; 20(3):314–320.

Moore KE, Murtaugh RJ. Pathophysiologic characteristics of hypovolemic shock, Vet Clin North Am Small Anim Prac, 2001; 31:1175.

Muir WW. Overview of shock. In proceedings of the 14th annual Kal Kan Symposium Emergency/Critical Care, Columbus, OH, 1990, p. 7.

Orton EC, Muir WW. Hemodynamics during experimental gastric dilitation and volvulus in dogs. Am J Vet Res, 1983; 44:1512–1515.

Rahilly L. Hypoalbuminemia: pathophysiology and treatment. Conference Proceedings, International Veterinary Emergency and Critical Care Symposium, 2006.

Rixen D, Siegel JH. Bench-to-bedside review: oxygen debt and its metabolic correlates as quantifiers of the severity of hemorrhagic and post-traumatic shock. Crit Care, 2005; 9(5):441–453. Epub 2005 Apr 20.

Rizoli SB. Crystalloids and colloids in trauma resuscitation: a brief overview of the current debate. J Trauma, 2003; 54 (Suppl):S82–S88.

Velasco IT, Pontieri V, Rocha E, Silva M. Hypertonic NaCl and severe hemorrhagic shock. Am J Physiol, 1980; 239:H664–H673.

Vercueil A, Grocott MP, Mythen MG. Physiology, pharmacology, and rationale for colloid administration for the maintenance of effective hemodynamic stability in critically ill patients. Transfus Med Rev, 2005; 19(2):93–109.

Walton RS. Polymerized hemoglobin versus hydroxyethyl starch in an experimental model of feline hemorrhagic shock. Proceedings IVECCS, 1996, San Antonio.

Wingfield WE, Betts CW, Rawlings CA. Pathophysiology associated with gastric dilatation-volvulus in the dog. JAAHA, 1976; 12:136–142.

9
NUTRITIONAL SUPPORT FOR THE CRITICALLY ILL FELINE PATIENT

Daniel L. Chan

Unique Features

1. A particular concern with hospitalized cats is the development of food aversion. For this reason, stressful means for nutritional support such as force feeding or syringe feeding are not recommended.
2. The importance of appropriate nutritional support in critically ill cats is highlighted by the development of hepatic lipidosis, which is usually secondary to another underlying condition and results from energy and protein deprivation. This is particularly true but not exclusively seen in obese cats.
3. Particular differences in the nutritional requirements of cats include a higher requirement for dietary protein (6 g of protein/100 kcal of food consumed) and strict requirements for taurine and arginine, explaining why enteral formulas designed for people are usually unsuitable for use in cats.

A. Importance of nutritional support
   a. Loss or decrease in food intake is often the first sign of illness in cats. An important consideration is that almost all diseases induce dramatic changes in energy and nutrient metabolism which puts critically ill patients at high risk for malnutrition and its subsequent complications. Whereas healthy animals primarily lose fat when fasted, sick or injured animals catabolize lean body mass when they are not provided with sufficient calories.
   b. Hospitalized cats are particularly stressed, which contributes to decreased food intake. Anorexia in cats can be particularly challenging to manage and if left untreated can have serious metabolic consequences.
   c. An important point to make is that successful management of anorexia in cats is to reverse the primary condition, rather than use appetite stimulants or simply encourage eating by offering "appetizing" food.
   d. The goals of nutritional support include correction of nutritional deficiencies and imbalances and provision of adequate energy substrates, protein, and micronutrients.
   e. Prevention of further catabolism of lean body tissue and reversal of metabolic derangements are other important goals of nutritional support.
   f. Because nutritional interventions are not without risk, appropriate nutritional assessment can help select which patients are most likely to benefit from nutritional support and to help minimize complications.
B. Indications for nutritional intervention

   a. Nutritional assessment identifies malnourished patients that require urgent nutritional support as well as those in which nutritional support is likely to be necessary to prevent malnutrition.
   b. Overt indicators of malnutrition include recent weight loss, poor haircoat quality, muscle wasting, signs of inadequate wound healing, hypoalbuminemia, and lymphopenia. However, these abnormalities are not specific to malnutrition and do not occur early enough in the process.
   c. Key factors to consider in the nutritional assessment include the following:
      i.   Anorexia lasting greater than 3 days
      ii. Serious underlying disease (e.g., severe trauma, sepsis, peritonitis, acute pancreatitis, burns)
      iii. Large protein losses (e.g., draining wounds, exudative effusions)
   d. Patients with obvious protracted disease courses in which the patient is likely to be hospitalized for over 5 days should be strongly considered to receive nutritional support.
   e. Nutritional assessment also identifies factors that can affect the nutritional plan, such as electrolyte abnormalities, hyperglycemia, hypertriglyceridemia, or comorbid illness such as significant hepatic, cardiac, or renal disease.
   f. Appropriate laboratory analysis (i.e., serum biochemical profile) should be performed in all patients in which nutritional support is being considered because abnormalities may influence the nutritional plan.
   g. Before commencing nutritional support, the patient should be rehydrated, adequately resuscitated, that is, cardiovascularly stable, and have significant electrolyte and acid base abnormalities addressed.
C. Determine the route of nutritional support
   a. If there are no signs of overt gastrointestinal dysfunction, for example, protracted vomiting or diarrhea that results in overt dehydration (>8%) or compromises intravascular volume status, the enteral route of delivery should be chosen.
   b. Enteral nutrition is the most practical, economical, and physiologically sound approach of delivering nutrients. Except for feeding tube problems, there are fewer complications associated with enteral nutrition compared with parenteral nutrition.
   c. Even when enteral nutrition does not completely meet all of the patient's energy and nutrient needs, delivery of food via the gastrointestinal tract is still beneficial in that it modulates gastrointestinal motility, immune function, and maintains the integrity of the intestinal barrier.
   d. For patients that cannot tolerate enteral feedings or in which there is concern for aspiration of food into the airways, for example, pharyngeal dysfunction or dyspnea, the parenteral route should be considered.
D. Enteral nutrition
   a. If the enteral route is chosen, the most appropriate type of feeding tube for that patient must be considered.
   b. Factors to consider in choosing a particular feeding tube include the anticipated duration of nutritional support, the need to circumvent certain segments of the gastrointestinal tract (e.g., pancreatitis, esophagitis), form of nutrition to be delivered (e.g, liquid diet vs. blenderized diet), suitability of the patient to withstand anesthesia, and clinician preference and experience.
   c. Feeding tube options
      i. Nasoesophageal tubes
         1. Technically, this is the simplest type of feeding tube to place (see figures 9.1 through 9.6).
         2. This is a good option if only a short (less than 3 days) course of nutritional support is anticipated.
         3. Patients that are unstable for anesthesia can have these tubes placed with minimal sedation if any is required and topical anesthetic instilled in nasal passages.
         4. Major limitations include using liquid diets only, patient discomfort, and requirement of Elizabethan collars.
         5. Most nasoesophageal feeding tubes in cats are either 3.5 Fr or 5 Fr tubes in size.

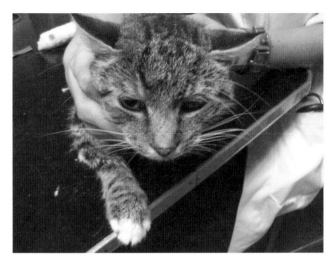

Fig. 9.1.   Underweight cat ready to receive placement of nasoesophageal tube.

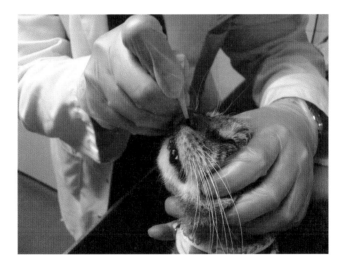

Fig. 9.2.   Placing local anesthetic nares. Note how the head is tilted straight up so that topical anesthetic will follow gravity into the nasal cavity.

6. Correct placement within the esophagus should be checked by either radiography, fluoroscopy, or end-tidal CO_2 measurement.
   a. Tubes placed within the esophagus should not yield appreciable CO_2 (fig. 9.6).
   b. The tip of the feeding tube should lie in the distal third of the esophagus and not directly within the stomach, as the lower esophageal sphincter may become irritated or incompetent.

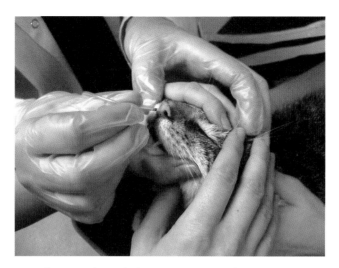

Fig. 9.3. Initial placement of nasoesophageal tube into nares. Note that initial placement should directed toward the ventromedial aspect of the nares.

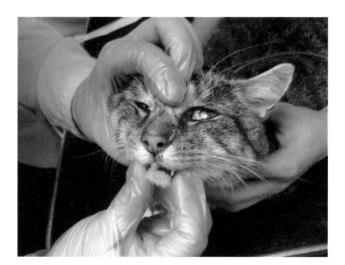

Fig. 9.4. Nasoesophageal tube has been placed the proper distance. Note how the exit of the tube is nearly flush with the lateral aspect of the nares and then is directed up toward the forehead between the eyes. The tube also could be directed to the lateral side of the face, but whiskers should be avoided as this will more likely cause irritation to the cat.

    ii. Esophageal tubes
        1. This is probably the most versatile and useful feeding tube for critically ill cats.
        2. It is relatively simple to place, requires only short anesthesia (should not be placed with sedation alone), and allows use of blenderized calorically dense diets.
        3. Most cats tolerate esophageal tubes without need of Elizabethan collars and can eat voluntarily with these tubes in place, compared with cats with nasoesophageal tubes, which may not have an interest in eating.

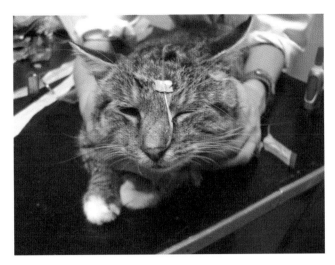

Fig. 9.5.   Tube is secured to skin using a tape butterfly and sutured or glued to the skin.

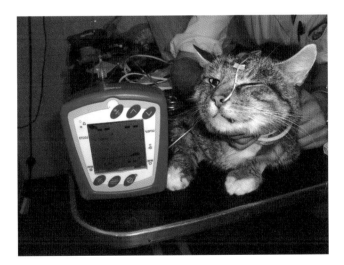

Fig. 9.6.   Attaching the end of the tube to the end tidal CO_2 monitor to evaluate for proper placement. CO_2 should not be detected if proper placement has occurred. If the tube is on the trachea or airways, CO_2 will be detected with respiration. Proper placement could also be confirmed by thoracic radiography. The tube should end in the distal third of the esophagus and should not enter the stomach.

    4. A full description of the technique in placing these tubes can be found in the caption for figures 9.7a through 9.7n.

    5. The positioning of the tube should be assessed via radiography, fluoroscopy, or end tidal CO_2 before use (see fig. 9.8).

       a. The distal tip should lie within the distal third of the esophagus.

    6. The most common sizes of esophageal feeding tubes for cats are 12 Fr and 14 Fr.

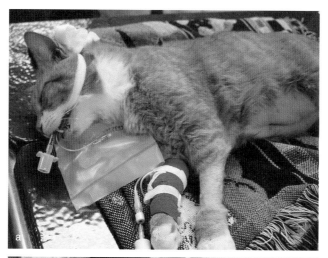

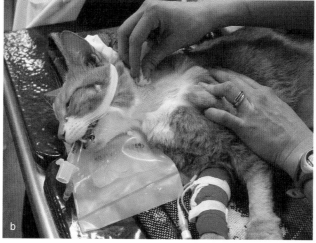

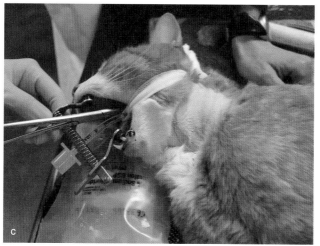

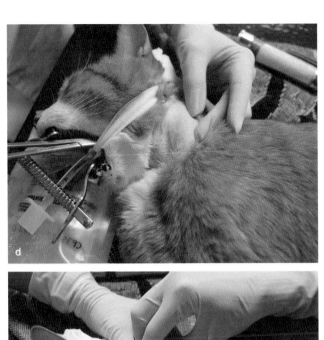

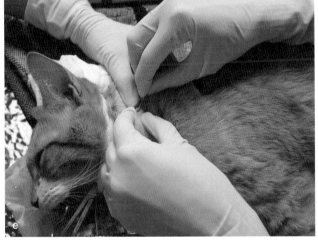

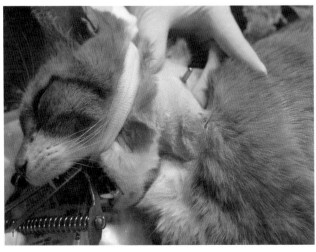

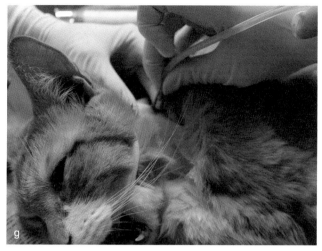

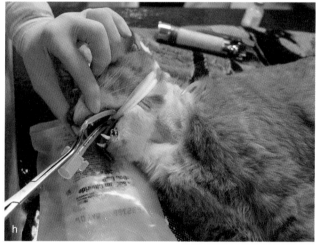

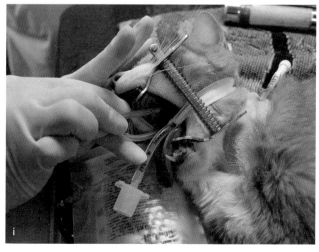

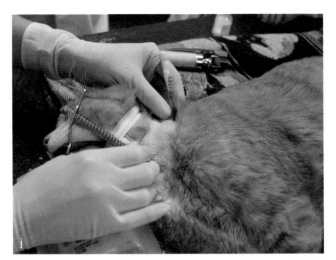

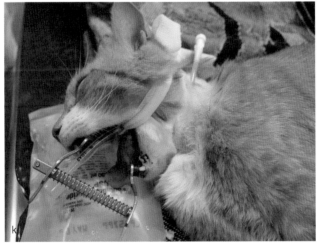

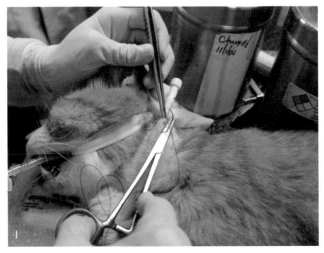

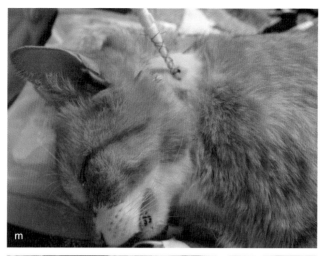

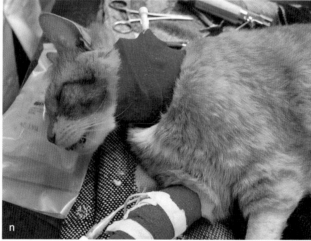

Fig. 9.7. a through n. Step-by-step technique for esophagostomy tube placement.

1. Proper placement of an esophagostomy feeding tube requires the distal tip to be placed in the distal esophagus at the level no farther than the ninth intercostal space. This may require premeasuring the tube. Rather than cutting the distal tip and creating a sharp edge, elongate the exit side hole using a small blade.
2. The patient should be anesthetized and preferably intubated. While in right lateral recumbency, the left side of the neck should be clipped and a routine surgical scrub is performed.
3. A curved Rochester carmalt is placed into the mouth and down the esophagus to the midcervical region. The jugular vein should be identified and avoided.
4. The tip of the carmalt is then pushed dorsally, pushing the esophagus toward the skin.
5. The tip of the carmalt is palpated over the skin to confirm its location, and an incision is made through the skin onto the tip of the carmalt in the esophagus. The mucosa of the esophagus is relatively more difficult to incise than the skin.
6. The tip of the instrument is then forced through the incision, which can be slightly enlarged with the blade to allow opening of the tips of the carmalt and placement of the esophagostomy tube within the tips.
7. The carmalt is then clamped closed and pulled from the oral cavity.
8. Disengage the tips of the carmalt, curl the tip of the esophagostomy back into the mouth, and feed it into esophagus. As the curled tube is pushed into the esophagus, the proximal end is gently pulled simultaneously. This will result in a subtle "flip" as the tube is redirected within the esophagus. The tube should easily slide back and forth a few millimeters, confirming that the tube has straightened.
9. Visually inspect the oropharynx to confirm that the tube is no longer present within the oropharynx.
10. The incision site should be briefly rescrubbed before a purse-string suture is placed, followed by a "Chinese finger trap," further securing the tube in place.
11. A light wrap is applied to the neck.

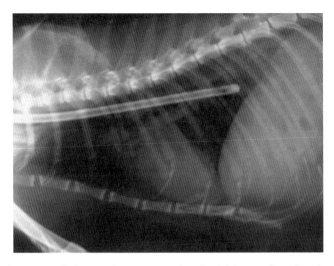

Fig. 9.8. Correct placement of the esophagostomy tube should be confirmed with either radiography or fluoroscopy.

    7. There is no minimal amount of time the tubes need to stay in place, and they can be pulled at any time. Tubes can remain in place for months, if necessary.

    8. The most common problems with esophageal feeding tubes are tube occlusion and cellulitis at the skin incision site.

  iii. Pharyngostomy tubes

    1. This is technically a slightly more difficult tube to place correctly, and associated complications are significant.

    2. Pharyngostomy tubes have been largely replaced by esophagostomy tubes and are not recommended.

  iv. Gastrostomy tubes

    1. Indications for placement of gastrostomy tubes (both percutaneous endoscopically guided [PEG] or surgically placed)

      a. Need for long-term nutritional support (greater than 4 weeks)

      b. Need to bypass the mouth, pharynx, or esophagus, for example, mandibular fractures or sites of radiation therapy

      c. Patients undergoing endoscopic evaluation

    2. Placement of gastrostomy tubes (typically 22–28 Fr tubes) allows feeding of various blenderized canned diets, which may not be amenable for feeding via other smaller tubes.

    3. Placement of these tubes requires full anesthesia and specialized equipment.

  v. Low-profile gastrostomy tubes

    1. These tubes are generally used to replace a long-standing gastrostomy tube with a more "cosmetic" tube when very long-term nutritional support is anticipated, for example, several months as in cases of patients undergoing chemotherapy.

    2. The decision to use these tubes is based mainly on practical and cosmetic reasons rather than medical reasons.

    3. In cats, replacement of a standard gastrostomy tube (in place for at least a month) with a low-profile gastrostomy tube requires general anesthesia.

  vi. Jejunostomy or jejunal tubes

    1. Placement of jejunostomy tubes is indicated when the patient necessitates abdominal surgery and there is a need to bypass a certain segment of the gastrointestinal tract.

2. A significant amount of technical expertise is required to place these tubes.
3. Major complications
   a. Tube dislodgement and leakage around stoma site, which can prove fatal due to septic peritonitis.
   b. Diarrhea
      i. Generally related to the composition or osmolarity of the diet, rather than being caused by the mode of feeding
4. Feeding via jejunostomy feeding tubes is best achieved using liquid diets designed for cats and administered as continuous infusions rather than bolus feeding.
5. A newer technique involves a "J-through-PEG" tube approach that circumvents the need for abdominal surgery or a jejunal incision.
6. These tubes are considerably more difficult to place and increase total anesthesia time dramatically.
7. J-through-PEG tubes are placed by threading a feeding tube through a PEG tube; the distal tip is placed within the jejunum with the aid of endoscopy. The jejunal tube is grasped with a biopsy wire and pushed through the pyrolus, and the procedure is repeated until approximately 20 cm of feeding tube is within the jejunum.

E. Parenteral nutrition (PN)
   a. PN should only be considered for patients with overt gastrointestinal dysfunction such as protracted vomiting, severe ileus, or diarrhea.
   b. Inappetance is not sufficient justification for PN.
   c. PN is usually a mixture of an amino acid solution with lipids and dextrose. Vitamins, trace minerals, and certain medications can be safely added to PN.
   d. General considerations for using parenteral nutrition include the following:
      i. Careful selection of patients most likely to benefit from this form of support
      ii. The ability to place appropriate catheters (double- or triple-lumen catheters)
      iii. The ability to safely compound and administer PN. Solutions are mixed aseptically, usually through intravenous filters, and administered continuously via infusion pumps.
      iv. Frequent monitoring for possible complications is imperative.
   e. Measures to reduce complications associated with PN include careful patient selection and conservative estimation of energy requirements.
   f. Partial parenteral nutrition (PPN; table 9.1)
      i. This type of PN refers to the administration of nutrients intravenously that are only capable of meeting some of the caloric and nutrient requirements of a patient.
      ii. This is designed for patients anticipated to return to enteral feeding within 3 days and for patients in which total parenteral nutrition (TPN) is not feasible, for example, when a central catheter cannot be placed.
      iii. Because PPN is a "less concentrated" form of PN, its osmolarity is considerably less (approx. 800 mOsm/L) than that of TPN (usually >1,200 mOsm/L) and could be administered peripherally, which explains why PPN is sometimes defined as "peripheral parenteral nutrition."
         1. The decrease in the osmolarity of the solution in PPN is achieved by the use of 5% dextrose as opposed to 50% dextrose. Additionally, the targeted amount of calories is between 65% and 80% of resting energy requirement with PPN.
      iv. PPN is perhaps associated with fewer complications as compared with TPN, and this may be related to the differences in total calories delivered, composition of solutions, or different patient populations.
      v. PPN can also be used to supplement cats that can only tolerate small amounts of enteral feeding.
      vi. As PPN is typically formulated with 5% dextrose, there is potential for fluid overload; the final volume of PPN should always be assessed for appropriateness for given patients.
   g. Total parenteral nutrition (TPN; table 9.2)

Table 9.1. Partial parenteral nutrition (PPN) calculations.

1. Calculate resting energy requirement (RER)
   RER = 70 × (current body weight in kg)$^{0.75}$ or
   RER = (30 × current body weight in kg) + 70
   RER = ____kcal/day
2. Calculate the partial energy requirement (PER)
   Plan to supply 70% of the animal's RER with PPN:
   PER = RER × 0.70 = ____kcal/day
3. Proportion of nutrient requirements according to body weight:
   (Note: for animals ≤ 3 kg, the formulation will exceed maintenance fluid
      requirements.)
      a. Cats 3–5 kg:
         PER × 0.20 = ____kcal/day carbohydrate required
         PER × 0.20 = ____kcal/day protein required
         PER × 0.60 = ____kcal/day lipid required
      b. Cats 6–10 kg:
         PER × 0.25 = ____kcal/day carbohydrate required
         PER × 0.25 = ____kcal/day protein required
         PER × 0.50 = ____kcal/day lipid required
4. Volumes of nutrient solutions required:
      a. 5% dextrose solution = 0.17 kcal/mL
         ____kcal carbohydrate required/day ÷ 0.17 kcal/mL = ____ mL/
         day dextrose
      b. 8.5% amino acid solution = 0.34 kcals/ml
         ____kcal protein required/day ÷ 0.34 kcal/mL = ____ mL/day
         amino acids
      c. 20% lipid solution = 2 kcal/mL
         ____kcal lipid required/day ÷ 2 kcal/mL = ___ mL/day lipid
         = ____ total mL of PPN to be administered over 24 hrs

Note: This formulation provides approximately a maintenance fluid rate.
Commonly used 8.5% amino acid solutions (i.e., Travasol) with electrolytes
contain potassium. The PPN solution made according to this worksheet will
provide approximately maintenance levels of potassium. Rates of other IV
fluids being concurrently administered should be adjusted accordingly.

i.   The indication for use of TPN in cats typically involves a case with overt and intractable gastro-
     intestinal dysfunction. These patients have severe vomiting, diarrhea, and/or malabsorptive condi-
     tions, and it is anticipated that enteral nutrition will not resume promptly.
ii. Patients with overt malnutrition, for example, greater than 15% loss of body weight, may not
     be adequately supported with PPN and may be best treated with TPN.
iii. Due to higher osmolarity and increased risk of thrombophlebitis, TPN usually requires central
     venous administration, that is, jugular catheters or femoral catheters threaded to caudal vena
     cava.
iv. In patients where placement of such catheters (e.g., double- or triple-lumen catheters) are not
     feasible, PPN may be the only option.
F. Calculation of caloric requirements
   a. The patient's resting energy requirement (RER) is the number of calories required for maintaining
      homeostasis while the animal rests quietly.

Table 9.2. Total parenteral nutrition (TPN) calculations.

1. Calculate resting energy requirement (RER)
   RER = 70 × (current body weight in kg)$^{0.75}$ or
   RER = (30 × current body weight in kg) + 70
   RER = _____kcal/day

2. Protein requirements   (g/100 kcal)
   Standard   6
   Reduced (hepatic/renal disease)   3–4
   Increased (excessive protein losses)   7–8
   (RER ÷ 100) × _____ g/100 kcal = _____ g protein required/day

3. Volume of nutrient solutions required
   a. 8.5% amino acid solution = 0.085 g protein/mL
      _____ g protein required/day ÷ 0.085 g/mL = _____ mL/day of amino acids
   b. Nonprotein calories:
      The calories supplied by protein (4 kcal/g) are subtracted from the RER to get total nonprotein calories
      needed.
      _____ g protein req/day × 4 kcal/g = _____ kcal provided by protein
      RER − kcal provided by protein = ___ total nonprotein kcal/day required
   c. Nonprotein calories are usually provided as a 50:50 mixture of lipid and dextrose.
      20% lipid solution = 2 kcal/mL
      To supply 50% of nonprotein calories
      _____ lipid kcal required ÷ 2 kcal/mL = ___ mL of lipid
      50% of dextrose solution = 1.7 kcal/mL
      To supply 50% of nonprotein calories
      ___ dextrose kcal required ÷ 1.7 kcal/mL = ___ mL of dextrose

4. Total daily requirements
   _____ mL of 8.5% amino acid solution
   _____ mL of 20% lipid
   _____ mL of 50% dextrose
   _____ total mL of TPN solution to be administered over 24 hrs

Note: Using a common 8.5% amino acid solution containing potassium (i.e., Travasol), TPN made according
to this worksheet will provide potassium at higher than maintenance levels. TPN for animals that are hyperkalemic
should be formulated using amino acid solutions without electrolytes. Rates of other IV fluids being concurrently
administered should be adjusted accordingly.

b. Estimation of energy requirements is calculated as follows:
    i.   RER = 70(body weight in kg)$^{0.75}$ or RER = 30(body weight in kg) + 70
c. Several factors impact the overall total energy expenditure, including level of activity and the effects
    of disease processes on metabolism.
d. Clinically, energy expenditure is difficult to measure; therefore, estimation of energy requirements is
    the standard for calculating nutritional support.
    i.   Formerly, there was an emphasis on adjusting energy expenditure by simply multiplying the RER
         with an arbitrary, extrapolated illness factor. More recently, this practice is purported to increase
         rates of complications without improving outcome. Therefore, recent recommendations propose
         initial caloric targets to be simply the estimated RER.

    e. One of the reasons for starting with RER is that the main purpose of nutritional support in critically ill patients is to support energy and substrate requirements, not result in immediate weight gain.

    f. Only after the patient is deemed to be recovering and tolerating feedings well should caloric targets be raised, usually by 10–20% increments if there is failure to gain weight.

G. Types of diets

    a. The choice of an appropriate enteral diet to be used for tube feeding depends on several factors:

       i. The underlying disease process and presence of comorbid conditions

       ii. The size and type of feeding tube placed

       iii. Access to veterinary specialized diets

       iv. Owner ability to obtain and administer prescribed diet

    b. Veterinary liquid diets

       i. There are only a few products commercially available that are suitable for cats.

         1. Human enteral formulas lack several key nutrients, such as arginine and taurine, which precludes recommending the use of such products.

       ii. These diets are ideal for cats that have nasoesophageal and jejunal tubes in place, although liquid diets can be used with any feeding tube.

       iii. In certain critically ill cats, a slow continuous infusion of liquid diets through nasoesophageal or esophagostomy tubes may be tolerated despite occasional vomiting. Infusion rates between 0.5 mL/kg/hr to 2 mL/kg/hr are recommended.

       iv. One of the major disadvantages of liquid diets is the high fat and protein content, which may not be appropriate for all patients (e.g., cats with steatorrhea or hepatic encephalopathy, respectively).

       v. The caloric density of most liquid diets is approximately 1 kcal/mL, which could translate to large volumes of the diet being necessary to meet energy requirements.

    c. Veterinary canned diets

       i. Placement of larger feeding tubes, for example, esophagostomy and gastrostomy tubes, allows feeding of more calorie-dense diets (some as high as 2 kcal/mL). This results in smaller volumes of food being administered at each feeding.

       ii. In addition to "critical care diets," almost any canned product can be prepared to make tube feeding amenable. This usually requires blenderizing a canned diet with a certain amount of water and sometimes straining the mixture through a sieve before being able to feed via feeding tubes.

       iii. Examples of how common veterinary diets can be modified to make them amenable for tube feeding are listed in table 9.3.

H. Role of appetite stimulants

    a. As appetite suppression is always a consequence of the underlying disease rather than the actual primary problem, the use of appetite stimulants is seldom recommended in the initial treatment of critically ill cats.

    b. The use of appetite stimulants while cats are hospitalized (e.g., diazepam) is usually ineffective and not recommended.

    c. The more appropriate use of appetite stimulants is when the patient is recovering from the underlying disease and has been discharged from the hospital.

    d. One of the main problems with the use of appetite stimulant is that while there may be a response to these drugs, adequate intake is seldom achieved.

    e. A commonly used appetite stimulant in cats recovering from illnesses is cyproheptadine administered orally at 2–4 mg q24h. This approach is not appropriate for severely ill hospitalized cats.

I. Monitoring and reassessment of the patient

    a. As with all interventions, it is important to emphasize the role of close monitoring of patients receiving nutritional support.

    b. Feeding tubes and PN catheters must be monitored for mechanical problems as well as infections at entry site. Catheter and feeding tube sites should be evaluated daily for signs of inflammation/infection.

Table 9.3. Enteral nutrition calculations for tube feeding.

1. Calculate resting energy requirement (RER)
   RER = 70 × (current body weight in kg)$^{0.75}$ or
   RER = (30 × current body weight in kg) + 70
   RER = _____kcal/day
2. Product selected: _____
   Caloric density of diet: _____ kcal/mL
3. Total volume to be administered per day
   Kcal required/day = ____mL/day
   Kcal/mL in diet
4. Administration schedule
   ½ of total requirement on Day 1 = ____mL/day (Day 1)
   Total requirement on Day 2 and beyond = ____mL/day (Day 2)
5. Feedings per day
   Divide total daily volume into 4–6 feedings (depending on patient tolerance for feedings)
   = ____feedings/day
6. Volume per feeding
   Divide total mL/day by the number of feedings per day
   = ____mL/feeding (Day 1)
   = ____mL/feeding (Day 2)
7. Diet options
   A. Nasoesophageal and jejunostomy tubes
      i.   Liquid diets only
      ii. CliniCare Canine and Feline Formula (1.0 kcal/mL)
      iii. Human liquid diets unbalanced for cats
   B. Esophagostomy and gastrostomy tubes
      i.   Eukanuba Maximum Calorie canned
           Supplies 2.1 kcal/mL straight from can but needs further dilution
           1 can + 50 mL water = 1.6 kcal/mL
           1 can + 25 mL water = 1.8 kcal/mL (for larger tubes)
      ii. Hill's a/d canned
           Supplies 1.3 kcal/mL straight from can but needs further dilution
           1 can + 50 mL water = 1.0 kcal/mL
           1 can + 25 mL water = 1.1 kcal/mL
      iii. Royal Canin Canine /Feline Recovery RS canned
           Supplies 1 kcal/mL straight from can but needs further dilution
           1 can + 25 mL water = 0.9 kcal/mL

   c. Recommended monitoring for patients receiving PN include frequent evaluation of heart rate, respiratory rate, temperature, blood glucose, blood urea nitrogen, and triglycerides. In particularly debilitated cats, monitoring of magnesium, potassium, and phosphorus is also recommended.
      i. Periodic nutritional reassessment can guide whether there should be an adjustment of nutritional support; for example, increase calories delivered by 20% if there is persistent weight loss in the face of nutritional support or decrease or stop delivery of nutrition if complications arise.

Recommended Reading

Chan DL. Nutritional requirements of the critically ill patient. Clin Tech Small Anim Pract, 2004; 19(1):1–5.

Crabb SE, Freeman LM, Chan DL, Labato MA. Retrospective evaluation of total parenteral nutrition in cats: 40 cases (1991–2003). J Vet Emerg Crit Care, 2006; 16(S1):S21–S26.

Freeman LM, Chan DL. Total parenteral nutrition. In DiBartola SP, ed, Fluid, Electrolyte, and Acid-base Disorders in Small Animal Practice, 3rd ed, pp 584–601. St. Louis: Saunders Elsevier, 2006.

Mazzaferro EM. Esophagostomy tubes: don't underutilize them! J Vet Emerg Crit Care, 2001; 11(2):153–156.

Mitchel K. Preventing and managing complications of enteral nutritional support. Clin Tech Small Anim Pract, 2004; 19(1):49–53.

Pyle SC, Marks SL, Kass PH. Evaluation of complications and prognostic factors associated with administration of total parenteral nutrition in cats: 75 cases (1994–2001). J Am Vet Med Assoc, 2004; 255(2):242–250.

10
RESPIRATORY EMERGENCIES AND PLEURAL SPACE DISEASE

Amy V. Trow, Elizabeth Rozanski, and Armelle de Laforcade

Unique Features
- Identification of the specific underlying cause will result in more effective therapy.
- Increased respiratory rate and effort due to pleural effusion should improve rapidly following thoracocentesis.
- The average cat thorax will contain 200–300 mL of effusion or air before respiratory distress will develop.
- Heart failure is less common than often believed.

I. Respiratory emergencies
   A. Triage
      a. Telephone triage
         i. If the owner reports any concern for ability to breathe, increased respiratory rate or effort, the patient should be brought in immediately for assessment.
         ii. Ensure that there is no closer appropriate facility.
      b. Waiting room triage
         i. Complaint of potential respiratory problems warrants immediate attention and movement of the patient to the treatment area.
         ii. Obtain brief history, specifically asking about signalment, rapidity of onset, cough, history of heart disease, asthma, trauma, or any other respiratory problems.
   B. Initial assessment (fig. 10.1)
      a. Complete physical examination is often not possible (or recommended) initially in cats with severe respiratory distress.
      b. Clinical signs of respiratory distress include rapid, shallow, or noisy breathing. Open-mouth breathing is occasionally present. Some cats demonstrate orthopnea, preferring to sit only in a sternal/hunched position. Cats will often have widely dilated pupils and may have excessive salivation. Cats with primary cardiac or pulmonary disease may have only been appreciated to be lethargic at home; however, following a car trip, they may demonstrate overt distress. Note that cats can have significant respiratory compromise primarily manifested only as increased respiratory rate until stressed, at which time full clinical signs of respiratory distress become evident.
      c. Assess whether the cat seems to be in immediate, life-threatening respiratory failure. Note cyanosis, gasping, pulmonary edema visible at nares, or rarely severe hypoventilation, recognized by intermittent apnea.

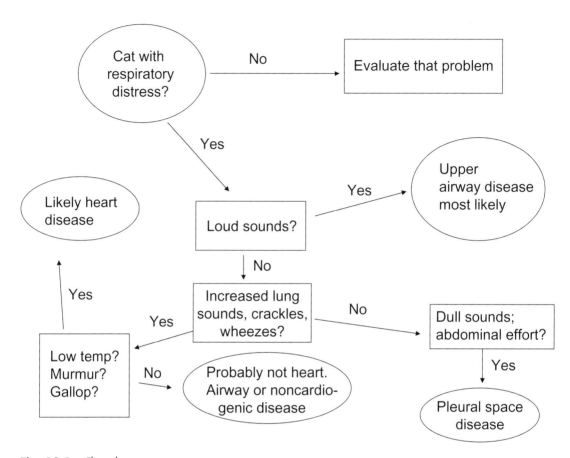

Fig. 10.1. Flow chart.

   d. If life-threatening state is assessed, cautiously sedate (if necessary) and intubate. Use of an opiod and a benzodiazepine is recommended, such as butorphanol 0.2 mg/kg and diazepam 0.4 mg/kg IV (medial saphenous vein often easiest). Propofol alone is a poor choice, due to its cardiovascular depressant properties. Maintain on 100% O_2 with manual positive pressure ventilation. Be prepared to suction any pulmonary edema.

   e. Allow the cat time (~10 minutes) to recover from the stress of transport in a low-stress environment with oxygen supplementation. Typically, an oxygen cage is used for this purpose, although the cat should be closely observed. Other options include an oxygen hood or flow-by administration of oxygen with a mask or oxygen line if the patient will tolerate it with minimal stress and movement. Prepare to intervene quickly (e.g., intubate or consider thoracocentesis if pleural space disease is suspected) if respiratory distress worsens.

   f. Observe the breathing pattern and effort.

   g. Proceed with physical exam. Assess for the following specifically:

      i. Increased respiratory rate and effort or, conversely, intermittent (or agonal) gasps. If agonal or intermittent apnea is present, begin CPR.

     ii. Evidence of abdominal or paradoxical breathing.

    iii. Upper airway noise/stertor/stridor; recall auscultation over trachea may help localize noisy breathing to upper airway.

    iv. Increased or decreased lung sounds

     v.   Crackles (fluid in alveoli, *not* specific for heart failure)

    vi.   Expiratory wheezes

   vii.   Compressibility of cranial thorax

       1.   Decreased compressibility may indicate a cranial mediastinal mass.

       2.   Older cats can normally often have a decreased compressibility and can confuse this diagnostic clue.

  viii.   Subcutaneous emphysema

    ix.   Heart murmurs

     x.   Gallop rhythms (may be best heard with the bell)

    xi.   Nasal discharge

   xii.   Cough (inducible with tracheal compression?)

  xiii.   Rectal temperature (typically low with heart failure)

  xiv.   Assess degree of hypoxemia with pulse oximetry; this is often unrewarding in cats with poor perfusion; prolonged efforts are not required.

  h. Attempt to localize the disease to the upper airway, lower airway, pulmonary parenchyma, or pleural space.

     i.   Loud, noisy breathing—upper airway

    ii.   Prolonged expiration with crackles and wheezes—lower airway

       1.   Cats with lower airway disease may also have an abdominal push at the end of expiration. Rarely, cats with severe lower airway disease (feline "asthma") may have decreased lung sounds due to air trapping and inability to expire air.

   iii.   Tachypnea with crackles or increased lung sounds—pulmonary parenchyma; most often cardiac. Pneumonia is very rare in cats.

   iv.   Rapid shallow breathing with abdominal component and decreased lung sounds—pleural space.

C. Loud breathing: suspect upper airway disease

  a. Dynamic extrathoracic obstructions (e.g., laryngeal paralysis, collapsing trachea—both rare in cats) may have noise only on inspiration, while fixed obstructions may have noise on inspiration and expiration.

     i.   Laryngeal tumors are the most common cause of fixed airway obstruction (fig. 10.2).

  b. Have a surgery pack and supplies available for emergency tracheostomy as well as a variety of sizes (2.0–5.0 mm ID) of endotracheal tubes (box 10.1).

  c. Sedation is helpful to place an IV catheter, although a complete oral exam may require brief anesthesia. Useful drugs include butorphanol (0.1–0.2 mg/kg IV) or hydromorphone/oxymorphone (0.05 mg/kg IV and diazepam 0.2 mg/kg IV). Propofol (2–8 mg/kg IV) is useful but may result in hypotension and apnea. Avoid ketamine, as altered laryngeal function is possible, which could lead to errors in interpretation.

  d. Use laryngoscope to visualize glottis. Assess first for a mass lesion; if no lesion is present, assess laryngeal function. Doxapram (0.5 mg/kg IV) is useful as a diagnostic adjuvant to temporarily stimulate respiratory efforts if laryngeal paralysis remains a concern.

  e. If a mass is present, intubation may be challenging. Smaller tubes, and careful observation of the air flow (may be visualized as bubbles through the distorted lumen) may permit capture of the airway. Excessive attempts to force an endotracheal tube into place will result in swelling and possible hemorrhage when a mass is present. However, successful intubation is ideal for patient care and complete evaluation.

  f. Consider a tracheostomy (if orotracheal intubation is not possible and the tracheostomy will bypass the obstruction) followed by a biopsy or debulking procedure. A biopsy without tracheostomy risks airway obstruction due to postprocedural swelling and bleeding. Informed client consent about the potential need as well as risks and benefits (see box 10.1) of a tracheostomy are warranted prior to proceeding with an oral examination.

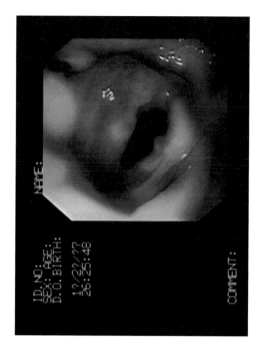

Fig. 10.2. Note the mass on this cat's right (upper) arytenoid.

Box 10.1. Tracheostomy.

i.   Make 2–3-cm incision on ventral aspect of neck, just caudal to thyroid cartilage.
ii. Separate the sternohyoideus muscles bluntly with hemostats and isolate the trachea. Stay on midline.
iii. Place stay sutures around adjacent cartilaginous tracheal rings if time allows, that is, if patient is not in severe distress due to tracheal obstruction. If patient requires immediate intubation via tracheostomy, place stay sutures after performing the tracheostomy.
iv. Once the trachea is visualized, incise the trachea between the third and fourth or fourth and fifth rings for about one-half circumference of the trachea. A longitudal (between rings) or a t-shaped incision are both acceptable.
v.   Place 3–4-mm endotracheal or tracheostomy tube into the tracheal incision and begin positive pressure ventilation. Do not inflate cuff unless cat is maintained on ventilator.
vi. Place stay sutures around adjacent cartilaginous tracheal rings. It is ideal to place sutures prior to incision, but in emergent situations, time may not allow that.

---

g. Tracheostomies may be lifesaving procedures but are associated with some risks, especially in cats. Specifically, due to the small size of the trachea and the general reactivity of the feline airway, the tube is at increased risk to get clogged with mucus or dislodged (see box 10.1). Cats with tracheostomy tubes in place should be carefully observed, and *all* personnel should be familiar with replacement of the tube. Additional recommendations include placement of a "trach kit" by the cage of the cat, which includes a new tube, Q-tips, scissors, syringe/needle, and propofol, so that valuable time is not lost gathering supplies in the event of a crisis.

D. Rapid, smooth, shallow breathing with crackles or harsh lung sounds suggests pulmonary parenchymal disease such as cardiogenic pulmonary edema (congestive heart failure), noncardiogenic pulmonary edema (secondary to choking/upper airway obstruction, electrocution, seizures or head trauma), endomyocarditis/inflammatory lung lesions, pulmonary hemorrhage (coagulopathy, neoplasia), contusions, infiltrative disease (bacterial pneumonia, fungal, toxoplasmosis, lymphoma), smoke, or other toxin inhalation.

   a. The most common parenchymal diseases in cats that present with respiratory distress are cardiogenic pulmonary edema or endomyocarditis/nonspecific inflammatory lung lesions.

   b. If cardiogenic pulmonary edema is suspected based on the rest of PE (e.g., heart murmur, gallop rhythm, low rectal temperature) and history, administer Furosemide (1–4 mg/kg IV or IM; avoid SQ as systemic absorption may be compromised with poor cardiac output). If pulmonary edema suspected, let cat rest in oxygen.

   c. Nitroglycerine paste may be used with very strong suspicion of heart failure based on auscultation of heart murmur, history of heart disease, pleural effusion, and/or cardiogenic pulmonary edema. Place ¼ inch topically; may be used for venodilation.

   d. If respiratory failure appears imminent, intubate patient for mechanical ventilation.
      i. Induction: Hydromorphone 0.05 mg/kg IV and Diazepam 0.2 mg/kg IV
      ii. Intubation: 3 or 4 endotracheal tube
      iii. Ventilation: ventilator, anesthesia machine, or ambu bag with 100% oxygen
         1. Start breathing for the patient at 10–20 breaths per minute. Inspiratory time should be about 1 second with an ideal inspiratory to expiratory ratio of 1:2.
         2. Minute ventilation (or oxygen flow) requirements are 150–250 mL/kg/min.
         3. Maintain airway pressure at <20 cm H_2O. Patients with severe parenchymal disease may require higher peak airway pressures, but higher peak airway pressures can be associated with development of a pnuemothorax, so use lowest pressure possible to maintain oxygen saturation >90%.
         4. PEEP (positive end expiratory pressure) valves may be helpful in keeping small airways and alveoli open and increasing oxygen saturation.
         5. A deep breath to 30 cmH_2O every half hour can help decrease small airway collapse also.
         6. Monitor pulse oximetry, end-tidal CO_2, and arterial blood gas if possible. Arterial blood gas sampling is very challenging in cats and often limited to anesthetized patients, and it is not indicated in awake feline patients with respiratory distress.
         7. Do tracheal wash while intubated to help with diagnosis if indicated.

   e. Once patient is stabilized, proceed with thoracic radiographs.
      i. With patchy or perihilar alveolar pattern +/- enlarged cardiac silhouette, continue treatment with oxygen and furosemide as needed and perform echocardiogram to determine cause of heart failure.
         1. Normal heart size in cats (use standard radiograph and vertebral heart size measurements; fig. 10.3): patient may still have heart disease due to concentric nature of hypertrophic cardiomyopathy.
      ii. With dorsocaudal alveolar pattern and low suspicion of cardiac disease, research possibility of noncardiogenic edema (determine if cat had experienced upper airway obstruction, head trauma, electrocution, or seizures). Continue supportive care with oxygen.
      iii. With diffuse alveolar pattern and no evidence for heart disease, test coagulation function, including prothrombin time, partial thromboplastin time, and blood smear for platelets. If coagulation function is normal and patient is assessed as stable, an endotracheal wash is recommended for further diagnostics.
         1. If endotracheal wash is not possible due to experience of clinicians or stability of cat, then empirical therapy with broad spectrum antibiotics and furosemide may be necessary until stabilization can be achieved. Intravenous formulations are recommended to minimize stress and ensure delivery. See table 10.1 for antibiotic recommendations.

E. Rapid shallow breathing with abdominal component and dull sounds; suspect pleural space disease.
   a. Differentials include congestive heart failure, trauma, chylothorax, pyothorax, diaphragmatic hernia, or malignant pleural effusion. In contrast to dogs, coagulopathy is rare. Heart failure is

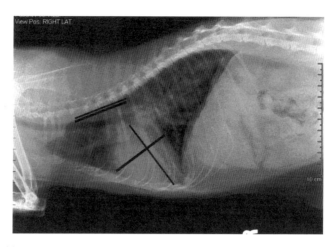

Fig. 10.3. Vertebral heart score (VHS) in cats. Measure both the long and short axis of the heart on a lateral thoracic radiograph. Then, starting at L4, measure caudally. Add these two numbers to give the VHS. The reference range is 7.5 ± 0.3 vertebrae (from Litster and Buchanan, JAVMA 2000; 216; 210–214).

Table 10.1. Recommendation for antibiotic therapy in possible respiratory disease.

Potentiated amoxicillin (Clavamox®)	10–15 mg/kg orally twice a day
Cephalexin	20 mg/kg orally twice a day
Doxycyline	5–10 mg/kg/day orally per day; follow tablets with syringe of water to try to prevent esophageal stricture
Enrofloxacin (Baytril®)	2.5–5 mg/kg/day orally or slow IV (off-label)
Ticarcillin/clavulanic acid	50 mg/kg IV three times a day

Note: Recall, cats are uncommonly affected with pneumonia; patchy infiltrates typically reflect another disease process. The specific antibiotic used should reflect clinician comfort, availability, cost, and degree of clinical illness. Other combinations are also effective. Oral therapy is contraindicated in cats with respiratory distress. Use parenteral therapy until respiratory distress is relieved.

   the most common cause of pleural effusion in cats presenting with respiratory distress followed by lymphosarcoma and chylothorax.
 b. If heart murmur/gallop and/or hypothermia present, administer furosemide 1–4 mg/kg IM or IV, not SC. Diuretics are much less effective against pleural effusion than pulmonary edema.
 c. If able, place IV catheter for venous access.
 d. Perform thoracocentesis (box 10.2) for diagnostic and therapeutic purposes. Thoracocentesis is a routine procedure with substantial benefits. However, complications are possible, specifically, iatrogenic pneumothorax and reexpansion pulmonary edema. Iatrogenic pneumothorax is most common in cats with chronic effusion; over time, the pleura become thickened and may be inadvertently torn by the thoracocentesis needle. In acute situations, the lung/pleural are rapidly self-sealing; however, in chronic situations the pleural thickening prevents adequate seal formation. In severe cases, thoracostomy tubes or even thoracic surgery may be required to prevent ongoing air leakage.
   i. Reexpansion pulmonary edema (NCPE) can be a complication of relief of chronic lung collapse due to effusion (table 10.2) or diaphragmatic hernia.

Box 10.2.   Thoracocentesis.
1. Clip area over sixth to eighth intercostal space. Perform a sterile prep over clipped area.
2. Attach butterfly needle (21 or 23 Ga) to extension set, followed by three-way stopcock and 12–30-mL syringe. Have collection container ready. In obese cats, a 1.5-inch needle or longer may be required.
3. Insert the needle through the chest wall. A distinctive "pop" may be appreciated by the more experienced operator.
4. Remove all fluid or air.
5. Determine the total protein of fluid and submit fluid for cytological analysis.
Note: A thoracostomy tube may be warranted in recurrent effusion or if a recurrent pneumothorax is present.

Table 10.2. Types of pleural effusion and associated diseases. (Most feline effusions are modified transudates.)

Type of Effusion	Protein Level	Cell Count	Other	Associated Diseases
Transudate	<2.5 g/dL	<1,000/μL	SG < 1.016	Heart failure, hypoalbuminemia (<1.5 gm/dL)
Modified transudate	>2.5 g/dL	1,000–8,000/μL		Heart failure, neoplasia
Chylous	>2.5 g/dL	1,000–22,000/μL	Triglyceride >100 mg/dL >2–3x that of serum	Heart failure, neoplasia, idiopathic, other
Exudate (septic or nonseptic)	>3.0 g/dL	>5,000/μL		Bacterial, FIP, fungal, protozoal, parasitic, neoplasia, immune-mediated
Hemorrhagic				Trauma, neoplasia, coagulopathy

ii. A thoracostomy tube may be warranted in recurrent effusion or if a recurrent pneumothorax is present (box 10.3). NCPE is potentially more likely with application of negative pressure to the pleural space via thoracostomy tube or when overenthusiastic ventilation is used. Lungs will gradually reinflate on their own; peak inspiratory pressure should be limited to 20 cmH$_2$0. Reexpansion pulmonary edema is characterized by decline in oxygen saturation, increased respiratory rate and effort, and/or crackles and harsh lung sounds.

F. Prolonged expiration, wheezes, cough
  a. Suggests lower airway disease, colloquially referred to as feline asthma.
  b. Administer dexamethasone 0.25–0.50 mg/kg IV or IM.
  c. Consider bronchodilator therapy with inhaled albuterol or subcutaneous terbutaline (0.01 mg/kg) or aminophylline. Administer sustained released theophylline (Inwood Laboratory), 20 mg/kg orally in the evening.
    i. If concurrent cardiac disease is suspected or can't be excluded, you may wish to avoid terbutaline due to beta effects, which could cause detrimental increase in heart rate.
  d. Most (all) lower airway disease cats should show prompt improvement following beta-2 (albuterol) and steroid therapy. Failure to improve within 8–12 hours should promote reconsideration of the diagnosis.

Box 10.3. Thoracostomy (chest) tube placement.
1. Establish vascular access first; gather supplies.
2. Preoxygenate for 5 minutes prior to anesthesia if possible; induce general anesthesia. Most clinicians prefer to place chest tubes in anesthetized cats unless their condition is moribund. Use cardioprotective anesthetic protocols and try to limit anesthesia time.
3. Intubate, ventilate, and maintain on 100% oxygen.
4. Monitor with continuous EKG, pulse oximetry, and assessment of anesthetic depth.
5. The cat may be placed in sternal or lateral recumbency at the operator's preference.
6. Sterily prepare the site, from 3rd to 13th rib, dorsal to ventral midline, and drape.
7. Have assistant pull skin from level of 4th rib cranially.
8. Make 1-cm incision cranial to rib at 7th, 8th, or 9th rib space.
9. Bluntly dissect with hemostats into pleural cavity or carefully use sharp dissection. Trochar use in cats can be challenging since their chests are so compressible—the chest often just collapses with pressure on trochar instead of puncturing chest cavity. Therefore, it is often easiest to perform a mini approach. Some clinicians prefer red rubber catheters for chest tubes in cats.
10. Once pleural space is punctured, start positive pressure ventilation (if not already performing).
11. Advance chest tube over trochar cranially.
12. Have assistant release skin to form subcutaneous tunnel to decrease risk of pneumothorax and infection.
13. Place purse-string suture around chest tube entrance into skin to secure tube location. Some clinicians also like to place suture through skin and around tube at midway point of subcutaneous tunnel for added security.
14. A bandage is often despised by the cat; a Tegaderm (3M, St. Paul, MN) is often adequate.
15. Attach adaptors and chest tube extension set with three-way stopcock and injection caps.
16. Evacuate and clamp tube for additional security in case adaptor, extension, or stopcock comes off.
17. Assure familiarity with chest tube care among all hospital personnel.

G. Hypoventilation
   a. Suggests brain, cervical spinal cord (diaphragmatic nerve damage), or lower motor neuron disease.
   b. Evaluate arterial PCO_2 or end-tidal CO_2; consider mechanical ventilation. Pulse oximetry is insensitive for determining hypoventilation, particularly in the face of supplemental oxygen. Additionally, end-tidal CO_2 analysis may provide a false sense of security, and normal values should *not* be taken to indicate that hypoventilation is not present.
   c. If severe altered mentation is present, in addition to careful monitoring and ventilatory support, consider the possible presence of cerebral edema and administer dexamethasone 0.25 mg/kg IV and mannitol 0.5–1.0 gram IV over 20 minutes (see chapter 25—General Approach and Overview of the Neurologic Cat and chapter 26—Neurologic Emergencies: Brain).

H. Further diagnostics for all conditions
   a. Chest radiographs are warranted. It is often still possible to interpret suboptimally positioned films. Set up the radiology suite prior to moving the cat from the oxygen cage. Set mas, kV, and plate and put pedal in easily accessible position if needed. Put on protective lead clothing before getting the patient to minimize patient time out of oxygen. Only one view at a time may be possible due to respiratory distress. Avoid laying cat on its back for ventral-dorsal view.
   b. Endotracheal wash
   c. Echocardiogram and ECG
   d. Thoracic ultrasound or CT scan for more detailed assessment of pulmonary parenchyma and pleural space.

I. Client education

      a. Respiratory distress is serious.

      b. Specific therapy is more likely to be effective than supportive care.

II. Pleural space disease

  A. Definition

      a. The area surrounding the lung lobes lined by parietal or visceral pleura depending on the surface against which the pleura rests

         i. Parietal pleura lines the body wall.

        ii. Visceral pleura lines the lungs and organs.

      b. Normally contains no more than 3–5 mL of a low-protein fluid

         i. Mostly lubricant function

  B. Clinical signs of pleural space disease

      a. Mild to severe depending on the volume of pleural effusion or severity of disease

      b. Mild tachypnea to overt respiratory distress

      c. Respiratory pattern

         i. Exaggerated inspiratory effort, abdominal component is often noted

        ii. The pattern of breathing can resemble signs of upper airway obstruction.

      d. Decreased lung sounds on thoracic auscultation

         i. Most pronounced ventrally with pleural effusion

        ii. Muffled heart sounds

  C. Types of pleural space disease

      a. Pleural effusion

         i. Abnormal accumulations of fluid in the pleural space

        ii. Classifications (see table 10.2)

           1. Transudate

              a. Protein <2.5 g/dL, nucleated cell count <1,000/μL

           2. Modified transudate

               a. Protein <2.5–3.5 g/dL, cell count <1,000–5000/μL

           3. Exudate (septic or nonseptic)

               a. Protein >3.5 g/dL, cell count >5,000/μL

           4. Chylous

               a. Protein >2.5, cell count >500/μL

               b. Gross appearance of milky white fluid (variable)

               c. Contains chylomicrons and lymph

               d. Does not clear upon centrifugation

               e. Pleural fluid triglyceride and cholesterol concentrations

                  i. Triglyceride concentration >100 mg/dL

                 ii. Triglyceride:cholesterol ratio <1

           5. Pseudochylous

               a. Grossly similar to chylous effusion

               b. Associated with chronic inflammatory conditions of the thoracic cavity

               c. Clears upon centrifugation

               d. Contains no chylomicrons

               e. Fluid is typically high in cholesterol but low in triglyceride

           6. Hemorrhagic

         iii. Diagnosis of pleural effusion

           1. Thoracic radiography images

               a. Small volume

                  i. Pleural fissure lines

               b. Large volume can be seen when fluid (pleural effusion) collects in fissures, which are the normal divides between lung lobes. Fissures are not normally visualized on radiographs but become apparent when filled with fluid.

          i.   Obscured cardiac silhouette

          ii. Rounded borders of lung lobes

          iii. Retraction of lung lobes from body wall

    2. Thoracic ultrasound images

       a. Fluid density (hypoechoic) surrounding lung lobes (see fig. 10.6)

       b. Lung lobes may appear to be floating

       c. Can help guide thoracocentesis

    3. Thoracocentesis (see fig. 10.4)

       a. 22-g needle with extension tubing and three-way stopcock

       b. Butterfly catheter often selected in cats

       c. 6th–10th intercostal space, aseptically prepared

       d. Often immediate improvement in clinical signs

       e. Complications

          i.   Pneumothorax with repeated thoracocentesis or chronic pleural disease

          ii. Pleural hemorrhage

  iv. Causes of pleural effusion

    1. Congestive heart failure (CHF)

       a. Common in older cats but can occur at any age

       b. Physical examination findings

          i.   Shortness of breath

          ii. Cardiac murmur or gallop

          iii. Distended jugular pulses

          iv. Hypothermia is common

       c. Diagnosis

          i.   Thoracocentesis

            1. Modified transudate or chylous effusion most commonly noted

          ii. Thoracic radiography

            1. Pulmonary edema or pleural effusion

            2. Enlarged cardiac silhouette

            3. Distended pulmonary vessels

            4. Better visualization of thoracic structures when performed after thoracocentesis

          iii. Echocardiogram

            1. Evidence of cardiomyopathy

              a. Hypertrophic cardiomyopathy (HCM) most common

              b. Intermediate, restrictive, or dilated cardiomyopathy also seen

            2. Left atrium distension supports a diagnosis of CHF

              a. May be less dramatic following multiple doses of furosemide

       d. Emergent therapy

          i.   Oxygen supplementation

          ii. Low-stress environment

          iii. Thoracocentesis (see fig. 10.4)

            1. Removal of as little as 50 mL can vastly improve respiratory distress.

            2. Large volume effusion often present (up to 350 mL)

            3. Both left and right side for best drainage

            4. Radiographs ideally taken following thoracocentesis

              a. Better visualization of cardiac structures

              b. Help rule out other causes of pleural effusion

                i. Cranial mediastinal mass

          iv. Furosemide

            1. Loop diuretic

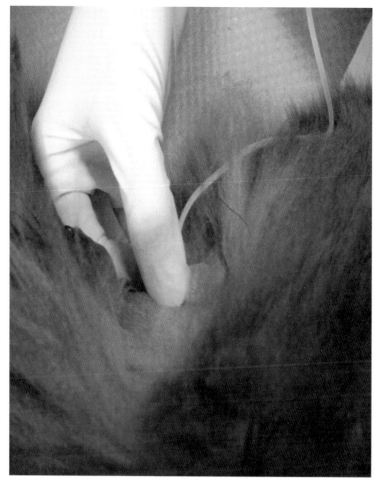

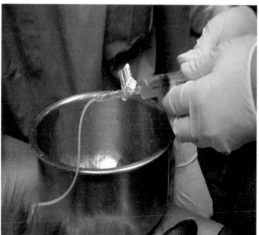

Fig. 10.4. Thoracocentesis performed in a cat with pleural effusion. Supplies include a 10–20-mL syringe, a three-way stopcock, and 19–21-ga butterfly needle. Aseptic technique is recommended.

        2. 2–4 mg/kg IM or IV
        3. Repeat
        4. Always provide bowl of water
        5. Avoid subcutaneous injection
           a. Questionable absorption due to lack of peripheral perfusion
     v. Nitroglycerine paste
        1. Venous vasodilator
        2. ¼-inch strip applied to ear pinna or groin (Clipping hair away at area of application may facilitate absorption.)
        3. Gloves must be worn for application.
        4. Efficacy questionable due to lack of peripheral perfusion
     vi. Nitroprusside
        1. Potent arterial and venous vasodilator
        2. Intravenous, continuous infusion
           a. Dose 0.5–2 µg/kg/min
        3. Rarely needed in the absence of severe pulmonary edema
           a. Most commonly used for several hours—up to 24 hours in cats
        4. Complications
           a. Extreme hypotension, may be fatal
              i. Blood pressure monitoring required
           b. Cyanide toxicity with extended use (>3 days)
     vii. Sedation, intubation
        1. Consider when clinical signs cannot be controlled with thoracocentesis, furosemide, and oxygen supplementation
        2. Control of airway
        3. Administration of 100% oxygen
        4. Sedative selection
           a. Minimal cardiovascular depression
           b. Diazepam (0.2–0.5 mg/kg)
           c. Hydromorphone (.05–0.2 mg/kg IV)
           d. Reversible
              i. Naloxone
2. Septic pleuritis (pyothorax, thoracic empyema)
  a. Definition
    i. Pleural accumulation of purulent exudates associated with bacterial infection
  b. Etiology
    i. Young cats
    ii. Access to outdoors, multicat household
    iii. Seasonal variation
      1. Most common in summer and fall months
  c. Causes of septic pleuritis
    i. Direct inoculation
      1. Penetrating bite wound 0.05 over thorax
        a. Often not documented
      2. Complications of thoracic trauma, surgery
    ii. Ruptured lung lobe abscess
    iii. Bronchopneumonia
    iv. Esophageal rupture
    v. Migrating foreign body
    vi. Parasitic migration

   d. Clinical signs
      i. Most common
         1. Tachypnea or dyspnea
         2. Reduced appetite
         3. Lethargy
      ii. Other clinical signs
         1. Hypersalivation
         2. Cough (rare)
         3. Ocular or nasal discharge
   e. Physical examination
      i. Tachypnea or dyspnea
      ii. Fever or hypothermia
      iii. Dehydration
      iv. Muffled heart sounds
      v. Poor body condition
      vi. Pale mucous membranes
      vii. Cardiovascular collapse possible
         1. Collapse
         2. Mentation changes
         3. Hypotension
         4. Tachycardia or bradycardia
   f. Diagnosis
      i. Clinical signs of systemic inflammation (SIRS)
         1. Not present in all cases
         2. Three of four criteria present
            a. Fever (>103.5°F) or hypothermia (<100°F)
            b. Tachycardia (>225 bpm) or bradycardia (<140 bpm)
            c. Tachypnea (>40 breaths/min)
            d. White blood cell count >19,500/μL, or <5,000/μL, or >5% bands.
      ii. Radiographic evidence of pleural effusion (fig. 10.5)
         1. Unilateral or bilateral effusion
            a. Most commonly bilateral
      iii. Thoracic ultrasound (fig. 10.6)
         1. Echogenic effusion
         2. Possible atelectasis or lung lobe abscess
      iv. Thoracocentesis
         1. Thick, malodorous fluid
            a. Red brown or cream colored
      v. Fluid cytology
         1. Septic suppurative inflammation (figs. 10.7 a, b)
            a. Primarily neutrophilic exudate
            b. Intracellular bacteria
         2. Suppurative inflammation
            a. Neutrophils only
            b. Filamentous organisms on cytology
               i. Nocardia, Actinomyces
      vi. Bacterial culture
         1. Infections often polymicrobial
            a. Anaerobes and facultative anaerobes
         2. Aerobic and anaerobic cultures recommended

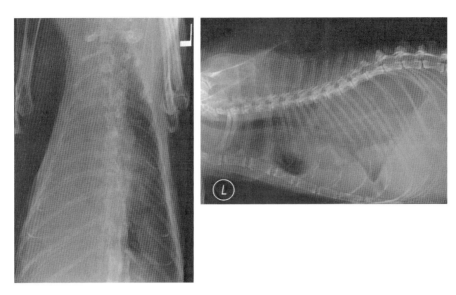

Fig. 10.5. Dorsoventral radiograph of a cat with unilateral pleural effusion. The cardiac silhouette is shifted to the left due to the effusion in the right hemothorax. There is flattening of the diaphragm consistent with increased volume within the thorax. The caudal aspect of the lung lobe margins are rounded, consistent with restrictive pleuritis.

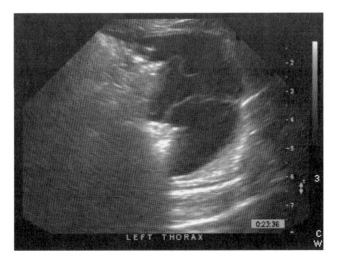

Fig. 10.6. Thoracic ultrasound image of a cat with severe pleural effusion. Note the echogenic nature of the effusion and the associated fibrin tags.

3. Most common infectious agents
  a. Aerobes
    i. *Pasteurella* spp.
    ii. *Actinomyces* spp.
  b. Anaerobes

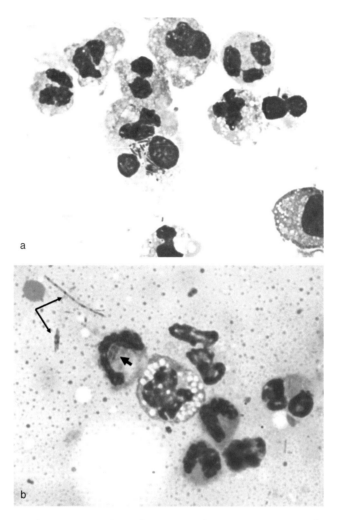

Fig. 10.7. a. Effusion cytology in a cat with pyothorax. Note the septic suppurative inflammation (predominance of neutrophils with intracellular bacteria). Here both intra- and extracellular bacteria along with degenerative neutrophils can be identified (photo courtesy of Dr. Joyce Knoll). b. Effusion cytology of a cat with pyothorax. Here intra- (thick arrow) and extracellular (thin arrows) filamentous rods are identified. These findings are consistent with either Actinomyces or Nocardia (photo courtesy of Dr. Joyce Knoll).

         i. *Bacteroides* spp.
        ii. *Peptostreptococcus anaerobius*
      iii. *Fusobacterium* spp.
      iv. *Clostridium* spp.
       v. *Porphyromonas* spp.
     vi. *Prevotella* spp.
  g. Treatment
    i. Oxygen supplementation
   ii. Antimicrobial therapy
      1. Broad spectrum, combination therapy
      2. Empiric pending results of culture and sensitivity

   3. Obligate anaerobes
      a. Ampicillin (2.2 mg/kg IV TID)
      b. Amoxicillin-clavulanic acid (13.75 mg/kg PO BID)
      c. Clindamycin (11 mg/kg IV BID, 5–10 mg/kg PO)
      d. Metronidazole (5–10 mg/kg) IV BID-TID
   4. Facultative anaerobes
      a. Amikacin (15 mg/kg IV SID) (Assure that renal function and perfusion are adequate.)
      b. Gentamicin (6 mg/kg IV SID) (Assure that renal function and perfusion are adequate.)
   5. Tailor antimicrobial to culture and sensitivity results
   6. Duration of therapy 4–6 weeks
iii. Fluid resuscitation
   1. Replacement fluid
      a. Lactated Ringer's or 0.9% NaCl
      b. Rate: 40–60 mL/kg/hr
      c. Reduce rate when endpoints are met
      d. Consider more gradual resuscitation in cats with known underlying cardiac diseaser (see chap. 8—Fluid therapy).
   2. Goals
      a. Improved mentation
         i. Alert or arousable, sternal recumbancy
      b. Normalization of blood pressure
         i. Systolic >100 mmHg using Doppler
      c. Normalization of heart rate
         i. HR 160–180 bpm
      d. Resolution of hyperlactatemia
         i. Lactate <2.5 mmol/L
iv. Drainage of pleural space
   1. Thoracostomy tubes preferred
      a. More complete drainage
      b. General anesthesia
         i. Control of airway (intubation)
      c. Bilateral tube placement for bilateral effusion
         i. 7th–8th intercostal space
      d. Median duration 5 days
   2. Intermittent drainage
      a. Thoracocentesis
   3. Pleural lavage (initially 2–3 times per day, and decrease frequency as fluid becomes more clear on initial aspiration or after initial flush drainage)
      a. 15–20 mL/kg warm saline
         i. Instill and drain
      b. Indications
         i. Effusion that is thick or containing solid particles
         ii. Persistent obstruction of thoracostomy tube
      c. Major complication: infection
v. Thoracotomy
   1. Rarely needed
   2. Persistent pleural fluid accumulation or cannot effectively drain with chest tubes due to loculation and compartmentalization of fluid

          3. Mass effect suggestive of abscess
          4. Advantage
            a. Complete exploration of thorax
            b. Complete drainage
          5. Disadvantage
            a. Increased length of hospitalization
            b. Increased cost of treatment
            c. Likely increased pain and morbidity
      vi. Prognosis
          1. 60–70% survival in treated cats
          2. Cost of care can be significant
   3. Chylothorax
     a. Definition
        i. Intrapleural accumulation of chylous fluid
          1. Lymph and chylomicrons
     b. Predispositions
        i. Older cats > younger cats
       ii. Purebreed cats overrepresented in some studies
          1. Siamese, Himalayans
     c. Causes of chylothorax
        i. Idiopathic
       ii. Cardiomyopathy and congestive heart failure
       iii. Neoplasia
       iv. Heartworm disease
       v. Thoracic lymphangiectasia
          1. Functional obstruction of lymphaticovenous junction
       vi. Trauma to the thoracic duct
       vii. Lung lobe torsion
      viii. Cranial vena caval obstruction
          1. Tumor
          2. Thrombus
          3. Granuloma (heartworm disease)
       ix. Diaphragmatic hernia
       x. Fungal infection
     d. Clinical signs
        i. Dyspnea and cough most commonly noted
     e. Diagnosis
        i. Thoracic radiography
          1. Radiographic evidence of pleural effusion
       ii. Thoracocentesis
          1. White or pink, opaque fluid
          2. Fluid analysis
            a. Pleural fluid triglyceride concentration > serum triglyceride concentration
            b. Pleural fluid cholesterol concentration:triglyceride concentration ratio <1
          3. Fluid cytology
            a. Primarily lymphocytes
            b. Ratio of neutrophils to lymphocytes may increase over time
     f. Treatment
        i. Medical management
          1. Low triglyceride diet

            a. Reduce chyle in thoracic duct

            b. Often poorly palatable

            c. Low caloric content

        2. Rutin (50–100 mg/kg BID or TID)

            a. Benzopyrone compound

            b. Stimulates uptake of chyle by macrophages

        3. Intermittent thoracocentesis

            a. Long-term effects

                i.   Restrictive pleuritis

                ii. Protein and electrolyte loss

                iii. Nutritional wasting

    ii. Surgical management

        1. Failure of medical management

        2. Persistent chylous effusion

        3. Mesenteric lymphangiography to highlight thoracic duct

        4. Thoracic duct ligation

            a. Most commonly performed

            b. Omentalization, advancement of omentum into thorax

            c. May enhance fluid absorption. Thoracic duct gluing has recently been described as another approach.

        5. Pleuroperitoneal shunts

        6. Pleurodesis

        7. Improvement in roughly 20–50% of cases

            a. 3–7 days following surgery

  4. Neoplasia

    a. Mediastinal or parenchymal in origin

    b. Mediastinal mass

        i.   Lymphosarcoma

        ii. Thymoma

            1. Must differentiate from lymphosarcoma

            2. Must be removed surgically

        iii. Branchial cyst

            1. Benign lesion

    c. Pulmonary parenchymal neoplasia

        i.   Pulmonary adenocarcinoma

    d. Other

        i.   Lymphangiosarcoma

        ii. Metastatic disease

    e. Clinical signs

        i.   Respiratory compromise

        ii. Regurgitation associated with mediastinal masses

            1. Likely esophageal compression

        iii. Weight loss

        iv. Lethargy, reduced appetite

    f. Diagnosis

        i.   Neoplastic cells noted on fluid cytology

            1. Lymphosarcoma most commonly noted

        ii. Reduced compressibility of the cranial thorax

            1. Mediastinal masses

        iii. Thoracic radiography

           1. Pleural effusion
           2. Mass effect cranial to the heart
       iv. Thoracic ultrasound
           1. Pleural effusion
           2. Mass effect cranial to heart
   g. Treatment
       i. Oxygen supplementation
       ii. Thoracocentesis
       iii. Exploratory thoracotomy
           1. Lung lobe resection
           2. Cranial mediastinal mass removal
       iv. Lymphosarcoma is more effectively treated with chemotherapy than with surgery.
  5. Diaphragmatic hernia
    a. Definition
       i. Protrusion of abdominal organs into thoracic cavity through the diaphragm
    b. Causes
       i. Most commonly traumatic
       ii. Peritoneopericardial
           1. Abnormal opening between the pericardial sac and the pleuroperitoneal membrane
           2. Congenital anomaly
    c. Clinical signs
       i. Respiratory distress
       ii. Vomiting
    d. Diagnosis
       i. Radiographs
           1. Inability to fully distinguish length of diaphragm
           2. Abdominal structures identified in thoracic cavity
              a. Liver, jejunum, stomach
           3. Enlarged cardiac silhouette
              a. Peritoneopericardial diaphragmatic hernia
       ii. Ultrasound
           1. Can be difficult to appreciate rent in diaphragm
           2. Abdominal structures identified in thoracic cavity
       iii. CT scan
           1. Not frequently required
    e. Treatment
       i. Oxygen supplementation
       ii. Exploratory laparotomy
           1. Manual reduction of abdominal organs
              a. Adhesions present with chronic hernias
       iii. Exploratory thoracotomy required in rare cases
    f. Complications
       i. Blood loss
       ii. Systemic inflammation
           1. Cardiovascular instability postoperatively
       iii. Ischemic, necrotic bowel
  b. Pneumothorax
    i. Definition
       1. Accumulation of air in the pleural space

    ii. Causes
      1. Trauma
      2. Penetrating thoracic wounds
      3. Iatrogenic secondary to thoracocentesis
        a. Uncommon in the dog but common in the cat with chronic pleural effusion
      4. Pulmonary parenchymal abnormality
        a. Ulcerated pulmonary mass, abscess
        b. Bleb or bulla
      5. Secondary to severe coughing from feline asthma/bronchial disease
      6. Secondary to tracheal laceration during endotracheal intubation
        a. Pneumomediastinum and subcutaneous emphysema often present
   iii. Clinical signs
      1. Acute onset severe respiratory distress
      2. Diminished bronchovesicular sounds on thoracic auscultation
   iv. Diagnosis
      1. Thoracic radiography images
        a. Lateral view
          i. Elevation of cardiac silhouette off sternum
        b. Ventral dorsal view
          i. Retraction of lungs from body wall
    v. Treatment
      1. Thoracocentesis
        a. May be sufficient for traumatic pneumothorax
      2. Thoracostomy tube placement
        a. If repeated thoracocentesis is required
        b. Continuous suction
        c. May take days for pneumothorax to resolve
      3. Exploratory thoracotomy
        a. If persistent despite repeated thoracocentesis
        b. If lung pathology is suspected
          i. Mass, bleb, bulla
      4. Airway capture if severe external wounds present
        a. Sedation, intubation
      5. Supportive care
        a. Pain medication
        b. Oxygen supplementation

Recommended Reading

Barr V, Allan G, Beatty J, et al. Feline pyothorax: a retrospective study of 27 cases in Australia. J Fel Med Surg, 2005; 7:211–222.

Brady C, Otto C, Van Winkle T, et al. Severe sepsis in cats: 29 cases (1986–1998). J Am Vet Med Assoc, 2000; 217:531–535.

Davies C, Forrester S. Pleural effusion in cats: 82 cases. J Small Anim Pract, 1996; 37:217–224.

Demetriou J, Ladlow J, McGrotty Y, et al. Canine and feline pyothorax: a retrospective study of 50 cases in the UK and Ireland. J Small Anim Practice, 2002; 43:388–394.

Fossum T, Forrester D, Swenson C, et al. Chylothorax in cats: 37 cases (1969–1989). J Am Vet Med Assoc, 1991; 198(4):672–678.

Fossum T, Jacobs R, Birchard S. Evaluation of cholesterol and triglyceride concentrations in differentiating chylous and nonchylous pleural effusions in dogs and cats. J Am Vet Med Assoc, 1986; 188(1):49–51.

Fossum T, Miller M, Rogers K, et al. Chylothorax associated with right-sided heart failure in 5 cats. J Am Vet Med Assoc, 1994; 1:84–89.

Kerpsack S, McLoughlin M, Birchard S, et al. Evaluation of mesenteric lymphangiography and thoracic duct ligation in cats with chylothorax: 19 cases (1987–1992). J Am Vet Med Assoc, 1994; 205(5):711–715.

LaFond E, Weirich W, Salisbury K. Omentalization of the thorax for treatment of idiopathic chylothorax with constrictive pleuritis in a cat. J Am Anim Hosp Assoc, 2002; 38(1):74–78.

Litster AL, Buchanan JW. Vertebral scale system to measure heart size in radiographs of cats. J Am Vet Med Assoc, 2000; 216:210–214.

Rooney M, Monnet E. Medical and surgical treatment of pyothorax in dogs: 26 cases (1991–2001). J Am Vet Med Assoc, 2002; 221:86–92.

Suess R, Flanders J, Beck K, et al. Constrictive pleuritis in cats with chylothorax: 10 cases (1983–1991). J Am Anim Hosp Assoc, 1994; 30:70–77.

Waddell L, Brady C, Drobatz K. Risk factors, prognostic indicators, and outcome of pyothorax in cats: 80 cases (1986–1999). J Am Vet Med Assoc, 2002; 221:819–824.

Walker A, Jang S, Hirsh D. Bacteria associated with pyothorax in dogs and cats: 98 cases (1989–1998). J Am Vet Med Assoc, 2000; 216:359–363.

11
UPPER AIRWAY DISEASE

April L. Paul and Elizabeth Rozanski

Unique Features
- Cats with respiratory distress are often fragile; proceed with caution.
- Supplemental oxygen and efforts to localize the source of the problem are warranted.
- Upper airway disease is characterized by loud breathing.
- Larygneal masses are not always cancer.

A. Physical examination
  a. Nose
    i. Nasal discharge
      1. Serous
        a. Clear, watery consistency
        b. Represents non-specific irritation of the nasal mucosa
      2. Mucoid
        a. Clear, thick consistency
        b. In response to chronic, noninfectious nasal disease
      3. Purulent
        a. Thick, white, yellow, or green, with ropey consistency
        b. Due to either primary or secondary bacterial or rarely fungal colonization
      4. Mucopurulent
        a. Mixture of mucoid and purulent discharges
        b. Common with chronic nasal disease where there is bacterial infection or a necrotic focus
      5. Sanguinous
        a. Blood is mixed with another discharge
        b. Indicates damage to the nasal mucosa or a coagulation defect (rare)
      6. Epistaxis
        a. Hemorrhage
          i. Head trauma
          ii. Coagulopathy (particularly thrombocytopenia/thrombocytopathia)
          iii. Nasal mass
          iv. Infection
    ii. Sneezing
      1. Acute (sudden onset; may be paradoxical)

       a. Environmental irritant (pollen, smoke, air freshener)

       b. Viral infection (often early)

       c. Foreign body

    2. Chronic (>2 weeks)

       a. Sinusitis

       b. Nasal tumor

       c. Nasal infection (bacterial, fungal)

  iii. Reverse sneezing—noisy, labored, inspiratory effort, possible orthopneic position with neck extension and elbow abduction (uncommon in cats)

  iv. Open-mouth breathing

    1. Will have pink mucous membranes

    2. Unable to breathe through nose, not respiratory distress

  b. Nasopharynx

    i. Auscultation

      1. Stertor—loud, coarse sound such as that produced by snoring or snorting

    ii. Referred upper airway sounds

  c. Laryngeal and pharyngeal disease

    i. Prolonged and labored inspiratory phase of respiration

    ii. Auscultation

      1. Referred upper airway sounds

      2. Stridor; high-pitched audible wheezing

      3. Relative decreased lung sounds possible (if upper airway obstruction)

  d. Trachea

    i. Cough—spontaneous or elicited on tracheal palpation

    ii. Airway obstructive breathing pattern—characterized by a slow inspiratory phase followed by a more rapid expiratory phase if problem is cervical trachea. If lower airways affected, then the reverse is true.

    iii. Loud rhonchi—rattling in the throat

    iv. Degree of respiratory distress reflects cause and severity

B. Differential diagnosis

  a. Nose

    i.   Feline upper respiratory tract complex

      1. Feline herpesvirus-1 (FHV-1), also called feline rhinotracheitis virus (FRV), feline calicivirus (FCV) and *Chlamydia psittaci*

      2. Opportunistic bacterial infections secondary to mucosal damage from above agents

      3. Pyrexia and anorexia

      4. Nasal discharge, sneezing, ulcerated nares, turbinate necrosis, severe conjunctivitis, and ulcerative keratitis

    ii. Mycotic infections

      1. *Cryptococcus neoformans*, other *Cryptococcus* spp. occasionally described

      2. Nasal discharge, pyrexia, anorexia

      3. Nose is often disfigured (roman nose), enlarged submandibular lymph nodes.

      4. Commonly feline leukemia positive

    iii. Neoplasia

      1. Adenocarcinoma, lymphosarcoma, squamous cell carcinoma of the nasal planum and undifferentiated carcinoma most common

      2. Locally invasive with variable metastatic potential

      3. May invade the cranial vault, which may or may not result in CNS signs, most often seizures and altered mentation

       4. Unilateral nasal discharge, sneezing epistaxis, epiphora, exophthalmus, facial deformity, pain, and neurologic signs

       5. Older animals

       6. Absence of airflow through one or both nostrils

       7. Deformation of the facial bones may be visible

    iv. Allergic rhinitis

       1. Serous to mucoid discharge

    v. Nasal polyps

       1. Inflammatory in nature

       2. Originate from the ethmoturbinates

    vi. Parasitic rhinitis

       1. *Cuterebra* spp.

    vii. Foreign bodies

       1. Inhaled or migrated from the external nares or oral cavity

       2. Serous to purulent discharge

       3. Sneezing/pawing at the face

    viii. Dental disease

       1. Tooth root abscess may cause nasal discharge.

       2. Oronasal fisula

b. Nasopharynx

    i. Nasopharyngeal polyp

       1. Proliferations of inflammatory tissue

       2. Extend via the eustachian tube from the middle ear, and may grow into the external ear canal, pharynx, and nasal cavity

       3. Young cats—average age is 3 years.

       4. May palpate mass in the soft palate (under anesthesia)

       5. Grossly the mass is pink, polypoid, often arising from a stalk.

       6. Stertorous breathing, upper airway obstruction, and serous-to-mucopurulent nasal discharge

       7. May see signs of otitis externa, head tilt, nystagmus, or Horner's syndrome

       8. May remove with gentle traction (50% recur) or via a ventral bulla osteotomy

    ii. Nasopharyneal stenosis or webbing

    iii. Grass or other foreign bodies

c. Larynx and pharynx

    i. Laryngeal paralysis—uncommon in cats

       1. Inspiratory stridor

       2. May be due to central and peripheral nerve disease or neoplasia, most often idiopathic

       3. Owner may notice change in meow.

    ii. Granulomatous/inflammatory laryngeal disease

       1. Irregular proliferation, hyperemia, and swelling of the larynx

       2. Upper airway obstruction

       3. Larynx appears grossly neoplastic

    iii. Neoplasia

       1. Squamous cell carcinoma most common, lymphoma and others reported

       2. Tumors originating in tissues adjacent to the larynx may compress or invade the larynx

       3. Respiratory noise—both with inspiration and expiration

       4. Inspiratory stridor and voice change initially, may progress to cyanosis, syncope

    iv. Foreign bodies

       1. Toys, plants, and cuterebra larvae

        2. May act as a valve and restrict inspiration
  d. Trachea
     i. Masses
        1. Intraluminal
           a. Neoplasia—uncommon
           b. Granulomas, abscesses, inflammatory polyps (fig. 11.1)
           c. Obstructive airway signs if impeding over half of the airway diameter (fig. 11.1)
        2. Extraluminal
           a. Causing compression of the trachea
     ii. Foreign bodies
        1. Large foreign bodies localize to the carina
     iii. Tracheal trauma
        1. Subcutaneous emphysema
        2. Respiratory distress if severe
        3. Tracheal perforation/tear (fig. 11.2)
           a. May be associated with intubation
     iv. Stricture or avulsion
     v. Tracheal collapse
        1. Rare in cats

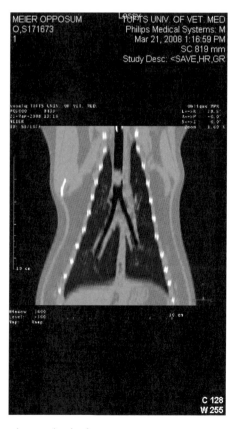

Fig. 11.1. CT image of a cat with a tracheal adenocarcinoma.

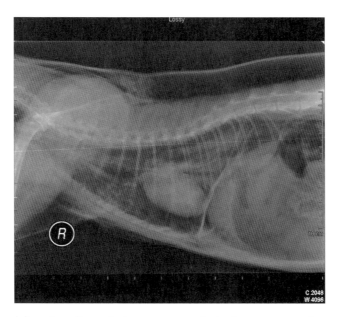

Fig. 11.2. This lateral thoracic radiograph demonstrates marked subcutaneous emphysema, as well as a pneumomediastium, pneumothorax, and pneumoretroperitoneum secondary to tracheal tear from intubation.

C. Diagnostics
    a. Nose
        i.   Routine hematology and biochemistry analysis
        ii. Coagulation profile for epistaxis; specifically platelet count
        iii. Smear of nasal discharge, most helpful in suspected Cryptococcus cases
        iv. Specific tests to identify the upper respiratory complex; rarely performed clinically unless a specific etiology is desired
            1. Fluorescent antibody testing on conjunctival scrapings, pharyngeal swabs, or tonsillar swabs
            2. Virus isolation on pharyngeal, conjunctival, or nasal swabs or on tissue specimens such as tonsillar biopsy specimens
            3. PCR of pharyngeal or ocular fluids
            4. Bacterial cultures from the oropharynx (generally not helpful)
            5. Serum antibody titers—rising titers over 2 to 3 weeks suggests active infection
        v. Diagnostic imaging
            1. Requires general anesthesia
            2. Radiography
               a. Two orthogonal views—lateral skull and a DV, dorsal ventral intraoral or occlusal or an oblique open-mouth view
               b. Assessment includes symmetry, bone, or turbinate destruction, masses, variations of opacity and soft tissue changes
               c. Interpretation can be difficult due to superimposition of structures
            3. Computed tomography (CT; fig. 11.3)
               a. Detailed view of the nasal cavity and paranasal sinuses with higher resolution and sensitivity
               b. Nasal discharge may be difficult to differentiate from soft tissue opacity

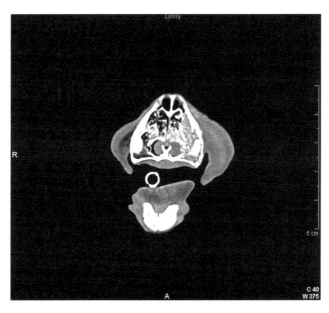

Fig. 11.3. The CT image showed a nasal mass on the left side of the nasal cavity. Note the asymmetry and bony destruction.

        4. Magnetic resonance imaging (MRI)
          a. Greater soft tissue resolution than CT or radiography
          b. Soft tissue opacities easily distinguished from nasal discharge
   vi. Rhinoscopy
        1. Allows direct evaluation of lesions and foreign bodies
        2. Collection of biopsy samples under visual guidance
        3. Can examine the pharynx above the soft palate with a flexible endoscope
  vii. Tissue biopsy
        1. Performed blind or with a scope
        2. Care must be taken not to penetrate the cribiform plate—the medial canthus of the eye is a general marker for maximal distance from the nares.
        3. Hemorrhage is a major complication.
          a. Pack the nasal cavity temporarily with cotton balls or gauze. Be sure to count the number that you place so they may all be accounted for at removal.
          b. Use of dilute epinephrine or phenylephrine applied locally may help to control hemorrhage.
          c. The ipsilateral carotid may be ligated if hemorrhage is not controlled.
 viii. Cytology
        1. Done by impression smears of biopsy samples
        2. Can be useful to detect the presence of fungal elements, tumor cells, type of inflammatory cells, and the presence of bacteria
   ix. Culture
        1. Normally the nasal cavity contains a mixed bacterial and fungal population.
        2. Bacterial culture is only considered significant if there is heavy growth of a single isolate.
        3. A positive fungal culture in a symptomatic cat is considered positive.
  b. Nasopharynx
   i. Radiography

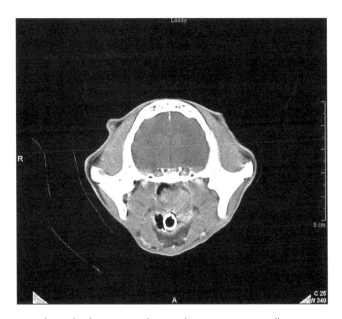

Fig. 11.4. This CT image showed a large mass, biopsied as a squamous cell carcinoma.

       1. Soft tissue opacity above the soft palate

       2. Evaluation of the osseous bullae to determine the extent of involvement

   ii. CT or MRI may be used for more advanced imaging, although direct visualization is more usual (fig. 11.4).

   iii. Gross visualization of a mass in the nasopharynx, nasal cavity, or external ear canal

   iv. Deep otoscopic examination

   v. Doxapram hydrochloride at 2.2 mg/kg IV may be used to stimulate laryngeal function under anesthesia when evaluating possible laryngeal paralysis.

  c. Larynx/pharynx

   i. Radiography

       1. May identify radiodense foreign bodies, soft tissue masses, and soft palate abnormalities

       2. Abnormal opacities may be misleading due to rotation of the head and neck.

   ii. Laryngoscopy and pharyngoscopy

       1. Anesthesia should be performed with short-acting injectable agents without prior sedation.

       2. Anesthesia titrated to allow visualization of the laryngeal cartilages with some jaw tone to evaluate for laryngeal paralysis

       3. Deeper anesthesia is required for thorough examination of the caudal pharynx and larynx.

       4. Biopsy specimens should be obtained from any lesions found on examination.

       5. The clinician should be prepared to perform a tracheostomy in any cat if a laryngeal mass is anticipated.

  d. Trachea

   i. Radiography

       1. Lateral and dorsoventral views

       2. Tracheal masses may decrease luminal size.

       3. May visualize radiopaque foreign bodies

       4. Hyperinflated lung may result due to air trapping caused by intrathoracic tracheal obstruction

      5. May reveal subcutaneous emphysema with tracheal tears (see fig. 11.2)

      6. Pneumomediastinum with a cervical or intrathoracic tracheal tear (see fig. 11.2)

  ii. Bronchoscopy

      1. Can be used to visualize tracheal masses, tracheal collapse, tears, and foreign bodies

      2. Useful for obtaining cytologic specimens of masses or obtaining biopsies

D. Treatment/prognosis

  a. Nose

    i.   Supportive care such as hydration and nutrition

    ii. Upper respiratory complex

      1. Vaporizers

      2. Antibiotic therapy if signs are severe or if there is evidence of secondary bacterial infection

      3. Amoxicillin (20 mg/kg q12h) Clavamox (10–15 mg/kg q12h) doxycycline (5–10 mg/kg q24h), or Azithromycin (5 mg/kg every other day) for 7–14 days

      4. Lysine (125–250 mg PO q12h, indefinitively)

      5. Prognosis is good.

    iii. Mycosis

      1. Amphotericin B, ketoconazole, itraconazole, fluconazole, and 5-flucytosine. Antifungal drugs should be used with caution and by individuals familiar with their possible side effects. For Cryptococcus, the preferred regime is typically fluconazole 2.5–10 mg/kg PO or 25 mg/cat PO q12h or 50 mg/cat PO once daily continued for 3–4 months after clinical cure. Amphotericin B is reserved for more resistant cases due to the side effects (renal failure).

      2. Prognosis is good if just nasal involvement. The costs of therapy can be quite high, and clients should be advised of this.

    iv. Neoplasia

      1. Surgical excision

      2. Radiation therapy

      3. Chemotherapy

      4. Prognosis is fair to poor. Tumor type influences prognosis.

    v.   Allergic rhinitis

      1. Remove the offending allergen.

      2. Antihistamines are variably effective. The most popular is chlorpheniramine (1–2 mg q12h). These may be continued as needed if the cat responds well. If there is no response, then the medicine should be discontinued.

      3. Glucocorticoids; prednisone or prednisolone, 1 mg/kg q12h for 5 days, then taper to lowest effective dose.

      4. Prognosis is excellent.

    vi. Nasal polyps

      1. Surgical removal

      2. Prognosis is good.

    vii. Foreign bodies

      1. Removal

      2. Prognosis is excellent.

  b. Nasopharynx

    i. Polyp

      1. Surgical excision

      2. Prognosis is excellent. Regrowth is possible if all abnormal tissue is not excised.

        a. A decrease in the incidence of regrowth has been reported in cats treated with a bulla osteotomy (versus simple polyp removal).

  c. Pharynx/larynx

    i.   Laryngeal paralysis

        1. Arytenoid lateralization; mildly affected cats may be treated avoiding stress. Some cats are evaluated only for increase in inspiratory noise without distress; in these cats surgery is not indicated due to the risk of aspiration pneumonia.

        2. Prognosis is fair; aspiration pneumonia is possible.

  ii. Granulomatous/inflammatory laryngeal disease

        1. Prednisone—5 mg/cat q12h for 30 days, then taper. Or as clinically indicated.

        2. Conservative excision of the tissue

        3. Prognosis varies depending on responsiveness to steroids and surgical resection.

  iii. Neoplasia

        1. Surgical excision

        2. Complete laryngectomy and permanent tracheostomy if highly invasive

        3. Prognosis is excellent for benign tumors and poor for malignant tumors.

  iv. Foreign bodies

        1. Removal

        2. May require temporary trachestomy if severe airway occlusion occurs

        3. Prognosis is excellent.

d. Trachea

  i. Masses

        1. May be removed via bronchoscopy

        2. Surgical removal or resection

        3. Chemotherapy depending on type

        4. Prognosis is guarded.

  ii. Foreign bodies

        1. May be removed via bronchoscopy

        2. Hold the cat upside down while under general anesthesia and gently but firmly tap the thorax.

        3. Surgical resection

        4. Prognosis is excellent although secondary tracheal stenosis is possible.

  iii. Tracheal trauma

        1. Cage rest for cats without respiratory distress

        2. Surgical repair

        3. Prognosis is fair to good.

12
LOWER AIRWAY DISEASE

Benjamin M. Brainard and Lesley G. King

A. Definitions: Lower airway disease
   a. Feline asthma: An inflammatory (usually allergic) disease of feline bronchi characterized by reversible bronchospasm and airway hyper-reactivity, epithelial edema, and mucous gland hypertrophy and hyperactivity.
   b. Bronchitis: A chronic, progressive inflammatory disease of the lower airways often clinically manifested as a cough.
   c. Bronchiectasis: Irreversible dilation of bronchi, occasionally congenital but more commonly seen as a consequence of chronic inflammatory or other bronchopulmonary disease.
   d. Chronic obstructive pulmonary disease: A sequela of chronic bronchitis denoting bronchial obstruction due to inflammation, edema, and mucus secretion, accompanied by early closure of small airways.
B. History, signalment
   a. Cats presenting with emergent lower airway disease may be of any age, although a predisposition for middle-aged to older female cats has been reported.
   b. Siamese and other oriental breeds are overrepresented.
   c. Common historical findings may include the following:
      i.   Introduction of new cats to the household
           1. Upper respiratory infections may be concurrent or may trigger clinical lower airway disease.
      ii. New construction or carpeting at home
      iii. A prior history of cough or an asthmatic episode
      iv. A change in seasons
           1. Increased airborne allergens
           2. Initiation of central heating
      v.   The aeroallergens associated with tobacco smoke may also cause exacerbations of allergic airway disease.
      vi. Some cats with lower airway disease may have sneezing episodes or nasal discharge in their history.
   d. The use of potassium bromide for control of seizures has been associated with the development of bronchial disease and coughing in cats.
   e. These historical findings and clinical presentations are common to a wide range of inflammatory diseases of the feline lower airway, which include allergic airway disease (classical asthma), chronic bronchitis, and even bronchiectasis. Individual cats may display features of more than one airway disorder.

C. Clinical signs, physical examination
  a. Respiratory pattern
    i. Because feline bronchial diseases are associated with bronchoconstriction and inflammation, the end result is a decrease in the diameter of the airways leading to the alveoli.
      1. Air flow into the alveoli is described by the Poiseuille equation, which relates flow to the radius of the airway to the fourth power.
        a. A 50% decrease in the bronchus diameter results in 1/16 of the normal flow through the airway.
      2. The airway diameter is slightly larger during inspiration because inspiratory muscle activity exerts radial traction on the small lower airways. During expiration the opposite forces are exerted, and there is early closure of narrowed small airways. Thus, while inhalation may sometimes be difficult in asthmatic cats, the majority of the dyspnea is expiratory.
        a. When observing the respiratory pattern in affected cats, the expiratory phase can be significantly longer than the inspiratory phase, but this may be difficult to discern clinically.
        b. Some cats display an increased effort at the end of expiration ("expiratory push") in an effort to complete the expiratory phase of respiration.
      3. Exhalation is usually prolonged in cats experiencing acute bronchoconstriction, and associated with recruitment and active effort by the muscles of the abdominal wall.
        a. Alveolar air trapping due to early closure of the small airways can lead to overinflation of the lungs.
        b. Some asthmatic cats may exhibit a barrel-shaped chest due to air trapping. In these instances minimal airway sounds are detectable on auscultation and the cat is in severe respiratory distress, but overall this manifestation is relatively rare.
        c. Excessive air trapping and barotrauma due to overdistended alveoli may eventually result in the development of emphysema and occasional instances of pneumothorax.
      4. Cats may present with clinical signs ranging from mild dyspnea to fulminant respiratory compromise and cyanosis.
  b. Auscultation
    i. The presence of wheezing sounds on exhalation, and occasionally on both inhalation and exhalation, is highly suggestive of bronchial disease. However, in most instances airway sounds are described as harsh or increased.
    ii. Cats may have a pronounced expiratory grunt.
    iii. If there has been lobar collapse, or if there is concurrent pulmonary parenchymal disease, focal crackles may be heard.
    iv. Dull sounds are ausculted in hemithoraces with pneumothorax, particularly dorsally rather than ventrally, as might be expected with pleural effusion.
  c. Cardiovascular
    i. Cats in respiratory distress due to bronchial disease are commonly tachycardic and hypertensive. In contrast, cats with congestive heart failure may be tachycardic or bradycardic and may be hypotensive.
    ii. Cardiac auscultation should be normal. The finding of a heart murmur or gallop rhythm should prompt suspicion of heart failure rather than bronchial disease.
    iii. ECG analysis may show sinus tachycardia, though if there is hypoxia, arrhythmias such as ventricular premature complexes may be seen. In cats with heart disease, arrhythmias or other abnormalities such as bundle-branch block may be observed. See chapter 17—Management of Life-Threatening Arrthymias.
D. Pathophysiology
  a. Bronchial disease, especially allergic bronchial disease, is multifactorial.
  b. Classically, an immune stimulus, usually in the form of aeroallergens, triggers Th2 cells (T-helper white blood cells, essential for antibody-mediated immunity).

     i. Th2 lymphocyte stimulation leads to allergen-specific IgE production, as well as chemoattraction of eosinophils, mast cells, and basophils.

     ii. IgE cross-linked to allergens binding to mast cells induces degranulation and subsequent airway hyperreactivity due to release of inflammatory mediators (e.g., serotonin, histamine, substance P).

     iii. Recruitment and degranulation of inflammatory cells cause thickening of the airway walls and contribute to bronchoconstriction and airway hyperreactivity.

     iv. Inflammation in the bronchial submucosa can cause hypersecretion of mucus by goblet cells.

     v. Chronic allergen stimulation can also lead to formation of circulating antigen-specific IgG and IgA.

  c. Chronic inflammatory disease such as bronchitis or bronchopneumonia may result in bronchiectasis, a relatively rare condition in cats.

     i. Widened bronchioles with abnormal bronchial epithelium interfere with mucociliary clearance mechanisms and may predispose to further chronic destruction of lung parenchyma by pneumonia.

  d. Histologically, cats with allergic or inflammatory bronchial disease have inflammatory cell influx into the bronchial mucosa and submucosa, causing edema and producing the characteristic radiographic pattern attributed to thickened bronchial walls. Other findings can include mucosal hyperemia, and hyperplasia of goblet cells and smooth muscle. Emphysema occurs in chronically affected cats due to obstruction of small airways and air trapping at the end of exhalation.

     i. Cats with bronchiectasis may also have endogenous lipid pneumonia or emphysema.

E. Diagnosis

  a. Compatible historical and physical examination findings

  b. Depending on the degree of dyspnea, it may not be appropriate to pursue radiographs on presentation if the cat is very unstable. Emergency treatment (see below) may be initiated based on physical examination findings and historical information. If the cat is extremely distressed and does not respond to initial management, it may be necessary to anesthetize, intubate, and ventilate it with 100% oxygen to safely perform diagnostic procedures.

  c. Radiography (figs. 12.1 a and b)

     i. Bronchial pattern, representing accumulation of inflammatory cells around the airways.

       1. Described as "doughnuts and train tracks," which are the end-on or cross-sectional views of the bronchial walls.

     ii. Bronchiectasis may be apparent in some cats with chronic bronchial inflammation. Bronchiectasis is characterized by variable radiographic patterns:

       1. Enlarged bronchi may appear cylindrical with an increased diameter and lack of tapering.

       2. Sacculated appearance

       3. Affected areas may be focal or diffuse

     iii. Hyperinflation of lungs

       1. Flattening of the diaphragm

       2. Borders of the lungs extend beyond the twelfth or thirteenth rib.

     iv. Collapse of the right middle lung lobe

     v. Pneumothorax (uncommon)

     vi. Aerophagia in severely dyspneic cats, causing a gas-filled stomach.

     vii. In some cats, especially those with concurrent pulmonary parenchymal disease, interstitial or mixed broncho-interstitial patterns may be seen.

  d. Complete blood count

     i. Peripheral eosinophilia is noted in about 20% of cats with bronchial disease, but can be seen with other respiratory diseases, systemic inflammation, or parasitic infection.

     ii. A stress leukogram may be present if the cat is distressed at the time of blood collection.

  e. Serum chemistry

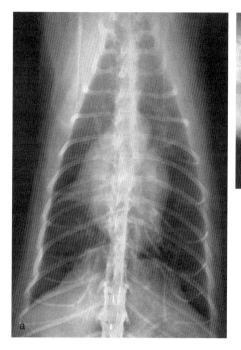
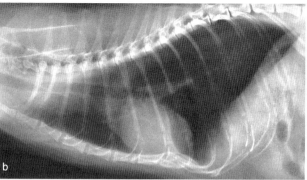

Figs. 12.1 a and b. Radiographs of a cat diagnosed with lower airway disease. See text for details of radiographic signs of lower airway disease.

    i. Should be normal in cats with uncomplicated bronchial disease.
    ii. Hyperglobulinemia may be present in some cats with chronic inflammation.
  f. Assessment for parasitic disease
    i. Fecal exam
      1. Baermann for detection of *Aeluorostrongylus*
      2. Zn-SO4 floatation for detection of eggs of *Capillaria* and *Paragonimus*
    ii. Heartworm serology
      1. Antibody serology is more accurate in cats (see chaps. 15 and 18)
F. Differential diagnoses
  a. Allergic bronchitis, asthma, chronic bronchitis, bronchiectasis
  b. Smoke inhalation (usually evident in history)
  c. Infections
    i. Bacterial
      1. *Bordetella bronchiseptica* has been isolated and may cause clinical disease in cats.
        a. May cause cough and bronchitis/bronchiolitis
          i. Acute history of a dry nonproductive cough, or cough elicited on tracheal palpation
        b. May cause severe fulminant bronchopneumonia
        c. Susceptibility
          i. Kittens and immunosuppressed cats may be more susceptible.
          ii. Cats housed in colonies with many individuals in close proximity or in multicat households may also be at increased risk.
      2. *Mycoplasma* sp. have been isolated from some cats presenting with lower airway disease; however, its significance in the lower respiratory tract is unclear.
      3. Pneumonia (see chap. 13)

    ii. Parasitic

       1. May induce eosinophil degranulation, causing bronchoconstriction, and the clinical signs of asthma.

       2. The most common species in the lungs include *Capillaria* and *Aelurostrongylus*.

       3. *Paragonimus* or *Ascaris* sp. may cause lower airway disease as the larvae migrate through the lungs.

   iii. Other infections

       1. Viral

          a. Some cats with acute viral upper respiratory infections (calicivirus or herpes virus) may have dyspnea and coughing as part of their clinical presentation.

       2. Fungal

          a. Histoplasma (*Histoplasma capsulatum*)

             i. Can cause granulomatous interstitial pulmonary lesions in susceptible cats.

             ii. Clinical signs include cough, dyspnea, fever, and lethargy.

          b. Cryptococcus (*Cryptococcus neoformans*)

             i. Commonly isolated from the nasal cavity and sinuses of cats, where it results in a granulomatous sinusitis

             ii. Rarely causes clinical signs of lower respiratory tract disease

          c. Other

             i. Coccidioides (*Coccidioides immitis*) is usually characterized by skin lesions (but may cause pneumonia) in cats.

             ii. Blastomycosis (*Blastomyces dermatitidis*) is rarely diagnosed in cats.

       3. Protozoal

          a. Although pneumonia caused by *Toxoplasma* commonly has an interstitial to alveolar pattern on radiographs, some of the initial clinical signs may mimic asthma.

  d. Neoplasia

     i. Neoplasms of the upper airways may present with coughing as the primary clinical sign, but dyspnea associated with extrathoracic upper airway obstruction would be expected to be primarily inspiratory.

    ii. Bronchial tumors

       1. Focal neoplasms that obstruct the trachea or bronchi may present with a clinical sign of coughing. Absorption atelectasis may occur if the neoplasm completely obstructs a bronchus.

       2. Carcinomatosis may occasionally be seen in bronchial walls, causing a bronchial pattern on radiographs, as well as characteristic clinical signs of dyspnea and coughing.

  e. Foreign bodies

     i. Typically, inhaled foreign bodies are more likely to cause upper airway obstruction associated with coughing and inspiratory dyspnea, rather than lower airway expiratory dyspnea. *Cuterebra* have been reported to cause tracheal obstruction.

  f. Chronic pleural effusion

     i. Cats with chylothorax may have a chronic cough due to fibrosing pleuritis of the parietal pleura after exposure to the chylous effusion.

       1. In these cats, lung lobe collapse and dyspnea will remain despite appropriate evacuation of the pleural effusion.

  g. Cardiac disease

     i. Heart disease rarely causes coughing in cats.

  h. Trauma

     i. Tracheal rupture secondary to blunt trauma can result in tracheal disruption just cranial to the carina. These cats may be presented with acute respiratory distress but may also have signs delayed by several days as fibrin and scarring cause narrowing at the site of the rupture.

G. Advanced diagnostic procedures
  a. Many diagnostic procedures require anesthesia, which may be challenging in cats with lower airway hyperreactivity. Any airway stimulation, such as placement of an endotracheal tube or instillation of saline for lavage, may stimulate further bronchoconstriction and a worsening of the cat's condition. Owners should be aware of these risks prior to performing anesthesia in asthmatic cats.
    i. Premedication/sedation is usually required, especially if there is no intravenous access.
      1. Ketamine
        a. In the absence of heart disease, a very useful premedicant and induction agent
        b. Results in bronchodilation, making it ideal for use in cats in asthmatic crises
        c. Induction doses can range from 3–7 mg/kg IV, and should always be combined with a tranquilizer such as a benzodiazepine (0.2–0.4 mg/kg IV).
      2. Halothane
        a. Bronchodilatory effect via relaxation of bronchial smooth muscle
        b. Not easily available currently; isoflurane may have similar properties but is more irritating to the bronchial mucosa, and the full effect may not be realized. Sevoflurane is less irritating to the respiratory tract and decreases airway resistance in anesthetized humans with chronic obstructive pulmonary disease.
        c. Arrhythmias may occur with halothane anesthesia in patients who have received large doses of sympathomimetic drugs for bronchodilation.
      3. Diazepam, midazolam
        a. Benzodiazepines combined with ketamine provide good sedation or anesthetic premedication.
      4. Narcotics may allow neuroleptanalgesia when combined with benzodiazepines and provide sedation in cats in which ketamine is contraindicated.
        a. Butorphanol may be administered at doses of 0.1–0.2 mg/kg.
        b. Butorphanol may have antitussive properties.
        c. Side effects include respiratory depression, and dyspneic animals should be monitored closely after administration.
      5. Drugs to avoid
        a. Beta-blockers
          i. May attenuate B2-induced bronchodilation and exacerbate clinical signs by causing bronchoconstriction
        b. Nonsteroidal anti-inflammatory drugs (NSAIDs)
          i. In humans, inhibition of cyclooxygenase with aspirin causes increased production of leukotrienes by inflammatory cells, which may worsen the asthmatic symptoms. It is unknown whether this is true in cats.
          ii. Contraindicated in animals that are receiving corticosteroids.
    ii. Cats should always be intubated for the duration of anesthesia, and care should be taken to ensure that they are adequately ventilating (either spontaneously or with assistance) with 100% oxygen during the diagnostic procedures. Ideally, these cats should be monitored with pulse oximetry and end-tidal capnography during anesthesia.
  b. Lung mechanics, pulmonary function tests
    i. May require anesthesia and special equipment.
    ii. Pulmonary function measurement may be more valuable as a measure of improvement in individual cats after treatment, as single measurements may be misleading.
      1. Increased lung resistance is expected in cats with bronchial disease
        a. Lung resistance testing can be used to determine the degree of bronchial hyperreactivity to various irritants such as methacholine, and also the response to selected bronchodilators.
      2. Changes in dynamic lung compliance may occur in cats with bronchopulmonary disease.

   a. Decreased lung compliance may occur if there is concurrent pulmonary disease.
   b. Emphysematous changes due to chronic asthma may cause an increase in dynamic lung compliance.
  3. Tidal breathing flow volume loops can be measured using a close-fitting face mask in awake cats, which can provide information about the extent of expiratory airway obstruction without the need for general anesthesia and intubation.
 iii. Whole-body plethysmography
  1. Allows noninvasive measurement of respiratory rate, tidal volume, peak inspiratory and expiratory flow rates, and inspiratory and expiratory time in the awake cat.
   a. Requires special equipment
   b. Can demonstrate a characteristic decrease in peak expiratory flow rates in cats with lower airway disease compared to normal cats
   c. Cats with bronchial disease may have prolonged expiratory times compared to normal cats.
 iv. Pulse oximetry
  1. Noninvasive way to estimate the percentage of oxygen-saturated hemoglobin (oxyhemoglobin)
  2. Related to the PaO_2 by the oxy-hemoglobin dissociation curve, but does not measure PaO_2 directly
  v. End-tidal capnography
  1. Sidestream adapters may be used to estimate partial pressure of exhaled carbon dioxide in awake patients; more accurate capnograms are obtained from intubated patients.
  2. Analysis of capnograms may give information on ventilatory parameters.
 vi. Arterial blood gas analysis
  1. Measures partial pressures of oxygen and carbon dioxide in arterial blood, in addition to the blood pH
   a. If animals have significant lower airway disease, the arterial partial pressure of oxygen (PaO_2) may be decreased.
   b. With significant lower airway disease, the arterial partial pressure of carbon dioxide ($PaCO_2$) may be increased.
   c. With less severe lower airway obstructive disease, the $PaCO_2$ may be decreased secondary to tachypnea.
  2. May be obtained from the metatarsal or femoral arteries
  3. Helps to quantify degree of oxygenation or ventilation disturbances and to monitor recovery
  4. Normal values (while breathing room air)
   a. PaO_2 = 80–100 mmHg
   b. $PaCO_2$ = 35–45 mmHg
 c. Endotracheal wash (ETW)
  i. The cat is intubated with a sterile endotracheal tube, and a sterile catheter (e.g., a red rubber urinary catheter) is passed through the endotracheal tube as far as possible into the lungs. Aliquots (each 5 mL) of nonbacteriostatic sterile saline are instilled into the airway and immediately aspirated using a syringe or suction trap. Yields are typically small (<1 mL) but can provide useful information for cytology and culture.
  ii. Cytology of ETW fluid. ETW is indicated for obtaining representative cytologic samples from the lower airway and is useful for distinguishing between infectious and inflammatory processes. Because it is a procedure that is performed blindly, the possibility of obtaining a less-diagnostic sample from an unaffected lung lobe exists.
  1. Eosinophils
   a. May be the predominant cell in 25%–30% of cats with feline asthma or bronchitis

        b. May also be isolated from ETW of normal cats

        c. In individual cats, eosinophils may correlate with severity of disease

    2. Neutrophils

        a. Consistent with lower airway inflammation

        b. With eosinophils, may be the predominant cell in feline asthma or bronchitis

    3. Mixed populations

        a. Some cats have mixed populations of eosinophils, neutrophils, and macrophages.

        b. Numbers of cells may correlate with the radiographic severity of the lesions.

        c. Lymphocytes are poorly represented in these mixed populations.

    4. Cytology may be normal in some cases, especially if the cat has been treated with corticosteroids prior to sampling.

    5. Increased amounts of mucus, produced by hypertrophied goblet cells, may be noted on ETW in cats with chronic bronchial disease.

  iii. Bacteriologic cultures

    1. Cultures from healthy and asthmatic cats can give similar results. Thus cultures may give misleading information unless there is heavy growth of a single species.

    2. *Mycoplasma* is a possible pathogen that has been isolated from the lower airways of asthmatic cats but is very difficult to culture.

  d. Bronchoscopy, bronchoalveolar lavage (BAL)

    i. Performed using a sterile bronchoscope. BAL allows samples to be obtained from the alveoli and distal airways.

    ii. Allows direct inspection of abnormal areas of the upper bronchial tree, more directed sample acquisition, and the potential to remove inspissated mucous plugs that might be causing bronchial obstruction.

    iii. Cytology is variable, depending on distribution of the lesion and recovery of sample.

      1. Cats with histologically confirmed lower airway disease may have alveolar cytology consistent with inflammation (e.g., neutrophils, eosinophils, and macrophages).

      2. The primary cells identified in BAL samples from healthy cats are pulmonary alveolar macrophages.

    iv. Bacterial and *Mycoplasma* culture may be performed, although even normal cats may have small numbers of bacteria in the lungs that may appear on culture.

H. Management of allergic and chronic bronchitis, feline bronchial asthma

  a. Emergent therapy (table 12.1)

    i. Oxygen

      1. Preferably via oxygen cage, to create an oxygen-rich atmosphere with minimal stress to the cat

      2. May also be administered via an e-collar with cellophane placed over the opening, with the oxygen tubing snaked under the collar, although this may be stressful

      3. If the degree of dyspnea is extreme, anesthesia and mechanical ventilation may be the only ways to adequately provide oxygen while treating the acute bronchoconstriction and confirm the diagnosis.

    ii. Corticosteroids

      1. Corticosteroids should be administered parenterally in an emergency situation.

        a. Dexamethasone sodium phosphate 0.2 mg/kg

          i. May be administered IV or IM

          ii. SQ administration may not be reliable, especially if the cat is clinically dehydrated.

          iii. Long-acting (depo preparations) steroids such as methylprednisone acetate are not recommended for management of acute dyspnea because of slower absorption.

      2. Inhaled corticosteroids may be useful in an emergency, especially if the cat has been on chronic therapy with an inhaler.

Table 12.1.   Emergency treatment of cats with dyspnea due to lower airway disease.

Drugs	MOAs	Doses	Contraindications and Adverse Effects	Expected Results
Oxygen	Increase alveolar PO_2	40–100% prn, via oxygen cage, mask, or hood; mechanical ventilation if no response to oxygen supplementation	Prolonged high FiO_2 (>60% for >8–12 hours) may predispose to oxygen toxicity	Decreased respiratory rate and effort, resolution of cyanosis
Dexamethasone sodium phosphate	Decrease inflammation in the airways	0.2–0.4 mg/kg IV, IM, SQ q12h	Relative risks of immunosuppression, GI ulceration, weighed against potential as a life-saving treatment	Gradual decrease in respiratory effort and rate
Prednisone sodium succinate	Decrease inflammation in the airways	1–3 mg/kg IV, IM	Relative risks of immunosuppression, GI ulceration, weighed against potential as a life-saving treatment	Gradual decrease in respiratory effort and rate
Terbutaline	Bronchodilation via β_2 agonism	0.01 mg/kg IV, IM, SQ q8 PRN	Contraindicated if the cat has heart disease or hypertension	Decreased respiratory rate and effort, relatively rapid onset
Albuterol	Bronchodilation via β_2 agonism	One puff (90–100 µg) q30min PRN up to 8 doses	Potentially distressing to the cat	Variable, depending on efficiency of drug administration
Aminophylline	Bronchodilation via phosphodiesterase inhibition	2–5 mg/kg slow, diluted, IV	Contraindicated if the cat has heart disease or hypertension	Less effective than terbutaline
Theophylline	Bronchodilation via phosphodiesterase inhibition	0.1 mg/kg slow, diluted, IV	Contraindicated if the cat has heart disease or hypertension	Less effective than terbutaline
Epinephrine	Bronchodilation via β_2 agonism	0.04 mg/kg IV, IM, SQ	Contraindicated if the cat has heart disease or hypertension	Used in extremis or if other bronchodilators are unavailable

a. Regular use of inhaled fluticasone for 7–10 days is necessary before seeing demonstrable effects in some cats.

b. Dosed at one puff (120–220 µg) every 12 hours × 1 month along with 7–10 days of oral steroid, tapering to q24h if tolerated and effective

c. Cats should be allowed to take 5–10 breaths from the mask and spacer after discharge of the puff of drug.

iii. Bronchodilators
   1. Injectable bronchodilators should be administered to cats exhibiting signs of bronchoconstriction.
      a. Nonspecific: bronchodilation is accompanied by generalized increases in sympathetic activity, including tachycardia and possibly hypertension.
         i. Methylxanthines such as aminophylline are available for injection but have a lower therapeutic index than terbutaline.
         ii. Vagolytics such as atropine are effective bronchodilators but may cause significant tachycardia.
         iii. Epinephrine (0.01–0.1 mg/kg IV, IM) can be given to extremely emergent cases but has significant alpha and β_1 agonist activity.
      b. Specific: β_2 agonists cause bronchodilation and vasodilation, with less effect on the β_1 receptors and therefore less tendency to cause tachycardia.
         i. Terbutaline (Brethine) is administered IV, IM, SQ at 0.01 mg/kg.
         ii. Clenbuterol is an available β_2 selective agonist but is orally administered and is therefore not applicable to emergency situations.
   2. Inhaled bronchodilators may provide immediate relief to some dyspneic cats if they tolerate use of a face-mask and spacer (fig. 12.2).
      a. Albuterol is a β_2 agonist; 90 μg (one puff) may be administered q30min up to three times, in combination with anti-inflammatory therapy and parenteral bronchodilators.
   iv. Antibiotics are rarely indicated as part of emergent therapy.
b. Chronic therapy (table 12.2)
   i. Corticosteroids are extremely important for chronic management of lower airway diseases caused by inflammation. Without adequate control of inflammatory processes, the disease may progress, eventually resulting in worsening clinical signs and irreversible damage to the lungs.
      1. Oral
         a. Prednisone
            i. Oral glucocorticoid of choice
            ii. Initially dosed at 1 mg/kg PO q12h, and then tapered to a lower dose based on individual response.

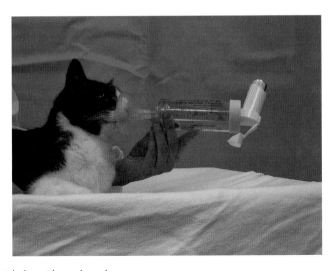

Fig. 12.2. Asthma inhaler with mask and spacer.

Table 12.2. Long-term treatment of cats with lower airway disease.

Drug	MOA	Dose	Contraindications	Expected Results
Prednisone	Decrease airway inflammation	1–2 mg/kg PO q12, gradual weaning to the lowest possible maintenance dose (e.g., 0.5 mg/kg PO EOD, depending on response)	May result in development of diabetes mellitus or other complications when used long-term	Maintenance free of clinical signs
Dexamethasone	Decrease airway inflammation	0.1–0.2 mg/kg PO q12, gradual weaning to the lowest possible maintenance dose (e.g., 0.05 mg/kg PO EOD, depending on response)	May result in development of diabetes mellitus or other complications when used long-term	Maintenance free of clinical signs
Methyl prednisone acetate	Decrease airway inflammation in cats who are unable to take inhaled or oral medications	1–3 mg/kg SQ q 4–8 weeks PRN	May result in development of diabetes mellitus or other complications such as heart failure when used long-term	Ideally, not a maintenance therapy, although some cats may only tolerate intermittent injection.
Fluticasone	Decrease airway inflammation	One puff (120–220 mcg) q12h × one month along with 7–10 days of oral steroid, tapering to q24h if tolerated and effective	Associated with fewer side effects than oral steroids, as long as cat tolerates administration	Maintenance free of clinical signs
Terbutaline	Bronchodilator	1.25–2.5 mg/cat PO q8–12h	May cause tachycardia at higher doses, avoid in cats with heart disease	Maintenance therapy
Theophylline	Bronchodilator	2–4 mg/kg PO q8–12h	May cause tachycardia at higher doses, avoid in cats with heart disease	Maintenance therapy
Aminophylline	Bronchodilator	2–5 mg/kg PO q8–12h	May cause tachycardia at higher doses, avoid in cats with heart disease	Maintenance therapy
Albuterol	Bronchodilator	One puff (90 µg) up to three times daily, may supplement in acute exacerbation	Less likely to cause adverse cardiac effects	Maintenance therapy

        b. Dexamethasone
           i. Initially dosed at 0.1 mg/kg PO q24h and tapered depending on response.
        c. Side effects include the possible development of diabetes mellitus, pancreatitis, and polyuria with polydypsia.
    2. Inhaled
        a. Fluticasone propionate
           i. To supplement or replace oral steroids
           ii. Works topically in the lungs, with minimal systemic absorption, thereby decreasing systemic side effects
           iii. Dosed at 1 puff (approximately 100 μg from the metered dose inhaler) once to twice daily, depending on severity of the asthma.
           iv. Administration is accomplished via a rebreathing chamber (e.g., Aerochamber), which holds the aerosolized drug while the cat takes 5–10 breaths via an attached soft face mask.
    3. Injectable
        a. Methylprednisone acetate ("Depo-medrol")
           i. If the owner has difficulty administering oral medications, corticosteroids can be administered by injection every 2–4 weeks.
           ii. Long-term use may result in side effects such as diabetes mellitus.
  ii. Bronchodilators
    1. Oral
        a. Terbutaline 1.25–2.5 mg/cat PO q8–12h
           i. Contraindications as listed above
        b. Theophylline 2–4 mg/kg PO q8–12h
           i. Available both in an instant-release (q6–8h administration) and a controlled-release (q12h) form
    2. Inhaled
        a. Albuterol: one puff (90 μg) up to three times daily, may supplement in acute exacerbation
  c. Other therapies
    i. Cyproheptadine
        1. Serotonin (5-HT) is a major product of eosinophils and mast cells in cats and is thought to be responsible for the majority of the airway reactivity seen in asthmatic cats.
        2. Administration of a 5-HT receptor blocker may help alleviate some of the bronchospasm. Experimentally, cyproheptadine appears to attenuate the severity of bronchoconstriction. However, when used as a single agent in a small clinical trial, it did not significantly attenuate the clinical signs.
        3. Dose 0.5 mg/kg, q8–12h, PO
    ii. Leukotriene inhibitors
        1. In human asthma, leukotrienes are important to the pathogenesis and clinical signs of asthma. The contribution of leukotrienes to feline asthma is unclear.
        2. One small clinical study in asthmatic cats did not show improvement when cats were treated with zafirlukast compared with prednisone alone.
        3. Thus, leukotriene inhibitors may not be useful as a monotherapy; however, they may be indicated as part of a treatment regime for asthmatic cats.
        4. Monoleukast (inhaled) and zafirlukast (oral) are two currently available leukotriene inhibitors.
        5. Zafirlukast (Accolate), 0.15–0.2 mg/kg, PO, q12–24h
I. Management of bronchiectasis
  a. Cats with bronchiectasis may be difficult to treat.

b. Treatment consists of symptomatic care for inflammatory airway disease as described above, using combinations of bronchodilators and antibiotics.

c. Due to inability to clear material from the lower airways, chronic pneumonia is common, and repeated courses of antibiotics may be indicated.

d. Corticosteroids may cause worsening of clinical signs in cats with bronchiectasis.

J. Management of smoke inhalation

  a. Smoke inhalation from house fires can cause damage to the respiratory tract by multiple mechanisms.

    i. Carbon monoxide (CO) is a byproduct of incomplete combustion that is produced in large quantities in structure fires.

      1. CO binds to hemoglobin with a significantly higher affinity (approx. 200 x) than oxygen, thus displacing O_2 from the molecule and decreasing tissue delivery.

      2. Carboxyhemoglobin is measured with a co-oximeter; pulse oximetry is not accurate (and consistently reads 85%).

      3. CO may also disrupt the utilization of oxygen by mitochondria.

        a. For this reason, carbon monoxide intoxication should be suspected when blood lactate is high despite adequate tissue perfusion.

      4. Delayed neurologic sequelae may also be recognized, presumed secondary to hypoxic brain damage.

    ii. Toxins from burning plastic and other household items may produce cyanide, which inhibits mitochondrial aerobic respiration.

    iii. Other toxins and irritants produced by combustion in structure fires

      1. Can cause direct irritation, which may result in reflex bronchoconstriction

      2. Specific toxins may interfere with the function of surfactant, decreasing the tidal volume.

    iv. Superheated air or steam may be inhaled and scald the entire respiratory tree.

      1. Thermal injuries to the respiratory mucosa include erythema, swelling, edema, and epithelial necrosis and sloughing.

    v. Animals that have been in fires may have been exposed to low fractional inspired concentrations of oxygen, combined with high inspired carbon dioxide concentrations, resulting in loss of consciousness.

    vi. In humans and mice exposed to smoke inhalation injury, histopathology of the lungs shows type II cell hypertrophy, with cytoplasmic blebbing and vacuolization. Additionally, mucosal hemorrhage and edema, with infiltration of macrophages and lymphocytes, is seen.

  b. Clinical signs in cats after smoke inhalation

    i. Tachypnea, open-mouthed breathing, vocalization, lethargy, and unconsciousness

    ii. A more severe clinical course may be seen in animals with evidence of both surface burns and respiratory distress.

      1. Physical examination may reveal increased upper airway noise (stridor) caused by laryngeal or pharyngeal edema.

      2. If bronchoconstriction is present, expiratory wheezes may be ausculted.

      3. Alternatively, if there is a component of lower airway disease, focal or diffuse crackles or harsh bronchovesicular sounds may be present.

  c. Diagnostic evaluation

    i. For animals in respiratory distress, as noted above

    ii. Co-oximetry may be of assistance in distinguishing the presence of methemoglobinemia or carboxyhemoglobinemia.

    iii. Pulse oximetry is inaccurate in the presence of met- or carboxyhemoglobin, and may overestimate the actual oxygen saturation.

    iv. Radiographs may show bronchial, alveolar, or interstitial patterns.

  d. Emergent therapy is geared toward support of the cat's oxygenation.

  i. Oxygen supplementation at high fractional inspired concentrations will help to clear carboxyhemoglobin.
     1. At least 2–4 hours of treatment have been recommended, more if indicated.
 ii. Bronchodilators are indicated if there is bronchoconstriction.
iii. If there is severe tissue edema in the upper airway, tracheostomy or mechanical ventilation may be indicated until resolution of the inflammatory changes.
 iv. Mechanical ventilation is occasionally indicated in animals that require high inspired oxygen concentrations, or in whom hypoventilation occurs.

Recommended Reading

Dye JA, McKiernan BC, Rozanski EA, et al. Bronchopulmonary disease in the cat: historical, physical, radiographic, clinicopathologic, and pulmonary functional evaluation of 24 affected and 15 healthy cats. J Vet Int Med, 1996; 10(6):385–400.

McKiernan BC, Dye JA, Rozanski, EA. Tidal breathing flow-volume loops in healthy and bronchitic cats. J Vet Int Med, 1993; 7(6):388–393.

Norris CR, Griffey SM, Christopher MM, et al. Thoracic radiography, bronchoalveolar lavage cytopathology, and pulmonary parenchymal histopathology: a comparison of diagnostic results in 11 cats. J Am Anim Hosp Assoc, 2002; 38:337–345.

Padrid PA. Feline asthma: diagnosis and treatment. Vet Clin North Am Small Anim Pract, 2000; 30(6):1279–1293.

13
PARENCHYMAL DISEASE

Deborah Silverstein

Unique Features
- Cats with pulmonary parenchymal disease and dyspnea rarely open-mouth breathe as dogs typically do. Cats most commonly exhibit tachypnea, nostril flaring, an increase in breathing effort, and reluctance to lie down.
- A perihilar interstitial-alveolar pattern is rarely seen on thoracic radiographs in cats with cardiogenic pulmonary edema. Instead, a patchy, diffuse interstitial infiltrate is commonly observed. Cardiomegaly and pulmonary venous distention are also frequently evident.

Differential Diagnoses
Pneumonia
Edema
Hemorrhage
Endogenous toxins
Inhaled toxins
Drug reaction
Neoplasia
Atelectasis
Accidental drowning/submersion
Pulmonary thromboembolism
Lung lobe torsion
General Diagnostic Plan
Venous blood gas +lactate
Pulse oximetry
Complete blood count, biochemical analysis, urinalysis
Three-view thoracic radiographs
+/− Computerized tomography
+/− Magnetic resonance imaging
Endotracheal wash with cytology and culture/susceptibility testing

A. Physical examination findings and clinical signs
  a. History
    i.   Exercise intolerance
    ii.   Shortness of breath
    iii. Lethargy
    iv. Coughing: Cats with parenchymal disease commonly have a history of and/or present with a soft, deep cough. They rarely have a hacking cough (more typical of large airway irritation).
    v.   Exposure (reside in or travel history) to area with fungal disease
    vi. +/– Vomiting, diarrhea
    vii. +/– Anorexia, weight loss
    viii. +/– Recent stressful event or corticosteroid treatment leading to immunosuppression
    ix. +/– Smoke or toxin exposure
    x.   +/– Exposure to colony situation
    xi. +/– Seizures, ataxia
    xii. +/– Pancreatitis
    xiii. +/– Recent anesthesia or prolonged recumbency
    xiv. +/– Recent trauma
    xv. +/– Recent accidental drowning or submersion injury
  b. Clinical signs (see Unique Features box)
    i.   Tachypnea
    ii.   Dyspnea
    iii. Cyanosis
    iv. Reluctance to lie down
    v.   Orthopnea
    vi. Lateral recumbency
    vii. Gasping/agonal breathing (prearrest)
    viii. +/– Fever
    ix. +/– Concurrent upper respiratory tract signs and/or nasal discharge
    x.   +/– Vague pain upon abdominal palpation
    xi. +/– Oral/ocular/nasal abnormalities (viral, fungal, parasitic disease)
    xii. +/– Skin lesions (poxvirus, coccidioidomycosis)
    xiii. +/– Peritoneal effusion (disseminated infectious or neoplastic disease)
    xiv. +/– Coma or seizures, gagging, foaming at mouth, rubbing eyes, soot on fur, smoky odor, skin burns (smoke or toxin exposure).
    xv. +/– Heart murmur, +/– gallop rhythm or irregular rhythm (cardiogenic pulmonary edema or endomyocarditis)
    xvi. +/– Decreased breath sounds ventrally (pleural effusion secondary to cardiogenic edema, neoplasia, bronchopneumonia, or hemorrhage)
    xvii. +/– Palpable thyroid nodule
    xviii. +/– Lameness (metastatic neoplasia)
  c. Auscultation
    i.   Normal tracheal breath sounds
    ii.   Loud breath sounds on inspiration +/– expiration
    iii. Adventitial breath sounds
        1. Inspiratory +/– expiratory crackles and/or wheezes
B. Differential diagnoses and most common etiologies
  a. Pneumonia
    i.   Bacterial/mycoplasmal/mycobacterial
        1. *Staphylococcus* spp.
        2. *Streptococcus* spp.

       3. *Escherichia coli*

       4. *Pseudomonas aeruginosa*

       5. *Bordetella bronchiseptica*

       6. *Pasteurella multocida*

       7. *Klebsiella pneumoniae*

       8. *Bacteroides fragilis*

       9. *Clostridium difficile*

     10. *Proteus mirabilis*

     11. *Capnocytophaga cyndegmi*

     12. *Chlamydia psittaci*

  ii. Viral

       1. Herpesvirus-1 (feline rhinotracheitis)

       2. Calicivirus

       3. Poxvirus

  iii. Protozoal

       1. Toxoplasmosis

  iv. Mycotic

       1. Histoplasmosis

       2. Blastomycosis

       3. Coccidioidomycosis

       4. Cryptococcosis (Abyssinian and Siamese breeds overrepresented)

       5. Aspergillosis

       6. Sporotrichosis

       7. Candidiasis

       8. Zygomycosis

       9. Penicilliosis

  v. Parasitic

       1. *Aelurostrongylus abstrusus*

       2. *Bronchostrongylus* spp.

       3. *Troglostrongylus* spp.

       4. *Capillaria aerophilia* (or *Eucoleus aerophilus*)

       5. *Paragonimus kellicotti*

       6. *Cuterebra* spp.

  vi. Lipid pneumonia

       1. Chronic forced mineral oil administration

  vii. Inflammatory

       1. Idiopathic hypereosinophilia syndrome

       2. Potassium bromide therapy

  viii. Usual interstitial pneumonia

       1. Idiopathic pulmonary fibrosis

b. Edema

  i. Cardiogenic (see chaps. 14—General Approach and Overview of Cardiac Emergencies and 15—Management of Specific Cardiac Diseases)

       1. Left-sided congestive heart failure

  ii. Noncardiogenic

       1. Acute respiratory distress syndrome (ARDS)

       2. Neurogenic pulmonary edema

       3. Upper airway obstruction

       4. Feline endomyocarditis

       5. Near drowning

    c. Hemorrhage
      i. Pulmonary contusions
      ii. Coagulopathy (i.e., anticoagulant rodenticide, liver dysfunction, biliary obstruction, thrombocytopathia, thrombocytopenia)
    d. Endogenous toxins
      i. Uremic pneumonitis
    e. Inhaled toxins
      i. Smoke or noxious gas inhalation
      ii. Prolonged oxygen therapy
    f. Adverse drug reaction
    g. Neoplasia
    h. Atelectasis
    i. Accidental drowning/submersion injury
    j. Pulmonary thromboembolism
    k. Lung lobe torsion
C. Diagnostic imaging
    a. Thoracic radiography and/or computerized tomography (CT) +/− magnetic resonance imaging (MRI)
      i. Combinations of interstitial and alveolar disease are typically evident in cats with pulmonary parenchymal disease. The distribution of infiltrates may assist in determining the underlying etiology.
      ii. Classically, cats with bacterial bronchopneumonia show cranioventral alveolar infiltrates, although patchy combinations of alveolar, interstitial, and bronchial disease may be present. Small pleural effusions may be present in severe cases (figs. 13.1 a, b, and c).
      iii. Diffuse or caudodorsal interstitial and/or alveolar infiltrates are typical of viral pneumonia or neurogenic pulmonary edema.
      iv. Pulmonary fungal disease may appear as interstitial, alveolar, bronchiolar, nodular, military, or mixed patterns. In addition, lobar consolidation, discrete nodules, or cavitary lesions, hilar lymphadenopathy, pleural effusion or thickening, and/or pneumothorax may be evident (figs. 13.2 a and b).
      v. The presence of a mediastinal shift, elevation of the hemidiaphragm, rearrangement of borders of inflated lung lobes, separation of the heart from the sternum, and asymmetry of the rib cage are consistent with atelectasis.
      vi. Pulmonary contusions appear as unilateral or bilateral patchy interstitial to alveolar infiltration. Animals with pulmonary contusions often have concurrent rib fractures, pneumothorax, and/or a diaphragmatic hernia. Pulmonary contusions are detected earliest using CT imaging. Additionally, the clinical radiographic signs of pulmonary contusions can often lag behind the clinical progression.
      vii. Pulmonary thromboembolism may have completely normal thoracic radiographs. Other reported abnormalities include pleural effusion, alveolar and interstitial pattern, and venous congestion.
      viii. Reported radiographic changes with idiopathic pulmonary fibrosis include dense patchy or diffuse interstitial, bronchiolar, and alveolar infiltration.
      ix. Cardiomegaly +/− pulmonary venous distention is common with cardiogenic edema. Cats typically have a more diffuse, patchy interstitial disease with cardiogenic pulmonary edema, *not* perihilar in distribution (see Unique Features box).
D. Additional diagnostic techniques
    a. Complete blood count, biochemical profile, urinalysis
      i. Leukocytosis or leukopenia +/− left shift may be seen with infectious or inflammatory diseases. Eosinophilia can be seen with parasitic disease, hypersensitivity reactions, or idiopathic hypereosinophililc syndrome.

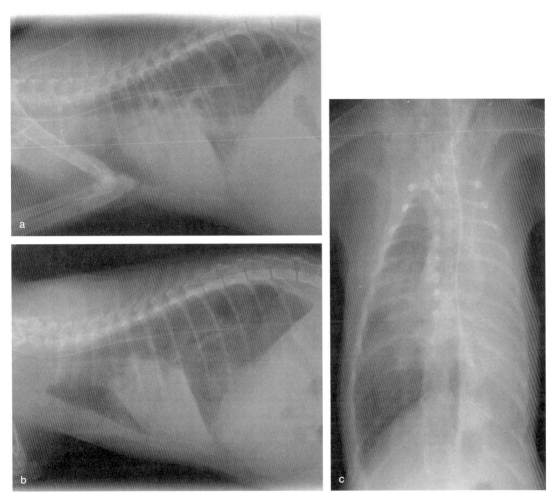

Figs. 13.1 a through c.   Severe aspiration pneumonia in a cat 1 week following anesthesia. There is consolidation and air bronchograms throughout the left hemithorax, the right caudal portion of the cranial lobe, and the right middle lung lobe.

    ii. Nonregenerative anemia may be seen with more chronic inflammatory, infectious, or neoplastic diseases.

    iii. Hypoalbuminemia and hyperglobulinemia are commonly seen with fungal disease. Hypercalcemia may also be present. Hyperbilirubinemia, increased alanine aminotransferase, alkaline phosphatase, and creatine kinase may be present in cats with *Toxoplasma gondii* due to infection in other organ systems.

    iv. Proteinuria may be seen in cats with *Toxoplasma gondii*.

  b. Pulse oximetry (SpO$_2$)

    i. Normal value 95–100% when breathing room air.

    ii. Values less than 93% indicate significant hypoxemia and warrant oxygen therapy.

  c. Fundic examination

    i. See chapter 37—Ocular Emergencies.

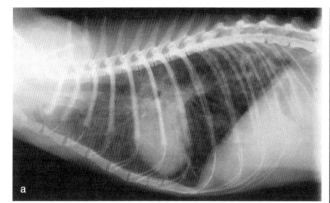
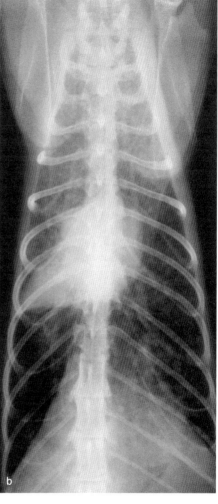

Figs. 13.2 a and b. Disseminated blastomycosis in a cat causing a diffuse bronchointerstitial pattern. Neoplasia should also be a rule-out based on these radiographs.

    d. +/– Arterial blood gas analysis or venous blood gas analysis and lactate
    e. Trans- or endotracheal wash or bronchoalveolar lavage
    f. Cytologic evaluation and culture/sensitivity should be done on fluid obtained +/– special staining for fungi (periodic acid Schiff, Gridley's fungal, Gomori's methenamine silver stain) and/or lipid (Sudan black, Sudan red, oil-red-O), +/– polarized light, +/– tissue chromatography.
       i. The presence of leukocytes with intracellular organisms confirms an infection.
    g. Lung aspirate with cytology +/– culture and sensitivity +/– special staining for fungi (periodic acid Schiff, Gridley's fungal, Gomori's methenamine silver stain) and/or lipid (Sudan black, Sudan red, oil-red-O), +/– polarized light, +/– tissue chromatography.
    h. Lung biopsy with cytology +/– culture and sensitivity +/– special staining for fungi (periodic acid Schiff, Gridley's fungal, Gomori's methenamine silver stain) and/or lipid (Sudan black, Sudan red, oil-red-O), +/– polarized light, +/– tissue chromatography.

    i. Immunohistochemistry or polymerase chain reaction testing for *Toxoplasma gondii* is available.

i. Serum toxoplasma titers

j. Fecal float, smear, Baermann to evaluate for evidence of parasitic infection

k. +/– serum FelV, FIV testing

l. +/– Heartworm testing

m. +/– Viral testing (virus isolation or immunochemistry on swabs of affected areas, polymerase chain reaction on respiratory samples)

n. +/– Serologic fungal testing (coccidioidomycosis and cryptococcus)

o. +/– Cerebrospinal fluid tap (*Toxoplasmosis gondii*)

p. +/– Co-oximetry to identify levels of carbon monoxide, methemoglobinemia, and/or cyanide intoxication in smoke or toxin inhalation victims

q. +/– Echocardiogram will help to identify pleural effusion and cardiomyopathy, respectively, in cats with cardiogenic pulmonary edema. Thyroid hormone levels should be checked in patients with suspected hyperthyroid induced cardiomyopathy.

r. Thoracic ultrasonography (identify coexisting pleural effusion, visualize pulmonary mass, lung lobe torsion)

s. +/– Thoracocentesis with cytology and culture

t. +/– Coagulogram, d-dimer, anticoagulant rodenticide serum levels, liver function tests, platelet function testing, thromboelastography in cats with suspected pulmonary thromboembolism or hemorrhage. Pulmonary angiography, computerized tomographic digital subtraction angiograph, and/or ventilation perfusion scanning may also prove helpful.

u. +/– abdominal ultrasound and/or skeletal radiographs (metastatic neoplasia, systemic infection)

E. General management of animals with pulmonary parenchymal disease

  a. Oxygen therapy PRN (via flow by, mask, hood, cage)

  b. Positive pressure ventilation if:

    i. PaO_2 <60 mmHg or SpO_2 <90% with oxygen supplementation

    ii. $PaCO_2$ >60 mmHg

    iii. Severe dyspnea with impending fatigue

  c. Fluid therapy

    i. Caution should be exercised since many parenchymal diseases cause vascular endothelial leakiness and predispose to fluid extravasation into the lungs (i.e., pulmonary contusions, ARDS)

    ii. Fluid therapy is contraindicated with cardiogenic pulmonary edema

F. Specific conditions (see table 13.1 for specific drug doses and details)

  a. Bacterial pneumonia

    i. Nebulization and coupage

    ii. Antibiotic therapy

      1. Empiric choices pending culture and susceptibility testing results include ampicillin/baytril, clindamycin/baytril, ampicillin/clavulanate, ticarcillin/clavulanate, cefoxitin, or a third-generation cephalosporin.

    iii. +/– Bronchodilator therapy

      1. Controversial benefit—may worsen V/Q mismatch

      2. Beta-2 agonists (i.e., terbutaline)

      3. Methylxanthines (i.e., theophylline, caffeine)

    iv. +/– Mucolytics

      1. Efficacy unproven

      2. N-Acetylcysteine

  b. Protozoal pneumonia

    i. *Toxoplasma gondii*

      1. Clindamycin hydrochloride

      2. Potentiated sulfonamides

Table 13.1. Drug table.

Drugs	Classes	MOAs	Side Effects	Contraindications or Precautions	Routes of Administration and Doses	General Uses
Aminophylline	Xanthine derivative	Competitive phosphodiesterase inhibition to increase cAMP, direct relaxation of smooth muscle in bronchi and pulmonary vasculature	CNS stimulation, gastric irritation, nausea, vomiting	1. Hypersensitivity to xanthines 2. Cardiac disease, gastric ulcers, hyperthyroidism, hypertension, renal or hepatic disease	5–10 mg/kg IV q6–8h	Feline asthma +/− atelectasis
Ampicillin +/− clavulanate	Aminopenicillin	Inhibit cell wall synthesis; addition of clavulanate will inhibit bacterial lactamase	Hypersensitivity, anorexia, vomiting, diarrhea	History of hypersensitivity	22 mg/kg IV or PO q8h	Broad spectrum infection
Amikacin	Aminoglycoside	Inhibit protein synthesis by binding 30S ribosomal subunit	Nephrotoxicity, ototoxicity, neuromuscular blockade, facial edema, hypersensitivity	Renal disease, dehydration, neuromuscular disease	15 mg/kg IV q24h	Gram negative infections
Amphotericin B	Polyene macrolide antifungal	Binds to sterols in cell membrane and alters permeability	Nephrotoxicity (less so with liposomal forms), anorexia, vomiting, hypokalemia, distal renal tubular acidosis, hypomagnesemia, phlebitis, cardiac arrhythmias, nonregenerative anemia and fever	1. Hypersensitivity 2. Renal disease	A 0.25 mg/kg in 30 mL D₅W IV over 15 minutes q48h (+/− additional therapeutics) B amphotericin B lipid complex (ABLC; Abelcet®) 1 mg/kg IV three days per week for a total of 12 treatments (cumulative dose of 12 mg). Dilute to a concentration of 1 mg/ml in dextrose 5% (D₅W) and infuse over 1–2 hours	Fungal infections

Drug	Class	Mechanism	Side effects	Contraindications	Dose	Indications
Azithromycin	Macrolide	Bind 50S ribosomal unit and inhibit bacterial growth	Hypersensitivity, diarrhea, vomiting, anorexia	1. Hypersensitivity 2. Hepatic disease	5–10 mg/kg IV or PO q24h	*Mycoplasma haemofelis*, *Toxoplasmosis*, broad spectrum bacterial infection
Cefoxitin	Cephamycin, 2nd-generation cephalosporin	Inhibit cell wall synthesis	Diarrhea, granulocytopenia, renal tubular necrosis, hypersensitivity	History of hypersensitivity, reduce dose with renal failure	30 mg/kg IV q6–8h	Broad spectrum infection
Cefotaxime	Aminothiazolyl cephalosporin, 3rd-generation cephalosporin	Inhibit cell wall synthesis	Diarrhea, granulocytopenia, renal tubular necrosis, hypersensitivity	History of hypersensitivity, reduce dose with renal failure	25–50 mg/kg IV q6–8h	Gram negative infections
Clarithromycin	Macrolide	Bind 50S ribosomal unit and inhibit bacterial growth	Hypersensitivity, diarrhea, vomiting, anorexia, pinnal erythema	History of hypersensitivity	7.5 mg/kg PO q12h	*Mycoplasma haemofelis*, *Toxoplasmosis*, atypical mycobacterial infections
Clindamycin	Lincosamide	Bind 50S ribosomal subunit	Gastroenteritis, hypersensitivity	History of hypersensitivity	10 mg/kg IV q8–12h	Anaerobic infections, *Toxoplasmosis*
Corticosteroids	Glucocorticoid	Many mechanisms	Polydipsia, polyuria, polyphagia with weight gain, diarrhea, depression, "Cushingoid" like signs	1. Hypersensitivity 2. Sepsis	Depends on formulation	Inflammatory disease, autoimmune disease
Enrofloxacin	Fluoroquinolone	Inhibit DNA gyrase	Vomiting, anorexia, ataxia, seizures, cartilage abnormalities, acute blindness, hypersensitivity	History of hypersensitivity, young animals, breeding or pregnant animals	5 mg/kg IV or PO q24h (diluted, off label use)	Gram + and − infections

(Continued)

Table 13.1. *Continued*

Drugs	Classes	MOAs	Side Effects	Contraindications or Precautions	Routes of Administration and Doses	General Uses
Fenbendazole	Benzimidazole anthelmintic	Interferes with microtubulin formation	Hypersensitivity, vomiting	None	50 mg/kg PO q24h for 10–14 days	Lungworms
Flucytosine	Fluorinated pyrimidine	Interferes RNA and DN synthesis	Vomiting, diarrhea, dose-dependent bone marrow suppression, oral ulceration, increased hepatic enzymes, CNS effects	1. Hypersensitivity 2. Renal impairment, preexisting bone marrow suppression, hematologic diseases, or receiving other bone marrow suppressant drugs	25–50 mg/kg PO q6h or 50–65 mg/kg PO q8h. Must be given with a polyene or azole antifungal agent	Cryptococcosis, Candidiasis/ candiduria
Furosemide	Loop diuretic	Increases renal excretion of water, sodium, potassium, chloride, calcium, magnesium, hydrogen, ammonium, and bicarbonate	Dehydration, electrolyte and acid/base imbalances, ototoxicity, gastrointestinal disturbances, hematologic effects (anemia, leukopenia), weakness and restlessness	1. Hypersensitivity 2. Severe dehydration 3. Furosemide should be used with caution in patients with preexisting electrolyte or water balance abnormalities, impaired hepatic function (may precipitate hepatic coma), and diabetes mellitus.	0.5–4 mg/kg IV or IM q1–2h in severe cases; 1–2 mg/kg PO q8–12h for maintenance	Cardiogenic pulmonary edema

Drug	Class	Mechanism	Adverse effects	Contraindications	Dose	Indication
Itraconazole	Triazole	Alter cell membrane and increase permeability	Anorexia, weight loss, vomiting, increased liver enzymes, depression	1. Hypersensitivity 2. Hepatic insufficiency 3. Achlorhydria/hypochlorhydria	10 mg/kg/day PO with food	Fungal infections
Ivermectin	Avermectin anthelmintic	Enhances release of GABA to paralyze parasite	Hypersensitivity, agitation, vocalization, anorexia, mydriasis, rear limb paresis, tremors, disorientation, blindness, headpressing, wall climbing, absence of oculomotor menace reflex, slow and incomplete pupillary light response	Hypersensitivity	0.4 mg/kg SQ once	*Aelurostrongylus abstrusus*, *Capillaria aerophilia*
Ketoconazole	Imidazole	Increase cell wall permeability and inhibit growth	Anorexia, vomiting, diarrhea, hepatic toxicity, thrombocytopenia, reversible lightening of haircoat, transient dose-related suppressant effect on gonadal and adrenal steroid synthesis	1. Hypersensitivity 2. Hepatic insufficiency 3. Thrombocytopenia **Cats may be especially sensitive to this drug.**	10–15 mg/kg PO q12h	Fungal infections
N-Acetylcysteine	Derivative of L-cysteine	Mucolytic	Nausea, vomiting	Hypersensitivity	70 mg/kg IV q6h (diluted, off label use)	Pulmonary consolidation
Terbutaline	Beta-2 agonist	Stimulation of B-2 receptors causes smooth muscle relaxation	Hypotension, tachycardia, tremors, CNS excitement, hypokalemia	1. Cats that are hypersensitive to terbutaline 2. Cardiac disease, diabetes, hyperthyroidism, hypertension, or seizure disorders	Asthma: 0.01 mg/kg SC q4h; 0.3–0.6 mg total dose or 0.03 mg/kg PO q8–12h Inhaler with spacer dose for asthma: Press inhaler twice and allow cat to take 5–7 breaths.	Feline asthma

(Continued)

Table 13.1. *Continued*

Drugs	Classes	MOAs	Side Effects	Contraindications or Precautions	Routes of Administration and Doses	General Uses
Praziquantel	Prazinoisoquinoline derivative anthelmintic	Unknown	Hypersensitivity, diarrhea, weakness, vomiting, salivation, sleepiness, transient anorexia, pain at the injection site	Hypersensitivity	23–25 mg/kg PO q8h for 3 days	*Paragonimus kellicotti*
Ticarcillin +/− clavulanate	Aminopenicillin	Inhibit cell wall synthesis; addition of clavulanate will inhibit bacterial lactamase	Hypersensitivity, anorexia, vomiting, diarrhea	History of hypersensitivity	50 mg/kg IV q6h	Broad spectrum bacterial infections
Trimethoprim sulfa	Potentiated sulfonamide	Inhibit bacterial thymidine synthesis	Anorexia, crystalluria, hematuria, leukopenia anemia	1. History of hypersensitivity 2. Hepatic disease 3. Blood dyscrasia 4. +/−Urolithiasis	15–30 mg/kg IV or PO q12–24h	Broad spectrum bacterial infections, Toxoplasmosis, Pneumocystis carinii, coccidia

        3. Pyrimethamine
        4. Minocycline
        5. Azithromycin
        6. Clarithromycin
        7. Topical, oral, or parenteral corticosteroids in cats with uveitis
  c. Mycotic pneumonia
    i. Nebulization and coupage
    ii. Polyene antibiotics
        1. Amphotericin B
           a. Lipid encapsulated form is less nephrotoxic.
        2. Hamycin
    iii. Azoles
        1. Ketoconazole
        2. Itraconazole
           a. Best tolerated "azole" in cats
        3. Fluconazole
    iv. Antimetabolites
        1. Flucytosine
    v. Chitin synthesis inhibitors
        1. Nikkomycin
        2. Lufenuron
           a. Published use in dogs only
  d. Parasitic pneumonia
    i. *Aelurostrongylus abstrusus*
        1. Often self-limiting
        2. Fenbendazole (extended regimen)
        3. Ivermectin
    ii. *Capillaria aerophilia*
        1. Fenbendazole
        2. Ivermectin
        3. Levamisole
    iii. *Paragonimus kellicotti*
        1. Praziquantel
        2. Fenbendazole
        3. Albendazole (careful of bone marrow suppression)
    iv. *Cuterebra* spp.
        1. Ivermectin
        2. +/– Corticosteroid therapy (anti-inflammatory regimen)
  e. Lipid pneumonia
    i. Exogenous lipid pneumonia
        1. Discontinue forced administration of petroleum products.
        2. Use of corticosteroids is controversial.
    ii. Endogenous lipid pneumonia
        1. Treatment of underlying disease, if present, and surgical removal of affected lung lobes (in humans since treatment of cat is not reported).
        2. Use of corticosteroids is controversial.
  f. Inflammatory
    i. Idiopathic hypereosinophilia syndrome
        1. Immunosuppressive corticosteroid therapy
        2. +/– Hydroxyurea therapy

      ii. Potassium bromide therapy
         1. Discontinue potassium bromide
         2. +/– Corticosteroid administration
  g. Usual interstitial pneumonia
      i. Idiopathic pulmonary fibrosis
         1. Drug therapy is typically unrewarding but has primarily included corticosteroids, bronchodilators, and antimicrobials.
         2. Cyclophosphamide has been used successfully in one cat.
  h. Edema
      i. Cardiogenic pulmonary edema (see chaps. 14—General Approach and Overview of Cardiac Emergencies and 15—Management of Specific Cardiac Diseases for further information)
         1. Furosemide
         2. +/– ACE inhibitor
         3. +/– Nitroglycerin
         4. +/– Nitroprusside
      ii. Noncardiogenic pulmonary edema
         1. +/– Diuretic therapy
         2. Correct underlying disease states
 i. Hemorrhage
      i. Pulmonary contusions
         1. Use of judicious intravenous fluids during resuscitation and maintenance is recommended.
         2. Treat associated thoracic and life-threatening injuries first.
         3. Analgesia PRN
         4. Avoid diuretics or prophylactic use of antibiotics or corticosteroids.
      ii. Coagulopathy
         1. Fresh frozen plasma (10 mL/kg) for prolonged PT, PTT, and/or ACT.
         2. Vitamin K_1 if indicated (anticoagulant rodenticide toxicity, liver disease, biliary obstruction).
            a. Dose: 2.5–5 mg/kg SQ or PO (with fatty meal) every 24 hours
            b. Caution: excessive vitamin K therapy in cats leads to oxidant injury to red blood cells and Heinz body anemia.
         3. Fresh whole blood or platelet-rich plasma for thrombocytopathia or severe thrombocytopenia (<20,000/μL)
 j. Endogenous toxins
      i. Uremic pneumonitis
         1. Correct uremia
 k. Inhaled toxins
      i. Smoke or toxin exposure (see chap. 12—Lower Airway Disease)
         1. Use of judicious intravenous fluids during resuscitation and maintenance is recommended.
         2. 100% oxygen for 4–6 hours to reduce the half-life of carbon monoxide
         3. Nebulization and coupage
         4. +/– Bronchodilators (reserved for cats with reflex bronchoconstriction (suspected in cats with audible or auscultable wheezes +/– hypercapnea)
         5. +/– Tracheostomy if severe upper airway obstruction
         6. +/– Treatment of ocular injuries
      ii. Prolonged oxygen therapy
         1. Decrease fraction of inspired oxygen to <60% after 4–6 hours
 l. Adverse drug reaction
      i. Discontinue drug
      ii. +/– Corticosteroids or epinephrine if needed

m. Neoplasia
   i. Surgical excision
   ii. Adjunctive chemotherapy +/– radiation therapy as indicated
n. Atelectasis
   i. Use adequate, not excessive concentrations of oxygen therapy since high inspired oxygen concentrations predispose to atelectasis.
   ii. If mechanical ventilation is required, the use of a recruitment or vital capacity maneuver may be beneficial. Positive end expiratory pressure will also help reduce atelectasis.
   iii. Aminophylline has proven helpful in humans with postoperative atelectasis.
o. Accidental drowning/submersion injury
   i. Use of judicious intravenous fluids during resuscitation and maintenance is recommended.
   ii. Correct acid/base abnormalities.
p. Pulmonary thromboembolism
   i. Identify underlying cause and treat it appropriately.
   ii. +/– thrombolytic therapy (streptokinase, urokinase, t-PA)
   iii. Anticoagulant therapy (i.e., aspirin, heparin, low molecular weight heparin, vitamin K antagonist)
q. Lung lobe torsion
   i. Cardiopulmonary stabilization
   ii. Surgical excision of affected lobe
   iii. +/– Thoracic duct ligation and subtotal pericardectomy PRN

14
GENERAL APPROACH AND OVERVIEW OF CARDIAC EMERGENCIES

Manuel Boller

Unique Features
- The most common clinical signs in cats with cardiac emergencies are respiratory distress, syncope, hind limb paresis, or a combination thereof.
- Pleural effusion often plays an important role in the etiology of respiratory distress in cats with left-sided congestive heart failure.
- Radiographic appearance of cardiogenic pulmonary edema in cats is widely variable; it can have a perihilar, caudal, or diffuse patchy distribution.

A. Signalment and history
- a. Breed predisposition
    - i. Dilated cardiomyopathy
        1. Oriental breeds (Siamese, Burmese, Abyssinian)
    - ii. Hypertrophic cardiomyopathy (HCM)
        1. Various breeds, including Maine Coon, American Shorthair, Persians, and possibly British Shorthair, Ragdoll, Norwegian Forest, Scottish Folds, and Turkish Van
- b. Age
    - i. HCM at any age (2 months to 19 years; mean 5 to 6 years)
- c. Sex
    - i. Male cats more frequently (4:1) affected with HCM.
- d. History
    - i. The cat may or may not have a history of heart disease (e.g., a previously ausculted murmur or gallop rhythm).
    - ii. A stressful event (i.e., anesthesia, surgery) within 3 months prior to occurrence of congestive heart failure is often reported in cats with endomyocarditis.
        1. Endomyocarditis is an inflammatory condition of the pulmonary vessels as well as the endocardium, and this may be the primary reason that these cats develop respiratory problems.
- e. Presenting complaint
    - i. Cats with heart disease present as emergencies due to congestive heart failure (CHF), low cardiac output heart failure (LOHF), or arterial (aortic) thromboembolism (ATE).
    - ii. Typical presenting complaints include
        1. Dyspnea, tachypnea

      2. Weakness, depression, collapse, syncope

      3. Sudden onset of paraparesis, paralysis, or pain

   iii. In contrast to dogs, coughing is an unusual finding in cats with CHF and should trigger investigation into other respiratory disease processes (i.e., feline bronchial disease).

B. Physical examination. Findings vary in accordance to whether the cat suffers from CHF, LOHF, ATE, or a combination of the above.

  a. Congestive heart failure (CHF):

     i. Mentation varies from anxiety to depression

     ii. Increased respiratory rate and/or effort

    iii. Open-mouth breathing

    iv. Cyanotic mucous membranes

     v. Lung auscultation

       1. Increased lung sounds

       2. Crackles with alveolar pulmonary edema

         a. Absence of crackles does not preclude a diagnosis of CHF.

       3. Dull lung sounds ventrally suggest presence of pleural effusion.

     vi. Heart auscultation

       1. Tachycardia

       2. Irregular heart rhythm; an electrocardiographic examination is necessary to reach a specific diagnosis.

       3. Positioning of stethoscope over 4th or 5th intercostal space or just to the right or left of the sternum allows best identification of heart murmurs in the cat.

       4. Muffled heart sounds with pleural effusion

       5. Gallop rhythm

         a. Consequence of an ausculted third (S3) or fourth (S4) heart sound and indicates heart disease in cats.

           i. S4: Atrial gallop. Indicates altered ventricular compliance as in HCM.

           ii. S3: Often heard in patients with dilative cardiomyopathy.

         b. Consider hyperthyroidism with abnormal cardiac auscultation (gallop rhythm or systolic murmur).

       6. Cardiac murmurs

         a. Systolic murmur in cats with dynamic left ventricular outflow obstruction or mitral valve regurgitation as can occur with ventricular concentric hypertrophy (e.g., HCM or hyperthyroidism)

         b. Soft systolic heart murmur may be present with dilative cardiomyopathy (i.e., due to annular ring enlargement and valvular regurgitation).

    vii. Pulse palpation

       1. Increased pulse rate

       2. Normal to weak femoral pulses

       3. Pulse deficits

       4. Irregular pulses

  b. Low cardiac output heart failure (LOHF)

     i. Depressed mentation and weakness as consequence of impaired cerebral blood flow and tissue perfusion (i.e., cardiogenic shock)

     ii. Increased respiratory rate +/− effort due to respiratory compensation for metabolic (e.g., lactic) acidosis

    iii. Cold extremities and decreased rectal temperature

    iv. Pale mucous membranes with prolonged capillary refill time

     v. Auscultation lungs

       1. No specific findings unless CHF concurrently present

2. Dull lung sounds with pleural effusion
vi. Auscultation heart
    1. Heart murmur and gallop rhythm possible
    2. Muffled heart sounds with pericardial effusion. (Clinically significant pericardial effusion is very rare in the cat. Muffled heart sounds are more commonly due to pleural effusion.)
    3. Heart rate may be increased, normal, or decreased
       a. Tachycardia
          i. Sinus tachycardia due to increased sympathoadrenergic tone
          ii. Supraventricular tachycardia, atrial flutter, or fibrillation
          iii. Ventricular tachyarrhythmias
       b. Bradycardia
          i. Sinus bradycardia with decompensated shock
          ii. First-, second-, or third-degree atrioventricular block (fig. 14.1)
          iii. Sinus arrest
vii. Pulse palpation
    1. Weak to absent femoral and/or metatarsal pulses
    2. High, low, or normal pulse rate
    3. Pulse deficits
    4. Regular, regularly irregular, or irregularly irregular pulse
c. Arterial thromboembolism (see chap. 16—Management of Thromboembolic Disease Secondary to Heart Disease)
    i. Cats are typically very painful, displaying excitement, vocalization, aggression, and open-mouth breathing (panting).

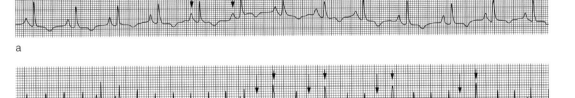

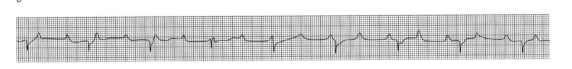

Fig. 14.1. Electrocardiograms (lead II) of cats with atrioventricular (AV) block.
a. First-degree AV block in a 15-year-old male castrated cat that was referred for a heart murmur and bradycardia. The PR-interval (arrows) measures 0.1 ms (normal 0.05–0.09 ms). 50 mm/s; 20 mm/mV.
b. Second-degree AV block in a 13-year-old male castrated cat with HCM, referred for a heart murmur and an irregular heart rhythm. Note the absence of QRS complexes after some of the P waves (long arrows). Ventricular beats are present as a consequence of an accelerated escape rhythm and fuse with the subsequent P waves (short arrows). 25 mm/s; 20 mm/mV.
c. Third-degree AV block in 17-year-old female cat presented for syncopical episodes. Note the complete dissociation of P waves and QRS complexes (escape beats). The ventricular heart rate is 95 beats per minute. 50 mm/s; 20 mm/mV.

     ii. Heart auscultation may reveal abnormalities suggestive for, but not proof of, heart disease, such as a heart murmur or gallop rhythm.

     iii. 40–60% of cats with ATE are in CHF at the time of presentation and show clinical signs accordingly (see above).

     iv. Neurological and musculoskeletal findings

        1. Any limb can be affected, but the hind extremities are involved in more than 90% of cases; thus, hind limb paresis or paralysis is observed most frequently.

        2. Typical clinical findings in the ischemic limb are the five P's:

          a. Pain proximal to desensitized area

          b. Poikilothermia: cold distal extremity

          c. Pulselessness: absence of femoral or radial pulse and absence of blood flow as determined with Doppler blood flow probe

          d. Pallor of the paw, if nonpigmented

          e. Paresis, lower motor neuron deficits

        3. The musculature in the affected limb may be firm and contracted, in the hind leg particularly the gastrognemic musculature.

        4. Deep pain in the distal extremity is absent in severe cases.

     v. Inadequate systemic perfusion or shock is frequently observed in affected animals.

        1. This may be due to the following:

          a. Left ventricular diastolic or systolic dysfunction associated with the underlying heart disease.

          b. Reperfusion injury leading to electrolyte abnormalities (hyperkalemia, hypocalcemia), impaired myocardial function, alterations in local and systemic vascular tone, and endothelial injury.

C. Differential diagnosis

  a. Congestive heart failure:

     i. Noncardiac causes of pulmonary gas exchange abnormalities, including pneumonia (bacterial, fungal, parasitic, viral), pulmonary neoplasia, heart worm disease, pulmonary thromboembolism, iatrogenic (excessive fluid administration), and others.

     ii. Lower airway disease: feline asthma, chronic bronchitis

     iii. Noncardiac causes of pleural effusion, including pyothorax, chylothorax, neoplastic effusion, and others.

  b. Low output heart failure:

     i. Noncardiac causes of low tissue perfusion or hypotension, including hypovolemic shock, SIRS/sepsis, and electrolyte abnormalities (hyperkalemia, hypocalcemia).

     ii. Noncardiac causes of syncope: vasovagal syncope, situational syncope, causes of transient loss of consciousness other than syncope (e.g., seizures, hypoglycemia).

  c. Arterial thromboembolism

     i. Other conditions leading to acute paraparesis, including spinal lymphosarcoma, spinal trauma, focal mengiomyelitis (FIP, toxoplasma, cryptococcus), discospondylitis, spinal ischemia (fibrocartilaginous embolism), and intervertebral disk disease

     ii. Noncardiac causes of thromboembolism, including tumor embolism, paraneoplastic thromboembolism, and other causes of hypercoagulability

  d. CHF, LOHF, and ATE in cats can be the sequelae of various types of heart disease, and an echocardiogram is required to differentiate between the different types, the most frequent being the following:

     i. Hypertrophic cardiomyopathy (HCM)

     ii. Restrictive cardiomyopathy

     iii. Unclassified cardiomyopathy

     iv. Dilated cardiomyopathy

     v. Endomyocarditis

     vi. Myocardial infarction

     vii. Primary mitral valve regurgitation

  e. The term *cardiomyopathy* generally applies to the presence of a primary myocardial disease, and other cardiac (e.g., aortic stenosis) or noncardiac causes (e.g., systemic hypertension, hyperthyroidism, taurine deficiency) have to be excluded prior to making that diagnosis.

D. Diagnostics and monitoring procedures

  a. Laboratory tests:

     i. Changes in CBC, serum biochemistry, and urine analysis may occur but are not specific for cardiac disease:

       1. Neutrophilia and less consistently lymphopenia and monocytosis may be present as a response to high serum cortisol and catecholamine levels (stress response).

       2. Stress hyperglycemia is common.

         a. In cats with ATE, blood glucose taken from the affected limb may be lower than that sampled from normal limbs.

       3. Azotemia is found as a consequence of inadequate effective circulating volume, chronic renal failure, or thromboembolic occlusion of the renal artery.

       4. Serum concentrations of enzymes associated with muscle injury (CK, AST > ALT; CK = creatine kinase, AST = aspartate aminotransferase, ALT = alanine aminotransferase) may be elevated in cats with ATE.

       5. Electrolyte abnormalities include

         a. Hyponatremia, which may occur in cats with LOHF. However, little data is available in this species.

         b. Changes that can occur in cats with ATE during reperfusion of the ischemic extremity include

           i. Hyperkalemia

             1. This may occur acutely, resulting in sudden death.

           ii. Ionized hypocalcemia secondary to hyperphosphatemia.

         c. Hypokalemia and metabolic alkalosis can occur with administration of loop diuretics (e.g., furosemide).

       6. Myoglobinuria may be present in cats with ATE during reperfusion.

     ii. Arterial blood gas analysis and pulse oximetry (SpO_2):

       1. Arterial blood gas collection in cats is technically difficult and very stressful and thus dangerous for the cat in respiratory distress. Therefore, this technique is rarely indicated in the clinical setting.

       2. Pulse oximetry (SpO_2) is clinically useful for objective assessment of the cat's oxygenation status.

         a. A lower than expected SpO_2 measurement supports the presence of a pulmonary gas exchange abnormality but is not specific for cardiogenic pulmonary edema as the etiology.

     iii. Venous blood gas analysis and acid-base status:

       1. Venous carbon dioxide partial pressure ($PvCO_2$) is typically decreased (due to hyperventilation) or normal in cats with CHF. An elevated $PvCO_2$ ($PvCO_2 > 45\,mmHg$) may indicate

         a. Upper or lower airway obstruction

         b. Respiratory fatigue with prolonged dyspnea

         c. Severe tissue hypoperfusion, for example, cardiogenic shock

       2. Metabolic acidosis may be present as a consequence of impaired tissue perfusion (lactic acidosis) and may indicate cardiogenic shock.

       3. An elevated blood lactate value ($>1.5\,mmol/L$) indicates anaerobic tissue metabolism and is most often the consequence of inadequate tissue blood flow; less frequently, it is the sequela

of arterial hypoxemia or other abnormalities. However, struggling can increase blood lactate levels in cats manifold; this effect has to be taken into account when interpreting lactate levels.

    a. In cats with ATE, venous lactate sampled from the affected (ischemic) limb is higher than that sampled from normal limbs.

  iv. Neurohumoral indices of heart disease:

    1. Circulating peptide hormones (natriuretic peptides) and proteins of the contractile apparatus of the cardiac myocytes (troponins) have been used to identify heart disease in people.

    2. While assays for brain natriuretic peptide, and to a lesser extent atrial natriuretic peptide, have been validated in dogs, data for the cat is currently lacking.

    3. Cardiac troponin I concentrations increase in cats with CHF due to HCM and may be helpful to identify heart failure as etiology of respiratory distress in the emergency situation.

      a. Most normal animals have levels below the threshold of detection of the assay, but normal values have to be established for each assay.

      b. A veterinary point-of-care assay is available for troponin I (cTnI catridge, i-STAT, Heska).

      c. Samples can be sent for analysis to

        i. New Bolton Center, Attn Heart Center, 382 West Street Road, Kenneth-Square, PA 19348; phone: (610) 444-5800, ext. 6359

        ii. At least 1 mL of heparinized plasma sent overnight on dry ice

        iii. Normal values: <0.03–0.16 ng/mL

b. Electrocardiography (ECG)

  i. Recording of an ECG is indicated in every patient in whom cardiac disease is suspected. The greatest value of the ECG consists of identification of arrhythmias and conduction abnormalities in regard to severity and necessity to treat (for details see chap. 17—Management of Life-Threatening Arrhythmias).

    1. An abnormal ECG can be present in an animal without heart disease and vice versa.

  ii. Continuous evaluation of the ECG is further indicated in all critically ill patients and in patients who may be predisposed to a malignant arrhythmia (e.g., thoracic trauma, shock, significant electrolyte and/or acid-base abnormalities, calcium gluconate administration, hypoxemia).

  iii. While various leads are routinely used for acquiring an electrocardiogram, Einthoven's bipolar three-lead system (I,II,III) suffices the needs of the emergency evaluation for most cases:

    1. Cat is positioned sternally and gently restrained.

    2. Adhesive electrode patches (Ambu Bluesensor N, Ambu A/S, Denmark) or blunted alligator clips can be used.

    3. One electrode is placed just proximal to the left and right olecranon and one just proximal to the left patella.

  iv. Normal ECG criteria (table 14.1) have been listed for cats.

Table 14.1. Normal values for heart rate, intervals between complexes, duration of P-QRS-T complexes, and heights of complexes.

Heart Rate (Beats per Minute)	120–240
P wave	Width: <0.04 secs; height: <0.2 mV
P-R interval	0.05–0.09 sec
QRS complex	Width: <0.04 secs; height: <0.9 mV
Q-T interval	0.07–0.20 sec; various w/heart rate
S-T segment	No depression or elevation
T wave	Positive, negative, or biphasic
Mean electrical axis	0° to +160°

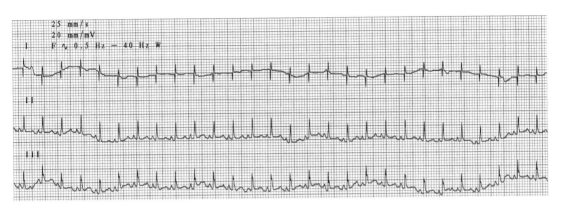

Fig. 14.2. Normal ECG cat, lead II, 25 mm/s; 20 mm/mV. The complexes are much smaller than in the dog, and P and T waves may become unidentifiable with only little baseline artifact being present. The T wave can be positive, negative, or biphasic. The heart rate is 214 beats per minute and the rhythm is sinus rhythm.

Table 14.2. Unique radiographic features in cats as opposed to dogs with congestive heart failure (CHF).

Feature	Cat	Dog
Distribution of pulmonary edema	Variable distribution; diffuse, patchy appearance of interstitial to alveolar infiltrates is common.	Predominantly perihilar interstitial to alveolar infiltrates; caudal and ultimately remaining lung lobes are involved with severe edema.
Pleural effusion	Common with left heart failure alone	Indicates right heart failure
Engorgement of pulmonary veins	Inconsistent finding: absence does not exclude presence of CHF.	Consistently present with CHF
Position of left atrium	Enlarged left atrium appears as prominent bulge at 2–3 o'clock position of VD thoracic radiograph; it is not prominent on laterolateral radiograph.	Left atrium is located between mainstem bronchi and not prominent on VD view; if enlarged, it appears prominent on laterolateral view.
Vertebral heart size	7.5 +/– 0.3 vertebrae on laterolateral radiograph	9.7 +/– 0.5 vertebrae on laterolateral radiograph

    v. Distinct characteristics of the feline versus canine ECG
        1. Sinus arrhythmia (also termed respiratory arrhythmia) is abnormal in cats.
        2. QRS configuration in cats is more variable than in dogs, and the R amplitude is usually low (figs. 14.2).
  c. Holter monitor
     i. A Holter monitor in cats is a device capable of continuously recording an ECG for 24–48 hours for later analysis.
    ii. The use of a Holter monitor allows identification and characterization of arrhythmias that occur only intermittently.
   iii. Further indications include
        1. Correlation of an arrhythmia with clinical signs (e.g., syncope)
        2. Evaluation of necessity for antiarrhythmic treatment
        3. Evaluation of the efficacy of an antiarrhythmic intervention
    iv. Due to the size of the recording device, cats have to be hospitalized for the duration of the recording process (fig. 14.3).

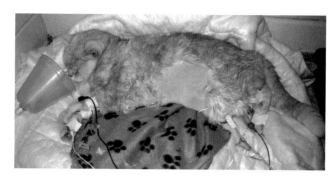

Fig. 14.3. Use of adhesive electrode patches taped in position on the distal extremities of the right and left front and left hind leg for continuous monitoring of a cat's electrocardiogram in an intensive care setting.

    d. Cardiovascular imaging
       i. Thoracic radiography (table 14.2, fig. 14.4)
          1. Heart size can be roughly assessed by using the thoracic vertebrae as a scale, starting at the 4th thoracic vertebra.
             a. On a lateral radiograph, the vertebral heart size (sum of short and long axes) measures no more than eight vertebrae in most normal cats (figs. 14.4 a and c).
             b. On a ventrodorsal view, the cardiac short axis measurement is less than four vertebrae in most normal cats (fig. 14.4b).
             c. Pericardial fat can mimic cardiomegaly.
          2. Absence of generalized cardiomegaly does not prove absence of heart disease (because of concentric hypertrophy). Heart size correlates best with dilated cardiomyopathy, followed by restrictive cardiomyopathy, unclassified cardiomyopathy, and HCM.
          3. Left atrial enlargement in cats can often not be identified on the lateral view due to its cranial position but appears as a bulge at the 2–3-o'clock position on the ventrodorsal view (fig. 14.5).
          4. Engorgement of pulmonary veins may be present in cats with CHF, but this is less consistently the case than in dogs (fig. 14.6).
          5. Pulmonary edema occurs with left-sided CHF and can have a perihilar location, can involve mostly the caudal lung fields, or have a more diffuse patchy appearance (fig. 14.7).
          6. Pleural effusion in cats is a frequent finding with left-sided CHF alone.
             a. This pleural effusion can be a modified transudate, pseudochylothorax, or a true chylothorax. Most commonly, it is a modified transudate.
       ii. Echocardiography
          1. Echocardiography is an essential tool to confirm and characterize heart disease in the cat. The diagnosis is made upon determination of wall thickness, chamber dimensions, cardiac valve function, and blood flow turbulence and velocities.
          2. Normal echocardiographic values for cats have been established (table 14.3) but are operator dependent.
          3. Decreased end-diastolic and -systolic volumes with a thickened left ventricular wall are typical for HCM. Increased end-diastolic and -systolic volumes with reduced thickness of the left ventricular wall are characteristic for dilated cardiomyopathy.
          4. The left atrium is almost always enlarged with left-sided CHF.

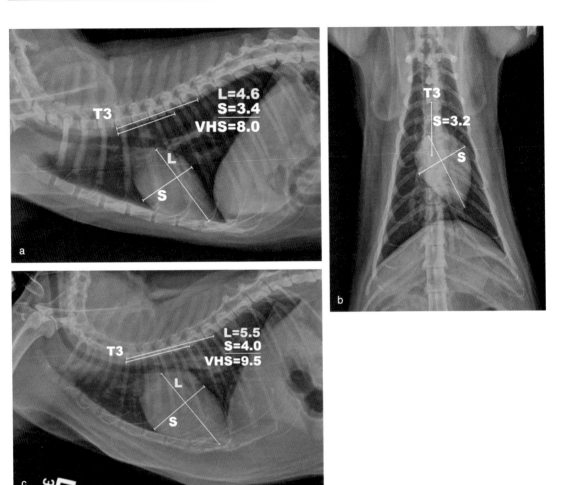

Fig. 14.4. Determination of the vertebral heart size.
a. Determination of the vertebral heart size on the lateral view in a cat with a normal thoracic radiograph: the long axis (L) that leads from the base of the heart (intersection of the trachea with the most ventral apical vein, just cranial to the bifurcation) to the apex of the heart, and the short axis (S) that runs perpendicular to the long axis and at the widest part of the heart. Both lengths of L and S are transferred to overlay the thoracic vertebrae starting at the cranial border of the fourth thoracic vertebra (T4). Summation of L and S leads to the vertebral heart size.
b. Determination of the short-axis cardiac dimension in the ventrodorsal view in the same animal. The short axis (S) runs perpendicular to the long axis (L) at the widest part of the heart. S is then compared to length of the vertebral body identical to the procedure described in 14.4a.
c. Determination of the vertebral heart size in an 1-year-old male castrated cat that presented with congestive heart failure secondary to hypertrophic obstructive cardiomyopathy.

5. Determining the ratio of the left atrial diameter to the aortic root diameter (LA-Ao ratio) facilitates objective judgment of left atrial size. LA-Ao ratio greater than 1.3 suggests left atrial dilation (fig. 14.8).

6. Spontaneous echo contrast ("smoke") in a dilated left atrium is thought to represent thrombus formation and occurs due to blood stasis in the large left atrium. Spontaneous echo contrast indicates an increased risk for thromboembolism (e.g., ATE).

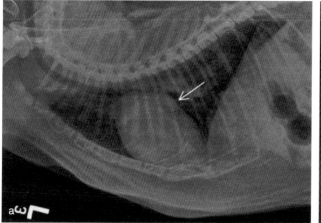
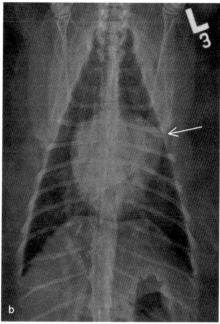

Fig. 14.5. Radiographic appearance of left atrial enlargement in an 11-year-old male castrated cat with hypertrophic obstructive cardiomyopathy.

a. A waistline (arrow) that is not normally visible indicates the presence of an enlarged left atrium.

b. Compared to the lateral view, the enlargement of the left atrium (arrow) is easier to detect on the ventrodorsal view and appears as a prominent bulge at a 2–3-o'clock position. This is not the case in the dog, where the left atrium is positioned between the mainstem bronchi of the caudal lung lobes.

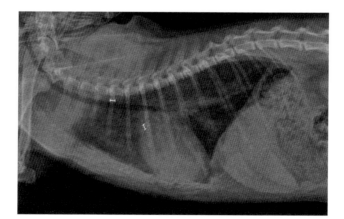

Fig. 14.6. Distension of pulmonary veins in cats is a less consistent marker for left heart failure than in dogs. However, the vessel size is assessed in an identical manner. On a lateral thoracic radiograph, the size of the pulmonary vein (vessel ventral to the bronchus; 5th intercostal space) is considered increased if it surpasses the diameter of the proximal 4th rib. This is the case in this 1-year-old male intact cat with hypertrophic cardiomyopathy.

176

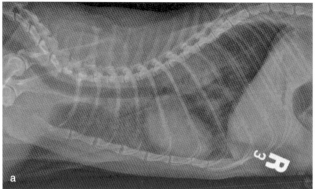

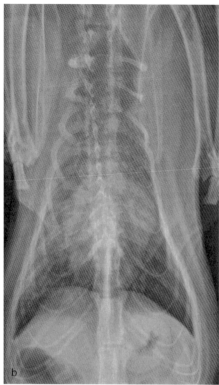

Fig. 14.7. Right lateral (a) and ventrodorsal (b) view of thoracic radiographs of a cat with congestive heart failure exemplifying the characteristic patchy appearance and diffuse distribution of cardiogenic pulmonary edema commonly seen in this species.

Table 14.3. Normal feline echocardiographic values (M-mode; *n* = 79).

Parameter	Mean ± SD	Range	95% CI
LVID$_d$(cm)	1.5 ± 0.2	1.08–2.14	1.46–1.54
LVID$_s$(cm)	0.72 ± 0.15	0.4–1.12	0.69–0.75
LVW$_d$(cm)	0.41 ± 0.07	0.25–0.6	0.39–0.43
LVW$_s$(cm)	0.68 ± 0.11	0.43–0.98	0.66–0.7
IVS$_d$(cm)	0.42 ± 0.07	0.3–0.6	0.4–0.44
IVS$_s$(cm)	0.67 ± 0.12	0.4–0.9	0.64–0.70
Ao	0.95 ± 0.14	0.6–1.21	0.91–0.98
LAD$_s$(cm)	1.17 ± 0.17	0.7–1.7	1.13–1.21
LA:Ao	1.25 ± 0.18	0.88–1.79	1.21–1.29
%FS	52.1 ± 7.11	40–66.7	50.51–53.69
Weight	4.7 ± 1.2	2.7–8.2	4.43–4.97

Modified from Drourr et al. JAVMA, 2005; 226(5):734–737.
LVID$_d$ and LVID$_s$ = Left ventricular internal dimension at end diastole and systole, respectively. LVW$_d$ and LVW$_s$ = Left ventricular wall at end diastole and systole, respectively. IVS$_d$ and IVS$_s$ = Interventricular septal thickness at end diastole and systole, respectively. Ao = Aortic root dimension. LAD$_s$ = Left atrial dimension at end systole. LA:Ao = Left atrium-to-aortic ratio. %FS = Percentage fractional shortening.

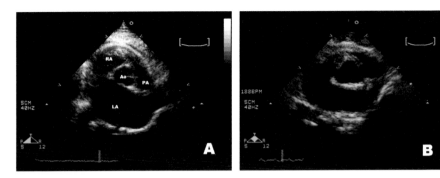

Fig. 14.8. Echocardiographic examination of the heart. Right parasternal short axis view at the level of the heart basis in a cat with hypertrophic obstructive cardiomyopathy (A) and in a cat with a normal heart (B). The left atrial size is markedly larger when compared to the aortic diameter in the cat with heart disease, leading to an increase in the LA-Ao ratio. LA = left atrium; RA = right atrium; Ao = Aorta; PA = pulmonary artery. (Images courtesy of Dr. Nick Russel.)

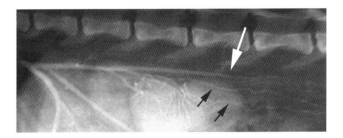

Fig. 14.9. Aortic angiogram of a cat with recurrent aortic thromboembolism (white arrow). Several collateral vessels (black arrows) have been forming as a result of the chronic occlusion of the distal aorta. (Image is courtesy of Dr. James Buchanan and the Veterinary Information Network [VIN.com].)

     7. Systolic anterior motion of the mitral valve describes the displacement of the anterior leaflet of the mitral valve into the left ventricular outflow tract during the rapid left ventricular ejection phase in cats with HCM. Consequences of systolic anterior motion of the mitral valve are dynamic stenosis of the left ventricular outflow tract and mitral regurgitation.

   iii. Angiocardiography

     1. Radiopaque dye is injected in a vessel or heart chamber, which allows visualization of these structures radiographically. It allows identification of vascular shunts, congenital cardiac anomalies, and valvular regurgitation and stenosis, including ATE (fig. 14.9).

     2. Administration of the contrast agent requires the following considerations:

       a. Contrast agents are hypertonic solutions: volume overload and pulmonary edema can occur.

       b. Renal failure can occur after repeated administration and in states of impaired renal blood flow.

  e. Central venous pressure

   i. The central venous pressure (CVP) is the intravascular pressure in the large thoracic veins and is typically measured at the junction of the cranial vena cava and the right atrium via a jugular catheter.

   ii. The CVP is normally used as a marker of intravascular volume status and preload.
   iii. If CVP is intended to serve as an index of cardiac preload, the end-diastolic pressure at end-expiration should be used.
   iv. A CVP of 0–3 mmHg (0–5 cmH$_2$O) is considered normal in a cat.
   v. In cats with heart disease that are in need of IV fluid therapy, the CVP is routinely measured to minimize the risk of causing cardiogenic pulmonary edema. An increase of the CVP above 5 mmHg (7 cmH$_2$O) suggests increased risk of fluid overload and consequent hydrostatic pulmonary edema.
   vi. Factors other than intravascular volume influence the CVP and have to be taken into consideration:
      1. Vascular tone
      2. Right ventricular compliance: myocardial disease (right-sided heart failure), pericardial disease, tamponade
      3. Tricuspid valve disease: stenosis, regurgitation
      4. Cardiac rhythm: atrial fibrillation, AV dissociation
      5. Intrathoracic pressure: pleural effusion (>20 mL/kg), tension pneumothorax, respiration, intermittent positive pressure ventilation, PEEP (positive end expiratory pressure)
f. Arterial blood pressure
   i. In cats, arterial blood pressure is best measured by Doppler sphygmomanometry (normal: 110–150 mmHg).
   ii. If trends are of importance, the same leg should be used for repeated measurements.
   iii. Doppler sphygmomanometry allows assessment of arterial blood pressure even in cats with severe hypotension; however, the correlation between Doppler blood pressure and arterial blood pressure can be affected by variables such as technique (e.g., pressure on transducer), arterial tone (e.g., hypothermia), blood pressure level, and others.
   iv. In cats with low output heart failure, blood pressure is often maintained due to counteracting neuroendocrine responses:
      1. Activation of the sympathoadrenergic system
      2. Activation of the renin-angiotensin-aldosterone system
      3. Secretion of other vasoactive hormones (vasopressin, endothelin)
   v. This has two clinical implications in this group of patients:
      1. A normal arterial blood pressure does not guarantee adequate cardiac output and tissue blood flow.
      2. Occurrence of hypotension indicates decompensation and requires immediate therapeutic intervention (see chap. 15—Management of Specific Cardiac Diseases).

15
MANAGEMENT OF SPECIFIC CARDIAC DISEASES

Mark A. Oyama

Unique Features
- Detection of heart murmurs, gallops, and other physical exam findings of early or mild heart disease in cats can be challenging.
- Chest radiographs are relatively insensitive in detecting heart enlargement in cats.
- Almost all forms of cardiomyopathy in cats result in diastolic heart failure.
- The mainstay of medical therapy in cats with heart failure is diuretics; long-term efficacy of ACE-inhibitors, beta-blockers, and calcium channel blockers is largely unknown.

I. General approach to feline heart disease
    a. The diagnosis and treatment of feline heart disease are challenging. The clinical signs associated with heart disease are often vague and nonspecific. In all but the most advanced cases, assessment of heart size and shape using thoracic radiography is difficult, and echocardiography is typically required for diagnosis. Treatment paradigms are controversial and unproven with respect to increased survival. The fragile clinical state of cats with severe congestive heart failure can hinder diagnostic and therapeutic efforts.
    b. Feline heart diseases can be classified as either primary or secondary.
        i. Primary diseases refer to those that occur in the absence of an identifiable etiology and are typically categorized based on their morphologic appearance. These diseases include hypertrophic, dilated, restrictive, and unclassified cardiomyopathy. Other less common conditions include endomyocardial fibroelastosis, arrhythmogenic right ventricular cardiomyopathy, and excessive left ventricular moderator band cardiomyopathy. These diseases are typically progressive and lead to clinical signs such as heart failure, fainting, or thromboembolism. In virtually all cases of primary disease, treatment is palliative.
        ii. Secondary diseases refer to those with a proven or strongly suspected etiology such as taurine deficiency, thyrotoxicosis, systemic hypertension, toxin (doxorubicin), and infiltrative (neoplasia). Cases of secondary heart disease are often relatively mild and may not be associated with cardiac clinical signs. In some cases (i.e., taurine deficiency, thyrotoxicosis), cardiac pathology is reversible if the underlying cause is successfully managed.
    c. Because most forms of feline heart disease primarily involve diastolic dysfunction, treatment is aimed at relieving signs of congestion, increasing the diastolic filling period, and improving ventricular relaxation.
    d. In cases of systolic dysfunction (i.e., dilated cardiomyopathy), treatment is aimed at relieving signs of congestion and improving contractility.

II. Clinical examination of patients with heart disease
    a. Common presenting complaints include the following:
        i. Tachypnea, dyspnea, inappetence, lethargy, posterior paralysis, or paresis.
        ii. Coughing, which is a common sign in dogs with congestive heart failure, is rare in cats.
        iii. Many patients with heart disease are asymptomatic and identified only after physical examination reveals a murmur or gallop heart sound.
    b. Physical examination findings
        i. Cardiac auscultation
            1. Systolic heart murmur heard along the sternal border
            2. Murmurs may be accentuated during periods of tachycardia.
            3. Diastolic gallop sound (typically due to a fourth heart sound)
            4. Arrhythmia
        ii. Pulmonary auscultation
            1. Increased bronchovesicular sounds
            2. Muffled lung and heart sounds (typical in cases of pleural effusion)
        iii. Jugular venous distension or pulses
        iv. Weak, irregular, or absent femoral pulses
        v. Signs of systemic thromboembolism (i.e., paresis)
    c. Clinical pathology
        i. In most cases, routine serum biochemistry, CBC, and urinalysis do not assist in the clinical diagnosis. These tests are often performed to screen for concurrent disease in geriatric patients or prior to pharmacologic intervention with agents such as diuretics or ACE-inhibitors.
        ii. Cardiac troponin, endothelin, and atrial and B-type natriuretic peptide concentrations are commonly increased in cats with primary and secondary cardiac disease.
        iii. Skeletal muscle enzymes (e.g., CPK) may be increased in cases of systemic thromboembolism.
        iv. Plasma or whole-blood taurine concentration should be determined in cats with poor systolic function (i.e., dilated cardiomyopathy).
        v. Fluid analysis of thoracic or abdominal effusion is commonly performed to screen for potential noncardiac etiologies (i.e., neoplasia, FIP, etc.).
    d. Electrocardiography
        i. In the emergency setting, ECG adds little to the diagnosis of a specific form of heart disease.
        ii. Occasionally, atrial or ventricular premature beats are identified.
        iii. Atrial fibrillation may be present in patients with severe disease.
        iv. Sustained episodes of ventricular tachycardia (>30 sec in duration) are uncommon.
    e. Thoracic radiography
        i. Useful in assessing cardiac size and shape, pulmonary parenchyma, pulmonary vessels, and the thoracic space.
            1. In cases of mild to moderate disease, thoracic radiographs are relatively insensitive and echocardiography may be required.
            2. The dorsoventral projection is the preferred view to assess left atrial size and shape.
        ii. Left-sided heart failure in the cat can result in pleural effusion, pulmonary edema, or both (fig. 15.1).
            1. In cases of severe pleural effusion, assessment of heart size and shape is difficult, and if suspected, therapeutic thoracocentesis should be performed prior to radiography.
            2. Distribution of pulmonary edema in cats is often multifocal and patchy and does not typically accumulate around the pulmonary hilus or in the caudodorsal lung fields as it does in the dog.
        iii. Cats with a fragile clinical presentation may not tolerate restraint for radiography, and the clinician should first attempt to stabilize these patients (see "III. Treatment of life-threatening heart failure" below).

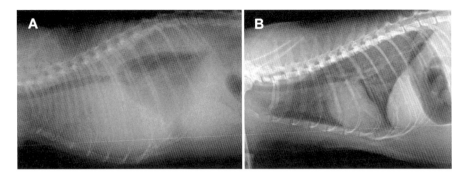

Fig. 15.1.   Lateral chest radiographs from two cats with hypertrophic cardiomyopathy demonstrating (A) pleural effusion; note the compression and rounding of the lung lobes in the dorsocaudal chest and loss of cardiac silhouette; this radiographic finding should initiate prompt pleurocentesis; and (B) pulmonary edema; note the hazy pulmonary pattern in the lung fields, enlarged pulmonary vessels, and enlarged cardiac silhouette. The large amount of air in the stomach is due to aerophagia secondary to severe respiratory distress.

    f. Echocardiography
        i. Useful in assessing cardiac structure and function and achieving a morphologic diagnosis. The echocardiographic examination typically concentrates on left ventricular and interventricular wall thickness, function, echogenicity, left atrial size, mitral valve motion and regurgitation, and presence of dynamic left ventricular outflow tract obstruction (fig. 15.2).
       ii. The typical echocardiographic features of the most common forms of feline cardiomyopathy are as follows. The author notes that disagreement exists regarding the appropriateness of considering restrictive and unclassified cardiomyopathy as two separate clinical diagnoses, rather than grouping them into a single "unclassified" category.
          1. Hypertrophic cardiomyopathy (HCM): idiopathic left ventricular concentric hypertrophy, left atrial enlargement, hyperechoic endocardium, and/or papillary muscles.
          2. Hypertrophic obstructive cardiomyopathy (HOCM): similar features as in HCM but also with systolic anterior motion of the mitral valve that creates a left ventricular outflow tract obstruction.
          3. Restrictive cardiomyopathy (RCM): left and right atrial enlargement, endocardial hyperechogenicity, occasionally bridging ventricular to septal bands of tissue, normal to mild degrees of ventricular hypertrophy, normal to mildly decreased systolic function, restrictive mitral inflow Doppler pattern.
          4. Unclassified cardiomyopathy (UCM): Displays various features of multiple forms of cardiomyopathy and used to describe cats whose cardiac morphology does not fit into any of the above categories.
          5. Endomyocardial fibroelastosis (EMF): widespread thickening and hyperechogenicity of the endocardial surface. Rare. Seen mainly in young Burmese or Siamese cats.
          6. Arrhythmogenic right ventricular cardiomyopathy: severe right atrial and right ventricular dilation, right ventricular aneurysmal dilations and dyskinesis, tricuspid regurgitation. Rare. Often misdiagnosed as congenital tricuspid valve dysplasia.
      iii. Cats with a fragile clinical presentation may not tolerate restraint for echocardiography and the clinician should first attempt to stabilize these patients (see "III. Treatment of life-threatening heart failure" below)
  III. Treatment of life-threatening heart failure (table 15.1)
    a. Regardless of etiology of the underlying cardiomyopathy, emergency treatment consists of an appropriate combination of diuretics, pleurocentesis, and supplemental oxygen (fig. 15.3).

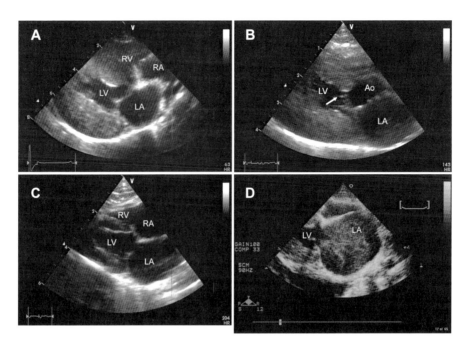

Fig. 15.2. Echocardiographic images from cats with cardiomyopathy. (A) Right parasternal long axis view of a cat with hypertrophic cardiomyopathy. Note the thickening of the ventricular walls and hyperechoic endocardial regions. (B) Right parasternal long axis view of a cat with systolic anterior motion of the mitral valve (arrow). The mitral valve has moved toward the interventricular septum, narrowing the lumen of the outflow tract. A hyperechoic region of the interventricular septum, likely due to repeated contact with the valve, is noted directly opposite the valve leaflet. Note the left atrial enlargement and thickening of the ventricular walls. (C) Right parasternal long axis view of a cat with restrictive cardiomyopathy. Note the enlarged right and left atria and relatively normal-appearing left ventricular wall thickness and chamber diameter. (D) Right parasternal long axis view of a cat with restrictive cardiomyopathy, severe left atrial enlargement, and spontaneous contrast within the atrial chamber. This finding is thought to represent a high risk for development of systemic thromboembolism.

   i. Diuretics
      1. Furosemide (1–2 mg/kg q1–2h IV, IM, SC as needed to alleviate respiratory distress).
      2. Response to diuretic therapy is monitored using respiratory rate and effort. Diuretic dose is sharply decreased once respiratory rate begins to decrease or is approximately 40 breaths/min (see "IV. Treatment of chronic heart failure" below).
      3. Overzealous diuretic therapy can precipitate or aggravate renal insufficiency. Thus, free-choice water is typically offered during acute treatment and the patient is monitored to ensure that urine is being produced.
      4. Mild increases in serum BUN (<60 mg/dL), creatinine (<2.5 mg/dL), and total solids are indications that effective diuresis is occurring.
         a. Supplemental parenteral fluids are not indicated unless cats demonstrate signs of low-output failure (i.e., hypotension), are severely dehydrated, cease taking in oral fluids, or are at high risk for acute renal failure due to preexisting renal insufficiency.
   ii. Pleurocentesis
      1. Most cats will tolerate pleurocentesis without chemical restraint.
      2. The author prefers use of a 21-gauge butterfly catheter.
      3. Typically, aspiration occurs over the 7th to 9th intercostal space.

Table 15.1. Commonly used drugs and doses in cats with heart failure.

Drugs	Indications	Mechanisms of Action	Adverse Effects	Dosages
ACE inhibitors	All forms of cardiomyopathy	Antagonize renin-angiotensin-aldosterone axis	Azotemia, hypotension	PO: enalapril, 0.5 mg/kg q12–24h; PO: benazepril, 0.25–0.5 mg/kg q24h
Atenolol	HCM, HOCM, RCM, UCM	Beta-blocker	Bradycardia, hypotension	PO: 6.25–12.5 mg/cat q12–24h
Digoxin	DCM, +/− RCM	Positive inotrope	GI upset, arrhythmias	PO: cats 1.9–3.2 kg, 0.031 mg/cat q72h; cats 3.3–6.0 kg, 0.031 mg/cat q24–28h; cats >6.0 kg, 0.031 mg/cat q12–24hrs
Diltiazem	HCM, HOCM, RCM, UCM	Ca-channel blocker	Bradycardia, hypotension, GI upset, inappetence	PO: Cardizem CD, 10 mg/kg q24h; PO: Dilacor XR, 30–60 mg/cat q12h; PO: diltiazem, 0.5–1.5 mg/kg q8h
Dobutamine	DCM	Sympathomimetic	Tachycardia, seizures	CRI: 2–10 µg/kg/min
Dopamine	DCM	Sympathomimetic	Tachycardia, vasoconstriction	CRI: 2–5 µg/kg/min
Esmolol	Ventricular or supraventricular tachycardia	Beta-blocker	Bradycardia	IV: 250–500 µg/kg slow bolus, 50–200 µg/kg/min CRI
Furosemide	CHF	Loop diuretic; for treatment of life-threatening heart failure, for treatment of chronic heart failure	Dehydration, hypokalemia	IV/IM/SC: 1–2 mg/kg q1–2h; PO/SC: 6.25–12.5 mg/cat q12–24hs
Hydrochlorothiazide	Refractory CHF	Distal tubule diuretic	Azotemia, hypokalemia	PO: 1–2 mg/kg q12–24 h
Hydrochlorothiazide/ Spironolactone	Refractory CHF	Distal tubule diuretic/ potassium-sparing diuretic	Azotemia, potassium imbalance	PO: 2.2 mg/kg q24h
Lidocaine	Ventricular arrhythmias	Na-channel blocker	Hypotension, seizures	IV: 0.25–0.75 mg/cat slow bolus
Propranolol	HCM, HOCM, RCM, UCM	Beta-blocker	Bradycardia, hypotension, aggravation of asthma or diabetes mellitus	PO: 5–10 mg/cat q8–12 h

Note: HCM = hypertrophic cardiomyopathy; HOCM = hypertrophic obstructive cardiomyopathy; RCM = restrictive cardiomyopathy; UCM = unclassified cardiomyopathy; DCM = dilated cardiomyopathy; CHF = congestive heart failure.

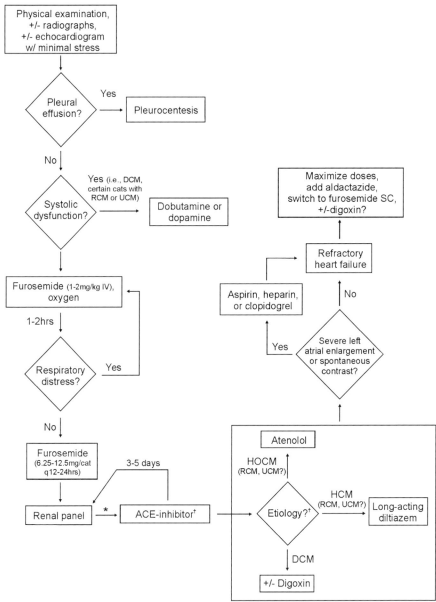

*Treatments beyond use of furosemide are of unknown and unproven efficacy.
†Recommendation of this treatment is based particularly on the author's experiences and preferences; clinical studies are required to document efficacy.

Fig. 15.3. Treatment algorithm for treatment of heart failure in cats. See text for further details and discussion.

    4. Pleurocentesis is an *essential* aspect of treatment in cats with effusions. Diuretic therapy alone is ineffective at significantly alleviating respiratory distress due to large accumulations of pleural effusion.
  iii. Supplemental oxygen
    1. Housing in an oxygen cage at 40% O$_2$ or greater.

     iv. Topical nitroglycerin paste (¼–½ inch topically on the inner pinna of the ear q6h) is occasionally administered but is of dubious efficacy.

     v. Cats with systolic dysfunction (i.e., DCM, some cases of UCM or RCM) benefit from intravenous inotropic support.

        1. Dobutamine (2–10 mcg/kg min CRI) is the preferred drug, seizures may occur.

        2. Dopamine (2–5 mg/kg/min CRI), excessive tachycardia may occur.

        3. Excessive tachycardia in cats with diastolic disease further impairs diastolic function and filling and should be avoided.

b. Confounding factors affecting emergency treatment

     i. Systemic thromboembolism (see section below)

     ii. Arrhythmias

        1. Ventricular premature beats are relatively common but often resolve once congestive heart failure is treated. Ventricular tachycardia is relatively uncommon. Standardized treatment recommendations are not available (see chap. 17—Management of Life-Threatening Arrhythmias).

           a. Beta-blockers

              i. Atenolol 6.25 mg PO q12–24h

              ii. Esmolol 250–500 µg/kg slow IV bolus, 50–200 µg/kg/min CRI

           b. Lidocaine (0.25–0.75 mg/cat slow IV bolus) may cause seizures.

        2. Atrial fibrillation is infrequently detected in cases with severe atrial enlargement, and treatment to slow the ventricular rate is considered.

           a. Beta-blockers (see "IV. Treatment of chronic heart failure")

           b. Calcium channel blockers (see "IV. Treatment of chronic heart failure")

           c. Digoxin is not commonly used due to high risk for toxicity.

IV. Treatment of chronic heart failure

a. Goals of treatment include alleviation of respiratory signs (i.e., congestive failure), prevention of syncope, sudden death, and systemic thromboembolism, and alleviation of left ventricular outflow tract obstruction caused by systolic anterior motion of the mitral valve. In cats with systolic dysfunction, positive inotropes are also used (see fig. 15.3).

b. Beyond diuretic therapy, the ideal treatment of feline cardiomyopathy has not been established. A combination of diuretics, beta-blockers or calcium channel blockers, and ACE-inhibitors is typically used.

c. Diuretics

     i. Furosemide (6.25 mg/cat PO q12–24h) is typically administered. The dose is tailored to the lowest dose required to control congestive signs. Thus, some cats can be maintained on 6.26–12.5 mg/cat PO every other day, while others will require 12.5 mg/cat q12–24h)

     ii. Periodic evaluation of renal function is recommended while receiving diuretics.

d. Beta-blockers

     i. Primarily used in cats with HCM and HOCM. Occasionally used in RCM, UCM, and EMF if cats are tachycardic. Atenolol (6.25–12.5 mg/cat PO q12–24h) or propranolol (5–10 mg/cat PO q8–12h) is used to slow heart rate, improve diastolic filling, and suppress ventricular arrhythmias.

     ii. Despite widespread use of beta-blockers, particularly in cats with concurrent left ventricular outflow tract obstruction (i.e., HOCM), long-term benefit is unproven.

     iii. Due to risk of bradycardia and hypotension, combination therapy with beta-blockers and calcium channel blockers is not recommended. The superiority of either treatment has not been rigorously established. Often, beta-blockers are chosen for cats with the obstructive form of hypertrophic cardiomyopathy, while calcium-channel blockers are chosen in cats without obstruction or in cats with restrictive/unclassified cardiomyopathy.

e. Calcium channel blockers

     i. Primarily used in cats with HCM and HOCM. Occasionally used in cats with RCM, UCM, and EMF.

       ii. Slow heart rate, improve diastolic filling, and theoretically improve diastolic relaxation. Long-acting formulations provide the advantage of longer dosing intervals.
          1. Cardizem CD (10 mg/kg PO q24h)
          2. Dilacor XR (30–60 mg/cat PO q12h)
       iii. Avoid concurrent use with beta-blockers (see above)
   f. ACE inhibitors
       i. The author uses ACE inhibitors in cats with any form of cardiomyopathy if they are concurrently receiving diuretic therapy.
       ii. Reduce activation of the renin-angiotensin-aldosterone axis, and theoretically ameliorate pathologic ventricular and coronary arterial remodeling and improve diastolic dysfunction. ACE inhibitors with high tissue penetration, such as benazepril, may be particularly advantageous.
          1. Enalapril (0.5 mg/kg PO q12–24h)
          2. Benazepril (0.25–0.5 mg/kg q24h)
       iii. Despite their vasodilatory capacity, ACE inhibitors do not significantly aggravate preexisting left ventricular outflow tract obstruction in cats with HOCM.
   g. Digoxin
       i. Use is restricted to cats with evidence of systolic dysfunction (i.e., DCM).
       ii. Risk of toxicity is relatively high, and stringent monitoring of patient's serum levels, appetite, and attitude is required.
       iii. Digoxin 0.031 mg/cat q72h in cats weighing 1.9–3.2 kg, 0.031 mg/cat q24–48h in cats weighing 3.3–6 kg, and 0.031 mg/cat q12–24h in cats >6 kg. The author rarely administers more than 0.031 mg/cat q24h.
   h. Taurine
       i. Supplementation (250–500 mg/cat q12h) is recommended in all cats with systolic dysfunction. Ideally, plasma or whole-blood taurine levels should be determined prior to supplementation, but the assay is not widely available.
   i. Antithrombotic therapy (see below)
V. Monitoring patients with chronic heart failure
   a. Owners are instructed to monitor patient appetite, activity level, respiratory effort, and rate.
   b. Adequate beta-adrenergic blockade is presumed if heart rate remains <150 bpm during in-hospital examination.
   c. Periodic evaluation of BUN, creatinine, and serum electrolytes is performed.
   d. Effective resolution of left ventricular outflow tract obstruction is accompanied by disappearance or reduction of heart murmur and resolution of systolic anterior motion of the mitral valve on echocardiographic examination. In some cases, this may be accompanied by partial or complete regression of left ventricular hypertrophy, and prognosis is favorable.
VI. Treatment of refractory or advanced heart failure
   a. In patients presenting with continued signs of congestive failure despite therapy, additional medications are required.
   b. Treatment strategies include increasing doses of existing therapy, prescribing additional classes of diuretics, altering route of furosemide administration, and addition of digoxin in cases of right-sided failure.
       i. Beta-blocker, calcium-channel blocker, and ACE-inhibitor therapy is maximized.
       ii. Hydrochlorothiazide (1–2 mg/kg q12–24h) is added to enhance diuresis. Alternatively, a combination of hydrochlorothiazide and spironolactone can be used (Aldactazide, 2.2 mg/kg q24h).
       iii. Route of administration of furosemide is changed from PO to SC. This strategy often permits a slight decrease in the dose as bioavailability is improved.
       iv. Digoxin (see above for dosages and precautions)
VII. Treatment and prevention of systemic thromboembolism

a. Systemic thromboembolism (STE) is a devastating complication of feline cardiomyopathy due to its acute onset, poor treatment options, high recurrence rate, and associated morbidity to the patient.

b. Etiology is likely a combination of blood stasis, local endothelial or endomyocardial injury, and hypercoagulability. The most common site of STE is the distal aorta (saddle thromboembolism).

   i. Echocardiographic evidence of severe left atrial enlargement or spontaneous contrast ("smoke") within the left atrium are considered risk factors for thrombus development.

c. Treatment of STE involves (1) promoting collateral circulation, (2) thrombolytic therapy, (3) anticoagulation, (4) alleviating patient pain and distress, (5) preventing recurrence, and (6) treatment of concomitant congestive heart failure. All aspects of treatment are challenging and prognosis is extremely guarded.

   i. Clinical signs of grave prognosis include evidence of multiple sites of STE (i.e., renal or mesenteric arteries), progressive loss of limb function/viability, coexisting refractory congestive heart failure or arrhythmias, hyperkalemia due to reperfusion injury, identification of intracardiac thrombus, severe hypothermia or cardiac shock, and owners who are unwilling to provide intensive and often frustrating long-term home care.

d. Approximately 50% of cats with STE are euthanized, 25% succumb during initial treatment in the hospital, and 25% are eventually discharged. Of the cats that leave the hospital, it is the author's experience that many are soon euthanized once owners attempt to provide extended home care. Other cats may recover enough function within several days to weeks to adequately ambulate and maintain an acceptable quality of life. Sloughing and necrosis of affected tissues can occur, and in these cases, amputation is the only remedy (fig. 15.4). Recurrence of thromboembolism or congestive heart failure is likely.

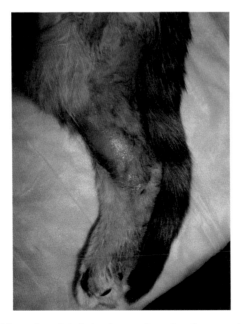

Fig. 15.4. Medial surface of the right pelvic limb of a cat 3 weeks after experiencing a saddle thrombus. Note the moist dermatitis and necrosis of superficial tissues indicating loss of viability and poor collateral circulation. Prognosis for limb salvage is grave, and eventual amputation is likely required should the owner choose to continue treatment.

    e. Specific therapy: see chap. 16—Management of Thromboembolic Disease Secondary to Heart Disease.

    f. Treatment of concurrent congestive heart failure

       i. Diuretics are used judiciously to avoid excessive dehydration, vasoconstriction, and compromise of collateral circulation.

    g. Supportive care

       i. Aggressive pain control is achieved during the initial episode using an appropriate combination of aspirin, morphine (0.05–0.1 mg/kg administered epidurally), oxymorphone (0.05–0.15 mg/kg IM or IV q6h) and butorphanol (0.02–0.4 mg/kg IM or SC q4h).

       ii. Promotion of collateral circulation is achieved by acepromazine (0.05–0.1 mg/kg IV), judicious fluid therapy, and maintenance of proper body temperature.

      iii. Nutritional support through a nasoesophageal feeding tube.

      iv. Prevention of self-mutilation using loose-fitting bandage material or an e-collar.

      v. Access to litter box, food, and water.

      vi. Physical therapy of the affected legs (i.e., massage or range of motion) is of questionable value and may precipitate patient discomfort or stress.

16
MANAGEMENT OF THROMBOEMBOLIC DISEASE SECONDARY TO HEART DISEASE

Amy J. Alwood

a. Arterial thromboembolism is an acute and potentially catastrophic syndrome that most commonly occurs in association with heart disease in cats (i.e., cardiogenic arterial thromboembolism; CATE). Other diseases associated with arterial thromboembolism include hyperthyroidism, neoplasia, and less commonly, sepsis or trauma. This chapter will focus on the approach to cardiogenic arterial thromboembolism, although the initial approach to arterial thromboembolism will be similar independent of the underlying cause or risk factors associated with thromboembolism.
b. The most common site(s) affected in CATE is the aortic trifurcation supplying the pelvic limbs. Partial or complete obstruction of flow in one or both femoral arteries leads to the common clinical signs of acute onset paresis of one or both hind limbs (more on clinical signs below). Other sites that may be affected either alternatively or concurrently include
   i. Left forelimb (brachial artery)
   ii. Right forelimb (brachial artery)
   iii. Mesenteric and/or renal arteries
   iv. Cerebral arteries
c. Clinical signs:
   i. Acute or peracute paresis of the affected limb(s), often severe enough to prevent walking. Patients often present dragging both hind limbs. A common presenting complaint may include an owner suspicious of a traumatic injury involving the spine or pelvis.
   ii. Tachypnea (which may represent pain or true respiratory compromise secondary to congestive heart failure)
   iii. Open-mouth breathing is fairly common in affected cats but in these patients can again represent either pain, behavioral distress, or true dyspnea.
   iv. Palpation of the affected limb(s) often reveals a cool extremity with absent or weak pulses.
   v. Upon inspection of the digital pads of the affected limbs, the clinician may find pale/cyanotic tissue corresponding with the severe compromise of primary circulation; however, this is not always readily appreciated despite significant obstruction of the main vessel(s). (The reader is reminded that collateral circulation preserves some flow to the affected limb even though the dominant supply may be occluded).
d. Triage/initial assessment
   i. Observation
      a. Cats with acute systemic arterial thromboembolism are distressed independent of true dyspnea. They are typically painful. Brief observation from a distance while providing oxygen via an

191

oxygen cage or flow-by oxygen can allow for initial assessment without adding to the stress that the patient is experiencing.

ii. Thoracic auscultation

a. Thoracic auscultation can be performed quickly and safely in most patients.

b. Initial auscultation should first include all regions of the thorax to detect any pulmonary crackles (suggesting pulmonary edema) or regions of diminished or dull lung sounds (suggesting possible pleural effusion).

c. Auscultation of the heart should assess rate and evaluate for the presence of a murmur or gallop.

iii. Peripheral circulation

a. Similar parameters should be assessed as with any routine triage: mucous membrane color, capillary refill time, and pulse quality as well as comparative assessment of temperature of the distal limbs.

b. Careful assessment of femoral pulses in both limbs as well as assessment of the distal pulses in all limbs is central to diagnosis of arterial thromboembolism. Additional information on diagnosis is provided below.

c. Observation of distal limbs should include assessment of the color of the digital pads—pale/gray coloration may be noted in the pads of affected limbs.

d. If assessment/definitive diagnosis is uncertain after routine physical examination, paired/comparative measurement of noninvasive blood pressure of a forelimb and hind limb can be performed (i.e., in a patient with a thrombus of the iliac artery; the BP would be expected to be obtained with relative ease in the forelimb and should be greater than that obtained in the hind limb. In many cases of distal iliac thrombembolism, a blood pressure (or pulsatile sounds with the Doppler) is not detectable in the affected limb[s]). Similarly, paired lactate measurements are sometimes evaluated. The measured lactate in the affected limb is higher than that in the unaffected limb. Similarly, blood glucose is often lower in the affected extremity than that in the normal extremity.

NOTE: THE AUTHOR DISCOURAGES USE OF DEEP CLIPPING OF THE TOENAIL TO ASSESS FOR LACK OF BLOOD FLOW. (The diagnostic tools listed above offer a less painful yet effective and sensitive means of diagnosis and should be chosen preferentially to deep nail clipping.)

iv. Further assessment of respiratory function

a. When possible, pulse oximetry provides more objective and detailed information about lung function; however, poor perfusion, especially in cases with concurrent heart failure, may make obtaining an accurate reading with pulse oximetry challenging.

b. Any cat showing signs of respiratory compromise should be given oxygen supplementation (see chap. 10).

e. Initial treatment

i. Oxygen therapy: Any cat showing signs of respiratory compromise should be given oxygen supplementation (see chap. 10—Respiratory Emergencies and Pleural Space Disease).

ii. Early use of analgesic therapy is encouraged. For specific recommendations and dosing, refer to the section below on comprehensive treatment.

iii. Diuretic therapy: An initial dose of 1–2 mg/kg (administered IV or IM) furosemide should be administered to cats with evidence of congestive heart failure (e.g., respiratory distress with increased lung sounds or pulmonary crackles).

f. Secondary assessment and comprehensive diagnostics

i. The secondary survey occurs after assessment and stabilization of the immediate and life-threatening conditions.

ii. Full physical assessment/examination with particular note of the following:

a. Thoracic auscultation

b. Pulse quality

      c. Careful assessment of the hind limbs for any muscle rigidity or contraction (particularly the gastrocnemius muscle in each leg can often be firm to palpation). Also note forelimb(s) for any postural changes/paresis.

      d. Rectal temperature

  iii. Clinical pathology/diagnostic samples

      a. Chemistry panel

      b. T4 and/or free T4

      c. CBC

      d. Urinalysis

      e. +/– Coagulation panel

      f. Thromboelastography

        1. Thromboelastography (TEG) is a specialized analysis of hemostasis utilizing citrated whole blood. This technology (which involves the instrument, a computer, and special software to process and translate results into a digital image) provides a global assessment of hemostasis (incorporating the effects of clotting factors, platelets, and fibrinolysis). TEG has gained interest in veterinary medicine in recent years because of its ability to assess hemostasis more comprehensively and because of its unique ability to identify hypercoagulable states. As such, TEG has the potential to be applied as a screening tool to cats known to have underlying heart disease in an attempt to identify degree of risk for thromboembolic disease. The application of TEG in veterinary medicine has recently been extended to use in feline patients. However, the necessity of performing the analysis on whole blood samples (citrated whole blood) within 30 minutes of sample collection requires that samples be collected and analyzed on site (remote sample submission is not possible). Currently, the presence of TEG analyzers is limited to a small number of academic or specialty veterinary institutions; hence, universal clinical use of TEG remains unlikely. As well, while research in this area is currently underway at multiple institutions, no data yet exists documenting the ability of TEG to distinguish which cats are at greater risk for clot events.

  iv. Imaging

      a. Chest radiographs are advised in all cases of suspected or confirmed CATE to evaluate or confirm the presence of congestive heart failure as well as potential identification of cardiomegaly (keeping in mind that many cats with cardiomyopathy will have no overt changes to the appearance of the cardiac silhouette on films).

      b. Echocardiogram: ultimately the performance of an echocardiogram allows confirmed diagnosis of underlying cardiac disease and the potential of a clot present in the left atrium.

      c. +/– Abdominal ultrasound is not an essential diagnostic in most cases but is sometimes utilized to sonographically confirm the presence of a thrombus at the aortic bifurcation or branching iliac arteries. More often it may be of value in cases suspected to have more extensive thrombosis involving the renal or mesenteric arteries.

g. Comprehensive treatment (short- and long-term)

  i. Continued diuretic therapy as needed for congestive heart failure (see chap. 15—Management of Specific Cardiac Diseases).

  ii. Continued oxygen therapy as needed.

  iii. Analgesia should be provided and may be selected from the following (see chap. 7—Pain Management in Critically Ill Feline Patients for more details):

      a. Buprenex 0.01–0.03 mg/kg IM or IV q6–8h

      b. Morphine 0.05–0.2 mg/kg IM or SQ q2–4h

      c. Fentanyl

        1. Injectable fentanyl: 4–10 µg/kg as initial IV bolus followed by a constant rate infusion at 4–10 µg/kg/hr.

2. Fentanyl patch placement (either 12.5 or 25 µg/hr based on patient size) may be considered for analgesia after initial patient stabilization and restoration of normal systemic circulation (use would not be advised for a patient in congestive heart failure as the impact of congestive failure on the pharmacokinetics of transdermal fentanyl has not been determined and the risk of ineffective analgesia exists).

   d. Butorphanol 0.2–0.4 mg/kg IM or IV q2–4h

   e. Hydromorphone 0.1–0.2 mg/kg IM or IV q2–6h

   f. NSAIDS SHOULD NOT BE USED ACUTELY DUE TO RISK OF RENAL INJURY.

iv. Anxiolytic therapy: administration of an injectable anxiolytic may be considered in addition to (but not as a replacement for) analgesic therapy.

   a. Diazepam or midazolam may be administered as intermittent IV injections at a dose of 0.2–0.5 mg/kg (an initial dose of midazolam IM may also be considered if IV access has not yet been achieved).

   b. Acepromezine may be administered by injection (IV or IM) in cardiovascularly stable patients (i.e., patients that are normotensive) at a dose of 0.005–0.02 mg/kg. It is thought that in addition to its anxiolytic effects, administration of acepromazine may also augment collateral circulation in the affected limb(s).

v. Monitoring

   a. Serial monitoring of electrolytes, renal values, and PCV/TS as an indicator of hydration status/fluid balance should be considered while patients are receiving acute/inpatient therapy. This is particularly true of patients receiving diuretic therapy for congestive heart failure or patients that are severely affected and where concern for ischemia-reperfusion injury exists.

     The majority of cases are treated supportively/symptomatically with secondary focus on complications. It is not common to pursue or attempt definitive treatment of the thromboembolism; however, several treatment options do exist but typically require or are most appropriately pursued at a secondary or tertiary referral center.

vi. Medical and surgical options for acute TE

   a. Pharmacologic thrombolytic therapy frequently has been considered for patients with CATE. Systemic administration of tissue plasminogen activator (tPA) and streptokinase have most commonly been reported. However, the use of these drugs remains a subject of continued debate as no convincing improvement in outcome has been seen, and in fact a higher risk of reperfusion complications, hemorrhage, or death may be associated with these drugs. At this time the author does not routinely advise the use of thrombolytic therapy.

   b. Interventional/catheter-assisted embolectomy has been reported, but while return of blood flow was achieved, there was no improved outcome in the cases treated with this specialized therapy. As with medical thrombolysis, this therapy is currently associated with a higher risk of complications and death.

   c. Surgical embolectomy is not considered a practical clinical therapy for CATE. In addition to the risk of complications (i.e., hemorrhage, reperfusion injury, embolism, and death), extended general anesthesia would be contraindicated for acute CATE patients.

vii. Prophylactic antithrombotic therapies: There are no antithrombotic therapies with proven benefit for treatment or prevention in cats with ATE. In addition, there are few therapies with known pharmacokinetics to guide dosing. However, it is important to consider antithrombotic therapy in cats affected with CATE and discuss options for future prophylaxis with owners.

   a. Heparins

     1. Unfractionated heparin (UFH) may be administered subcutaneously for future prophylaxis. Prior to initiation of UFH therapy, a baseline-activated partial thromboplastin time (aPTT) should be obtained. A dose of 250 IU/kg SQ q6h has been shown to achieve the desired prolongation of PTT (1.5–2 times patient baseline) in healthy cats in an experimental setting. However, the actual dose found to be effective in individual cats with illness may vary; hence,

the dose administered to a patient will likely need to be adjusted based on serial monitoring of aPTT (anticipate a dosing range of 150–300 IU/kg SQ q6–8h in most clinical circumstances). If acute therapy (with rapid onset of effect) is desired, IV administration of the initial dose (200–250 IU/kg IV once) followed by intermittent SQ administration may be pursued. Administration of the initial UFH dose intravenously may be of particular benefit to hemodynamically unstable patients in congestive heart failure. Note: If baseline (pretreatment) coagulation analysis identifies a mild prolongation of PT or aPTT, more conservative dosing (25% reduction of initial dosing recommendations) may be considered, and closer monitoring of clotting times would be advised. If moderate to severe prolongation of clotting time(s) is noted, repeat analysis in 12–24 hours may be warranted prior to initiating heparin therapy.

2. Dalteparin (Fragmin) is a low-molecular-weight heparin (LMWH) that has a longer half-life than UFH when administered to people. Recent studies would suggest this is not true in normal cats; however, many veterinarians still find this heparin appealing for the potential benefit in prophylaxis and the need for less frequent monitoring compared to UFH. Dosing is species-specific and currently limited to subcutaneous administration. Recommended dosing is 150 IU/kg SQ q4–6h. Baseline PT and aPTT may be obtained prior to initiating therapy to confirm clotting times are normal prior to administering an antithrombotic agent, but baseline values are not part of monitoring of LMWHs. Monitoring is recommended but requires measurement of anti-Xa levels (inhibition of the activity of activated Factor X) with a specialized and standardized assay requiring submission of samples to the Comparative Coagulation Laboratory of Cornell University. Routine monitoring is based on peak anti-Xa activity levels (drawn 2 hours after drug administration) with the goal of achieving values between 0.5 and 1.0 IU/mL. Steady-state effect with low molecular weight heparins may not be achieved until 48–72 hours of use, so unless concern for excess drug effect exists, monitoring is not advised until 2–3 days after initiating treatment. Dalteparin is not commonly used by the author due to its short half-life and the need for frequent administration. Some specialists do advocate for reduced dosing and less frequent administration of dalteparin in cats (i.e., 100 IU/kg SQ q12h); however, pharmacokinetic studies in normal cats would suggest lower dosages, and less frequent administration may be inadequate. In general, there is uncertainty about the optimal use of dalteparin in cats with CATE and its efficacy at any dose. Cost and availability can be a significant limiting factor for use of this medication long-term.

3. Enoxaparin (Lovenox) is another LMWH with a slightly longer half-life in cats (relative to dalteparin) and is the author's preferred LMWH choice for cats. Recommended dosing is 1.25 mg/kg SQ q6h (in some cases, it may be possible to adjust frequency of administration to q8h for long-term therapy). As with dalteparin, cost and availability may be a limiting factor for some clients and their patients, and therefore some specialists advocate for reduced dosing and less frequent administration (i.e., 1 mg/kg SQ q12h, but as with dalteparin, pharmacokinetic studies in normal cats would suggest lower dosages, and less frequent administration may be inadequate). Also, monitoring should be considered, and the recommendations for monitoring of enoxaparin are the same as those described above for dalteparin.

b. Warfarin has been reported previously but is uncommonly used due to the challenges of appropriate dosing and the risk of serious bleeding complications. If warfarin is to be used, it would be advised to pursue such treatment with the involvement of a specialist experienced with the use of this antithrombotic therapy.

1. Standard dosing recommendations of 0.06–0.09 mg/kg PO q24h necessitate compounding of the medication since tablets CANNOT be split (the medication is not evenly distributed within a standard tablet, and administration of a portion of a tablet will result in erratic and

unsafe dosing). Daily monitoring is necessary when initiating therapy, with less frequent monitoring being possible long-term. Monitoring requires establishment of an international normalized ratio (INR) with an established laboratory, and while prolongation of prothrombin time is seen with this therapy and is incorporated within the determination of a lab's INR, simple use of PT prolongation as a monitor of therapy would be considered below the standard of care.

    c. Primary platelet antagonists

        1. Aspirin (chronic): 0.5–1 mg/kg or 5 mg/cat q72h (Note: This is the advised dosage of aspirin for clot prevention in cats as it is believed to be effective while limiting side effects; however, it requires the use of a compounding pharmacy, and as a result some veterinarians and/or clients may prefer the use of 20 mg aspirin q72h [¼ of an 81-mg tablet].)

        2. Clopidogrel, an oral antiplatelet agent (chronic): 18.75 mg (¼ of a 75-mg tablet) q24h

        3. While some specialists will consider concurrent use of aspirin and clopidogrel, generally use of either aspirin or clopidogrel would be the standard approach to antiplatelet/antithrombotic therapy. Monitoring of platelet antagonists is not readily performed in the clinical setting and is generally limited to academic institutions with specific platelet function analysis available (i.e., PFA-100, TEG with Platelet Mapping, Verify Now). The author would caution against concurrent use of aspirin *and* clopidogrel at this time unless appropriate platelet function analysis indicates that an individual cat is in fact resistant to standard, single-agent therapy.

  viii. Physical therapy/convalescence

    a. Passive range of motion exercises should be performed several times daily in all patients as soon as their comfort allows.

    b. Bladder care: periodic bladder expression or assistance with litter box use may occasionally be needed early on in some cases.

h. Short-term complications or sequelae

  i. Ischemia-reperfusion (IR) injury: While uncommon unless thrombolytic therapy is utilized, it still can occur in cases treated with supportive care alone, particularly in cases that achieve rapid recovery of circulation. Primary features of ischemia-reperfusion injury include development of metabolic acidosis and hyperkalemia. Marked elevation of potassium levels, which have the potential to cause significant arrhythmias, are of greatest clinical concern. Hence, regular ECG analysis or continuous ECG monitoring may be considered. As well, periodic evaluation of electrolytes (and venous acid-base status) may be considered every 12–24 hours to monitor for early signs of IR injury.

  ii. Delayed onset of congestive heart failure

  iii. Organ failure secondary to extensive thrombosis or IR injury

i. Prognosis

  i. Numerous studies have documented that both short-term and long-term prognoses are negatively affected by the presence of concurrent congestive heart failure in cats with CATE.

  ii. Survival to hospital discharge: in addition to the presence of congestive heart failure, several characteristics have been associated with short-term survival

    a. Single-limb involvement favors hospital discharge.

    b. Presence of motor function (in the affected limb[s]) favors hospital discharge.

    c. Hypothermia: While hypothermia is common in cats presenting acutely, a single study evaluating 127 cats identified a 50% probability of survival in cats with a body temperature of 98.9°F. In this same study, a body temperature of 96°F appeared to be associated with only a 25% probability of survival.

  iii. Recovery of limb function should be anticipated in most cats but occurs over days to weeks, or in some cases even months.

  iv. Long-term complications/risk of recurrence

a. It is important to note and communicate to cat owners that progression of heart disease, future episodes of congestive failure, and euthanasia related to these factors are much more likely to influence long-term survival and complications than the thromboembolic event itself or recurrence of thromboembolic disease. However, repeat clot events do occur in about 25% of cases. (For further information on survival in cats with heart disease, readers may also refer to chap. 15—Management of Specific Cardiac Diseases.)
b. Complications in the affected limb(s) are in fact uncommon, but limb contracture, self-trauma, and tissue/limb necrosis may occur in a minority of cases (approximately 10–15% of cases).

17
MANAGEMENT OF LIFE-THREATENING ARRHYTHMIAS

Meg M. Sleeper

Unique Features

Clinically relevant arrhythmias are less common in cats than dogs. Ventricular tachycardias are the most common necessitating therapy. Highlights:

- Cats are more sensitive to the neurotoxic effects of lidocaine, and care should be taken when using this medication in cats. If seizure activity does occur, diazepam should be administered for control.
- Vagal maneuvers are not always effective, but the technique should be a first-line approach in cats presenting with rapid tachycardias that are narrow or wide complex in QRS morphology.
- B adrenergic blockers, while primarily for supraventricular tachycardias, may also be beneficial in some cats with ventricular tachycardia.

A. Overview
  a. Feline arrhythmias are similar to those seen in dogs, but they occur less commonly.
  b. Arrhythmias can be secondary to primary heart disease or due to extracardiac disease.
  c. All cats presenting with arrhythmias should be screened for the following abnormalities. Correction of the underlying disease often results in abolition of the arrhythmia.
      i. Hyperthyroidism may be associated with sinus tachycardia, atrial, ectopy, and/or conduction disturbances. Electrocardiographic (ECG) changes are most common with severe thyroid hormone elevations or chronic disease.
      ii. Hyperkalemia may be associated with atrial standstill or sinoventricular rhythms. Urethral obstruction is the most common cause, but hyperkalemia can also be caused by acute renal failure or reperfusion following arterial thromboembolic disease. Classic ECG changes associated with hyperkalemia include
          1. absent or flattened P waves
          2. widened QRS complex
          3. tall, or spiked, T waves
B. When to treat
  a. Arrhythmias are clinically relevant when they cause hemodynamic consequences (such as systemic hypotension) or degenerate into unstable forms (i.e., rapid ventricular tachycardia with R on T; fig. 17.1). In these scenarios they should be treated, but otherwise therapy is not recommended.
  b. The clinical signs most frequently associated with feline arrhythmias are lethargy, syncope, weakness, or sudden death. Additionally, in some cases the arrhythmia may contribute to decompensation of congestive heart failure.

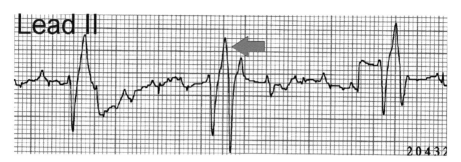

Fig. 17.1. Lead II strip from a cat run at 25 mm/sec and 20 mm/mV. Note the several ventricular premature complexes (VPCs) that are wider and taller than the normal sinus beats. In the middle of this ECG strip, two closely coupled VPCs occur. In this couplet, the QRS from the second complex occurs nearly on top of the preceding T wave (arrow), a phenomenon called "R on T."

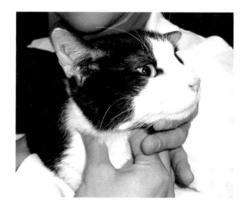

Fig. 17.2. Vagal stimulation using the carotid body massage technique.

   c. Antiarrhythmic pharmacodynamic/kinetic studies have rarely been performed in cats, and most of the medication protocols are anecdotal. Therefore, it is important to be cautious when using these medications in cats and start with a low dose, titrating upwards if necessary.

C. Diagnosis

   a. The ECG is recorded with the feline patient restrained in right lateral recumbency. However, in dyspneic cats, stress must be avoided and the ECG can be recorded with the cat standing or in sternal recumbency.

   b. When the arrhythmia or clinical signs are intermittent, definitive diagnosis may require the use of ECG telemetry, a 24-hour Holter monitor, or even an event monitor. There are many different Holter and event monitors available on the market, and several companies will rent devices.

   c. Vagal maneuvers can be useful diagnostically or therapeutically when a tachycardia is present, but the maneuvers should be avoided if AV block or significant bradyarrhythmias are present. Vagal stimulation can be achieved with ocular pressure (retropulsing the globes), carotid sinus massage (fig. 17.2), or stimulation of a gag reflex. The sinus and AV nodes are particularly sensitive to vagal tone, so vagal stimulation results in slowing of the sinus node discharge rate and prolonged AV nodal conduction time (and refractoriness). During a tachycardia requiring the AV node as part of its circuit, brief AV block will result in termination of the tachycardia. With atrial tachycardia, if transient AV block can be achieved, the atria will continue to rapidly fire; however, some of these P waves will not conduct (physiologic AV block).

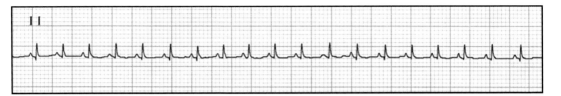

Fig. 17.3.   Normal sinus rhythm from an adult cat in right lateral recumbency. Note the regular RR intervals and the normal (narrow) QRS morphology (paper speed 25 mm/sec; 20 mm = 1 mV).

   d. The rapid heart rate and low-voltage ECG complexes can make interpretation of feline ECGs challenging (see fig. 17.3).
     i. Use of calipers or ECG rulers are very helpful for interval measurement.
     ii. Magnification of the ECG (2x normal gain or 20 mm/mV) is helpful.
     iii. Minimize artifact (ensure lead wires are not touching, an alcohol-soaked cotton ball placed near the cat's nose may stop purring, etc.).
     iv. Use multiple leads for complete assessment of ECG wave morphology.
D. Treatment of specific arrhythmias
  a. Tachycardias and premature complexes
    i. Supraventricular—the site of origin is proximal to the bundle branches (atrial or AV nodal). Therefore, the QRS morphology is normal unless a concurrent ventricular conduction abnormality is present.
      1. Isolated supraventricular premature complexes are common with primary heart disease or extracardiac disease, but sustained supraventricular tachycardias (SVT) are rare in cats.
      2. Sinus tachycardia, an accelerated sinus rate due to elevated adrenergic tone, is considered a normal physiologic response; however, in some patients (particularly hyperthyroid patients) sinus tachycardia can be rapid enough to negatively affect cardiac output warranting therapy (heart rates ≥250 bpm).
      3. Similarly, sustained rapid rates due to SVT often result in poor ventricular filling and cardiac output, especially when primary heart disease is present. As the heart rate gets faster, impairment is more likely.
      4. Atrial fibrillation occurs when significant structural heart disease leads to heart enlargement in the cat. QRS complex morphology may be non-uniform due to varying AV nodal and ventricular conduction.
      5. Ventricular pre-excitation
        a. An accessory pathway allows a supraventricular impulse to bypass the AV node and activate ventricular tissue earlier than would be expected if the impulse traveled through the AV node. This phenomenon results in a shorter than normal PR interval (fig. 17.4). The QRS duration may be increased (as in figure 17.4) or normal.
        b. Most affected cats have no clinical signs; however, AV reentrant or reciprocating tachycardias can occur rarely.
      6. Treatment of supraventricular tachycardias (table 17.1)
        a. Vagal maneuvers may abolish the tachycardia or reveal underlying P waves (the maneuver can be diagnostic as well as therapeutic).
        b. Negative chronotropes that slow conduction through the AV node are all potentially effective for treating SVT; however, *digoxin should be avoided in cats with hypertrophic cardiomyopathy or if an accessory pathway is suspected.*
        c. For reciprocating tachycardias characterized by a re-entrant circuit, if vagal maneuvers are ineffective, they should be followed by diltiazem and repeated vagal maneuvers. If

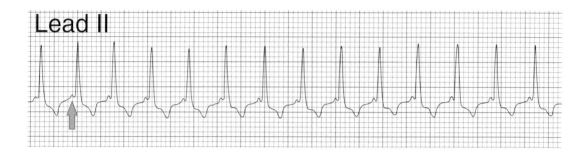

Fig. 17.4. Note the short PR interval (arrow) in this cat with ventricular preexcitation (paper speed 25 mm/sec; 20 mm = 1 mV).

unsuccessful, add antiarrhythmic agents that suppress conduction in abnormal pathways (i.e., procaineamide).

  i. Calcium channel blockers
    1. Diltiazem is used most widely in veterinary medicine.
    2. Dose: 1.0–2.5 mg/kg PO q8h; 0.1–0.2 mg/kg as a slow IV bolus, then 2–6 μg/kg/min IV CRI; Dilacor XR: 30–60 mg PO q24h per cat
  ii. Beta adrenergic blockers
    1. Atenolol is cardiac specific and used most frequently in cats for chronic use.
      a. Dose: 6.25–12.5 mg PO q12–24h
      b. Less likely to cause bronchoconstriction or vasoconstriction than propranolol
    2. Propranolol is not cardiac specific, but it is available in an injectable form.
      a. Dose: 0.02–0.06 mg/kg IV over 5–10 minutes
      b. Start with low dose and titrate to effect; taper dose when discontinuing therapy; reduce dose with liver disease; beware possible bronchoconstriction
    3. Esmolol is an ultra-short-acting beta-adrenergic blocker with effects lasting for only minutes.
      a. Dose: 50–100 μg/kg IV bolus every 5 minutes up to a maximum of 500 μg/kg; 50–200 μg/kg/min CRI
      b. Useful for SVT which does not respond to vagal maneuvers or diltiazem; usually switch to atenolol for chronic therapy
  iii. Digoxin
    1. Dose: 0.005–0.01 mg/kg q24–48h
    2. Digoxin is excreted renally, so lower dose with renal disease
    3. Steady state is attained after 7–10 days (therefore, it is not a good drug for acute therapy but is used for chronic therapy). Therapeutic range is 0.5–2.0 ng/mL.
    4. Dose on lean body weight and avoid elixir form in cats.
    5. Signs of toxicity: anorexia, vomiting, diarrhea
ii. Ventricular ectopy
  1. Ventricular ectopy is the most common feline arrhythmia.
  2. The origin or focus is distal to the bundle of His, and the QRS morphology is wide and bizarre (fig. 17.5).
  3. Ventricular ectopy can be associated with primary heart disease or extracardiac disease.
  4. Intermittent ventricular premature complexes (VPC) which are not associated with clinical signs do not necessitate treatment. However, when frequent enough to cause hemodynamic impairment, such as systemic hypotension, syncope, weakness, and so on, therapy is indicated.
  5. Treatment (table 17.2)

Table 17.1. Drugs for treatment of feline cardiac supraventricular tachycardias.

Tachycardias	Drug Classes	Mechanisms of Actions	Side Effects	Contraindications or Precautions	Routes of Administration and Doses
Dilitiazem	L-type calcium channel blocker	Slows AV node conduction and inhibits cardiac and vascular smooth muscle contractility	CV: Modest peripheral vasodilation and negative inotropic effect	Bradycardia, overt congestive heart failure, hypotension	7.5 mg/cat TID PO or 30–60 mg/cat extended release formula q12–24 h; 0.1–0.2 mg/kg IV bolus (over 1 min) followed by 2–6 μg/kg/min IV
Atenolol	Beta-blocker	β_1-selective beta adrenergic blocker	CV: Bradycardia, negative inotropic effect, hypotension Neuro: lethargy	Bradycardia, asthma (less than nonselective blockers), overt congestive heart failure; renal disease	6.25–12.5 mg PO q12–24h (drug of choice for tachycardias associated with hyperthyroidism)
Esmolol	Beta-blocker	Ultra-short-acting β_1-selective beta adrenergic blocker	CV: Bradycardia, negative inotropic effect, hypotension	Bradycardia, overt congestive heart failure; use caution with asthma and/or diabetes	50–100 μg/kg IV every 5 min (over 1 min) as needed up to 500 μg/kg max. 50–200 μg/kg/min CRI
Propranolol	Beta-blocker	Nonselective β receptor blocker	As for cardioselective beta-blockers and also potential bronchoconstriction	Bradycardia, asthma, diabetes, renal and/or hepatic disease	0.01–0.06 mg/kg IV over 1 min; up to a maximum of 1 mg/kg
Digoxin	Cardiac glycoside	Antiarrhythmic effect due to parasympathetic stimulation	GI: anorexia, nausea, diarrhea, vomiting Neuro: depression CV: rarely arrhythmogenic	Toxicity potentiated by electrolyte disturbances, thyroid disorders, and hypoxia. Typically contraindicated in cases of hypertrophic cardiomyopathy or existing bradycardia.	0.005 mg/kg PO q24–48h (12 depending on serum digoxin level) Dose on lean body weight. Do not use elixir in cats. Therapeutic range is 1–2 ng/mL 6–8 hours after administration.

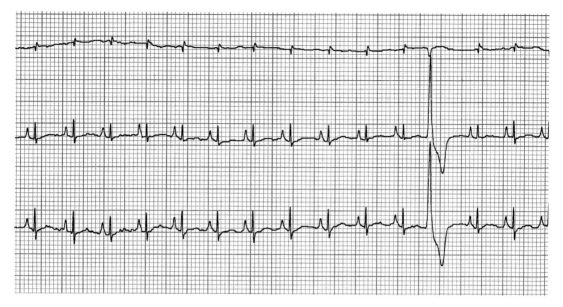

Fig. 17.5. Normal sinus rhythm with a VPC (wide and bizarre in appearance compared with the normal sinus beats (paper speed 25 mm/sec; 20 mm = 1 mV).

     a. Acute therapy
       i. Sodium channel blockers
         1. Lidocaine
           a. Dose: 0.25–0.75 mg/kg IV over 5 minutes
           b. Cats are more sensitive to neurologic toxic effects than dogs (seizures), which can be controlled with diazepam.
         2. Procainemide
           a. Dose 3–8 mg/kg IM q6–8h
           b. Reduce dose with renal or liver disease
           c. A sign of toxicity is 25% prolongation in QRS interval
       b. Chronic therapy
         i. Beta adrenergic blockers
           1. Atenolol (see above)
         ii. Sodium channel blockers
           1. Procaineamide
             a. Dose: 3–8 mg/kg PO q6h
             b. Reduce dose with renal or liver disease
             c. A sign of toxicity is 25% prolongation in QRS interval
         iii. Class III antiarrhythmics
           1. Sotalol
             a. Dose: ⅛ of 80 mg tab PO q12h
             b. Reduce dose if bradycardia and/or weakness develop
  b. Bradyarrhythmias
     i. AV block
       1. Advanced second- or third-degree (complete) AV block (fig. 17.6) can result in intermittent or continuous bradycardia. However, in many cats, the heart rate is fairly normal and there are no clinical signs.

Table 17.2. Drugs for treatment of feline cardiac ventricular tachycardias.

Tachycardias	Drug Classes	Mechanisms of Actions	Side Effects	Contraindications or Precautions	Routes of Administration and Doses
Lidocaine	Class IB ventricular antiarrhythmic	Sodium channel blocker	GI: nausea, vomiting CV: hypotension Neuro: seizures Drug level may be increased with concurrent administration of cimetidine or other antiarrhythmics	Cats are sensitive to neurotoxic effects and deserve caution. Diazepam will control secondary seizures.	0.25–0.5 mg/kg IV (over 1 min); CRI at 10–20 µg/kg/min
Procaineamide	Class IA ventricular antiarrhythmic	Sodium channel blocker	CV: proarrhythmic potential, hypotension GI: vomiting, diarrhea Neuro: seizure potential	Second- or third-degree AV block (unless paced), hypotension	3–5 mg/kg PO q8h; 1–2 mg/kg IV (over 1 min); CRI at 10–20 µg/kg/min CRI
Sotalol	Mixed class III ventricular antiarrhythmic and β-blocker	Potassium channel blocker and β-blocker	CV: myocardial depression, bradycardia GI: vomiting Neuro: lethargy	Overt congestive heart failure, asthma, bradycardia; lower dose with renal disease.	2 mg/kg PO q12–24 h

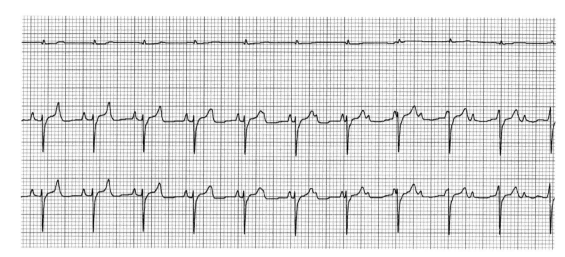

Fig. 17.6. Complete heart block from an adult cat in right lateral recumbency. Note the varying PR interval that suggests ventricular activation is not associated with atrial activation (P waves; paper speed 25 mm/sec; 20 mm = 1 mV).

2. Possible clinical signs include lethargy, episodic weakness, syncope, inappetance, and respiratory distress.
3. First-degree AV block (PR intervals of >.09 s) is common in cats but requires no specific therapy. Iatrogenic block can be caused by digoxin, beta adrenergic blockade, or calcium channel blockers and suggests dose reduction.
4. Treatment (when clinical signs such as syncope or weakness are present)
5. Acute management (table 17.3)
   a. Sympathomimetics
      i. Dobutamine
         1. Dose: 2–10 µg/kg/min IV (titrate up to effect)
         2. Preferable to dopamine if cat in congestive heart failure; inotropic effect is dose dependent; less arrhythmogenic than most other catecholamines; monitor for arrhythmias and/or hypotension. Dobutamine has been reported to cause seizures in cats.
      ii. Isoproterenol
         1. Dose: 0.04–0.09 µg/kg/min IV (titrate up to effect); 10 µg/kg IM or SQ q6h
         2. Hypotension is possible, but vasodilatory effect is usually offset by increased heart rate.
   b. Parasympatholytics are worth trying but rarely increase AV conduction significantly.
      i. Atropine
         1. Dose: 0.01–0.04 mg/kg IV, IM; 0.02–0.04 mg/kg SC q6–8h
            a. When given IV may transiently worsen bradyarrhythmia; more potent chronotropic effect than glycopyrrolate
      ii. Glycopyrrolate
         1. 0.005–0.01 mg/kg IV or IM; 0.01–0.02 mg/kg SC
         2. Longer duration of action with less chronotropic effect than atropine
6. Chronic management
   a. Long-term control necessitates a permanent pacemaker.
      i. Occasionally these arrhythmias are short lived and a temporary pacemaker is supportive until a sinus rhythm returns.

Table 17.3. Drugs for treatment of feline cardiac bradyarrhythmias.

Bradycardias	Drug classes	Mechanisms of Actions	Side Effects and Drug Classes	Contraindications or precautions	Routes of administration and doses
Dobutamine	Synthetic beta-adrenergic stimulating agent	Mixed $\beta_1 > \beta_2$–α agonist	CV: proarrhythmic potential GI: nausea, vomiting Contraindicated when HCM is present	Less arrhythmogenic than most catecholamines. Use with caution and monitor for arrhythmias and hypotension.	3–10 µg/kg/min IV titrate upward to effect
Isoproterenol	Synthetic sympathomimetic	Pure β ($\beta_1 > \beta_2$) agonist	CV: proarrhythic potential, hypotension GI: vomiting Neuro: weakness	Hypotension; ventricular arrhythmias	0.01–0.08 µg/kg/min IV titrate up to effect
Terbutaline	Synthetic sympathomimetic	β_2 agonist	CV: hypotension, tachycardia Neuro: tremors, CNS excitement Transient hypokalemia possible	Cats hypersensitive to terbutaline; caution in cats with myocardial disease, hyperthyroidism, hypertension, seizure disorders; decrease dose with renal disease.	0.625–1.25 mg/cat q8–12h PO 0.01 mg/kg SQ; IM
Atropine	Anticholinergic	Competitively inhibits acetylcholine	CV: tachycardia GI: decreased motility, dry secretions More potent chronotropic effect than glycopyrrolate	May transiently worsen bradyarrhythmia. Contraindicated with glaucoma, hypersentitivity, GI obstruction	0.01–0.04mg/kg IV, IM, SQ q6–8h
Glycopyrrolate	Anticholinergic	Competitively inhibits acetylcholine	CV: tachycardia GI: decreased motility, dry secretions	Longer duration of action with less of a chronotropic effect than atropine	0.005–0.01 mg/kg IM, IV 0.01–.02 mg/kg SQ
Theophylline	Xanthine deriviative	Phosphodiesterase inhibitor (increases cAMP)	CV: tachycardia Neuro: CNS stimulation Resp: bronchodilation (mild signs usually resolve after several days of medication)	Patients hypersensitive; use caution if hyperthyroidism, severe heart disease, hypertension; dose on lean body weight	4 mg/kg PQ q12h PO (extended release formula)

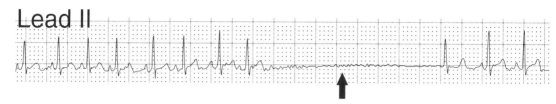

Fig. 17.7. Sinus arrest in a cat. Note the pause in the rhythm (no P or QRS depolarizations), which lasts almost 2 seconds (paper speed 25 mm/sec; 20 mm = 1 mV).

   ii. Sinus node disturbances
     1. Sinus arrest is the complete lack of atrial activation for one or more beats (fig. 17.7). Sinus bradycardia occurs when the sinus node pacemaker discharge rate is slower than normal (<140 bpm).
     2. These arrhythmias can commonly occur with extracardiac disease (respiratory, CNS, gastrointestinal, etc.).
     3. Associated clinical signs are rare, but lethargy or weakness is possible.
     4. An atropine response test will help determine if the bradycardia is due to elevated vagal tone (0.04 mg/kg atropine IV or IM should result in a sinus tachycardia greater than 220 bpm if the bradycardia is secondary to vagal influence).
     5. Treatment (only if symptomatic)
       a. Parasympatholytics if atropine response test suggests vagal tone is abnormally high and atropine is likely to be effective
         i. Atropine
         ii. Glycopyrrolate
         iii. Propantheline bromide
       b. Pacemaker if the patient is clinical
         i. Typically exhibited signs include: weakness, exercise intolerance, syncope, overt congestive heart failure
     6. Permanent pacemaker implantation
       a. Prior to implantation, the patient should be thoroughly assessed to exclude possible underlying disease as a cause of the arrhythmia.
         i. Complete blood count, chemistry panel, urinalysis
         ii. A 24-hour Holter monitor may be necessary if the arrhythmia is not evident on the resting ECG.
         iii. Thoracic radiographs and echocardiography are performed to evaluate underlying heart disease.
       b. Implantation
         i. In cats, an epicardial lead is usually placed via a lateral thoracotomy, caudal median sternotomy, or a ventral abdominal transdiaphragmatic approach.
         ii. The lead is implanted in an avascular site on the left ventricular apex and the pulse generator is optimally placed on the flank in a subcutaneous pocket.
     7. Temporary pacemakers
       a. Temporary pacemakers are often placed in cats for heart rate control during implantation of the permanent pacemaker and are particularly useful in cats that do not respond to positive chronotropic agents (isoproternol, atropine).
       b. In these situations, the temporary pacemaker can be placed in an emergency setting and kept in place for 24–48 hours until the permanent pacemaker can be placed.

18

LESS-COMMON CARDIAC CONDITIONS: HEARTWORM, SYNCOPE, PERICARDIAL DISEASE, BACTERIAL ENDOCARDITIS, AND DIGITALIS TOXICITY

Jamie M. Burkitt

Unique Features
I.   Feline heartworm infestation
     a. Relatively rare compared to dogs
     b. Low worm burden (~1–3 worms/cat)
     c. Diagnostic tests:
        i. False negatives are common due to low worm burden, all-male infestation, and the fact that cats are rarely microfilaremic.
     d. Treatment
        i. Cats should NOT be treated with adulticides, sudden worm dieoff can result in severe reactions.
II. Pericardial effusion
     a. Pericardial disease causing tamponade in cats is relatively rare compared to this condition in dogs.
     b. Hemangiosarcoma is a rare cause of pericardial effusion in cats.
     c. Causes of pericardial disease are more varied in cats compared to dogs.
III. Bacterial endocarditis
     a. Rare in dogs but even more rare in cats.
     b. *Bartonella hensalae* as a cause for endocarditis is being recognized now in cats.

A. Heartworm infestation
   a. Heartworm infestation is less common in cats than in dogs due to the species' inherent resistance to infection. The causative agent in the United States is *Dirofilaria immitis*. The parasite is introduced when a mosquito carrying *D. immitis* bites a cat, transmitting larvae. Larvae mature into adult worms over about 3–4 months, at which time they arrive and attach in the pulmonary arteries. Because cats are small, they are usually infected with only 1–3 adult heartworms; therefore, cats may have an infection with only male worm(s), which can affect testing for the disease (see below). Clinical signs are most likely to manifest in cats during initial worm migration into the pulmonary arteries or at death of the worm(s). Heartworm lifespan in cats is 2–3 years.
   b. History—Veterinarians in endemic areas should ask about use of heartworm preventative. Historical complaints in cats with heartworm infestation may include:

     i. Respiratory: tachypnea, dyspnea, and coughing
     ii. Gastrointestinal: vomiting
     iii. Rarely: syncope, neurologic signs, embolic events, caval syndrome
  c. Physical examination—Findings are nonspecific and may include tachypnea, dyspnea, increased breath sounds, or a right-sided heart murmur if worms are disrupting the tricuspid valve.
  d. Diagnosis of heartworm infestation in cats can be challenging. The clinician must have an increased index of suspicion in geographic areas where heartworm is common in dogs. The combination of chest radiographs, serology (both antibody and antigen), and echocardiography is the most reliable method. Cats are rarely microfilaremic, so blood evaluation for larvae is very insensitive.
     i. Feline heartworm antibody test—Once thought highly sensitive, it is now known to be only 32–89% sensitive in clinically infected cats. Therefore, false negative tests are possible. Detects exposure to both male and female larvae; not specific for current, adult infection.
     ii. Heartworm antigen test—Highly sensitive for infection with adult female heartworm(s). However, because cats are usually infected with only 1–3 worm(s), cats may have active adult infection and a negative antigen test. A positive test indicates active infection.
     iii. Chest radiographs—Most changes are related to the appearance of the pulmonary arteries. Prominent, tortuous, and truncated pulmonary artery appearance, best visualized on the dorso-ventral view, are consistent. The heart usually looks normal. There may be an increased bronchointerstitial pulmonary pattern.
     iv. Echocardiography—The worm's body wall may be visualized as two highly echogenic (white), parallel, linear artifacts in the right ventricular outflow tract or pulmonary arteries (fig. 18.1). They can be seen as far proximal as the vena cavae. This technique is relatively sensitive in the hands of an experienced ultrasonographer.
  e. Treatment—Cats should NOT be treated with adulticides, as sudden worm dieoff can be associated with severe inflammatory and embolic complications. All cats with significant clinical signs should be treated supportively with oxygen, bronchodilators, and/or IV fluids as indicated.
     i. Conservative management: In clinically normal cats, specific treatment may not be necessary. Cats should be monitored periodically for disease resolution as the worm(s) dies. In cats showing clinical signs, standard medical treatment is corticosteroids. Prednisolone 2 mg/kg/day tapered to 0.5 mg/kg/every other day for 2 weeks, then discontinued after another 2 weeks is one empirical regimen. Reevaluation should be performed, and the treatment regimen repeated as needed.

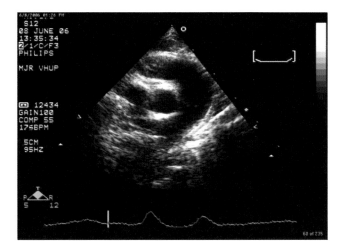

Fig. 18.1. Short-axis view of heartworms and the main pulmonary artery trunk and right ventricle of a cat.

ii. Definitive treatment: Surgical removal of heartworm(s) can be performed, either by right jugular venotomy for forceps or brush retrieval, or by thoracotomy.

f. Prognosis for cats with heartworm varies significantly. Many cats have occult, subclinical infections and clear the infection on their own without treatment or obvious untoward effects. Other cats die as a result of pulmonary inflammation or embolic disease.

B. Syncope

a. Syncope is rare in cats. It is defined as a temporary decrease or loss of consciousness and postural tone. It is always a sign of another primary disease rather than a definitive diagnosis. Therefore, the primary underlying disease must be found and treated appropriately to resolve the syncopal events. Syncope happens when oxygen or energy substrate (i.e., glucose) delivery to the brain is inadequate. Syncopal events generally last ≤10 seconds and are not usually preceded or followed by abnormal behaviors. Cats can experience syncope during exercise or at rest, depending on the underlying etiology and its severity.

b. Etiologies

i. Cardiac abnormalities are common underlying causes of syncope. Such cardiac causes include:

1. Tachyarrhythmias, as seen in hypertrophic cardiomyopathy. Very high heart rates prevent adequate diastolic chamber filling, which leads to decreased stroke volumes and poor cardiac output (see chap. 17—Management of Life-Threatening Arrhythmias).

2. Bradyarrhythmias (see chap. 17—Management of Life-Threatening Arrhythmias) such as high-grade second-degree AV block or third-degree AV block. Primary conduction disturbances are rare in cats. Bradyarrhythmias caused by metabolic disease (hyperkalemia of urethral obstruction or renal failure) are unlikely to lead to syncope before the primary disease causes other significant clinical signs.

3. Pericardial tamponade. Tamponade causes decreased venous return to the right atrium, and can therefore lead to poor cardiac output. Causes of pericardial tamponade are discussed in a later section.

4. Heartworm infestation. The worm(s) may intermittently obstruct the main pulmonary arteries, leading to periods of poor cardiac output.

ii. Respiratory disease sufficient to cause hypoxemia can cause syncope, though syncope in the absence of significant dyspnea is very unlikely.

iii. Metabolic causes such as hypoglycemia, anemia, or electrolyte abnormalities may cause syncope. Hypoglycemia or anemia can lead to decreased brain function due to decreased neuronal energy production, and electrolyte aberrations can cause neural conduction abnormalities, but cats with these conditions generally have persistent neurologic dysfunction rather than intermittent syncope or evidence of the underlying metabolic cause.

c. Differential diagnoses—Occasionally (extremely rare) primary neurologic disease can produce clinical signs indistinguishable from syncope. Examples include atypical (flaccid) grand mal seizures, petit mal or "absence" seizures, and narcolepsy. Primary neurologic events may be preceded and followed by pre- and postictal phases, respectively, whereas syncopal events generally are not. Neurologic events may be of minutes' duration and often include urination, defecation, or tonic limb movements or postures.

d. Historical findings—Clients report short periods of collapse and unresponsive mentation that resolve spontaneously. Syncopal episodes may happen only during exercise or during normal, quiet activity. They may occur very infrequently or multiple times a day.

e. Physical examination findings may be normal or may reveal signs of the cardiac, respiratory, or metabolic diseases listed above. Unfortunately, it is uncommon for patients to experience syncopal events during the short time period of examination.

f. Diagnosis of the underlying cause of syncope may be difficult. In some patients, an underlying etiology is never found. It is important to search extensively for the underlying cause (the most common cause is cardiac disease), however, as it may lead to death without appropriate treatment. The diagnostic database includes:

i. Clinicopathologic database. Complete blood count, chemistry panel with glucose and electrolytes, T4, heartworm test (see above section for details), and urinalysis

ii. Electrocardiogram. A standard three-lead ECG can be used for basic evaluation. The ECG should be studied for intermittent or persistent brady- or tachyarrhythmia.

iii. Chest radiographs. Radiographs should be evaluated for cardiac and vascular size and shape, and pulmonary parenchymal markings.

iv. Echocardiography. Cardiac ultrasound may reveal structural heart disease such as HCM that can be associated with tachyarrhythmias or bradyarrhythmias leading to syncope.

v. Complete neurologic exam to help differentiate syncope from neurologic events

vi. Outpatient heart rhythm monitoring is often necessary to diagnose primary conduction abnormalities causing syncope, since these rhythms may be intermittent and thus absent during hospital evaluation. Traditionally, 24- to 48-hour continuous ECG monitoring has been performed using Holter monitors, but they must be worn by the patient and are bulky for cats. Another option is the cardiac event monitor, which is smaller and can be worn for a longer period of time. The event monitor records and stores the ECG for only a short period of time prior to and after an event; it stores a limited number of event recordings. The owner must activate the recorder when an event is witnessed, so this method works best for cats that are well supervised.

g. Treatment—The treatment of syncope is based on appropriate treatment of the underlying disease.

i. Cardiac diseases

1. Tachyarrhythmias should be treated to improve cardiac output (see chap. 17—Management of Life-Threatening Arrhythmias). Cats with HCM may require heart rate reduction to improve diastolic filling even if their heart rate is normal (See chapter 15—Management of Specific Cardiac Diseases). Prognosis depends on the underlying cause of the tachyarrhythmia.

2. Bradyarrhythmias severe enough to cause syncope (i.e., high-grade, second-degree to third-degree AV block) are usually unresponsive to anticholinergics. However, cats with clinical bradyarrhythmia should receive an atropine challenge (see chap. 17—Management of Life-Threatening Arrhythmias). Most patients with severe bradyarrhythmias require permanent pacemaker implantation. Transvenous and surgical implantation techniques have been used successfully in cats. Prognosis with successful artificial pacing is good.

3. Pericardial tamponade (extremely rare in cats) due to pericardial effusion requires timely pericardiocentesis. See section below regarding management.

4. Treatment of heartworm infestation in cats is usually conservative. Adulticides are generally considered too risky in cats due to the likelihood of worm embolism into the pulmonary arteries after treatment. See section above on specific treatments for heartworm infestation in cats.

ii. Respiratory and metabolic diseases should be treated as indicated.

iii. Prognosis—Short-term prognosis for the patient with syncope is guarded; decreased cerebral function can be life threatening and the patient may die if the diagnosis is not readily made and treatment initiated. The long-term prognosis for syncope depends on the underlying etiology, and therefore varies from very good to grave.

C. Pericardial disease

a. Pericardial disease is uncommon in cats, and it is rarely clinically significant. Pericardial disease becomes clinically significant when high pressure within the pericardial sac impedes right atrial filling (cardiac tamponade) resulting in decreased cardiac output and increased venous pressures. Thus, when clinically apparent, pericardial disease causes clinical signs of right heart failure and/or decreased cardiac output. A small volume of fluid within the pericardium can cause tamponade when the fluid accumulates acutely; a large fluid volume may not lead to tamponade if it develops over a long period of time, allowing for stretching of the pericardial sac.

b. Etiologies

    i. Pericardial effusion is fluid accumulation within the pericardial sac. Etiologies in cats include neoplasia (especially lymphoma), septic exudate, feline infectious peritonitis, primary heart disease such as HCM, fluid overload, and hemorrhage.

    ii. Peritoneopericardial diaphragmatic hernia (PPDH) is usually a congenital abnormality in which the peritoneum is continuous with the pericardial sac. The most common herniated organ is the liver. Because it is a congenital abnormality and the pericardium is likely chronically stretched, PPDH does not usually cause clinically evident cardiac tamponade. PPDH is an incidental finding in many cases.

    iii. Restrictive pericardial disease is rare in cats. It can be idiopathic or due to a chronic inflammatory process. Restrictive pericardial disease can cause tamponade.

  c. Historical findings vary by etiology and severity of disease and include dyspnea, tachypnea, anorexia, lethargy, and collapse. PPDH may be associated with gastrointestinal signs due to incarceration of the abdominal organs within the pericardial sac, or PPDH may become clinically evident as a result of abdominal straining from intestinal disease or parturition. Cats with tamponade may develop abdominal distention due to ascites.

  d. Physical findings in cats with pericardial disease vary by etiology and severity of cardiac compromise. Findings may include

    i. Dyspnea, tachypnea

    ii. Muffled heart sounds. In the case of PPDH, heart sounds may be asymmetrically muffled. Small volumes of acute effusion may cause tamponade in the absence of muffled heart sounds.

    iii. Muffled breath sounds if right heart failure and subsequent pleural effusion develop.

    iv. Hepatomegaly, ascites, and jugular venous distention can be seen if right heart failure has developed.

    v. Pulsus paradoxicus (variable pulse quality with respiration—weaker pulses on inspiration) is not commonly appreciated in cats with pericardial disease as it is in dogs.

  e. Diagnostic evaluation includes the following:

    i. Chest radiographs. Significant pericardial effusion or PPDH with herniated organs will cause an enlarged, globoid cardiac silhouette.

    ii. Acute accumulation of a small pericardial effusion or restrictive pericardial disease will not cause an obvious change to cardiac silhouette, although a distended caudal vena cava should be noted on the lateral view. If pleural effusion is present, it may obscure the cardiac silhouette and prevent accurate diagnosis of pericardial disease; pleurocentesis should be performed and thoracic radiographs performed thereafter to evaluate the cardiac silhouette.

    iii. Electrocardiography. Pericardial effusion is associated with low-voltage QRS complexes and electrical alternans (alternating size of the R-wave) on ECG, although the latter is rarely detected. This finding must be interpreted with caution in cats, which normally have low voltage QRS complexes compared to dogs.

    iv. Echocardiography. Definitive diagnosis of pericardial effusion or PPDH with herniated organ(s) is made by echocardiography. Pericardial effusion is visualized as anechoic fluid within the pericardial sac (fig. 18.2). Tamponade is present if the right atrium moves inwardly (collapses) during diastole.

    v. Contrast peritoneogram may aid in the diagnosis of PPDH. If contrast media injected into the peritoneal cavity appears within the pericardial sac, a PPDH is present though false negatives can occur (figs. 18.3 a and b).

      1. Positive contrast peritoneogram technique

        a. Dilute iodinated contrast material to 25% concentration with normal saline into appropriately sized syringe (~10-mL syringe).

        b. Inject diluted contrast material into abdominal cavity near umbilicus using a 220-gauge needle (avoid falciform fat).

        c. Wait 5 minutes and perform whole body lateral radiograph.

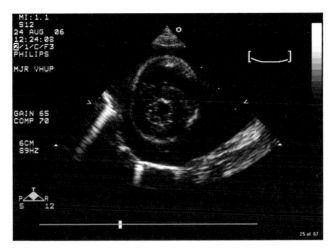

Fig. 18.2. Short-axis view of a cat with pericardial effusion. Note the fluid-filled, anechoic region surrounding the heart.

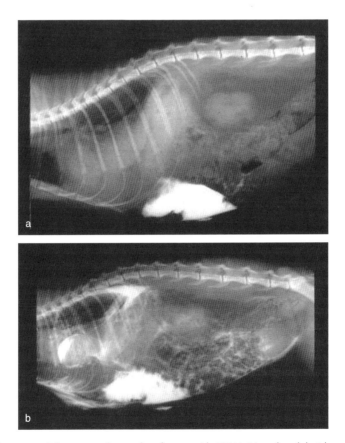

Fig. 18.3 a and b. Lateral thoracic radiographs of a cat with PPDH. Note the globoid appearance to the heart and loss of a complete outline of the cranial aspect of the diaphragm. Also note how the positive contrast agent injected into the abdomen has leaked into the thoracic cavity.

      vi. Cytologic analysis of pericardial fluid should be performed. See treatment section below for centesis technique. Cytologic analysis may reveal the underlying cause (neoplastic cells in fluid, septic exudates) or may be suggestive of the underlying etiology (high-protein exudates in FIP, low-protein transudates with primary heart disease or fluid overload). Biochemical analysis of pericardial fluid is unlikely to lend significantly to the diagnosis.

  f. Treatment for pericardial disease is specific to the underlying etiology.

      i. Pericardiocentesis is performed to remove fluid from the pericardial sac. Most cats do not require sedation for this procedure; it may be performed in sternal or lateral recumbency. Continuous ECG should be performed to monitor for arrhythmias associated with catheter insertion. An 18-gauge, over-the-needle catheter should be inserted aseptically into the pericardium via the right or left 4th or 5th intercostal space. Chest radiographs or echocardiography can be used to determine the ideal rib space for catheter insertion. Once fluid appears in the stylet hub, the flexible catheter is advanced into the pericardial space and the stylet removed. If arrhythmias are noted, the catheter should be repositioned to decrease epicardial contact until the arrhythmia resolves. The catheter should be attached to flexible tubing and a 20-cc syringe for fluid withdrawal. Fluid analysis should include a total protein, cell count, and cytology evaluation.

      ii. Definitive treatment for PPDH requires surgery for hernia reduction and herniorrhaphy. Cats with clinical signs referable to PPDH should be treated supportively with oxygen therapy and IV fluids as indicated prior to surgical repair. Owners of cats with incidental diagnosis of PPDH may or may not elect surgical repair. However, organs can herniate in previously clinically "silent" cases, leading to acute cardiac tamponade and death. This latter event occurs more commonly in cats straining due to gastrointestinal disease or during parturition.

      iii. Definitive treatment of restrictive pericardial disease requires total or subtotal pericardectomy. Cats should be treated supportively with oxygen and IV fluids as indicated prior to the thoracoscopic or surgical pericardectomy.

  g. Prognosis for the cat with pericardial disease depends largely on the underlying disease, and on the performance of definitive treatment in the case of PPDH.

D. Bacterial endocarditis

  a. Bacterial endocarditis is rare in cats. Information on the disease in cats is very limited. Endocarditis usually manifests as infection of the valves on the left side of the heart. In dogs, the aortic valve is the most commonly affected. In the few reports of bacterial endocarditis in cats either the aortic valve, mitral valve, or both have been affected. In dogs, many different bacteriologic agents have been associated with endocarditis, most commonly *Staphylococcus aureus*, *Streptococcus* spp., *E. coli*, *Bartonella* spp., and others.

  b. Predisposition—Most people with bacterial endocarditis have a predisposing cardiac lesion. This is not the case in cats. Most veterinary patients' endocarditis lesions occur on previously normal valves. It is unclear whether other factors such as severe dental disease or dermatologic disease predispose to bacterial endocarditis. Diseases leading to immune compromise such as diabetes mellitus may predispose cats to development of endocarditis, but the literature does not support a connection.

  c. Historical findings in cats with endocarditis are usually those of left-sided congestive heart failure, including dyspnea, tachypnea, and lethargy. Other reported clinical signs in cats include coughing, anorexia, and hemoptysis.

  d. Physical examination findings may include the following:

      i. Signs referable to cardiac disease or failure, such as a heart murmur often loudest on the left side, tachycardia, dyspnea, tachypnea, and lethargy

      ii. Signs referable to sepsis, which in cats include hypo- or hyperthermia, bradycardia, poor mental responsiveness, pale mucous membranes, and poor pulse quality

  e. Diagnostic tests should include the following:

    i. Thorough historical and physical review. The presence of a new heart murmur and clinical signs of sepsis are consistent with the diagnosis.

    ii. CBC, chemistry panel, urinalysis. A complete blood count may reflect the septic process; however, an inflammatory leukogram was not a consistent finding in cats with endocarditis in the literature. The chemistry panel and urinalysis are important to rule out other, more common causes of sepsis and to determine if other organs (kidneys, liver) are affected.

    iii. Chest radiographs. Chest radiographs may reveal left-sided heart enlargement and/or evidence of congestive heart failure (pulmonary edema, pleural effusion).

    iv. Blood cultures. Aseptic collection and handling technique is imperative, and samples from at least 2–3 vessels should be submitted. Blood cultures are not very sensitive or specific for bacterial endocarditis. Collecting blood cultures prior to antibiotic administration may increase the diagnostic yield but should not be allowed to significantly delay institution of antibiotic therapy. Urine culture may be an alternative or an adjunct to blood cultures in diagnosing the specific bacteria responsible for the infection.

    v. Echocardiography. Demonstration of a vegetative, destructive, and/or thickened valvular lesion on echocardiography. Pericardial effusion has also been reported in cats with infective endocarditis.

  f. Treatment includes the following:

    i. Supportive care. Appropriate supportive care measures, including oxygen therapy, vasoactive agents, and intensive nursing care will likely be required. Intravenous fluids should not be used in animals in left-sided congestive heart failure and should be used judiciously in cats predisposed to it by endocarditis.

    ii. Antibiotic therapy. Empirical, injectable, broad-spectrum antibiotic therapy should be instituted as soon as possible. Combinations such as a potentiated beta-lactam antibiotic (i.e., ticarcillin-clavulonate) and a fluoroquinolone (i.e., enrofloxacin) would be appropriate. Once blood or urine culture and sensitivity results are available, antibiotic therapy should be tailored appropriately.

    iii. Treatment for congestive heart failure, if present. Oxygen therapy and diuretics are the cornerstone of management. See chapter 15—Management of Specific Cardiac Diseases.

  g. Prognosis is poor to grave. All feline cases reported in the literature either died or were euthanized within 11 months of diagnosis.

E. Digitalis toxicity

  a. Intoxication with digoxin or other cardiac glycosides is uncommon in cats. Glycoside intoxication in cats usually occurs secondary to digoxin therapy. The drug has a narrow margin of safety, with signs of toxicity seen at <10 times the standard therapeutic dosage. Due to cats' discerning behavior, accidental ingestion of digoxin medication is rare. Many plants contain cardiac glycosides, including oleander and yellow oleander, laurel, dogbane, foxglove, lily-of-the-valley, some milkweed plants, and *Kalanchoe* spp. The toxins of *Bufo* spp. toads also contain cardiac glycosides, which can enter through cats' oral mucous membranes.

  b. Pathophysiology—Digoxin inhibits Na+/K+ ATPase pumps throughout the body. The heart is the targeted therapeutic organ; digoxin is used to increase contractility and slow heart rate, particularly in cats with DCM. Therapeutic index is small with significant individual variation. Intact females are resistant to toxicity. Approximately 45% of digoxin is excreted unchanged in the urine; therefore, cats with renal disease may be predisposed to toxicity. The remainder appears to be excreted in the bile.

  c. History—Most cats with digitalis toxicity will be those purposely medicated with digoxin. Other exposures (ingestion of owner medication, toxic plants, or *Bufo* toads) are rare. The earliest clinical signs of toxicity are GI disturbance such as vomiting, diarrhea, or anorexia. Advanced clinical signs include GI signs and those of dysrhythmia (weakness, collapse, dyspnea).

  d. Physical examination findings may include nonspecific abnormalities of the gastrointestinal system; cardiac arrhythmias may be noted. Cardiac glycosides can lead to a variety of rhythm disturbances.

e. Definitive diagnosis of digoxin toxicity is by a combination of historical known or suspected exposure, physical examination, and the following:

i. Serum digoxin levels should be measured. The toxic plasma concentration in cats was 2.4–2.9 ng/mL in one small experimental study. Contact your local reference or toxicologic laboratory for sample collection and handling procedures. Even if the patient has a digoxin level within the reference interval, digoxin toxicity is still possible due to significant individual variation in susceptibility to toxicity as well as electrolyte disturbances, particularly hypokalemia. Hypokalemia lowers the threshold for digoxin toxicity.

ii. ECG. All patients with suspected cardiac glycoside intoxication should have continuous ECG monitoring. These toxins can cause a variety of dysrhythmias.

iii. Full minimum database (PCV, TS, BUN, Glucose, Na+, K+, Cl–, Mg++, blood gas) should be performed to rule out other causes of gastrointestinal disturbance and/or arrhythmia at presentation followed by CBC, chemistry panel, urinalysis, chest radiographs, abdominal imaging, and echocardiography if the underlying cause has not been determined.

f. Treatment

i. Digibind is an immune Fab antidote for digitalis toxicity. The product contains Fab fragments from ovine antidigoxin antibodies. The fragments bind digoxin and other cardiac glycosides, removing them from the Na+/K+ ATPase. The dosage to use is derived from the serum digoxin concentration. However, in veterinary medicine these results are unlikely to be rapidly available. Therefore, it is recommended to initiate treatment with one vial of Digibind and monitor for efficacy, but the safety of this medication has not been fully evaluated in cats. Additionally, this medication is extremely expensive.

ii. Withhold digoxin therapy until serum levels are available.

iii. Antiarrhythmic therapy as indicated. See chapter 17—Management of Life-Threatening Arrhythmias.

iv. Supportive care as indicated for gastrointestinal signs.

g. Prognosis for long-term recovery is good if the patient survives the initial toxic crisis.

Recommended Reading

Bolton GR, Powell W. 1982. Plasma kinetics of digoxin in the cat. Am J Vet Res, 1982; 43(11):1994–1999.

Borgarelli M, Venco L, Piga PM, et al. Surgical removal of heartworms from the right atrium of a cat. J Am Vet Med Assoc, 1997; 211(1):68–69.

Brady CA, Otto CM, Van Winkle TJ, King LG. Severe sepsis in cats: 29 cases (1986–1998). J Am Vet Med Assoc, 2000; 217(4):531–535.

DeFrancesco TC, Atkins CE, Miller MW, et al. Use of echocardiography for the diagnosis of heartworm disease in cats: 43 cases (1985–1997). J Am Vet Med Assoc, 2001; 218(1):66–69.

Erichsen DF, Harris SG, Upson DW. Therapeutic and toxic plasma concentrations of digoxin in the cat. Am J Vet Res, 1980; 41(12):2049–2058.

Glaus TM, Jacobs GJ, Rawlings CA, et al. Surgical removal of heartworms from a cat with caval syndrome. J Am Vet Med Assoc, 1995; 206(5):663–666.

Gwaltney-Brant SM, Rumbeiha WK. Newer antidotal therapies. Vet Clin Sm Anim, 2002; 32(2):323–339.

Hawe RS. Bacterial endocarditis: a review. Vet Med Sm Anim Clin, 1980; 75(10):1569–1579.

Kittleson MD. Infective endocarditis (and Annuloaortic Ectasia). In Kittleson MD, Kienle RD, eds, Small Animal Cardiovascular Medicine, pp 402–412. St. Louis: Mosby, 1998.

Nelson CT, McCall JW, Rubin SB, et al. 2005 Guidelines for the diagnosis, prevention, and management of heartworm (Dirofilaria immitis) infection in cats. Vet Parasitol, 2005; 133(2–3):267–275.

Peterson EN, Moise NS, Brown CA, et al. Heterogeneity of hypertrophy in feline hypertrophic heart disease. J Vet Int Med, 1993; 7(3):183–189.

Reimer SB, Kyles AE, Filipowicz DE. Long-term outcome of cats treated conservatively or surgically for peritoneopericardial diaphragmatic hernia: 66 cases (1987–2002). J Am Vet Med Assoc, 2004; 224(5):728–732.

Rush JE, Keene BW, Fox PR. Pericardial disease in the cat: a retrospective evaluation of 66 cases. J Am Anim Hosp Assoc, 1990; 26(1):39–46.

19
DIAGNOSTIC EVALUATION OF GASTROINTESTINAL CONDITIONS

Daniel Z. Hume

Unique Features
- The sublingual space should be examined for string foreign bodies.
- Cats less frequently exhibit abdominal pain associated with pancreatitis and septic peritonitis compared to dogs. However, it has been reported that septic cats may exhibit nonspecific abdominal pain despite the absence of abdominal disease.
- Reactive feline mesothelial cells do not often exhibit cellular characteristics of malignancy. Therefore the presence of cells with these characteristics should prompt the consideration of a cancerous process.

I. Clinical signs, diagnosis
  A. Oral examination
    1. A thorough oral examination should be performed on all cats. The sublingual space should be examined for string foreign bodies (fig. 19.1). Ptyalism and icterus may be present in cats with hepatobiliary disease. Oral ulcers may be present in association with renal disease or viral disease. Advanced dental disease is a frequent cause of anorexia in the feline patient.
  B. Abdominal auscultation
    1. Abdominal auscultation is frequently unrewarding in the evaluation of emergent gastrointestinal disease and is probably more important in the serial evaluation of the hospitalized patient.
  C. Abdominal palpation
    1. Careful and thorough abdominal palpation is paramount in the physical examination in cats presenting for signs of gastrointestinal disease. The loose abdominal musculature of a cat makes abdominal palpation relatively easy and often helps in the diagnosis. The liver margins should not extend past the last rib and any enlargement should prompt suspicion of hepatobiliary disease. The location and severity of any abdominal pain should be noted. Cats less frequently exhibit abdominal pain associated with pancreatitis and septic peritonitis compared to dogs. However, it has been reported that septic cats may exhibit nonspecific abdominal pain despite the absence of abdominal disease. The large and small intestines should be carefully palpated for thickness, symmetry, masses, or focal pain. Constipation or obstipation is often diagnosed based on a physical examination. The anus should be visually examined. Gentle digital rectal examination is mandatory in any cat presenting for tenesmus or constipation.
II. Diagnostic and monitoring procedures
  A. Survey abdominal radiographs

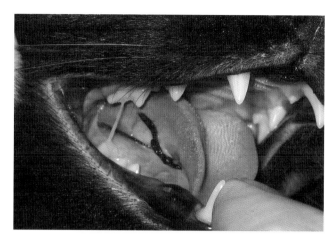

Fig. 19.1. String foreign body under the base of the tongue. (Courtesy of Dan Hume, MJR-Veterinary Hospital at the Univeristy of Pennsylvania.)

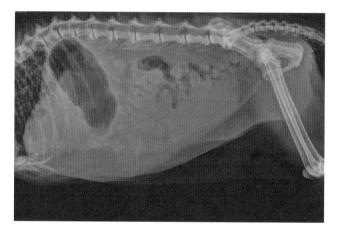

Fig. 19.2. Lateral radiograph of a cat with carcinomatosis secondary to pancreatic carcinoma. Note the ground-glass appearance to the cranial abdomen. (Courtesy of Anthony J. Fischetti, Animal Medical Center.)

1. Decreased abdominal serosal detail is compatible with abdominal effusion or peritonitis, though this finding is also seen in young patients, thin patients, or poor radiographic technique. A "ground glass" appearance to mid-abdomen may be seen in patients with carcinomatosis (fig. 19.2).
2. Moderate to severe gas or fluid enlargement of small intestine may be seen with small intestinal mechanical obstruction. Normal bowel diameter is ≤12 mm or less than twice the height of the central portion of a lumbar vertebrae (figs. 19.3 and 19.4).
3. A soft tissue tubular structure with an oblong, tapering gas bubble ("bullet" sign or "snakehead" sign) may be seen in animals with intussusceptions.
4. Intestinal plication and tear-drop–shaped luminal gas bubbles may be seen with a linear foreign body (fig. 19.5).
5. Although extremely rare in cats, compartmentalization of the stomach and pyloric displacement occur with a gastric dilation-volvulus (right lateral projection).

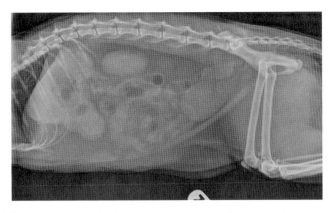

Fig. 19.3. Lateral abdominal radiograph of a cat with a mechanical intestinal obstruction secondary to a foreign body. Note the two populations of small bowel (one population of normal diameter and one distended population with a diameter >12mm. (Courtesy of Anthony J. Fischetti, Animal Medical Center.)

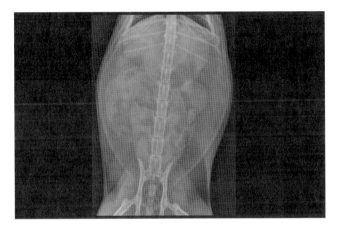

Fig. 19.4. VD abdominal radiograph of a cat with a mechanical intestinal obstruction secondary to a foreign body. Note the two populations of small bowel (one population of normal diameter and one distended population with a diameter >12mm. (Courtesy of Anthony J. Fischetti, Animal Medical Center.)

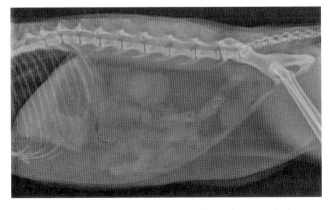

Fig. 19.5. Lateral abdominal radiograph of a cat with a mechanical intestinal obstruction secondary to a linear foreign body. Note the bunched or plicated small intestine. (Courtesy of Anthony J. Fischetti, Animal Medical Center.)

6. Animals with pancreatitis may have increased opacity, granularity, and decreased detail in the right cranial quadrant, along with an increase in the gastroduodenal angle.

B. Esophagram

1. Indicated for the evaluation of esophageal causes of gastrointestinal signs (e.g., regurgitation weight loss).

2. Diseases include esophageal strictures, masses, foreign bodies, and esophageal motility disorders.

3. Barium is contraindicated and nonionic, iodinated contrast preferred if esophageal perforation is suspected or possible.

4. Obtain orthogonal survey radiographs prior to initiation of ANY contrast study.

5. Administer 5–7 mL of 60% barium sulfate suspension or barium paste (or 5–10 mL of solution of 50:50 nonionic iodinated contrast media to water.

6. Lateral projection of the neck and a lateral and V/D projection of the thorax are immediately obtained.

7. The study can be repeated with barium-soaked kibble if warranted.

8. The caudal third of the esophagus normally has a herringbone appearance given the smooth muscle composition of the feline esophagus in that region.

C. Upper and lower GI series

1. Indications for upper GI study
   a. Survey radiographs are not definitive.
   b. Intestinal obstruction (stricture, foreign body, mass) is suspected.
   c. For the evaluation GI transit time
   d. GI ulcers and other mucosal irregularities

2. Barium is contraindicated and iodinated contrast preferred if GI perforation is suspected. Barium is generally preferred over iodinated contrast material because barium is more opaque, not absorbed, and adheres better to abnormal mucosa.

3. Obtain orthogonal survey abdominal radiographs prior to initiation of the contrast study.

4. Administer 12–20 mL/kg of 30% barium solution (or 600–800 mL/kg of iohexol diluted with water to obtain a volume of 10 mL/kg) via nasogastric or orogastric tube.

5. At time zero, four-view abdominal radiographs are taken allowing for visualization of all regions of the stomach.

6. Right lateral and V/D radiographs are obtained at 15 minutes, 30 minutes, and 60 minutes.

7. Radiographs should be taken every 30 minutes until the contrast reaches the colon and the stomach does not contain a pool of barium.

8. If a colonic abnormality is suspected, the radiographs should continue until the barium has completely emptied the colon.

9. Normal gastric emptying time with liquid 30% barium is 15–60 minutes but can take up to 17 hours with food, depending on size, shape, pH, and fiber content of the food.

10. Normal small intestinal transit time with liquid barium 30% is 30–60 minutes but can take as long as 3–4 hours.

D. Pneumocolonography

1. May be used to distinguish between normal gas or feces-filled large intestine and a small intestine dilated with gas. This is particularly useful in cats suspected of having a GI obstruction.

2. Obtain orthogonal survey abdominal radiographs prior to initiation of the contrast study to allow comparison with the contrast enhanced films.

3. Administer 20–30 mL of air into the rectum using a red rubber catheter or an oral dosing syringe.

4. Immediately after insufflation, a right lateral film should be taken. A ventral/dorsal film and opposite lateral film may be taken if enough air remains. The procedure may be repeated if additional air is needed for orthogonal views.

E. Fecal examination

1. Fecal parasitology
    a. Fecal flotation is indicated to find cysts, oocysts, and ova in feces.
    b. Techniques utilizing centrifugation methodology consistently recover more eggs than other methods.
    c. Zinc sulfate flotation of three separate samples procured at least 48 hours apart is the preferred floatation technique for *Giardia* cyst detection (fig. 19.6).
2. Fecal cytology
    a. Direct wet preparation
        1. A small amount of fresh feces is mixed with a drop of saline.
        2. Motile trophozoites of *Giardia* spp. and *Tritrichomonas foetus* may be visualized.
    b. Stained preparations
        1. Diff-Quick or Wright's stain may be used.
        2. The smears may be evaluated for increased number of white blood cells, presence of a monomorphic bacterial population, *Clostridial* endospores, or spiral-shaped bacteria consistent with *Campylobacter* spp.
        3. It is important to note that the diagnostic utility (low sensitivity and specificity) of fecal cytology in the diagnosis of bacterial causes of diarrhea is low and there is poor correlation with other more definitive diagnostic tests and that these organisms may be present and visualized in both health and disease.
3. Other fecal tests
    a. *Clostridium* spp.
        1. Tests are available for the determination of fecal enterotoxin (*Clostridium perfringens*) and toxin (*Clostridium difficile*) quantification.
        2. Submit 0.5–1.0 gram of feces.
        3. May be considered useful in cats with acute onset hemorrhagic diarrhea, diarrhea developing during hospitalization, or diarrhea in which another cause cannot be identified.
    b. *Tritrichomonas*
        1. A commercially available culture pouch (InPouch, Biomed Diagnostics, White City Oregon) is available that specifically augments the growth of *Tritrichomonas spp.* This technique has been shown to increase the diagnostic yield compared to direct wet mounts.
        2. A sensitive, inexpensive PCR test is also available (North Carolina State University, Texas A&M GI Lab).
    c. *Giardia*
        1. Snap ELISA (IDEXX Laboratories, Inc., Westbrook, Maine) and several direct immunofluorescence tests are available.
F. Diagnostic peritoneal lavage
    1. Indicated in animal with suspected abdominal disease in which simple abdominal or 4-quadrant paracentesis has been unsuccessful.
    2. Diagnostic peritoneal lavage is more sensitive than paracentesis in the diagnosis of abdominal disease.
    3. Procedure
        a. Local and systemic sedation and analgesia are indicated (e.g., lidocaine 1%, butorphanol 0.25–0.5 mg/kg, diazepam 0.25–0.5 mg/kg)
        b. Clip and aseptically prepare an area approximately 10 cm × 10 cm centered on the umbilicus.
        c. Place animal in lateral recumbency.
        d. Gently insert a 20–22-gauge, over-the-needle catheter or peritoneal dialysis catheter into the abdominal cavity near the umbilicus and direct the catheter caudally.
        e. If no fluid is noted after removal of the stylet, infuse sterile, warmed crystalloid fluid (20–22 mL/kg) over approximately 5 minutes; remove catheter.

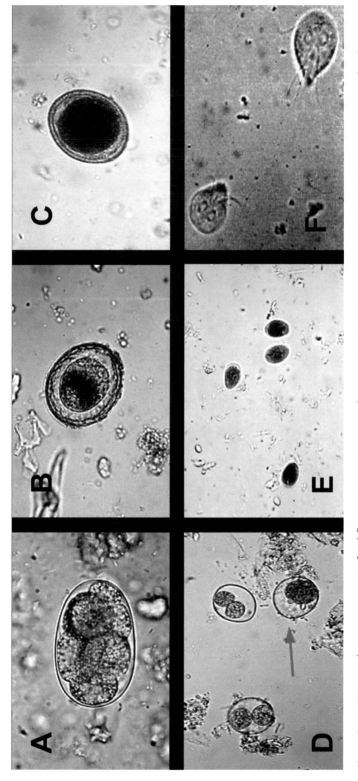

Fig. 19.6. (A) *Ancylostoma* sp. eggs in fecal float (40x); (B) *Toxascaris leonina* (10x); (C) *Toxocara* sp. egg (10x); (D) *Isospora* sp. unsporulated oocyst—arrow (40x); (E) *Giardia* cysts (40x) F. *Giardia* trophozoites (100x). (Courtesy of the Laboratory of Parasitology, University of Pennsylvania School of Veterinary Medicine.)

      f. Roll the animal from side to side and gently massage the abdomen to help distribute the lavage fluid throughout the abdomen.

      g. Repeat a simple or four-quadrant paracentesis.

G. Abdominal ultrasound

  1. An abdominal ultrasound is an invaluable imaging modality in cats with gastrointestinal abnormalities. Considerable expertise and experience is required to properly perform and interpret abdominal ultrasonography. The use of abdominal ultrasonography in the emergency room setting is usually limited to identification of abnormal fluid accumulation. Studies have shown minimal training is necessary in order to become proficient at detecting free abdominal fluid.

  2. It may be used to evaluate the architecture and size of the abdominal viscera, identify and procure samples of abdominal fluid, and aid in the diagnosis of many abdominal diseases.

  3. May be used alone or in combination with survey abdominal radiographs to confirm a gastrointestinal foreign body or obstruction.

H. Specific blood tests

  1. Serum trypsin-like immunoreactivity (fTLI)

      a. Species specific—0.5 mL fasting (12–18 hours) nonhemolyzed serum

      b. This assay detects both trypsinogen and trypsin, but trypsin should only be present in the serum when there is pancreatic inflammation.

      c. A low value ($\leq 8.0\,\mu g/L$) is diagnostic for exocrine pancreatic insuffiency.

      d. Serum TLI is increased in approximately 30–40% of cats with pancreatitis.

      e. Serum TLI may be increased with small intestinal disease and severely decreased renal function.

  2. Feline pancreatic lipase immunoreactivity

      a. Species specific—0.5 mL fasting (12–18 hours) nonhemolyzed serum. No special handling needed (Texas A&M GI Lab, College Station, TX).

      b. This assay detects lipase specifically released from the pancreas.

      c. The most sensitive (up to 100%) and specific (up to 100%) test for diagnosing feline pancreatitis

      d. An elevated value ($>12\,\mu g/L$) is consistent with pancreatitis.

  3. Cobalamin (vitamin B12)

      a. 0.5 mL fasting nonhemolyzed serum. No special handling.

      b. Cobalamin is a vitamin absorbed in the distal small intestine (specifically in the ileum).

      c. A decreased value may be seen in cats with small intestinal bacterial overgrowth, diseases affecting the distal small intestine, and exocrine pancreatic insuffiency.

  4. Folate

      a. 0.5 mL fasting nonhemolyzed serum. No special handling.

      b. Folate is absorbed in the proximal small intestine.

      c. Folate may be produced by bacteria, and the serum folate concentration may be increased with small intestinal bacterial overgrowth.

      d. Serum folate concentration may be decreased in cats with abnormalities in small intestinal absorption.

  5. Bile acids

      a. The bile acids are secreted in the bile primarily to facilitate fat absorption and are subsequently reabsorbed in the ileum and transported in the portal blood to the liver, where they are extracted by hepatocytes and resecreted in bile.

      b. The fasting serum total bile acid concentration is a reflection of the efficiency and integrity of the enterohepatic circulation.

      c. Pathology of the hepatobiliary system or the portal circulation results in increased serum bile acids prior to the development of hyperbilirubinemia.

      d. In the absence of hyperbilirubinemia, serum bile acids are a sensitive and specific measure of hepatobiliary function.
   6. Serum albumin
      a. Albumin may be reduced with decreased production or increased loss.
      b. Cats with protein-losing enteropathies may have a decreased albumin.
   7. Serum globulins
      a. Globulins may be decreased in cats with protein-losing enteropathies.
      b. Globulins may be increased in cats with infectious, inflammatory, or neoplastic diseases.

I. Endoscopy
   1. Indicated for the evaluation of chronic gastrointestinal diseases, which can cause chronic vomiting, chronic diarrhea, melena, weight loss, hematochezia, and hematemesis. Diseases may include inflammatory bowel disease, gastrointestinal neoplasia, ulcers, lymphangiectasia, and foreign bodies.
   2. May be used for removal of esophageal and gastric foreign bodies

J. Abdominocentesis
   1. Indicated in any cat with an abdominal effusion of unknown etiology
   2. Abdominocentesis *may be* contraindicated with a suspected increased bleeding problem.
   3. Greater than 5 mL/kg needed for successful tap using a single-hole needle or catheter
   4. Increased yield with ultrasound guidance
   5. Paracentesis
      a. The cat is placed in lateral recumbency and the area clipped and aseptically prepared.
      b. 20–22-gauge hypodermic needle or over-the-needle catheter is gently inserted near the umbilicus.
      c. Fluid is allowed to drip into sample tubes or gentle aspiration with a syringe.
      d. An increased yield can be obtained utilizing a catheter with side holes or a peritoneal dialysis catheter.
   6. Four-quadrant paracentesis
      a. Four quadrants are sampled as described above for simple abdominocentesis.
      b. Samples taken from an imaginary square centered over the umbilicus with the corners of the square being approximately 4–6 cm from the umbilicus
         1. Right cranial quadrant
         2. Right caudal quadrant
         3. Left cranial quadrant
         4. Left caudal quadrant

K. Abdominal fluid analysis
   1. Assess packed cell volume (PCV), total protein (TP), and total nucleated cell count TNCC).
      a. Transudate: total nucleated cell count (TNCC) <1,500 cells/µL, TP <2.5 g/dL
      b. Modified transudate: TNCC 1,000–7,000 cells/µL, TP 2.5–7.5 g/dL
      c. Exudate: TNCC >5,000 cells/µL, TP >3.0 g/dL (table 19.1)
   2. Perform aerobic and anaerobic bacterial culture as indicated.
   3. Cytology
      a. Cytologic evaluation involves a subjective description of fluid, determination of the type of inflammatory infiltrate, presence and degree of nuclear degeneration/toxicity and microorganisms, plant or food material, bile pigments, and/or evidence of criteria of malignancy. A direct smear is often used to gauge the cellularity of the fluid. In samples with a low to moderate cellularity, examination of a centrifuged sediment sample may increase the sensitivity of detecting bacteria or malignant cells.
      b. A large number of degenerative neutrophils may indicate a significant inflammatory or infection process and should prompt the clinician to consider exploratory laparotomy even in the absence of intracellular bacteria.

Table 19.1.   Effusion types.

Effusion Type	Total Protein (g/dL)	Total Nucleated Cell Count (cells/µL)	Examples
Transudate	<3.0 g/dL	<1,500 cells/µL	hypoalbuminemia right heart failure portal hypertension (prehepatic and hepatic) neoplasia lymphatic obstruction
Modified transudate	3.0–5.0 g/dL	1,000–7,000 cells/µL	neoplasia chylous effusion portal hypertension (posthepatic)
Exudate	>3.0 g/dL	>5,000 cells/µL	pancreatitis, FIP, uroabdomen, bile peritonitis, neoplasia, septic peritonitis

    c. The presence of intracellular bacteria (within neutrophils and macrophages) is diagnostic for a septic intra-abdominal process, and emergency exploratory laparotomy is indicated.

    d. Reactive feline mesothelial cells do not often exhibit cellular characteristics of malignancy. Therefore, the presence of cells with these characteristics should prompt the consideration of a cancerous process.

    e. Bile pigments may also be seen on cytologic evaluation in cats with bile peritonitis. Bile pigment may be found either intracellular or extracellular. Bile pigment ranges in color from a dark yellow to green brown with Romanowsky-type stains.

4. Bilirubin measurement

    a. A fluid bilirubin concentration >2 times the serum bilirubin collected at the same time is supportive of a diagnosis of bile peritonitis.

5. Creatinine measurement

    a. An abdominal fluid creatinine >2 times the serum creatinine collected at the same time is supportive of uroabdomen. The serum creatinine should be greater than normal.

    b. This difference is not noted in all patients with an uroabdomen.

6. Potassium measurement

    a. In cats, potassium in the fluid >1.9 times the serum potassium collected at the same time is supportive of an uroabdomen.

    b. This difference is not noted in all patients with an uroabdomen.

7. Glucose measurement

    a. A peritoneal effusion with glucose levels <50 mg/dL is suggestive of a septic peritoneal effusion.

    b. A blood-to-peritoneal glucose difference >20 mg/dL is suggestive of a septic peritoneal effusion.

8. Lactate measurement

    a. The use of peritoneal fluid lactate concentration and blood to fluid lactate difference has not been shown to be accurate in detecting septic peritoneal effusions in cats.

Note: The clinician should take into account the whole clinical picture (signalment, history, physical examination findings, and diagnostic results) prior to making a diagnosis. Caution should be used against making a diagnosis based on an isolated parameter or value. Additional studies are needed to further validate the use of glucose and lactate in the diagnosis of a septic abdomen.

Recommended Reading

Bonczynski JT, Ludwig LL, et al. Comparison of the peritoneal fluid and peripheral blood ph, bicarbonate, glucose, and lactate concentration as a diagnostic tool for septic peritonitis in dogs and cats. Vet Surgery, 2003; 32:161–166.

Wallack ST. The Handbook of Veterinary Contrast Radiology. San Diego: San Diego Veterinary Imaging, 2003.

Walters JM. Abdominal paracentesis and diagnostic peritoneal lavage. Clin Tech Small Anim Pract, 2003; 18(1):32–38.

20
GENERAL APPROACH TO THE ACUTE ABDOMEN

Sara Snow and Matthew W. Beal

Unique Features
- Cats presenting with acute abdominal illness may or may not demonstrate abdominal pain.
- Early nutritional support is critical in cats with acute abdominal illness.
- The diagnostic and therapeutic value of abdominal exploration in cats with acute abdominal illness should not be overlooked.
- Cats that are septic may exhibit pain on abdominal palpation in the absence of abdominal disease.

Introduction

Acute abdomen refers to the rapid onset of abdominal pain. Acute abdomen is most often a sign of significant and potentially life-threatening abdominal disease but may also be a manifestation of minor intra-abdominal disturbances, or even disease outside the abdomen (box 20.1). The following pages will focus on the pathophysiology of abdominal pain as well as physical examination, diagnostic workup, differential diagnoses, and emergency stabilization and management of the cat with acute abdomen.

1. The perception of abdominal pain
   a. Stimulation of nociceptors (sensory neurons) in and around the abdominal wall is responsible for the initiation of abdominal pain.
      i. Nociceptors have unmyelinated (C-polymodal fiber/CPM fiber) or thinly myelinated (Aδ-fiber) axons that are critical in the perception of acute abdominal pain in patients with intra-abdominal pathology.
      ii. Aδ-fiber nociceptors specialize in the detection of dangerous mechanical and thermal stimuli, such as those associated with abdominal wall injury or surgery.
      iii. CPM fiber nociceptors respond to strong mechanical and chemical stimuli such as stretch, tension, inflammatory mediators, and ischemia. These fibers mediate dull visceral pain associated with the parenchymal organs of the abdomen. Visceral pain is poorly localized, and patients demonstrating this type of pain might appear restless and ambulatory in an effort to relieve discomfort.
      iv. Both Aδ and CPM fibers mediate somatic pain arising from the abdominal wall or surgery. Somatic pain is a sharp pain that can be localized to a specific area and may be immobilizing for the patient.
      v. Various mechanical forces, inflammatory mediators, ischemia, and chemical irritants can activate nociceptors.

Box 20.1. Common causes of acute abdomen in cats.

Gastrointestinal System
- Foreign body
- Obstruction
- Perforation
- Ischemia
- Neoplasia
- Gastroenteritis, colitis
- Intussusception
- Ileus

Urogenital System
- Urethral/ureteral obstruction
- Disruption of ureter, bladder, urethra, renal pelvis
- Pyelonephritis
- Urolithiasis
- Acute renal disease
- Neoplasia

Pyometra

Peritoneum
- Septic peritonitis
- Hemoperitoneum
- Feline infectious peritonitis
- Disseminated neoplasia

Hepatobiliary
- Cholangiohepatitis
- Biliary obstruction
- Cholecystitis
- Neoplasia

Pancreatic
- Pancreatitis
- Neoplasia

Body Wall
- Penetrating injury
- Hernia

Referred Pain
- Intervertebral disc disease
- Spinal neoplasia
- Pelvic trauma

---

    vi. Nociception is initiated by various stimuli that activate the peripheral nerve terminals of nociceptors. Conscious perception of pain will occur when action potentials generated in the periphery travel via the spinothalamic and spinoreticulothalamic tracts to the thalamic nuclei and finally, the cerebral cortex.

  b. Referred pain presents as abdominal pain when the source of pain is a site at the periphery that shares a common nociceptive segment.

    i. Thoracolumbar spinal pain and neoplasia may be causes of referred abdominal pain in the feline patient.

2. Complete physical examination of the feline patient with acute abdomen is critical to the rapid identification of specific intra-abdominal injury or disease.

  a. Initial evaluation will focus on the major body systems and will trigger initiation of treatment for immediately life-threatening problems.

b. Abdominal palpation is performed to localize abdominal pain and narrow differential diagnoses. It should be noted that not all cats will demonstrate pain on abdominal palpation even in the presence of significant intra-abdominal disease. In addition, cats that are septic may exhibit pain on abdominal palpation in the absence of abdominal disease.
  i.   Dissemination of abdominal pain
      1. Focal abdominal pain
          a. Small bowel obstruction
          b. Foreign body
          c. Mild pancreatitis
          d. Intussusception
          e. Focal neoplastic disease
      2. Regional abdominal pain
          a. Pyometra
          b. Moderate to severe pancreatitis
          c. Regional septic peritonitis
          d. Pyelonephritis
      3. Diffuse abdominal pain
          a. Generalized septic peritonitis
          b. Generalized chemical peritonitis
          c. Generalized neoplastic disease
          d. Diffuse gastroenteritis (example: feline panleukopenia)
  ii. Anatomic location
      1. Cranial abdomen
          a. Hepatobiliary disease
          b. Pancreatitis
          c. Gastric and cranial duodenal disease
      2. Midabdomen
          a. Splenic disease
          b. Diseases involving the bowel
      3. Caudal abdomen
          a. Genitourinary disease
          b. Conditions affecting the distal colon
      4. Dorsal abdomen/retroperitoneum
          a. Renal and ureteral disease
          b. Retroperitoneal disease or injury
c. Miscellaneous physical examination considerations for abdominal assessment
  i.   Assessment of organ size
  ii. Assessment for the presence of intra-abdominal masses
  iii. Visual inspection
      1. Abdominal distention
      2. Bruising may suggest intra-abdominal disease.
          a. Periumbilical bruising suggests peritoneal disease or injury; however, thrombocytopenia/thrombocytopathia should also be considered.
          b. Inguinal or perineal bruising suggests retroperitoneal disease or injury.
  iv. Gentle ballottement for assessment of a fluid wave
  v.   Other physical considerations
      1. Oral examination, including assessment of the sublingual region for a linear foreign body, should always be performed (figs. 20.1a and b.). This is best accomplished by placing the index finger on the mandibular incisors to open the mouth while pushing upward with the thumb in the intermandibular space to elevate the tongue.

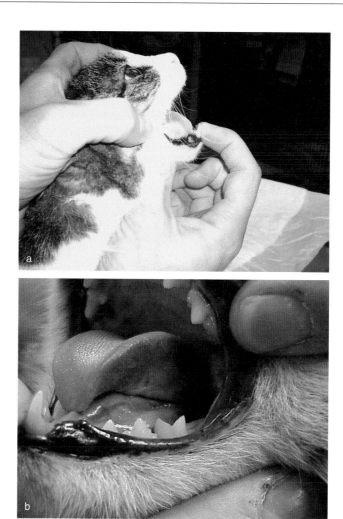

Fig. 20.1 a and b. a. Technique for evaluation of the sublingual region in a cat. Place the index finger on the mandibular incisors to open the mouth while pushing upward with the thumb in the intermandibular space to elevate the tongue. b. Linear foreign body anchored under the tongue in a cat.

    2. Spinal palpation should also be undertaken as spinal pain is frequently mistaken for abdominal pain (please see above).

    3. Rectal examination is indicated with the utilization of a sedative protocol in cats with history and physical examination suggesting large bowel obstruction, hematochezia, or straining to defecate.

3. Stabilization of the patient with acute abdomen should focus on restoring abnormalities identified in the major body systems assessment.

   a. Vascular access is critical for the delivery of fluids and blood products.

     i. Peripheral venous access initially

     ii. Central venous access will facilitate monitoring of CVP, delivery of nutritional support, and the reliable sampling of blood for diagnostic purposes. Assessment of primary and secondary hemostatic potential with PT, aPTT, and platelet count should be considered prior to central venous catheter placement.

b. Blood should be collected for a minimum database including packed cell volume, total solids, venous blood gas, electrolytes, blood glucose, and blood urea nitrogen (BUN).

c. Blood may also be collected for a complete blood count, serum biochemical profile, blood type, and coagulation profile (or activated clotting time).

    i. It is not necessary to run all of these samples on every patient; however, early sample collection prevents the need for repeated venipuncture and minimizes patient discomfort.

d. Urine should be collected via cystocentesis early in the course of therapy.

    i. Urine specific gravity is most useful prior to the initiation of fluid therapy to assess urine-concentrating ability.

    ii. A urine sample should be saved for culture prior to the institution of antibiotic therapy.

    iii. Caution using cystocentesis in potentially coagulopathic cats.

e. The fluid therapy plan should initially be focused on restoring intravascular volume deficits. The fluid therapy plan may later focus on rehydration, maintenance, and management of ongoing fluid losses. For a more in-depth discussion of fluid therapy, please refer to chapter 8—Fluid Therapy.

f. Antibiotics should be instituted immediately in patients that demonstrate evidence of sepsis, severe sepsis, or septic shock.

    i. Current evidence in human literature suggests that the early institution of antibiotic therapy within 1 hour of the recognition of severe sepsis may improve survival.

    ii. Fluid or tissue samples for culture and cytology should be obtained prior to the institution of antibiotic therapy if possible. However, antibiotic therapy should not be delayed if said samples cannot be easily acquired (see below).

    iii. Empiric antibiotic therapy should be based on underlying disease process, cytological examination of infected fluids and tissues, and Gram staining of these specimens.

4. Abdominal effusion is a common clinical finding in cats presenting with acute abdomen. Retrieval of fluid from the abdomen for subsequent analysis and culture is essential for accurate determination of the disease etiology. Fluid cytology and analysis provides information that is essential in determining whether medical or surgical management is most appropriate.

a. The accumulation of abdominal effusion is the result of changes in Starling's Forces, lymphatic drainage, or most often, a combination thereof.

b. A sample of abdominal fluid may be obtained through abdominocentesis, ultrasound-guided abdominocentesis, or diagnostic peritoneal lavage (DPL).

    i. To obtain a sample of abdominal effusion through abdominocentesis, the patient should be placed in left lateral, clipped, and aseptically prepared (fig. 20.2).

        1. A site that is 1–2 cm caudal to the umbilicus and 1–2 cm left of midline is chosen for sampling.

        2. Abdominocentesis is performed using a needle and syringe advancing in 1–2-mm increments in a direction perpendicular to the skin, the subcutaneous tissues, and the abdominal wall.

        3. The syringe should be aspirated intermittently as it is advanced through the body wall.

        4. Abdominal fluid sample handling

            a. Aliquot placed in EDTA tube for cytological analysis

            b. Aliquot placed in a tube for serum determinations (red top) chemical analysis if desired

            c. Aliquot placed in sterile tube and saved for culture if indicated based on cytological analysis or chemical analysis

            d. Aliquot of hemorrhagic samples placed in serum tube to evaluate for clotting. Samples retrieved from the abdominal cavity (rather than the spleen or other vascular structure) will generally not clot unless the hemorrhage is peracute.

    ii. When single-quadrant abdominocentesis is unsuccessful, four-quadrant abdominocentesis may be performed.

        1. With this technique, abdominocentesis is repeated in areas 1–2 cm cranial and lateral to the umbilicus and caudal and lateral to the umbilicus.

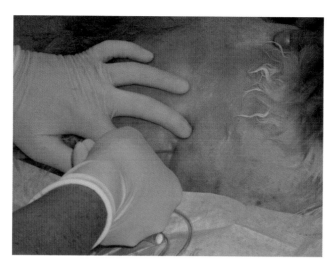

Fig. 20.2. Abdominocentesis in a cat.

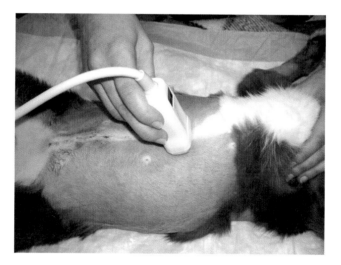

Fig. 20.3. Evaluation of the subxyphoid region in the cat using ultrasonography for the identification of peritoneal fluid accumulations.

iii. Ultrasonography may be used for the identification and retrieval of abdominal fluid accumulations. Four anatomic locations that can be quickly imaged with both longitudinal and transverse views are listed below (figs. 20.3 and 20.4).
   1. Subxyphoid
   2. Right flank
   3. Left flank
   4. Prepubic
iv. Abdominal paracentesis and DPL with a peritoneal dialysis catheter is a more sensitive method for the detection and collection of intra-abdominal fluid and the detection of intra-abdominal disease.

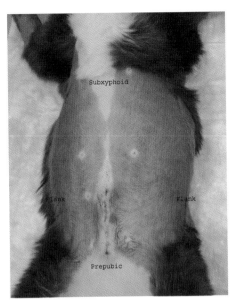

Fig. 20.4.   Longitudinal and transverse ultrasonographic images may be collected in the subxyphoid, right and left flank, and prepubic regions for the identification of intraabdominal fluid accumulations.

1. This procedure is performed with the patient heavily sedated and in dorsal recumbency.
2. The urinary bladder should be emptied manually or with a urinary catheter to minimize the likelihood of inadvertent puncture.
3. The abdomen is aseptically prepared and a local anesthetic (lidocaine) is infused just caudal to the umbilicus to include all planes of the body wall.
4. A 1- to 2-cm skin incision is made, and blunt dissection is performed to allow visualization of the linea alba (figs. 20.5a and b).
5. The linea is grasped with forceps and a 0.5-cm stab incision is made into the abdomen with the sharp edge of the blade pointing outward (figs. 20.5c and d).
6. A peritoneal dialysis or other multifenestrated catheter is placed and directed toward the pelvic inlet (fig. 20.5e).
7. Free-flowing fluid may be collected from the catheter or a syringe may be attached to retrieve a fluid sample (fig. 20.5f).
8. With this catheter in place, DPL may be performed in cats suspected to have focal abdominal effusion and in which the aforementioned techniques are unsuccessful in retrieving a fluid sample. DPL is the more sensitive test for the identification of serious abdominal injury or disease when compared with abdominocentesis. In DPL, lavage fluid contacts all peritoneal surfaces and the fluid retrieved is representative of what is happening throughout the peritoneum (fig. 20.5g).
9. DPL utilizes warm 0.9% sodium chloride (20–22 mL/kg) that is introduced, and then collected through a peritoneal dialysis catheter.
10. The collected fluid sample will be diluted, which will preclude significant biochemical testing.
11. The authors find DPL to be most useful for ruling in or out septic peritonitis in patients presenting with acute abdomen.

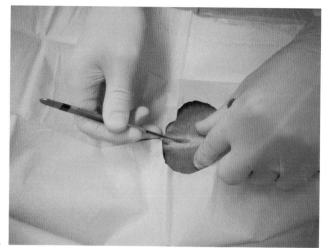

a

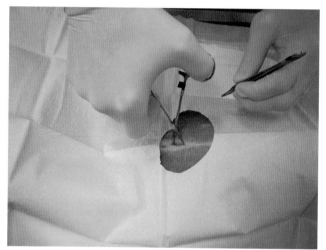

b

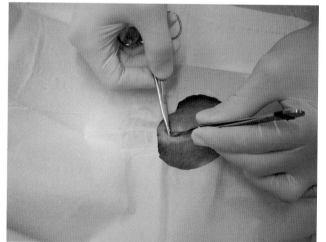

c

236

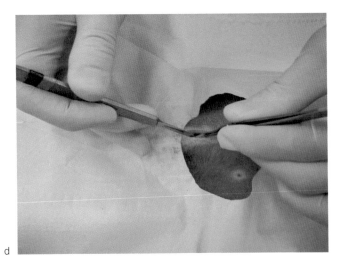

d

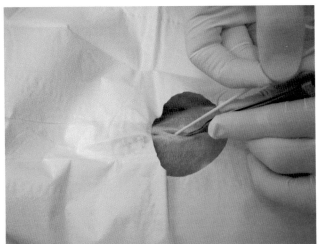

e

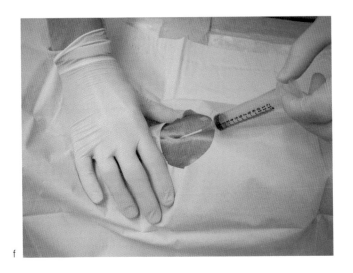

f

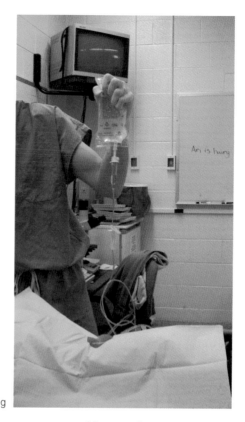

Figs. 20.5 a–g. Steps for diagnostic peritoneal lavage. The patient is positioned in ventrodorsal recumbency and the head is located to the right. Please refer to p. 235 for a description of these procedures.

5. Cytological and chemical fluid analysis should be conducted on abdominal fluid samples.
   a. Characterization of the fluid sample through total cell count and total protein concentration in concert with cytological evaluation can aid in the diagnosis of underlying illness.
      i. A transudate contains less than 1,000 cells/μL and less than 2.5 g/dL protein. Transudates accumulate in response to changes in hydrostatic pressure or colloid osmotic pressure. Transudates are associated with hypoproteinemia, or lymphatic or venous congestion. Transudates are not generally associated with acute abdominal pain unless associated with acute portal hypertension.
      ii. A modified transudate contains greater than 1,000 cells/μL and/or a protein concentration greater than 2.5 g/dL. Modified transudates may result from the chronic transudation of fluid and increased venous hydrostatic pressure. Modified transudates may be associated with cardiac disease, vascular insult, inflammation or torsion of an organ, and leakage of a sterile irritant such as urine. Macrophages or mesothelial cells represent the predominant cell types in these effusions.
      iii. An exudate contains greater than 5,000 cells/μL with greater than 3.0 g/dL protein. Exudates accumulate in association with chemotaxis of inflammatory cells, altered vascular permeability, organ inflammation, leakage of plasma proteins, rupture of a visceral organ or vessel, exfoliation of neoplastic cells, leakage of chylous fluid, and leakage of bile or urine. Any cell type may be present; however, exudates typically contain a high number of neutrophils.

    iv. A septic effusion is exudative due to the presence of bacterial agents. Septic fluid contains an increased number of neutrophils and macrophages with free and phagocytosed bacteria. There are numerous causes for septic effusion, including abdominal wall penetration or rupture of a visceral organ, internal abscessation, hematogenous spread, or surgical entry.

  b. Direct smears of the fluid sample may be diagnostic; however, centrifugation with subsequent cytological examination will allow the clinician to review a greater number of nucleated cells.

  c. Cytological evaluation can aid in the differentiation between septic and nonseptic peritonitis and is the test of choice for diagnosing acute septic peritonitis.

    i. Causes of nonseptic peritonitis in cats include FIP, pancreatitis, neoplasia, bile peritonitis, uroperitoneum, and hemorrhage.

    ii. Cytological evaluation is considered to be 57–87% diagnostic for acute septic peritonitis. The presence of phagocytosed bacterial agents is critical in making this diagnosis.

    iii. Acute septic peritonitis is always a surgical emergency and should proceed following rapid medical stabilization.

    iv. The presence of gold-green-blue phagocytosed bile pigment may be noted in abdominal effusion associated with bile peritonitis. Bile peritonitis is relatively uncommon in cats.

6. Biochemical analysis of undiluted abdominal effusion is an important diagnostic tool to aid in the identification of the origin of the cause of acute abdominal illness. Results of biochemical analysis of abdominal fluid should always be interpreted in concert with cytological findings.

  a. The diagnosis of uroperitoneum can be made based on evaluation of the ratio of abdominal fluid creatinine and potassium concentration to that of the peripheral blood.

    i. A creatinine level of the abdominal fluid twice that of peripheral blood is a highly sensitive and specific indicator of uroperitoneum.

    ii. A potassium concentration of the abdominal fluid 1.9 times greater than that of peripheral blood is also supportive of uroperitoneum in cats.

    iii. A positive diagnosis of uroperitoneum should prompt further diagnostic testing through contrast radiography to determine the site of urine leakage.

      1. A retrograde urethrocystogram will identify urethral or bladder disruption.

      2. An excretory urogram will identify kidney, renal pelvis, ureteral, and possibly bladder disruption. Patients should be volume resuscitated prior to intravenous iodinated contrast agent administration. Prolonged renal excretion of contrast media has been associated with renal damage in humans; therefore, excretory urography should be considered cautiously in patients with evidence of dehydration and azotemia.

        a. An enema to empty the large bowel will facilitate visualization of the ureters and ureterovesicular junction. This may or may not be feasible in the critically ill patient.

        b. Water-soluble, sterile iodinated contrast agent equivalent to 400–800 mg iodine/Kg body weight is injected intravenously. Nonionic agents are preferred due to a lower incidence of side effects.

        c. Right lateral and VD radiographs are taken at times 0, 5, 20, and 40 minutes. Oblique views at 20 and 40 minutes may facilitate visualization of the ureters.

        d. Creating a pneumocystogram will facilitate visualization of ureters emptying into the bladder.

        e. Side effects of administration of iodinated contrast medium include hypotension, vomiting, hives, and acute renal failure.

  b. The ratio of bilirubin concentration of abdominal effusion to peripheral blood may be useful in the diagnosis of bile peritonitis.

    i. A ratio greater than 2.0 may be a sensitive indicator of bile peritonitis. However, further investigation is warranted to identify the overall utility of this ratio.

  c. The utility of amylase and lipase measurements in abdominal fluid has yet to be adequately investigated.

d. The measurement of glucose gradients between abdominal fluid and blood has been found to be a quite sensitive (86%) and highly specific (100%) test for the diagnosis of septic peritonitis in cats.
  i. An abdominal fluid glucose 20 mg/dL lower than blood glucose in the cat supports a diagnosis of septic peritonitis. This has been demonstrated when glucose concentrations were measured with a Vet Test 8008 Analyzer (Idexx Laboratories Inc., Westbrook, ME) and has not been demonstrated with the use of glucometers or other laboratory equipment used for chemistry and blood gas analysis. It should be noted that highly cellular nonseptic abdominal fluids may also demonstrate a large glucose gradient (>20 mg/dL). Further evaluation of animals with highly cellular nonseptic effusions will be beneficial to definitively evaluate the utility of the glucose gradient for the diagnosis of septic peritonitis. A definitive diagnosis of septic peritonitis, however, should be based on integration of cytological, biochemical, and imaging findings.
7. Diagnostic imaging is a valuable resource for identification of the underlying cause of acute abdomen in cats. Prior to any imaging, the patient should be stable, calm, and pain free.
  a. Abdominal radiography is a valuable tool for evaluation of cats with acute abdominal pain. It is important that image quality allow for the assessment of all intra-abdominal structures and the surrounding tissues.
  b. A significant percentage of cats presenting with acute abdomen have ingested foreign material. Upper gastrointestinal studies are the most appropriate diagnostic test to rule out gastric and small bowel obstruction.
    i. 30% barium sulfate suspension can be administered via nasogastric tube at a dose of 10 mL/kg in cats with no evidence of gastrointestinal disruption. In cases where gastrointestinal perforation is suspected, an iodinated contrast medium may be used at a dose of 2 mL/kg diluted in 8 mL/kg of water. However, if gastrointestinal disruption is suspected, an indication for surgery may be sought through acquisition of abdominal fluid.
      1. Lateral and ventrodorsal radiographic views may be taken at 0, 15, 30, 60, 90, 120, or 180 minutes after administration.
      2. Normal gastrointestinal transit time is anywhere from 1 to 2 hours in cats but can be increased to 3 to 4 hours (but can vary depending on other factors [see chap. 19—Diagnostic Evaluation of Gastrointestinal Conditions]).
  c. Thoracic radiography is indicated in any patient with acute abdomen in concert with history or physical evidence of cardiorespiratory disease or decreased oxygen indices.
    i. Due to the high incidence of cardiomyopathy in the cat population, thoracic radiographs may be indicated in all cats presenting with acute abdomen and critical illness because of the fluid loading that is often necessary in this patient population.
    ii. Acute lung injury (ARDS) can occur secondary to numerous conditions associated with acute abdomen.
    iii. Thoracic radiographs should be evaluated for evidence of neoplastic disease in all geriatric patients.
  d. Abdominal ultrasound may also be useful in the search for an underlying cause of acute abdomen in the cat. Abdominal ultrasound should be considered complimentary to rather than a substitute for abdominal radiography.
    i. The diagnostic utility of ultrasound is very operator dependent, and misdiagnosis is common when performed by individuals without appropriate training and experience.
8. Abdominal exploration is often the definitive diagnostic and therapeutic tool for the feline patient with acute abdomen (box 20.2).
  a. Surgical exploration is indicated based on a presumptive diagnosis through findings from history, physical examination, and diagnostic testing.
    i. When a diagnosis has not been established, surgical exploration is indicated in patients with persistent symptoms of acute abdominal pain.
    ii. Grossly "negative" abdominal exploration may have important diagnostic value after biopsies are taken.

Box 20.2.   Common surgical conditions associated with acute abdomen in cats.
- GI foreign body
- Intussusception
- Gastrointestinal perforation
- Biliary obstruction
- Septic peritonitis
- Hemoperitoneum
- Uroperitoneum
- Pyometra
- Penetrating injury
- Body wall hernia/disruption
- Abdominal neoplasia

---

iii. Problems identified during abdominal exploration may be definitively treated. Due to the high incidence of infiltrative small bowel disease in the feline population, biopsies should be taken of all grossly abnormal tissues and of all small bowel segments in cats with a history of vomiting and diarrhea without an obvious cause. Mesenteric lymph node biopsies should also be performed in these patients.

iv. Biopsies of the large bowel are indicated only in patients with gross evidence of pathology or a history of large bowel disease such as large bowel diarrhea.

b. Evaluation of a patient with any wounds over the abdomen should always include surgical exploration of those wounds following abdominal radiography.

  i. Wound probing with a blunt instrument is not an accurate tool for identifying penetrating injury because of the ability of skin and subcutaneous and body wall muscle layers to move over one another.

  ii. All bite wounds should be surgically explored (and opened) to facilitate adequate exposure for complete exploration, debridement, lavage, and establishment of drainage.

  iii. Wounds that penetrate the abdominal cavity warrant ventral midline abdominal exploration from xyphoid to pubis.

    1. Intra-abdominal injuries are identified and treated.

    2. Body wall repairs are performed from the abdomen.

    3. Aggressive lavage is performed, culture is taken, and closed suction drainage (Blake Drain; Ethicon Inc., Somerville, NJ; figs. 20.6 a and b) is established in all cases of penetrating injury. Although not all cases may require ongoing drainage, the infected nature of penetrating wounds makes early drainage important. Drains may be removed when abdominal fluid production decreases to <5–7 mL/kg/day.

    4. External wounds are then definitively managed. Definitive management includes debridement, lavage, and establishment of drainage.

  iv. Nonpenetrating wounds may result in severe intra-abdominal injury from crushing and shearing injury. The author has found laparoscopy to be a rapid, minimally invasive yet highly diagnostic tool for abdominal exploration in these types of cases. Surgical abdominal exploration may be warranted in cases where laparoscopy is not available. A proactive philosophy to approaching these patients is important. Cats will not experience serious morbidity from a negative abdominal exploration; however, failure to identify serious intra-abdominal injury can result in serious morbidity or mortality.

c. Analgesia is an important consideration for cats with acute abdominal pain.

  i. Appropriate analgesia will facilitate both diagnostics and therapeutics (see chap. 7—Pain Management in Critically Ill Feline Patients).

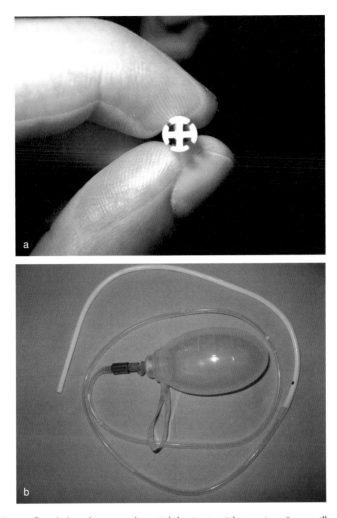

Figs. 20.6 a and b. T-fluted closed suction drain (Blake Drain; Ethicon, Inc. Somerville, NJ).

  d. Early enteral nutritional support is important to rapidly meet caloric needs in critically ill patients
     (see chap. 9—Nutritional Support for the Critically Ill Feline Patient).
     i. Anesthesia events common to the management of cats with critical illness offer the opportunity
        for the placement of nasoesophageal, esophagostomy, gastrostomy, nasojunostomy, gastrojeju-
        nostomy, or surgical jejunostomy feeding tubes.
     ii. Nasoesophageal/nasogastric, esophagostomy, or gastrostomy tubes are good choices for feline
        patients that are not vomiting.
        1. Nasoesophageal or nasogastric tubes are quick and easy to place and are excellent for short-
           term nutritional support in the feline patient.
        2. Esophagostomy tubes are preferred to endoscopic gastrostomy tubes due to a perceived lower
           complication rate. These tubes are excellent for longer-term nutritional support.
     iii. Gastrostomy tubes offer a means of both feeding and gastric decompression.
     iv. Nasojejunostomy, jejunostomy, or gastrojejunostomy tubes bypass the stomach and are indicated
        in patients with persistent vomiting (such as in cats with pancreatitis) or decreased gastric
        motility.

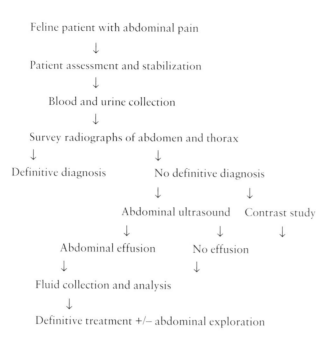

Feline patient with abdominal pain
↓
Patient assessment and stabilization
↓
Blood and urine collection
↓
Survey radiographs of abdomen and thorax
↓   ↓
Definitive diagnosis   No definitive diagnosis
↓   ↓
Abdominal ultrasound   Contrast study
↓   ↓   ↓
Abdominal effusion   No effusion
↓   ↓
Fluid collection and analysis
↓
Definitive treatment +/− abdominal exploration

Fig. 20.7 Approach to acute abdomen.

Summary

Acute abdomen is a common clinical complaint identified in feline patients. Successful management results from rapid stabilization of major body systems, early identification of underlying disease, and timely definitive therapy.

References

Aumann M, Worth LT, Drobatz KJ. Uroperitoneum in cats: 26 cases (1986–1995). J Am Anim Hosp Assoc, 1998; 34:315–324.

Baker R, Lumsden JH. Pleural and peritoneal fluids. In Baker R, Lumsden JH, eds, Color Atlas of Cytology of the Dog and Cat, pp 159–164. St. Louis: Mosby, 2000.

Beal MW. Approach to the acute abdomen. Vet Clin North Am Small Anim Pract, 2005; 35(2):375–396.

Bonczynski JJ, Ludwig LL, Barton LJ, et al. Comparison of peritoneal fluid and peripheral blood pH, bicarbonate, and lactate concentration as a diagnostic tool for septic peritonitis in dogs and cats. Vet Surg, 2003; 32:161–166.

Dellinger RP, Carlet JM, Masur H, et al. Surviving sepsis campaign guidelines for management of severe sepsis and septic shock. Crit Care Med, 2004; 32(3):858–873.

Dillon AR, Spano JS. The acute abdomen. Vet Clin North Am Small Anim Pract, 1983; 13:461–475.

Heuter KJ. Excretory urography. Clin Tech Sm Anim Pract, 2005; 20:39–45.

Mazzaferro E. Triage and approach to the acute abdomen. Clin Tech Small Anim Pract, 2003; 18(1):1–6.

Mueller MG, Ludwig LL, Barton LJ. Use of closed-suctioned drains to treat generalized peritonitis in dogs and cats: 40 cases (1997–1999). J Am Vet Med Assoc, 2001; 219(6):789–794.

Shelly SM. Body cavity fluids. In Raskin RE, Meyer DJ, eds, Atlas of Canine and Feline Cytology, pp 187–205. Philadelphia: Saunders, 2001.

Woolf CJ. Pain: moving from symptom control toward mechanism specific pharmacologic management. Ann Intern Med, 2004; 140:441–451.

21
MANAGEMENT OF SPECIFIC GASTROINTESTINAL CONDITIONS

Anne Marie Corrigan and Douglass K. Macintire

Unique Features

1. The feline esophageal muscle layer contains more smooth muscle compared with dogs (the proximal two-thirds are striated muscle and the distal one-third is smooth muscle; the canine esophagus contains striated muscle throughout).
2. High doses of enrofloxacin may cause blindness in cats.
3. Esophageal hairballs occur relatively commonly in cats compared with dogs.
4. String foreign bodies under the tongue are relatively common, and this site should be consistently evaluated in vomiting or anorexic cats with acute onset of clinical signs. Additionally, string foreign bodies can be found protruding from the anus. Passage this far does not assure absence of GI obstruction and the necessity for surgery.
5. Cats with similar diseases that cause vomiting in dogs tend to not vomit as prolifically as dogs do.
6. Triaditis (pancreatitis, inflammatory bowel disease, and cholangiohepatitis) is relatively unique to cats compared with dogs.
8. Cats are more sensitive to the colloidal effects of oxyglobin compared with dogs, and administration of large volumes should be done with caution.
9. Loss of appetite in cats can result in clinically significant hepatic lipidosis compared with dogs.
10. Acute vomiting due to benign gastritis anecdotally seems to be less common in cats compared with dogs.

Complete physical exam, history, and evaluation of clinical signs and test results are necessary to adequately diagnose and treat any gastrointestinal disease in cats.

Many diseases will respond to therapeutic trials without having a primary diagnosis; however, for recurrent, complicated, or severe diseases, a working knowledge of the appropriate disease process will assist in selecting the appropriate medical, nutritional, or surgical choices in a timely manner. Initial emergency database is indicated for most conditions; however, more complete blood work will be indicated for many diseases, as well as for anesthesia preparedness. Drug recommendations are made in the appropriate paragraphs, but all dosages are listed in the table at the end of the chapter.

A. Regurgitation
  a. Key points and rule-outs
    i. The feline esophageal muscle layer contains more smooth muscle compared with dogs (the proximal two-thirds are striated muscle and the distal one-third is smooth muscle; the canine esophagus contains striated muscle througout).
    ii. Must identify passive versus active expulsion of food to differentiate from vomiting.

           1. Many owners will not specify vomiting versus regurgitation. Most will consider the cat to be vomiting.

      iii. Possible causes include

           1. Esophagitis causing esophageal motor dysfunction or stricture formation

              a. Causes of esophagitis include profuse vomiting, ingestion of caustic substances, gastric contents pooling in the esophagus during general anesthesia, hiatal hernia, and lodging of doxycycline tablets.

              b. Esophageal obstruction/stricture

                  i. Esophageal foreign body, previous trauma, mediastinal mass, esophageal neoplasia, previous esophagitis, and persistent right aortic arch.

              c. Esophageal motility disorder (megaesophagus)

                  i. Neuromuscular disease (generally will see other signs of muscular weakness), active esophagitis, lead toxicity, hypokalemia, organophosphate toxicity

                  ii. Inherited esophageal motility disorder (Siamese cats)

                  iii. Paraneoplastic megaesophagus

      iv. The primary cause needs to be identified to prevent recurrence after therapy.

    b. Diagnostics

      i. Radiographs (cervical and thoracic), fluoroscopy, and contrast studies are beneficial; it is also helpful to monitor for common associated conditions such as aspiration pneumonia or neoplasia.

      ii. Endoscopy may be indicated to evaluate mucosal surfaces, identify foreign bodies or strictures. May also be utilized for therapeutic balloon dilation.

    c. Therapeutics

      i. Elevated feedings, frequent small calorie-dense feedings, the Bailey Chair, or holding upright after feedings for 10–15 minutes, feeding tubes to bypass or rest a dilated esophagus. Balloon dilation while under anesthesia if stricture present

           1. The Bailey Chair may work well in dogs, but cats may not tolerate it or may not intake food in the appropriate position.

    d. Drugs

      i. Omeprazole (0.7 mg/kg PO q24h)

      ii. H_2 blockers (Famotidine 0.5 mg/kg PO, SC, IM IV q12–24h, Ranitidine 2.5 mg IV q12h or 1–2 mg/kg PO q8–12h)

      iii. Sucralfate (0.25–0.5 g PO as slurry q8–12h)

      iv. Cisapride (2.5 mg PO <10-lb cat, 5 mg PO >10-lb cat q8h, give 30 minutes prior to meal) or metoclopramide (0.2–0.4 mg/kg PO or SC q8–12h or 1–2 mg/kg per day CRI infusion) to increase lower esophageal sphincter tone (30 minutes prior to feeding—the prokinetic aspects may not be particularly beneficial).

      v. Pain management for severe esophagitis (see chap. 7—Pain Management in Critically Ill Feline Patients).

      vi. Broad spectrum antibiotic therapy if aspiration pneumonia present

           1. Ampicillin 22 mg/kg IV q8h for gram positive bacteria combined with a gram negative coverage antibiotic—aminoglycoside or fluoroquinolone

           2. Gentamicin 6 mg IV q24h (avoid in cats that are dehydrated, have decreased blood pressure or perfusion, or have renal compromise)

           3. Enrofloxacin 2.5 mg/kg q12h or Marbofloxacin 5 mg/kg q24h

B. Esophageal foreign body

    a. Key points

      i. Historical observation of foreign body ingestion, recent hairballs, ptyalism, or dysphagia

      ii. Ensure careful palpation on left side of neck for the presence of a mass, swelling, or pain in the cervical esophagus.

b. Diagnostics/therapeutics
   i. Radiographs or fluoroscopy
     1. Pay particular attention to thoracic inlet, heart base, and diaphragm, which are common areas for foreign body lodgment
     2. Note the mediastinum for fluid or air, which may indicate tracheal or esophageal perforation.
     3. Subcutaneous air or pneumothorax indicate possible esophageal perforation.
   ii. Use caution with contrast agents if perforation is suspected.
     1. If perforation is a significant possibility, then consider an iodated contrast material.
   iii. Endoscopy with removal and evaluation of mucosal surface damage.
     1. If further damage may occur to esophagus with removal with the endoscope, then consider advancement of the foreign body to stomach and surgical gastrotomy for removal.
   iv. Surgical repair of esophagus if perforation is present
   v. Placement of an esophageal or gastric feeding tube should be considered at this time. If mucosal damage is present, monitor the cat for future complications such as stricture formation (1–3 weeks) or perforation.
c. Drugs
   i. Sucralfate slurries (0.25–0.5 g PO q8–12h) after removal to assist in mucosal protection and healing
   ii. H_2 blockers or omeperazole if esophagitis is a concern, consider therapeutics listed above for regurgitation.
C. Gastric foreign body/intestinal foreign body/obstructions/intussusception
a. Key points
   i. Historical, clinical signs, radiographic, or ultrasound diagnosis.
     1. Vomiting and anorexia are the most common clinical signs.
     2. Gastric foreign bodies can cause intermittent vomiting/anorexia until they pass into the small intestine; can cause obstruction and then signs become more persistent.
   ii. Always check under tongue for a string if any foreign body or obstruction is suspected.
     1. Occasionally, string will be found protruding from the anus. This does not rule out the possibility of intestinal obstruction.
   iii. Consider toxin ingestion and monitor for complications, for example, zinc and lead (see chap. 39—Toxicological Emergencies).
   iv. Gastric/high intestinal obstructions tend to have more acute presentations. Lower intestinal obstructions may present with more chronic onset and may include foreign bodies, tumors, and intussusceptions.
   v. Extraluminal (adhesions and strangulations) as well as intramural diseases (FIP, fungal infections, and neoplasia) also occur.
   vi. If severe ileus is present, monitor closely for endotoxemia, bacterial translocation, or septic shock.
     1. Severe ileus is primarily characterized by absence of borborygmi on abdominal auscultation and uniformly dilated small intestinal loops on abdominal radiographic evaluation.
b. Diagnostics/therapeutics
   i. Perform blood work to identify metabolic derangements that can be addressed before or during surgery. High obstructions are often characterized by hypochloremia, hypokalemia, and metabolic alkalosis, although severe vomiting from any cause can result in this constellation of electrolyte and acid/base changes.
   ii. Abdominal radiographs with characteristic patterns—severely dilated bowel loops proximal to foreign body or obstruction, bunched intestines seen with linear foreign bodies, loss of abdominal detail seen with perforation, radiodense metallic foreign body seen with lead or zinc

     iii. Abdominal ultrasound is especially beneficial for visualizing intussusceptions—can appear as oval masses, target-shaped masses, or thickened intestines with too many layers .

     iv. If plain radiographics are questionable for the diagnosis of intestinal foreign body obstruction, then consider repeating plain abdominal radiographs in 2–3 hours. If intestinal pattern still indicates the same local bowel distention, then intestinal obstruction is more likely.

     v. Positive-contrast upper GI study is the noninvasive gold standard for ruling out intestinal obstruction if plain radiographs are questionable for the diagnosis.

     vi. Definitive treatment

         1. Endoscopic examination and removal (for gastric foreign bodies)

         2. Exploratory laparotomy and correction, removal, and intestinal resection if necessary.

     vii. Initiate IV fluid therapy to correct dehydration and any acid base or electrolyte disturbances.

  c. Drugs

     i. Sucralfate, H_2 blockers, and omeprazole (see drug table at end of chapter).

  d. Nutritional support

     i. Rest damaged mucosa and gastrotomy/enterotomy site 12–24 hours and reintroduce food in liquid or slurry form. Caloric requirements are calculated at $30 \times BW$ (kg) + 70. Begin with one-third of caloric needs on day 1, increasing to full dose by day 3 (see chap. 9—Nutritional Support for the Critically Ill Feline Patient).

         1. Monitor for hypophosphatemia in cats that have been off feed. Signs of hypophosphatemia include weakness, lethargy, altered mentation/seizures, and hemolysis.

         2. If ileal resection is performed, cobalamin supplementation 250–500 ug SQ or IM every 1–2 weeks may be necessary; use injectable form, not a multivitamin.

D. Inflammatory bowel disease (IBD)

  a. Key points

     i. One of the most common causes of chronic vomiting and diarrhea in cats.

     ii. Historical findings may range from acute to chronic and from mild to severe.

     iii. Physical examination findings can include any GI signs, as well as nonspecific findings such as lethargy, anorexia, and weight loss.

     iv. Rule out systemic disease such as FIV, FeLV, hyperthyroidism, parasites, food allergies, and lymphosarcoma.

  b. Diagnostics

     i. Blood work to assess hydration status and anesthesia preparedness

     ii. Gastric and intestinal biopsies via endoscopy, colonoscopy, or surgical exploratory

     iii. The laparotomy increases diagnostic power over endoscopy by obtaining full-thickness biopsies.

  c. Therapeutics

     i. Supportive care depending on severity of presenting signs

     ii. Hypoallergenic or low-additive diet and immunosuppressive therapy are the mainstays of IBD therapy.

     iii. Prednisolone or prednisone (see table 21.1 at end of chapter for doses and adjustments depending on severity) and metronidazole

         1. For more severe or resistant disease, chlorambucil can be added to corticosteroids for enhanced immunosupression.

         2. Methylprednisolone injections can be administered every 2–4 weeks if owners are unable to administer pills or liquid.

         3. Budesonide is a locally acting steroid, with low systemic effects, which might be promising in diabetic cats with IBD.

E. Gastric ulceration

  a. Key points

i. Predisposing factors include shock, mast cell tumors and other neoplasia, NSAIDs, renal failure, liver disease, gastric foreign bodies, sepsis, ischemia/infarction, and trauma.

ii. Patients may present with hematemesis (coffee grounds or frank blood), melena, anemia, and may present with uremia and oral ulceration if concurrent with renal disease.

iii. Complications can include perforation and peritonitis, coagulopathies, and DIC.

b. Diagnosis

   i. Fine-needle aspirates of lymph nodes, spleen, or masses, thoracic radiographs, buffy coat smear, abdominal ultrasound, and a diligent search for tumors are utilized to find evidence of mast cells or other neoplasia.

   ii. Serial PCVs or CBCs to monitor for anemia and regenerative response. If severely anemic, pRBC, whole blood, or oxyglobin transfusion may be required for stabilization.

     1. Whole blood use (recipient wt [kg] × 60) × (desired HCT—HCT of recipient/donor HCT in anticoagulant).

     2. For pRBC use half the calculated dosage listed immediately above.

     3. Monitor closely for vomiting, fever, or other transfusion reactions.

     4. Oxyglobin use 5–20 mL/kg IV, but use caution as oxyglobin acts as a colloid, and pulmonary edema and pleural effusion are relatively common side effects. Give small doses of 2–4 mL/kg/hr and monitor for sign of fluid overload (pulmonary edema/pleural effusion).

   iii. Endoscopy or abdominal exploratory with gastrotomy and biopsy samples are definitive diagnostics.

   iv. Perforation will require surgery to repair the defect and flush abdominal cavity to decrease complications from peritonitis.

c. Therapeutics

   i. Fluid therapy and gastric protectants: sucralfate, H_2 blockers, omeprazole.

   ii. Antibiotic therapy for *Helicobacter* spp. if indicated (after histologic evaluation and other causes for vomiting have been ruled out, including amoxicillin, metronidazole, and Pepto-Bismol). Treat for 5–7 days and reevaluate. Some animals may need longer trials.

   iii. Metoclopramide as a prokinetic and antiemetic if indicated

   iv. Iron supplementation if chronic microcytic hypochromic anemia. Although blood transfusion is an excellent source of iron.

F. Acute vomiting

a. Key points

   i. Many causes should be considered, including disorders of the central or peripheral nervous systems, and GI, renal, hepatic, and systemic inflammatory diseases.

   ii. Ensure vomiting versus regurgitation and check under tongue for string foreign body.

     1. Vomiting is an active process with abdominal contractions and preliminary signs, while regurgitation a passive one usually with no preliminary signs.

b. Diagnostics

   i. Initial database can include PCV/TS, glucose, BUN, and urine specific gravity, but due to the variety of systemic causes, a more complete workup is usually indicated and includes CBC with a blood smear, chemistry, and urinalysis. One venipuncture would be less stressful for the cat.

   ii. Other diagnostics may include fecal examination, abdominal radiographs, abdominal ultrasound, endoscopy with biopsies, or surgical exploratory with biopsies.

   iii. The primary rule-outs on an emergency basis for acute vomiting are gastrointestinal obstruction, septic peritonitis, and gastrointestinal ischemia or rupture.

c. Therapeutics

   i. Even if the correct diagnosis is not identified, therapeutics are aimed at supportive care, correcting dehydration, metabolic derangements, and gastritis. Positive responses may be seen within 24–48 hours if the condition is self-limiting and relatively benign.

    ii. Antiemetics and prokinetics may mask primary cause and could be dangerous if foreign body or obstruction have not been ruled out.

    iii. Treatment includes IV fluids, antiemetics, (phenothiazines, metoclopramide [also has the benefit of preventing ileus], Meclizine if vestibular cause), and anthelmintics.

    iv. Diet recommendations

       1. If the cat will eat, a bland diet such as cottage cheese and rice, lean cooked hamburger and rice, or lean chicken and rice can be fed within 24–48 hours.

       2. Force-feeding is not recommended for anorexic cats.

       3. Trickle feeding through NE tube, esophagostomy, or jejunostomy tube can nutritionally support the cat and prevent hepatic lipidosis (see chap. 9—Nutritional Support for the Critically Ill Feline Patient).

       4. Partial or total parenteral nutrition may be indicated when oral feeding is not an option and cannot be instituted within 3–5 days.

G. Acute diarrhea

  a. Key points

    i. Differentiate between large and small bowel, localized versus diffuse disease, and evaluate systemic effects such as dehydration, electrolyte disturbances, or sepsis.

       1. Large-bowel diarrhea is characterized by small-volume bowel movements that occur frequently and with urgency. Straining and mucus are also frequent with occasional fresh blood.

       2. Small-bowel diarrhea tends to be less frequent with larger volumes.

    ii. Rule-outs include parasitism, dietary changes or indiscretion, drug side effects or intoxication, IBD, LSA or other neoplasia, and fungal, protozoal, and bacterial infections.

  b. Diagnostics

    i. Minimum database (PCV, TS, blood glucose, BUN) to evaluate for hydration status if acute or mild, or complete blood work (CBC, chemistry screen) if more severe or chronic disease

    ii. Obtain a fecal sample for flotation, direct smear, or culture if indicated. Advanced diagnostics may include CBC, chemistries, blood gases, cobalamin, folate, feline pancreatic lipase immunoreactivity (fPLI), abdominal radiographs, and ultrasound.

  c. Therapeutics

    i. Administer fluids with KCl supplementation if necessary to rehydrate and maintain the cat during diagnostics.

    ii. Diet modification—including NPO for 24 hours and then a reintroduction with a bland diet for 3–5 days.

  d. Drugs

    i. May include sucralfate, H_2 blockers, omeprazole, and metoclopramide if necessary

    ii. Immunosuppressive therapy for IBD

    iii. Antibiotics are indicated if there is a clear indication of infection or sepsis risk, including fever, neutrophilia or neutropenia, bloody stool, and shock.

       Symptomatic therapies may often mask underlying causes and decrease one's ability to monitor progress and therapeutic response.

H. Acute pancreatitis

  a. Key points and rule-outs

    i. Common associated diseases include cholangiohepatitis, hepatic lipidosis, IBD, trauma, and toxoplasmosis.

    ii. Triaditis includes concurrent pancreatitis, cholangiohepatitis, and IBD.

    iii. Cats can present with a variety of signs. General malaise, weight loss, anorexia, dehydration, hypothermia, and icterus are common.

    iv. Differentials include foreign bodies, IBD, gastroenteritis, intussusceptions, infections (panleukopenia), neoplasia, and cholangitis.

       1. These can progress to more severe conditions such as hepatic lipidosis, septic shock, and DIC.

    v.   Cats are much less likely to vomit with pancreatitis than dogs.

    vi.   Siamese cats may be predisposed.

b. Diagnostics

    i.   Complete blood work and urinalysis to assess systemic responses to disease and to have baseline data for therapeutic monitoring.

    ii.   Amylase and lipase have not proven helpful in the diagnosis.

    iii. The fPLI serum test is appropriate for diagnosis and monitoring therapy.

    iv. Other laboratory changes are variable: dehydration, early (neutrophilia with a left shift) or late (decreased WBC) signs of inflammation, elevated liver enzymes, hypocalcemia due to fat saponification, and hyper- or hypoglycemia.

    v.   Radiographic appearance may range from no signs to loss of cranial abdominal detail (ground glass), and/or duodenal gas.

    vi.   Chest radiographs may identify diffuse infiltrates (ARDS), pleural effusion, and/or aspiration pneumonia.

    vii. Abdominal ultrasound is excellent for evaluating any concurrent liver disease and may identify hypoechoic masses in cranial abdomen, cysts, abscesses, free abdominal fluid, and may allow for evaluation of the pancreas and gall bladder.

    viii. Abdominocentesis if indicated; cytology usually reveals an exudative effusion that is aseptic. Monitor for signs of diabetes mellitus; insulin therapy may have to be instituted.

c. Therapeutics

    i.   Most are aimed at supportive care and fluid and electrolyte deficit correction.
Begin crystalloid fluid therapy with KCl supplementation.

        1. If rapid resuscitation is required to treat shock or poor perfusion, KCl supplementation should be delayed until after the initial fluid bolus has been administered.

    ii.   Pain medication such as buprenorphine, oxymorphone, or fentanyl

    iii. Antibiotic therapy to prevent bacterial translocation (cats have a higher bacterial count in duodenum compared with dogs), enrofloxacin (caution with high doses), cefazolin, or a combination of ampicillin and enrofloxacin are recommended in cats with fever and more severe disease.

        There is some controversy surrounding reintroduction of food. If the cat will eat, a low-fat feline diet can be fed within 24–48 hours.

        1. Force-feeding is not recommended for anorexic cats as this may result in food aversion.

        2. Trickle feeding through NE tube, esophagostomy, or jejunostomy tube can nutritionally support the cat and prevent hepatic lipidosis.

        3. Partial or total parenteral nutrition may be indicated when oral feeding is not an option (consider restricted lipid content; see chap. 9—Nutritional Support for the Critically Ill Feline Patient).

    iv. Other medications of value include antiemetics such as metoclopramide, cobalamin, and oral pancreatic enzymes.

    v.   Surgical exploratory may be indicated for abscesses, peritonitis, bile duct obstruction, and jejunostomy tube placement.

    vi.   Complicated or severe cases may benefit from plasma transfusions 5–20 mL/kg IV, hetastarch or dextran 20 mL/kg/day IV, or oxyglobin 5–20 mL/kg/IV to assist in oxygen delivery to damaged tissues.

        1. Caution should prevail with aggressive oxyglobin administration as fluid overload is a relatively common side effect. Try 2–4 mL/kg doses over 1 hour and evaluate response and evidence of fluid overload (pulmonary edema, pleural effusion, persistent increase in central venous pressure).

d. Complications may include renal failure, diabetes mellitus, DIC, ARDS, cardiac arrhythmias, bile duct obstruction, vitamin K responsive coagulopathies, hypokalemia, hypophosphatemia, and death in severe cases.

    e. The prognosis depends on the severity of disease and complications such as concurrent disease states, and on possible sequelae such as chronic pancreatitis, hepatic lipidosis, exocrine pancreatic insufficiency, and rarely, diabetes mellitus.

I. Acute stomatitis/oral ulcers

    a. Key points

       i. Frequent problem in cats, and it is common for this to progress and involve many sites, including tongue, gingiva, lips, periodontal membranes, and glossopalatine folds.

       ii. Rule-outs include severe dental disease, immune-mediated diseases, immunodeficient diseases, and infectious diseases, including bacterial and viral diseases (most commonly calicivirus), metabolic diseases (most commonly uremia), neoplasia, nutritional disorders, toxic/caustic, diabetes mellitus, and trauma (including foreign bodies and electrical cord burns).

    b. Diagnostics

       i. Due to the wide variety of causes, a detailed history including onset and duration must be evaluated.

       ii. Clinical signs usually associated with oral disease, including anorexia, dysphagia, halitosis, and ptyalism

       iii. Physical exam to try and identify if localized disease or oral manifestation of systemic disease, as well as a careful oral exam to identify and describe all inflamed areas

       iv. If the cat is particularly painful or fractious, sedation/anesthesia is indicated, and while under, culture swabs (usually not diagnostic, but sensitivity will help pick antibiotics that are efficacious), scrapings, or biopsy samples are necessary to identify cause or cellular infiltrate via cytology.

       v. Blood work to identify underlying causes including CBC-leukocytosis for chronic infection or inflammation, eosinophilia-eosinophilic granuloma complex, FIV/FeLV testing, serum chemistries, and urinalysis to assess kidney function and test for diabetes mellitus

       vi. Cytology or histopathology of oral samples

       vii. Dental radiographs to assess alveolar bone and possible tooth root disease

    c. Treatment

       i. Identification of primary cause necessary for appropriate long-term therapy

       ii. Adequate nutrition and hydration must be managed—soft foods, vitamin supplementation, and fluid therapy. Additional conservative therapeutics includes full dental prophylaxis, followed with daily oral antiseptic rinses, fluoride gel, lidocaine gel, and wax coatings.

       iii. Feeding tube placement indicated for severe inflammation, pain, or prolonged anorexia

       iv. Antibiotic therapy to control secondary infections (clindamycin 5–11 mg/kg PO q12h); bacteria are rarely primary causes.

       v. Culture and sensitivity will aid in selection of appropriate drugs; common choices include amoxicillin/clavulanic acid, clindamycin, azithromycin, and doxycycline.

       vi. Immunosuppressive therapy is indicated for eosinophilic granulomas.

       vii. Antifungal therapy if indicated; antivirals: interferon-α for retroviruses (efficacy questionable) or immunosuppressive or anti-inflammatory therapy, but only after trying antibiotics. This is beyond the scope of emergency medicine and the reader is referred to more appropriate internal medicine/infectious disease texts.

       viii. Bovine lactoferrin for calicivirus, although this is experimental and clinical efficacy and safety has not been established

       ix. More veterinarians are finding that partial (molars and premolars) or complete tooth extractions are the only ways to halt the progression of lymphocytic or plasmacytic gingivostomatitis.

J. Large-bowel diarrhea—colitis

    a. Key points

       i. This is often acute and self-limiting.

       ii. Clinical signs include small-volume, frequent bowel movements often with straining, mucus, and occasionally fresh blood.

    iii. History must include diet, previous anthelmintic therapy, frequency and amount of defecation, the presence of blood or mucus, and duration of clinical signs.

    iv. Chronic disease can be associated with decreased appetite, weight loss, and lethargy.

    v. Parasites, including *Trichomonas*, *Cryptosporidium*, *Giardia*, *Coccidia*, whipworms, hookworms, and roundworms can cause large-bowel diarrhea.

  b. Diagnosis

    i. Physical exam often normal, palpation may be painful.

    ii. Digital rectal examination should be performed to rule out rectal strictures, masses, or other abnormalities.

    iii. Collect feces for floatation, smear, and culture if necessary.

    iv. Complete blood work and further diagnostics for severe or complicated disease.

    v. Colonoscopy or exploratory laparotomy with biopsies will provide the definitive diagnosis.

K. Therapeutics

    i. Symptomatic therapy includes crystalloid fluid therapy to restore and maintain hydration.

    ii. Dietary manipulations may include high-fiber diets (commercial brand or by adding psyllium, bran, or canned pumpkin pie filling 1–4 tsp/meal).

    iii. Hypoallergenic diets may benefit more chronic inflammatory disease.

    iv. The appropriate use of anthelmintics, antiparasitics, and antibiotics, commonly beginning with metronidazole and fenbendazole

    v. Immunosuppressive therapy such as prednisone should be reserved for definitively diagnosed inflammatory colitis that is unresponsive to the above therapeutics.

    vi. Sulfasalazine—must use caution in cats as they are more sensitive to salicylates than dogs and may become acidotic; reserve use for complicated or recurrent cases and monitor for vomiting, diarrhea, and anemia.

L. Constipation/obstipation/megacolon

  a. Key points

    i. Tenesmus in middle-aged to older cats is commonly idiopathic megacolon (dilation and hypomotility).

    ii. Other rule-outs: dietary indiscretion (less common in cats), neoplasia, dyschezia, neurologic disease, trauma/previous pelvic fractures, dehydration (especially with chronic renal failure), and strictures.

  b. Diagnostics

    i. Abdominal palpation and radiographs are useful for identifying the primary cause during or after treatment.

      Blood work will help assess hydration status and anesthesia preparedness as well as any other diseases.

  c. Therapeutics

    i. Administer fluid therapy and electrolyte replacement as needed for rehydration.

    ii. Enemas using 5–10 mL/kg warm water or saline with K-Y jelly, along with manual fecal removal using gentle digital manipulation

      1. Do not use commercial Fleet enemas as hyperphosphatemia and hypocalcemia will result.

    iii. If obstipated, administer fluid therapy to rehydrate for 12–24 hours before attempting manual removal. Manual removal often requires general anesthesia.

    iv. Utilize oral stool softeners or laxatives: lactulose or docusate sodium. Cisapride is used for its prokinetics effects.

      1. Avoid use until pelvic fracture or other obstructions have been ruled out and manual evacuation completed.

    v. Feed high-fiber or low-residue diet. The addition of Metamucil (1–4 g every 12–24 hours mixed with wet food) or pumpkin filling may be beneficial in stimulating motility via increasing output, reducing stool density, and increasing bulk.

      vi. Hairball laxatives are not usually beneficial, except in mild cases.

     vii. For complicated or unresponsive cases, a subtotal colectomy should be considered, along with lifelong lactulose.

M. Hepatic encephalopathy

  a. Key points

    i. Porto-systemic shunts—usually extrahepatic in cats (look for copper eyes and ptyalism), end-stage liver disease, and severe acute liver disease are all possible causes.

    ii. The toxins involved in the development of CNS signs are complex and multiple; they are probably produced by abnormal metabolism of neuroactive agents and are often due to hepatic dysfunction and gastrointestinal tract bacterial metabolite production. These may include ammonia, excitatory and inhibitory neurotransmitter imbalances, the production of false neurotransmitters, and mercaptans.

    iii. Complicating factors include high-protein meals/gastrointestinal bleeding, neoplasia, corticosteroids, and infections with concurrent tissue catabolism.

    iv. Presenting signs may range from ptyalism to seizures and coma. Gastrointestinal and renal signs are also common.

    v. Avoid benzodiazepines, barbiturates, and acepromazine.

  b. Diagnostics

    i. Blood work

      1. CBC—mild anemia

      2. Serum chemistry—liver-specific findings common, low BUN, hypoalbuminemia, hypoglycemia, hypocholesterolemia, possibly elevated liver enzymes

      3. Urinalysis may show ammonium biurate crystals, hematuria, pyuria, isosthenuria.

    ii. Liver function tests, resting ammonia, and bile acids

    iii. Radiographs may show microhepatica for chronic liver disease or PSS, hepatomegaly for acute liver disease, and renomegaly in some cats due to the trophic effects of ammonia.

    iv. Abdominal ultrasound may identify urate urolithiasis, a shunting vessel, and allow evaluation of liver echotexture; portal scintigraphy is also helpful in identifying shunts.

    v. Definitive diagnosis is usually based on liver biopsy or identification and repair of a shunting vessel. Portal hypertension is the most common postsurgical complication.

  c. Therapeutics

    i. Initially directed toward supportive care while trying to identify cause

    ii. Fluid therapy, low-protein diet, oral antibiotic therapy options include neomycin, amoxicillin, and metronidazole.

    iii. If ammonia levels are high, use oral lactulose to help reduce ammonia.

      1. Lactulose retention enemas (warm saline, lactulose 10 mL/kg 1 : 3 dilution retained for 15 minutes) or betadine (10 mL/kg 1 : 10 dilution retained for 15 minutes) can be used to decrease the ammonia levels if the cat is seizuring or comatose.

    iv. If a shunt is suspected or identified, surgical exploratory and shunt repair with an ameroid constrictor is the treatment of choice. Many cats may have a persistent shunt, and continued medical therapy may keep them free of clinical signs.

N. Acute hepatic failure

  a. Key points

    i. Regardless of cause, hepatic necrosis can follow any insult.

    ii. Common causes include toxins (aflatoxins, pesticides, and many cleaning products), drug exposure (acetaminophen, diazepam, glipizide, and griseofulvin), and infectious disease (leptospirosis, although extremely rare in cats), sepsis, FIP, fungal disease, bacterial cholangiohepatitis, and toxoplasmosis).

    iii. Prognosis will vary depending on cause, ability of liver to regenerate, and previous hepatic insult.

    iv. Presenting signs can range from lethargy and anorexia to shock, DIC, and CNS signs. Common signs include dehydration, anorexia, vomiting, diarrhea, and icterus.

  b. Diagnosis

    i. History of toxin or drug exposure, CBC, chemistry, urinalysis

    ii. Elevated liver enzymes, hyperbilirubinemia, and hypoglycemia

      1. Extremely high liver enzymes are expected with acute hepatic necrosis that results in liver dysfunction.

    iii. Elevated bile acids (only run if not icteric) or elevated ammonia

    iv. WBC can vary depending on stage and severity of disease.

    v. Coagulation abnormalities occur with liver failure and DIC.

    vi. Radiographs may show mild hepatomegaly or microhepatica with chronic disease or shunting. Abdominal ultrasound may indicate hepatic necrosis (hypoechoic foci) or lipidosis (diffuse hyperechogenicity); mixed patterns can indicate neoplasia or cholangiohepatitis.

  c. Therapeutics

    i. Crystalloid fluid therapy with acetate buffer instead of lactate (Normosol-R or Plasmalyte) with potassium supplementation to correct dehydration and electrolyte imbalances

    ii. Colloids may be necessary if hypoproteinemia in present, especially with more chronic or severe disease.

    iii. Monitor glucose and supplement as necessary. Hypoglycemia treated with 0.5–1 mL/kg IV of 50% dextrose (dilute 1:4) and then 2.5–5% in fluids.

    iv. Broad-spectrum antibiotics may be necessary if there is evidence of sepsis: ampicillin in combination with an aminoglycoside or a fluoroquinolone

    v. Blood products if necessary, heparin therapy (controversial), and antidote therapy for intoxications should be used when indicated.

    vi. Nutritional support with a liver diet such as Hill's L/D if anorexic for more than 24–48 hours.

      1. If anorexic, a feeding tube may be necessary (see chap. 9—Nutritional Support in Critically Ill Feline Patents).

O. Cholangiohepatitis

  a. Key points

    i. Complex disease state in cats may include local diseases such as cholangitis, hepatitis, and pancreatitis.

    ii. Clinical signs include anorexia, vomiting, diarrhea, weight loss, and possibly icterus.

    iii. Causes include immune or local inflammatory disease, neoplasia, infectious disease including toxoplasma, FIP, and bacterial; oftentimes the diagnosis is idiopathic.

    iv. Definitive diagnosis is provided by liver biopsy and histologic evaluation.

      1. Histologic findings include suppurative and/or lymphocytic/lymphoplasmacytic cellular infiltrates, or fibrosis with more chronic disease.

  b. Diagnostics

    i. Blood work, including CBC (neutrophilic leukocytosis), serum chemistry with elevated liver enzymes and bilirubin, elevated globulins, and urinalysis identifying bilirubinuria

    ii. Coagulation profile may be abnormal.

    iii. Radiographs may identify an enlarged liver or loss of cranial abdominal detail if pancreas is involved.

    iv. Abdominal ultrasound can identify enlarged liver, also useful to evaluate gall bladder and common bile duct size and patency, as well as pancreas and duodenum (inflammation of either can cause secondary bile duct obstruction).

    v. If the disease is nonsuppurative, aggressive diagnostics should be performed, such as ultrasound-guided liver biopsy, culture of bile, or exploratory surgery with appropriate sampling. If an infectious cause can be ruled out, immunosuppressive therapy may be efficacious.

   c. Therapeutics
      i. Fluid therapy and nutritional support are necessary to correct hydration, electrolytes, and acid/base abnormalities as well as prevent hepatic lipidosis.
      ii. If improvement does not occur with supportive care and therapy, liver aspirate or biopsy are indicated to help diagnose and better treat, either ultrasound guided or during an abdominal laparotomy.
      iii. Ursodeoxycholate after bile duct obstruction is ruled out
      iv. Sam-E is indicated to help support the liver.
      v. Long-term antibiotic therapy, best if chosen on culture and sensitivity of biopsy or gall bladder aspirate
         1. Common choices include amoxicillin/clavulanic acid, enrofloxacin, or cephalosporins for 8 weeks.

P. Rectal prolapse
   a. Key points
      i. May be complete or incomplete, depending on how many layers of the rectal wall are everted
      ii. Owners may report tenesmus, diarrhea, or other signs of intestinal disease. It is also seen with stranguria, chronic FLUTD, and in reproductive diseases such as dystocia.
      iii. Manx cats have predisposition.
         Intussusception (with obstructive pattern associated) must be ruled out and differentiated from true rectal prolapse. Perform a careful rectal exam to determine extent and layers involved in prolapse.
         1. A lubricated blunt probe will not pass lateral to rectal prolapse, but will if colonic or ileoce-cocolic intussusception and prolapse.
   b. Therapeutics
      i. Identify and treat the predisposing cause, GI or genitourinary tract disease.
      ii. Assess the prolapse: Is the tissue viable or necrotic?
         1. Black or purple rectal tissue suggests necrosis and may have to be resected.
      iii. Conservative therapy for viable prolapse includes anesthesia and analgesics, warm saline with dextrose or hypertonic fluids that will clean, warm, and moisten the tissues and allow for reduction of edema.
         1. Gently reduce the tissues and place a loose purse-string suture in anus (a 3-cc-size syringe case will allow for proper sizing) with nonabsorbable suture, and place patient on stool softeners and a low-residue diet. Purse-string suture can be removed in 10–14 days.
         2. Tilting the body such that the anus is higher than the head may facilitate reduction of the prolapsed tissue. Use caution and watch ventilation and blood pressure when putting the cat in this position.
         3. Occasionally ice packs placed on the prolapsed tissue may reduce swelling and inflammation and facilitate reduction of the prolapsed tissue.
      iv. If the tissue is not reducible or viable, then surgical correction is indicated.
      v. Colopexy to prevent recurrent prolapses plus amputation of necrotic tissue if necessary and aggressive antibiotic therapy
      vi. Surgical complications include recurrence, stricture, and stenosis.

Q. Peritonitis—septic, aseptic, FIP, bile
   a. Key points
      i. Primary or secondary causes possible for peritonitis
      ii. Complication anticipation will be the key to adjusting therapies and diagnostics.
      iii. Cytology and fluid analysis will help differentiate underlying etiology.
   b. Diagnosis
      i. Blood work for patient assessment and anesthesia preparedness

  ii. Four-quadrant abdominocentesis using sterile technique, ultrasound-guided aspirate, or diagnostic peritoneal lavage will allow you to identify the effusion type and allow for appropriate therapeutics.

  iii. Cytology and chemistry of sample will allow for differentiation for the types of peritonitis.

   1. Bile peritonitis—bile crystals (gold to green) on cytology, chemistry will show more elevated bilirubin in effusion than in serum.

   2. Septic—suppurative effusion with intracellular bacteria, degenerate neutrophils, low glucose in aspirate, and elevated lactate may also indicate septic effusion.

    a. A blood-to-abdominal-fluid glucose difference of >20 mg/dL was 86% sensitive and 100% specific for a diagnosis of septic peritonitis in cats. The blood-to-fluid glucose difference was more accurate for a diagnosis of septic peritonitis than peritoneal fluid glucose concentration alone. Further studies will be required to determine the ability of this diagnostic tool to differentiate a sterile but severely inflammatory peritonitis versus a septic peritonitis.

   3. FIP–pyogranulomatous effusion usually characterized by a high total protein of moderate to severe cellularity

  iv. Surgical exploratory is indicated in all cases with intracellular bacteria or bile peritonitis.

   1. Surgical exploratory may also be indicated in cases with degenerate neutrophils with no intracellular bacteria or in a decompensating patient where peritonitis is suspected but abdominocentesis is negative. This will allow for diagnostics as well as therapeutics such as identifying an underlying cause, obtaining biopsy samples, flushing abdomen, correcting any abnormalities, and removing any necrotic tissue or blood clots.

   2. Rarely, no obvious surgically correctable underlying cause for septic peritonitis can be found.

 c. Therapeutics

  i. Initiate fluids and broad spectrum antibiotic therapy pending culture and sensitivity results.

   1. Commonly used combination therapy including a cephalosporin with metronidazole or an aminoglycoside (caution with dehydration or azotemia)

   2. Another common and effective combination in cats with poor renal perfusion or azotemia is intravenous ampicillin and intravenous enrofloxacin, +/– intravenous metronidazole.

  ii. Monitoring for hydration status, blood pressure, and urine output to assess perfusion

  iii. Pain medication is warranted and necessary in cats with septic peritonitis. Choose cardiovascular-sparing pain medications (see chap. 7—Pain Management in Critically Ill Feline Patients).

R. Mesenteric thrombosis

 a. Key points

  i. May be secondary to arterial thrombus associated with underlying cardiac disease or other diseases that result in hypercoagulability (see chap. 29—Hematologic Emergencies: Bleeding). Will often present with an acute onset of vomiting, bloody diarrhea, anorexia, shock, and pain.

  ii. This disease holds a very poor prognosis.

 b. Diagnostics

  i. Blood work to assess electrolytes and anesthesia preparedness

  ii. Abdominal radiographs and ultrasound may reveal dilated gas-filled loops of bowel with reduced motility. However, not diagnostic for mesenteric infarction.

  iii. Auscultation, ECG, and echocardiography should be performed to identify underlying cardiac disease.

  iv. A complete blood count, serum chemistry profile, and thyroid level should be done to investigate other disease processes.

  v. Thoracic radiographs may be helpful to identify any pulmonary, cardiac, or vascular abnormalities.

Table 21.1. Drug chart.

Drugs	Classes	MOAs	Side Effects
Amoxicillin	Aminopenicillin	Bactericidal, inhibits mucopeptide synthesis	Mostly GI, rare hypersensitivities
Amoxicillin/clavulanic acid	Aminopenicillin/ beta-lactamase inhibitor	Bactericidal, inhibits mucopeptide synthesis/ irreversibly binds betalactamases	Mostly GI, rare hypersensitivities
Ampicillin	Aminopenicillin	Bactericidal, inhibits mucopeptide synthesis	Mostly GI, rare hypersensitivities
Aspirin-acetylsalicylic acid	NSAID	Analgesia, anti-inflammatory and antiplatelet effects	Gastric irritation, blood loss, hypersensitivity reactions, acidosis
Azithromycin	Macrolide antibiotic	Inhibits bacterial protein synthesis—bacteriostatic	GI distress
Bethanechol	Cholinergic agonist	Muscarinic receptor agonist	Parasympathetic activation
Budesonide	Locally acting steroid	Glucocorticoid, high first pass effect, low systemic levels, still suppresses HPA	HPA suppression
Buprenorphine	Partial opiate agonist	mu receptor partial agonist: 30x more potent than morphine	CV and resp. depression
Butorphanol	Partial opiate agonist/ antagonist	kappa and sigma agonists, mu antagonist—4–7x more potent than morphine	mild sedation
Cefoxitin	2nd-generation Cephalosporin B-lactam antibiotic	Bacteriocidal—inhibit cell wall synthesis	GI distress hypersensitivity, thrombocytopenia, diarrhea
Chlorambucil	Cell cycle nonspecific alkylating agent	DNA crosslinking immunosupressant and antineoplastic	Myelosuppression—anemia, thrombocytopenia, leukopenia, possible teratogen
Clindamycin	Lincosamide antibiotic	Binds 50S ribosomal subunit—inhibits peptide bond formation	Gastroenteritis
Cisapride	Substituted piperidinyl benzamide	GI prokinetic	May impair absorption of other drugs due to decreased GI transit time
Cobalamin	Vitamin B12	Replacement for decreased GI absorption	Pain at injection site
Docusate sodium	Stool softener	Surfactant stool softener	Cramping, diarrhea, GI mucosal damage
Doxycycline	Tetracycline antibiotic	Bacteriostatic—inhibits bacterial protein synthesis	Esophageal strictures, vomiting

258

Contraindications and Precautions	Routes of Administration and Doses	General Uses
In animals with history of allergic reactions to beta lactam antibiotics	22 mg/kg PO q12h 2–3 weeks	For helicobacter infection with metronidazole, clarithromycin, and possibly Pepto-Bismol
In animals with history of allergic reactions to beta lactam antibiotics	62.5 mg/cat PO q12h	Urinary tract, skin, and soft tissue infections
In animals with history of allergic reactions to beta lactam antibiotics	10–20 mg/kg PO q12h 20–30 mg/kg PO q8h 20–40 mg/kg IV q6–8h	Gram + infections Gram − infections For sepsis
Cats very sensitive; caution with dosing	5 mg/ CAT PO q72h	Antithrombotic dose often used with hypertrophic cardiomyopathy
Caution in hepatic disease	5–10 mg/kg PO q24h for 3–5 days or 5 mg/kg PO q24h for 2 days then every 3–5 days for a total of 5 doses	Stomatitis, upper respiratory infections
Outflow obstruction	1.25–7.5 mg/day divided q8h	Bladder palpation often For dysautonomia
GI ulcers, active infections	1 mg/cat PO q24h	For IBD in diabetic cats, may be promising
CNS and hepatic dysfunction, biliary tract disease	0.005–0.01 mg/kg IM, IV, SQ q6–12h Can also be given orally/transbuccally	Pain management
Renal disease, liver disease, Addison's, CNS	0.1–1 mg/kg IM, IV, SQ q1–3h	Antiemetic—decreased sensitivity of vomiting center to chemical stimuli, anxiolytic Mild pain management
Decrease dose in renal failure	25–30 mg/kg IV q8h	For peritonitis and sepsis
Caution with other myelosuppressives	0.05–0.1 mg/lb/day (can decrease to EOD if side effects) in conjunction with prednisolone at 1 mg/lb/day Or 0.07–0.15 mg/lb q72h	IBD, adjunctive treatment of FIP, pemphigus, severe feline eosinophilic granuloma complex
Caution in severe renal or hepatic disease	11–33 mg/kg PO q24h 12.5 mg/kg PO or IM q12h	Dental infections Anaerobic infections Toxoplasmosis
Caution with GI obstruction Decrease dose in hepatic failure Drug interaction with cimetidine	2.5 mg/ <10-lb cat PO q8h 5 mg/>10-lb cat PO q8h Give 30 minutes before meal	Constipation/obstipation or megacolon Use in conjunction with stool softeners and a bulk laxative
None reported	Injectable 250 µg SC q7d for 6 weeks then q14d for 5 more doses, then once monthly.	For ileal resection
Caution with preexisting electrolyte disturbances	2 mg/kg PO q24h	Stool softener
Do not use in pregnant or nursing animals	5 mg/kg PO q12h followed by at least 6 mL of water, or choose a liquid formulation	For susceptible infections

Table 21.1. *Continued.*

Drugs	Classes	MOAs	Side Effects
Enrofloxacin	Flouoroquinolone antibiotic	Inhibits DNA gyrase	Blindness with high doses in cats. Caution in young animals—cartilage defects
Famotidine	H₂ histamine receptor blocker	Reduces gastric acid production	Give slow IV—may cause bradycardia Hypersensitivity
Fenbendazole	Benzimidazole	Microtubule assembly inhibitors	Vomiting; monitor for reactions to rapid antigen release from dying parasites
Fentanyl	Opioid analgesic	mu receptor agonist	Respiratory depression and bradycardia
Ferrous sulfate	Oral iron supplement	Iron supplementation	GI upset. Can be very toxic if overdosed
Heparin and low molecular weight heparin	Anticoagulants	Depending on size fraction and dose many different coagulation effects	Bleeding and thrombocytopenia
Interferon alfa-2a	Cytokine-antiviral	Antiviral, immunomodulating, and antiproliferative effects	Uncommon: malaise, fever, allergic reations, myelotixicity, myalgia
Lactoferrin	Cytokine	Immunomodulatory	Not reported
Lactulose	Disaccharide laxative and blood ammonia reducer	Osmotic laxative and colonic acidifier which allows for ammonia trapping	Flatulence, gastric distension diarrhea and dehydration
Lomotil—diphenoxylate, Imodium—loperamide, codeine	Antidiarrheal opiates	Mu agonist, decreases peristalsis	Excitation, constipation
Marbofloxacin	Fluoroquinolone antibiotic	Inhibits DNA gyrase	Seizures, GI distress, drug interactions
Meclizine	Piperidine derivative, antiemetic and antihistamine, antispasmodic and local anesthetic effects	Not completely understood, central anticholinergic and CNS depressant activity	Sedation, dry mucous membranes, tachycardia, CNS stimulation possible
Methylprednisolone	Glucocorticoid	4–5x more potent than hydrocortisone	Cushing's-like: PU, PD, PP
Metoclopramide	Para-aminobenzoic acid derivative	Increases LES tone Prokinetic Antiemetic	Frenzied behavior or disorientation, constipation
Metronidazole	Nitroimidazole antibacterial and antiprotozoal	Bacteriocidal; proposed MOA is disrupting DNA and nucleic acid synthesis, antiprotozoal activity not understood	Neurotoxicity, lethargy, weakness, neutropenias, hepatotoxicity, hematuria, anorexia, nausea, vomiting, and diarrhea

Contraindications and Precautions	Routes of Administration and Doses	General Uses
Caution with renal, or hepatic insufficiency and dehydration	5 mg/kg per day q24 h or divided q12h until 3 days beyond clinical signs	For susceptible infections
Cardiac, hepatic, or renal disease—consider reduced dose	0.5 mg/kg PO, SC, IM IV q12–24h	For GI diseases, regurgitation, or other esophageal disease, vomiting, gastric ulceration
Not FDA approved, but many reports of use and no contraindications reported	50 mg/kg PO q24h for 5 days	Ascarids, hookworms, strongyloides, *Taenia* spp., lungworms, and *Giardia*
Severe cardiovascular, respiratory, or CNS disease. Rashes at site of patch placement	1–2 µg/kg IV bolus, then 0.017–0.33 µg/kg/min CRI IV or a 25 µg/h transdermal patch	For <5 kg can cover a portion of a 24 µg/h patch with liner—do not cut patch
Urine retention and dysphoria		
Hemosiderosis, hemochromatosis, hemolytic anemial or hypersensitivity	50–100 mg/cat PO q24h	For iron deficiency anemia
Hypersensitivity, cautious use with renal dysfunction	Heparin 250–375 U/kg SQ q6–8h Lovenox (Enoxaparin) 1.25–1.5 mg/kg SC q6h	For thromboembolic disease Research pending
Caution in severe cardiac, pulmonary, and CNS disorders, autoimmune diseases	30 U/cat PO q24h 7 days on 7 days off	For retroviral infections, stomatitis
Not reported	40 mg/kg or one 350-mg capsule opened into mouth	For stomatitis
Use caution in diabetic patients	0.25–1 mL/cat PO q8–12h Or 1 mL/4.5 kg q8h then PRN Goal 2–3 soft stools per day	For PSS, constipation Hepatic encephalopathy
Constipation, hypersensitivity, renal disease, concurrent MAOI use, toxin ingestion, CNS injury, respiratory compromise, hepatic disease	Wide variety: 0.04 mg/kg, 1 mg/cat, ONLY for a maximum of 3 days	Adverse reactions and lack of safe dosing information restricts use in cats
Young/growing animals due to cartilage effects, caution in hepatic or renal insufficiency	5 mg/kg PO q24h	Susceptible infections
Bladder neck obstruction, severe cardiac failure, angle-closure glaucoma	12.5 mg per cat PO once daily 4 mg/kg PO once a day	For vestibular disease/ vomiting As antiemetic
Hyperglycemia, insulin resistance, immunosuppression, weight gain, hepatomegaly, thin hair coat, PU/PD	20 mg SQ or IM per cat q 2 weeks for 2–3 doses then every 4–6 weeks as needed for control	For IBD if owners cannot administer pills or liquid
GI hemorrhage, obstruction or perforation	0.2–0.4 mg/kg PO, SC q8–12h 1–2 mg/kg per day CRI	As antiemetic and prokinetic
Metabolized by the liver, may need to dose reduce with hepatic dysfunction, hypersensitivity	10–15 mg/kg PO q12–24h	For susceptible infections, and antibiotic responsive diarrhea, anaerobic and protozoal infections

Table 21.1. *Continued.*

Drugs	Classes	MOAs	Side Effects
Omeprazole	Substituted benzimidazole	Proton pump inhibitor	GI distress hematologic abnormalities, urinary tract infections, proteinuria, other CNS disturbances
Ondansetron/Dolasetron	5-HT$_3$ receptor antagonist	Antiemetic when other drugs will not work	Sedation, lip licking, head shaking
Oxymorphone	Semi-synthetic opiate	Mu agonist	Ataxia, hyperesthesia, behavior changes
Pepto-Bismol bismuth subsalicylate	GI protectant	Not completely understood	Dark color stools—do not confuse with melena Radio-opaque
Phenothiazine Chlorpromazine Prochlorperazine	Phenothiazines	Low dose inhibits chemoreceptor trigger zone High dose depresses vomiting center	Sedation, significant hypotension, cardiac rate abnormalities, hypo- or hyperthermia; may cause extrapyramidal effects at high doses in cats
Prednisone/Prednisolone	Corticosteroid	Anti-inflammatory and immunosuppressant	Hyperglycemia, insulin resistance, immunosuppression
Psyllium Metamucil	Hemicellulose mucilage	Bulk laxative	Flatulence, fecal impaction, or obstruction
Ranitidine	H$_2$ histamine receptor blocker	Reduces gastric acid production	Give slow IV—may cause bradycardia Hypersensitivity
S-adenosyl-methionine (SAMe)	Nutraceutical	Naturally occurring molecule—essential in liver biochemical pathways	Very safe, rare vomiting
Sucralfate	Aluminum complex of sucrose sulfate	Unknown, forms protective barrier at ulceration sites	Constipation, hypophosphatemia
Sulfasalazine	Sulfa derivative	Exact mechanism unknown	Anorexia, vomiting, anemias
Ursodeoxycholate acid/ Ursodiol	Bile acid	Increases bile flow	

Contraindications and Precautions	Routes of Administration and Doses	General Uses
Hepatic or renal disease	0.7 mg/kg PO q24h	Most potent gastric acid inhibitor, may increase liver enzymes
Caution with use in cats Do not use in nursing animals Very expensive	0.22 mg/kg PO q8–12h 0.1–0.15 mg/kg slow IV push q6–12h PRN	Good for chemotherapy-induced nausea
Respiratory, cardiovascular, and CNS depression	0.1–0.2 mg/kg IV, SQ, IM q4–8h	Pain management
Do not use frequently or in high doses, do not use in pregnant or nursing animals, renal disease Separate from tetracyclines by 2 hours	0.25 mL/kg/ PO q4–6h Kitten dose 1–2 mL 3–4 times a day	Elimination prolonged in cats; care should be taken.
Hypovolemia, dehydration, hypotension	0.5 mg/kg IV, IM or SC q6–8h 0.5 mg/kg SC or IM q8h; ensure adequate hydration.	Most effective central-acting antiemetic in cats regardless of cause
Systemic infection, cardiac disease	Mild IBD 1–2.2 mg/kg divided q12h for 2–4 weeks then 50% decline at 2-week intervals depending on severity of signs, may be 2–3 months for q48h or q72h or 3–6 months before discontinuation Severe 2–4 mg/kg divided BID for 2–8 weeks or until clinical signs resolve, 1–2 mg/kg dose may be necessary for months to years	IBD, Eosinophilic granuloma complex, lymphocytic plasmacytic stomatitis
Fecal impaction, intestinal obstruction	1–4 tsp/meal	Increases dietary fiber, good for IBD, diarrhea, can also use canned pumpkin pie filling
Cardiac, hepatic or renal disease— consider reduced dose	2.5 mg/kg IV q12h 1–2 mg/kg PO q8–12h	For GI diseases, regurgitation or other esophageal disease, vomiting, gastric ulceration As prokinetic to increase colonic motility
Give on an empty stomach	18 mg/kg rounded to closest pill size, usually one 90-mg tablet PO q24h 200 mg/cat PO q24h	Adjunctive treatment for liver disease chronic hepatitis
Need to use as a slurry if esophageal irritation or inflammation	0.25–0.5 g, PO q8–12h can be diluted 1:5 as a slurry	Binds to injured gastroesophageal mucosa Neutralizes acid Inactivates pepsin Adsorbs bile acids and pancreatic enzymes Stimulates local cytoprotective prostaglandins
Liver, renal or hematologic diseases	5–7 mg/kg PO q24h for 14 days	Caution in cats; monitor for vomiting, diarrhea, and anemia
Aluminum-containing antacids	10–15 mg/kg PO q24h	Mix with food

      vi. Definitive diagnosis will only be provided by surgical exploratory. All other diagnostic findings are supportive but not necessarily specific or necessary for mesenteric thrombosis. The decision for surgical exploratory is based on clinical suspicion and accumulation of diagnostic evidence.

    c. Therapeutics

      i. Crystalloid fluid therapy to maintain perfusion, prevent more ischemic damage, and stabilize before or during surgical identification and resection of damaged bowel loops, followed by copious abdominal lavage

      ii. Use caution if underlying heart disease is present. Placement of a central line to monitor CVP may be indicated.

      iii. Ischemic injury may cause gastrointestinal sloughing, protein loss, and bacterial translocation.

      iv. Broad-spectrum combination antibiotic therapy (see septic peritonitis discussion above)

      v. Anticoagulant therapy with heparin or aspirin may be indicated postoperatively to prevent additional thromboembolic episodes (see chap. 16—Management of Thromboembolic Disease Secondary to Heart Disease).

S. Dysautonomia

    a. Key points

      i. Also known as Key-Gaskell syndrome, usually associated with megaesophagus, esophageal hypomotility, mydriasis, constipation, and regurgitation

      ii. May present with mydriatic pupils, KCS, and occasionally anisocoria

      iii. This disease carries a guarded to poor prognosis, with 20–40% of affected cats likely to recover. Recovery may take up to 12 months, and often the patient may not completely recover.

    b. Diagnosis

      i. Suggestive clinical signs and physical exam findings that include a generalized loss of both sympathetic and parasympathetic nervous systems

    c. Therapeutics

      i. Supportive care includes fluid therapy, artificial tears, parenteral nutrition, feeding tube placement, or elevated feedings.

      ii. Parasympathomimetic therapy with bethanechol or metoclopramide, bladder palpation, and expression

      iii. Close monitoring is necessary; many animals may become resistant to therapy and need dose adjustments.

T. Intestinal parasites

    a. Key points

      i. Roundworms, hookworms, coccidia, toxoplasmosis, protozoans, trichomonads, and cestodes are all common intestinal parasites.

      ii. Clinical signs may range from none to severe chronic anemia, and sepsis.

        1. Clinical signs may be more severe in kittens or immunocompromised cats.

    b. Diagnosis

      i. Fecal examination including direct smear, floatation, and culture if necessary

      ii. *Giardia* can be identified with zinc sulfate flotation.

      iii. Trichomonads identified on direct exam, special stains to differentiate from *Giardia*, if clinical may have other intestinal disease or immunodeficiency.

    c. Therapeutics

      i. Empirical therapy is commonly attempted with fenbendazole or pyrantel pamoate; if tapeworms are visualized, use praziquantal and discuss flea treatments with owners.

      ii. For severe infections, hospitalization with fluid therapy and supportive care is indicated while waiting for more complete diagnostics.

      iii. Antibiotics commonly used empirically are clindamycin and metronidazole.

      iv. Tricomonad therapeutics are currently under research. Some cats have responded to ronidazole at 30–50 mg/kg PO q12h, but neurologic side effects have been noted during clinical use.

References

August JR. Consultations in Feline Internal Medicine, vol. 5. Elsevier Saunders, 2006.

Carmichael D. Feline gingivostomatitis: how to relieve the oral discomfort. Vet Med, 2006; 101(2):76–78.

Colopy-Poulsen, Danova, Hardie, Muir. Managing feline obstipation secondary to pelvic fracture. Compendium, Sept 2005; 662–669.

Ettinger, Feldman. Textbook of Veterinary Internal Medicine, 5th ed. W.B. Saunders, 2000.

Gookin J, Copple C, Papich M, Poore M, Levy M. Efficacy of Ronidazole in vitro and in vivo for treatment of feline *tritrichomonas foetus* infection. ACVIM 23rd Annual Veterinary Medical Forum Abstract Program. J Vet Int Med, 2005; 19(3):436.

Kyles, Hardie, Mehl, Gregory. Evaluation of ameroid ring constrictors for the management of single extrahepatic portosystemic shunts in cats: 23 cases (1996–2001). J Am Vet Med Assoc, 2002; 220(9):1341–1347.

MacIntire DK, Drobatz KJ, Haskins SC, Saxon WD. Manual of Small Animal Emergency and Critical Care Medicine. Lippincott Williams & Wilkins, 2005.

Morgan RV, Bright RM, Swartout MS. Handbook of Small Animal Practice, 4th ed. W. B. Saunders, 2003.

Norsworthy GD, Crystal MA, Grace SF, Tilley LP. The Feline Patient: Essentials of Diagnosis and Treatment, 2nd ed. Lippincott Williams & Wilkins, 2003.

Patsikas MN, Papazoglou LG, Papaioannou NG, Savvas I, Kazakos GM, Dessiris AK. Ultrasonographic findings of intestinal intussusception in seven cats. J Feline Med Surg, 2003; 5(6):353–343.

Plumb DC. Veterinary Drug Handbook, 4th ed. Iowa State Press, 2002.

Tams T. Handbook of Small Animal Gastroenterology, 2nd ed. W. B. Saunders, 2003.

22
DIAGNOSTIC EVALUATION, MONITORING, AND THERAPEUTIC TECHNIQUES FOR THE UROLOGIC SYSTEM

Simon W. Tappin and Andrew J. Brown

Unique Features
- The most common cause of acute renal failure in cats is urethral obstruction.
- Feline urine is normally very concentrated; specific gravity values below 1.035 represent suboptimal concentration.
- Struvite crystals are a normal finding in feline urine, but numbers increase with storage and infection.
- Stress can elevate serum glucose levels above the renal threshold leading to glucosuria.
- Bilirubin is not normally found in feline urine and reflects icterus.

I. Clinical signs and diagnosis
   A. **Uremia** refers to the clinical and clinicopathologic abnormalities that occur secondary to renal failure.
   B. **Clinical signs** are nonspecific and vary between patients. Signs result from the accumulation of solutes within the blood that would normally be excreted by the kidneys. Cats may be presented for vomiting, nausea, anorexia, hypersalivation (due to either uremia or oral ulceration), diarrhea, weight loss, changes in drinking habits, hiding, lethargy, or straining.
   C. **Physical examination** findings may include depression, pale mucous membranes, dehydration, poor pulses, tachycardia, bradycardia, hypothermia, cachexia, oral ulceration, abnormal kidney size, painful abdomen and/or kidneys, and an absent or large firm bladder.
   D. **Clinicopathologic** abnormalities include **azotemia** (accumulation of nitrogenous compounds in the blood), elevated BUN (blood urea nitrogen) and serum creatinine, hyperkalemia or hypokalemia, hyperphosphotemia, nonregenerative anemia, and metabolic acidosis.
   E. **Diagnosis** is made using the above clinical and clinicopathologic findings. Classification into primary renal, prerenal, and postrenal azotemia is useful to guide further diagnostics, therapy, and prognosis.
      i. Prerenal
         a. Secondary to decreased renal perfusion (see chap. 3—Shock)
            i. Hypovolemic shock (decreased circulating volume)
            ii. Cardiogenic shock (ineffective circulating volume)
            iii. Distributive shock (inappropriate dilatation or constriction of the afferent and/or efferent arterioles)

   b. Clinical signs usually result from inadequate systemic perfusion rather than the subsequent uremia.
   c. Urine specific gravity (pre-fluids) should be maximally concentrated (>1.050) unless concentrating ability is impaired (e.g., glucosuria, diuretic administration).
   d. Blood urea nitrogen (BUN) will increase prior to, and to a greater degree than, serum creatinine.
   e. Unless primary renal damage has occurred, prerenal azotemia is reversible with restoration of renal perfusion.
   f. In the presence of primary renal dysfunction (when >25% of tubules are still functioning normally), azotemia may occur with just a mild decrease in renal perfusion.
 ii. Primary renal (see chap. 24—Acute Intrinsic Renal Failure)
   a. With normal renal perfusion, azotemia occurs when less than 25% of renal tubules are functioning.
   b. Can be classified to guide prognosis:
      i.   Acute renal failure
      ii. Chronic renal failure
      iii. Acute on chronic (see chap. 23—Urologic Emergencies: Ureter, Bladder, Urethra, GN, and CRF)
   c. Clinical signs will result from azotemia, electrolyte abnormalities, anemia, and metabolic acidosis.
 iii. Postrenal (see chap. 24)
   a. Impaired renal excretion secondary to rupture of or obstruction to:
      i.   Ureters
      ii. Bladder
      iii. Urethra
   b. Leakage from the urinary tract leads to resorption of urinary solutes and azotemia.
   c. Obstruction of the urinary tract leads to reduced glomerular filtration rate and azotemia.
   d. Physical examination findings will depend on site of obstruction or rupture.
   e. Patient stabilization (e.g., correction of hypovolemia and hyperkalemia) important before invasive diagnostic and therapeutic procedures are performed
   f. Azotemia typically reversible unless prolonged obstruction, which can lead to irreversible tubular damage
   g. The most common cause of acute renal failure in cats is urethral obstruction.
II. Diagnostic and monitoring procedures
  A. Urethral catheterization
    i. Indications
      a. To collect a urine sample
      b. To monitor urine output
      c. To relieve urethral obstruction
      d. To keep the bladder empty and facilitate healing
      e. To act as a urethral stent and allow healing after trauma
      f. To perform retrograde contrast radiography of the lower urinary tract
   ii. Considerations
      a. The cat must be sedated or anaesthetized for catheterization.
      b. The catheter should be placed as aseptically as possible (sterile gloves, hair clipped as needed, and the area surgically scrubbed). The prepuce or vestibule should be flushed with dilute povidone iodine solution or similar.
      c. Catheters should be long, soft, and sterile. Red rubber catheters (Tyco Healthcare Group LP, Mansfield, MA) are commonly used for indwelling catheters. Polypropylene Tom Cat catheters (Tyco Healthcare Group LP, Mansfield, MA) are more rigid and useful to relieve

urethral obstruction. They should NOT be used as an indwelling catheter, as their rigid construction can lead to bladder wall irritation. Diameter depends on patient size (3.5–5 French). A wire stylet may aid placement of a red rubber catheter in a female, but caution should be used to avoid iatrogenic urethral injury.

d. A closed collection system should always be used for indwelling catheters. The bladder should be allowed to empty under gravity. The collecting system should have enough slack to prevent its interfering with the cat's movement. It should be attached to the tail to prevent trauma to the anchor sutures. Sterile collection systems are commercially available; however, sterile tubing and an empty intravenous fluid bag may also be used.

e. After placement, an Elizabethan collar should be fitted to prevent the cat's removing the catheter.

iii. Technique

a. Male

   i. The tom is positioned in lateral or dorsal recumbency.
   ii. For the right-handed operator, the left thumb and forefinger are used to extrude the penis by pushing the prepuce cranially.
   iii. The catheter is well lubricated (with sterile water-soluble lubricant) and inserted into the penile urethra.
   iv. The penis is then extended caudally to align the penile and membranous urethra while the catheter is gently advanced.
   v. Once in the bladder, urine will appear at the hub and advancement is ceased.
   vi. The catheter is sutured to the prepuce using holes in the catheter hub or using a tape butterfly.
   vii. If resistance is felt, the catheter should not be forced as this may lead to urethral trauma. Instillation of sterile saline will allow dislodgment of urethral material.

b. Female

   i. The urethral opening lies in a depression in the ventral vaginal wall approximately 1cm from the vulva. This depression helps guide the catheter allowing "blind" catheterization
   ii. The queen is usually placed in lateral or sternal recumbency. However in difficult cases dorsal recumbency may aid placement.
   iii. For the right handed operator, the left hand is used to grasp and gently extend the vulva
   iv. The catheter is well lubricated (with sterile water-soluble lubricant) and gently guided along the ventral vestibule floor which commonly results in placement.
   v. A small speculum or sterile otoscope can help identify the urethral orifice.
   vi. Once in the bladder urine will appear at the catheter hub. Advancement is ceased and the catheter is secured as above.

iv. Concerns

a. Iatrogenic urinary tract infection

   i. Avoid by aseptic catheter placement and management of the collection system
   ii. Prophylactic systemic antibiotics or flushing the catheter with antibiotic/antiseptic solutions are not advised as these can increase the risk of resistant urinary tract infections.
   iii. Urine culture and sensitivity should be performed 24–48 hours following catheter removal.

B. Cystocentesis

i. Indications

a. To collect a urine sample without contamination from the lower urinary tract
b. To help localize the source of hematuria, bacteriuria, or pyuria to the upper or lower urinary tract
c. Therapeutic bladder decompression due to urethral obstruction, when urethral catheterization is not possible. Repeated decompression via cystocentesis in the obstructed cat is not

recommended, and placement of a cystostomy tube for continuous bladder evacuation should be considered until urethral patency is attained.

  ii. Considerations
      a. Ultrasound guidance may be useful in obese cats or when the bladder is small.
  iii. Technique
      a. The cat is restrained in lateral recumbency by an assistant. Sedation or anesthesia is not normally needed but should be considered in the fractious patient.
      b. For diagnostic sample collection a 1–1.5-inch, 22-gauge needle and 2–10-mL syringe will allow adequate sample collection.
      c. The skin on the caudal ventral abdomen is clipped and aseptically prepared.
      d. With one hand the bladder is immobilized, and with the other the needle (with syringe attached) inserted through the abdominal wall into the bladder.
      e. The most common site for cystocentesis is ventrally; however, ventrolateral or dorsal approaches may be considered. The ideal site for bladder compression is just cranial to the urethral junction, as this will allow drainage without multiple insertions as the bladder empties.
      f. Where possible, the needle should enter the bladder wall at a 45-degree angle. This reduces the possibility of leakage postprocedure by passing through different bladder layers at slightly different points.
      g. Once in the bladder, urine will appear in the syringe hub and gentle aspiration will yield a sample. The needle and syringe can then be gently withdrawn.
      h. For therapeutic bladder decompression, the needle is connected via an intravenous extension set to a 20-mL syringe and three-way tap. As the syringe fills, the three-way tap allows the syringe to be repeatedly emptied into a collection bowl until the bladder is empty.
  iv. Concerns
      a. A severely distended bladder wall may be compromised, leading to rupture on cystocentesis.
      b. Hemostatic disorders are a contraindication to cystocentesis.
      c. Tracking of neoplastic cells along the needle paths has been reported.
C. Routine urinalysis
  i. Routine urinalysis involves the measurement of specific gravity, dipstick evaluation. and sediment analysis.
      a. Specific gravity
          i.   Specific gravity reflects the solute concentration of urine and should be measured using a refractometer before therapy begins.
          ii. Glucosuria and proteinuria will elevate specific gravity by approximately 0.005 per gram of glucose or protein.
          iii. Urine with a specific gravity of 1.008–1.012 is regarded isosthenuric as it has the same solute concentration as the glomerular filtrate.
          iv. Urine with a specific gravity <1.008 is regarded as hyposthenuric and has been actively diluted.
          v.   Urine specific gravity >1.012 is regarded as hypersthenuric; however, feline urine is usually concentrated (SG >1.035); values below this may reflect poor renal concreting ability or polydipsia.
      b. Dipstick evaluation
          i.   Urine pH
              1. Normal pH for feline urine is 5–7.5
              2. Acidic urine may reflect a high protein diet, catabolic state, or metabolic or respiratory acidosis.
              3. Alkaline urine may reflect the presence of urease positive bacteria, respiratory or metabolic alkalosis, postprandial alkaline tide, or prolonged exposure to room air.

ii. Glucose
1. Glucose appears in the urine if the renal threshold is exceeded (250–350 mg/dL). This can occur with diabetes mellitus and stress.
2. Primary glucosuria occurs secondary to tubular dysfunction, and glucosuria will be seen with normal blood glucose concentrations.
iii. Ketones
1. Ketones are not normally present in feline urine and reflect changes in fatty acid metabolism.
2. Acetone and acetoacetate react with the nitroprusside agent on dipsticks; however, beta hydroxybutyrate does not. Beta hydroxybutyrate can be oxidized to acetoacetate using 1–2 drops of hydrogen peroxide.
iv. Occult blood
1. Hemoglobin, myoglobin, and erythrocytes all cross-react with dipstick reagents. Results must therefore be interpreted in conjunction with a spun-down urine sample. Sediment analysis will reveal intact red cells when hematuria is present, whereas examination of the supernatant will confirm pigmenturia.
v. Bilirubin
1. Bilirubin is not normally found in feline urine and when present reflects elevated serum bilirubin.
2. Bilirubinuria occurs prior to hyperbilirubinemia.
c. Urine sediment analysis
i. Urinalysis should be performed as promptly after collection as possible. Cells and casts will degenerate, bacteria may grow, and crystals may form or dissolve.
ii. The sample should be evaluated with its collection method in mind. For example, a catheterized sample may contain epithelia cells as a result of urethral trauma, and a cystocentesis sample may contain red blood cells as a result of trauma.
1. White blood cells
a. Occasional white blood cells are normal (0–8/hpf in voided samples, 0–5/hpf in catheterized samples, 0–3/hpf in cystocentesis samples).
b. Increased white blood cells (pyuria) indicate urinary tract inflammation.
2. Red blood cells
a. Occasional red blood cells are normal (0–8/hpf in voided samples, 0–5/hpf in catheterized samples, 0–3/hpf in cystocentesis samples).
b. Increased red blood cells (hematuria) indicate urinary tract inflammation or hemorrhage.
3. Bacteria
a. The bladder is normally sterile, but increasing numbers of commensals will be found along the lower urinary tract.
b. If visual numbers are present, they are usually significant and should be accompanied by an active sediment.
c. Care needs to be taken to differentiate stain precipitate and contaminants.
4. Crystals
a. Struvite crystals ("coffin lids") are normal in feline urine but increase in number with infection and precipitate if urine is stored.
b. Oxalate crystals:
i. Monohydrate crystals ("picket fence" or "dumbbell") are rarely seen except in animals that have ingested ethylene glycol.
ii. Dihydrate crystals ("Maltese cross" or "envelope") can be seen in normal cats, but large numbers can be associated with ethylene glycol intoxication.
c. Urate stones (thorn apples) are suggestive of liver dysfunction
5. Casts

      a. Casts are cylindrical concretions formed in the renal tubules.

      b. They consist of cells, proteins, and cellular debris.

      c. Hyaline casts may be seen due to normal sloughing of tubular epilethial cells (<2 per low-power field). This may increase after exercise. Hyaline casts consist partly of protein; hence numbers may increase with glomerular nephritis and amyloidosis.

      d. Granular casts reflect precipitation of filtered proteins or cellular degeneration. Occasional granular casts may be seen in normal cats (<2 per low-power field); however, large numbers suggest tubular degeneration or necrosis.

      e. Fatty casts contain lipid granules and can be seen with nephrotic syndrome or diabetes mellitus.

      f. White cell casts suggest pyelonephritis.

      g. Waxy casts are uncommon and reflect degeneration of granular casts. They are seen mainly with chronic renal failure.

      h. Hemoglobin and myoglobin casts suggest hemoglobinuria and myoglobinuria.

D. Urine culture and sensitivity

    i. Although urinalysis and clinical signs may suggest a urinary tract infection, a positive urine culture is needed to confirm the diagnosis and differentiate the condition from other causes of feline lower urinary tract disease.

    ii. Urinary tract infections occur when sterile areas of the urinary tract are colonized by bacteria. This is more common in females, animals with poor concentrating ability, or when glucosuria is present.

    iii. *Escherichia coli* is the most commonly isolated organism. *Staphylococcus*, *Streptococcus*, *Klebsiella*, *Proteus*, and *Pseudomonas* species are also reported.

    iv. Urine should be collected for culture by cystocentesis to avoid contaminants. Culture of catheterized and voided samples frequently results in false positive results.

    v. Urine should be cultured as quickly as possible, as bacterial numbers change rapidly once the sample had been collected. If immediate culture is not possible, transporting in boric acid tubes is recommended and the sample refrigerated is a culture swab. Bacterial concentrations above 1,000 colony-forming units per milliliter of urine are considered significant growths.

    vi. Treatment should be based on sensitivity results, and determining the minimum inhibitory concentration may help in resistant or recurring cases.

E. Urine protein–creatinine ratio

    i. The urine protein–creatinine ratio (UPC) allows quantification of urine protein loss and is indicated in the investigation of renal failure (acute and chronic) as well as hypoalbuminaemia.

    ii. Protein loss is corrected for urine concentration by correlating it to the urine creatinine concentration. The results of UPC ratios correlate well with 24-hour urine protein excretion.

    iii. Normal feline UPC values are <0.4 (cats fed high-protein diets can have higher values, so fasted samples are desirable).

    iv. Inflammation and blood contamination can increase urine protein content; thus, the UPC ratio should be interpreted in conjunction with a sediment examination and urine culture. The true extent of blood contamination on the feline UPC ratio is unknown. However, studies with canine urine revealed that urinary albumin concentrations do not change until urine becomes grossly hematuric, and the maximal change in UPC seen was an increase of 0.4.

F. Fractional clearance/excretion of electrolytes

    i. The renal tubules are responsible for the secretion and resorption of filtered electrolytes. Fractional clearance of electrolytes can therefore be used to investigate tubular function by comparing them to the excretion of creatinine, which is excreted at a constant rate.

    ii. Fractional clearance of electrolyte $x = (U_x V/P_x) / (U_{cr} V/P_{cr}) = (U_x P_{cr}) / (U_{cr} P_x)$

      a. U_x = Urine concentration of x

      b. P_x = Plasma concentration of x

c. U_{cr} = Urine concentration of creatinine

d. P_{cr} = Plasma concentration of creatinine

e. V = Urine volume over time period of test

iii. Normal values for feline fractional clearance of electrolytes

    a. Sodium <1%

    b. Potassium <6%

    c. Chloride <1.3%

    d. Phosphate <73%

iv. Fractional excretion of sodium

    a. Renal failure

       i. Fractional excretion of sodium increases with renal failure (>1%) due to decreased tubular function

       ii. Fractional excretion of sodium decreases with prerenal azotemia (<1%) to conserve sodium and prevent further volume depletion

    b. Hyponatraemia

       i. An increased fractional excretion of sodium indicates that renal loss of sodium is contributing to the hyponatraemia (e.g., reduced aldosterone secondary to ACE inhibitor administration, loop diuretics increasing sodium excretion, increased ANP, or tubular disease).

       ii. A decreased fractional excretion of sodium indicates that the kidneys are attempting to conserve sodium (through the actions of aldosterone and angiotensin II) and suggests an extrarenal cause (e.g., gastrointestinal tract loss through vomiting or diarrhaea)

v. Fractional excretion of potassium

    a. Renal insufficiency and loop diuretics may cause potassium wasting (fractional excretion >10%). Supplementation should be considered to prevent clinical signs of hypokalaemia.

G. Abdominal ultrasound

    i. Abdominal ultrasound allows noninvasive imaging of the urinary tract, revealing shape, size, and structure of the kidneys and lower urinary tract.

    ii. This can usually be achieved when conscious, but sedation should be considered in fractious cats.

    iii. Hair needs to be clipped from the viewing area, and alcohol followed by ultrasound gel applied.

       a. Kidney

          i. The feline kidneys can usually be imaged with the transducer placed on the ventral abdominal wall, with the cat in lateral recumbency. In some cases, moving the cat to dorsal recumbency or placing the transducer directly over the area of the kidney (just caudal to the last rib on the left and level with the last two ribs on the right) may help.

          ii. The normal kidney has a smooth, well-defined outline and measures approximately 3–4.3 cm in length.

          iii. Ultrasound allows the differentiation of the cortex, medullar, and renal pelvis. The normal feline kidney is less echogenic than liver or spleen, with the renal medulla appearing less echogenic than the cortex due to its higher water content. In normal cats, the relative difference in echotexture between the cortex and medulla can vary due to differences in the fat content of the proximal tubular cells.

          iv. Hydronephrosis and marked dilation of the renal pelvis is seen with ureteral obstruction, whereas mild pelvic dilation can be seen with pyelonephritis or intravenous fluid therapy.

          v. Renal calculi (of all types) appear echogenic and cast acoustic shadows.

          vi. Renal cysts appear as discrete rounded anechoic areas. Infarcts, abscesses, and neoplastic lesions have variable appearances.

          vii. Diffuse parenchymal diseases do not usually change ultrasound appearance until the disease is relatively advanced; a normal ultrasound therefore does not rule out renal disease.

        viii. Ethylene glycol toxicity leads to the deposition of calcium oxalate crystals within the kidney, which appears more hyperechoic than the liver or spleen.

        ix. The medullary rim sign (a hyperechoic band at the corticomedullary junction) is not specific for renal disease in the cat, as mineralization of the basement membrane causes the same effect in normal cats.

  b. Ureters

      i. Ureters are not normally seen on ultrasound evaluation due to their small size.

      ii. Periodic jets of urine may be seen entering the bladder (especially using color flow Doppler) and can be useful when searching for ectopic ureters.

      iii. Ureteral dilation (hydroureter) is caused by ureteral obstruction and is usually accompanied by dilation of the renal pelvis. The ureter can then be traced medially and caudally from the renal pelvis toward the trigone of the bladder.

      iv. Doppler examination can help distinguish dilated ureters from vascular structures.

      v. Ureteral calculi may be identified as focal areas of echogenicity that are usually associated with acoustic shadowing.

  c. Bladder

      i. The bladder is imaged via a ventral abdominal approach, which gives information about size, shape, integrity, wall thickness, and luminal content.

      ii. The normal bladder wall is smooth with well-defined layers. A full colon may indent the dorsal bladder wall.

      iii. Inflammation may increase wall thickness, and neoplasia may form focal masses.

      iv. Calculi may be seen as echogenic masses that cast acoustic shadows.

H. Plain radiography

  i. Abdominal radiography allows noninvasive imaging of the urinary tract, revealing shape, size, and structure of the kidneys and the bladder.

  ii. Radiographs may be achieved when conscious, but sedation should be considered in fractious cats.

  iii. Conventionally, projections are right lateral and ventrodorsal (VD).

    a. Kidneys

      i. Both kidneys are normally visible ventral to L3, with the right silhouette slightly cranial to the left.

      ii. Normal kidneys should be 2.4–3 times the length of L2.

      iii. Enlarged kidneys may displace other abdominal structures (e.g., in the lateral projection right renomegaly may depress the duodenum, whereas left renomegaly may depress the descending colon. In VD the colon may be deviated medially by renal enlargement).

      iv. Renal enlargement may be due to neoplasia, acute nephritis, hydronephrosis, FIP, porto vascular abnormalities, polycystic kidney disease, or a hematoma.

      v. Reduced renal size usually results from end-stage chronic renal disease, although it can occur due to renal hypoplasia.

    b. Ureters

      i. Ureters are not normally seen on plain radiographs.

      ii. Ureteroliths may be seen on lateral and VD projections, but are generally best visualized on lateral radiographs.

    c. Bladder

      i. Bladder varies with the volume of urine it contains.

      ii. Bladder wall thickness cannot be assessed on plain radiographs (ultrasound or contrast studies are needed).

      iii. Gas bubbles may be seen in the dependent portion of the bladder; these may be secondary to catheterization or cystocentesis.

      iv. Gas in the bladder wall is called emphysematous cystitis and is often secondary to diabetes mellitus.

    v. Radiodense mineralized calculi may be seen in the dependent portion of the bladder. The type of calculi present cannot be determined by radiography. Radiolucent calculi may not be visualized without ultrasound or contrast studies.

I. Contrast cystogram
- i. Indications
  - a. Identification and evaluation of bladder shape, size, position, and integrity
  - b. Identification and evaluation of urethral position and integrity
  - c. Investigation of persistent feline lower urinary tract disease
- ii. Technique
  - a. If possible, the cat should be fasted for 12–24 hours.
  - b. A cleansing enema should be administered 2–3 hours prior to the procedure, although it may not be required for primary assessment of bladder integrity.
  - c. Ideally, general anesthesia should be considered (as urethral catheterization is required).
  - d. Plain survey radiographs (lateral and ventrodorsal) should be taken to evaluate the urinary tract prior to urethral catheterization and the administration of contrast.
  - e. A sterile urethral catheter should be placed (as described above) and the bladder emptied of urine.
  - f. Several contrast techniques are available, and the technique chosen will depend on the information required. For example, to check bladder integrity, instilling a small volume of water-soluble iodine media may be sufficient, whereas for diagnostic evaluation of FLUTD, a combination of techniques will be required for thorough evaluation of the lower urinary tract.
    - i. Pneumocystogram
      - a. Air is injected to fill the bladder until moderate resistance is felt or the bladder is moderately distended on abdominal palpation (approx. 50 mL air).
      - b. A lateral radiograph is taken centered at the bladder neck and a ventrodorsal view taken if needed.
    - ii. Positive contrast cystogram
      - a. Dilute 5–10% water-soluble iodinated contrast medium is instilled into the bladder until it is moderately distended on abdominal palpation or until resistance is felt (approx. 50 mL).
      - b. Positive contrast cystography gives good mucosal detail; however, calculi and small intraluminal lesions may be masked by the contrast.
    - iii. Double contrast cystogram
      - a. 5–10 mL of 20% water-soluble iodinated contrast medium is instilled into the bladder followed immediately with air (the bladder is distended as described above).
      - b. Contrast media highlights the mucosal surface, and the small pool of contrast that forms in the dependent part of the bladder will highlight calculi or small masses in that area.
    - iv. Positive contrast urethrogram
      - a. The urinary catheter is withdrawn to the proximal part of the penile urethra.
      - b. 5 mL of 20% water-soluble iodinated contrast medium is injected.
      - c. A lateral radiograph is taken at the end of the injection centered at the bladder neck.
      - d. This allows evaluation of urethral integrity and diameter.
- iii. Concerns
  - a. Care needs to be taken to not rupture the bladder due to overdistension.
  - b. Air embolism as a result of a pneumocystography is rare but has been reported as a fatal complication. The use of nitrous oxide or carbon dioxide reduces the risk of fatal embolization, as they are rapidly dissipated due to higher solubility when compared with room air.

J. Intravenous urography
- i. Indications

      a. Identification and evaluation of renal shape, size and position

      b. Identification and evaluation of ureter integrity and course (e.g., to evaluate potential obstruction or avulsion)

      c. Investigation of urinary incontinence or upper urinary tract hematuria or pyuria

  ii. Technique

      a. If possible, the cat should be starved for 12–24 hours.

      b. A cleansing enema should be administered 2–3 hours prior to the procedure.

      c. Ideally, general anesthesia should be performed.

      d. Plain survey radiographs (orthogonal views lateral and ventrodorsal) should be taken to evaluate the urinary tract prior to the administration of contrast.

      e. A rapid bolus of 600–800 mg/kg of iodinated contrast medium should be given intravenously and a ventrodorsal radiograph taken immediately. Further films should be taken at 1, 5, 10, 15, and 20 minutes.

      f. Initial films should be taken in the ventrodorsal position, progressing to lateral views once adequate opacification is achieved. Oblique views may also be helpful.

  iii. Concerns

      a. Intravenous urography is contraindicated in dehydration, decreased glomerular filtration rate, hypovolemia, and hyperosmolar states.

      b. A diagnostic study requires adequate glomerular filtration rate.

      c. Renal failure is reported as a consequence of intravenous urography in people with renal insufficiency. Fluid diuresis after the procedure is therefore suggested.

      d. Adverse reactions include retching and vomiting. Hypotension is also reported in some patients.

      e. Contrast media increases urine specific gravity measurements.

      f. Contrast media may inhibit the growth of bacteria, thus interfering with urine culture and sensitivity.

K. Antegrade pyelography image

  i. Indications

      a. Allows identification and evaluation of ureteral size and position

      b. Allows diagnosis and localization of ureteral obstruction

  ii. Considerations

      a. Requires skilled ultrasonographer

      b. Plain radiographs and ultrasound evaluation should be performed prior to antegrade pyelography.

      c. Antegrade pyelography allows ureteral evaluation in patients with compromised glomerular filtration rate and avoids the potential nephrotoxicity associated with systemic contrast administration.

  iii. Technique

      a. If possible, the cat should be fasted for 12–24 hours.

      b. A cleansing enema should be administered 2–3 hours prior to the procedure.

      c. General anesthesia should be performed.

      d. The kidney of interest is immobilized so it lies directly under the skin, and the area over the kidney to be aspirated is clipped and aseptically prepared.

      e. Under ultrasound guidance, a 2.5-inch 25-gauge spinal needle is inserted into the renal pelvis.

      f. An extension set is attached and urine is aspirated for culture and cytology.

      g. An equivalent volume of ionic iodinated contrast media is then instilled slowly into the renal pelvis.

      h. The contrast is then followed using fluoroscopy or multiple radiographs, with filling defects revealing obstruction.

  iv. Concerns

       a. Hemorrhage or trauma to the renal pelvis

       b. Nondiagnostic study due to leakage of contrast media

L. Computer tomography (CT)

    i. CT is used as an adjunct to other imaging modalities.

    ii. CT contrast studies are especially useful in the diagnosis of ureteral obstruction and ectopic ureters.

    iii. General anesthesia is required.

M. Renal biopsy

    i. Indications

       a. Allows a definitive histopathological diagnosis and should be considered when this information is likely to change patient management (e.g., diagnose neoplasia, differentiate ARF from CRF, guide likely outcome of continued therapy).

       b. Definitive diagnosis allows an accurate prognosis to be given.

       c. Repeated biopsies may yield information about the response to treatment.

    ii. Considerations

       a. A renal biopsy should not be performed until a thorough less-invasive diagnostic investigation has been performed.

       b. Platelet numbers, buccal mucosal bleeding time, and a coagulation profile should be checked before biopsy, as uremia can cause thrombocytopathia and an increased risk of hemorrhage.

    iii. Technique

       a. Fine needle aspiration (FNA)

         i. The cat is sedated and percutaneous aspirates are taken for cytological evaluation.

         ii. Ultrasound guidance is advantageous, as it allows accurate needle placement and monitoring of any postaspiration complications, such as hemorrhage.

         iii. FNAs are useful for the diagnosis of diseases where cells aspirate easily, for example, renal lymphoma or inflammatory conditions; however, they can give inconclusive results.

         iv. The kidney of interest is immobilized so it lies directly under the skin (if using ultrasound guidance, this is best done by an assistant).

         v. The area over the kidney to be aspirated is clipped and aseptically prepared.

         vi. A 1-inch, 22-gauge needle is inserted gradually into the kidney and sequentially moved back and forth through the renal cortex.

         vii. Using an air-filled syringe, the contents of the needle can be deposited onto a slide and smears made for cytological evaluation.

         viii. Repeat sampling with aspiration of the syringe can be performed if the cell harvest is poor or for FNAs of more solid tissue (e.g., a focal mass).

       b. Tru-cut biopsy

         i. Tru-cut biopsy will yield tissue for histopathology and culture. It is more invasive than an FNA but yields information about tissue structure.

         ii. Good sedation or general anesthesia is required.

         iii. The area is clipped and aseptically prepared as for FNAs.

         iv. With the kidney immobilized, the Tru-cut needle (18 g) is then advanced into the renal cortex.

         v. Biopsies should be taken at parallel to renal pelvis to avoid the ureter and renal vessels.

         vi. Once collected, the sample should be fixed in formalin and sent for histopathology.

         vii. Coagulopathies, pyelonephritis, and hydronephrosis are considered contraindications to Tru-cut biopsy.

       c. Surgical biopsy

         i. Surgical biopsies yield the largest volume of tissue for histopathology and therefore allow the most accurate diagnoses to be made.

  ii.   Obtaining surgical biopsies requires general anesthesia and exploratory laparotomy or laparoscopy.
iv. Concerns
  a. Complications are rare but include:
      i.   Leakage of urine, for example, uroperitoneum
      ii. Hemorrhage (gross or microscopic)
      iii. Spread of infection, for example, leakage of infected urine from pyelonephritis or rupture of a renal abscess
      iv. Possible seeding of neoplastic cells along the biopsy path
v.   Histopathological interpretation
  a. Good prognostic signs include tubular regeneration and an intact basement membrane
  b. Poor prognostic signs include tubular necrosis, basement membrane disruption, and interstitial mineralization.
N. Interpretation of urine output
  i.   Normal urine output is 1–2 mL/kg/hr.
  ii.   Oliguria is urine output <0.5 mL/kg/hr.
  iii. Anuria is the complete absence of urine production.
  iv.   Urine production must be interpreted in conjunction with intravascular volume status.
  v.   Urine output is a function of renal perfusion and renal function.
        a. If renal perfusion decreases, then glomerular filtration will decrease, leading to reduced urine output.
        b. Mean arterial blood pressure needs to be >60 mmHg to maintain renal perfusion. Mean pressures <60 mmHg or systolic pressure <80 mmHg will therefore lead to progressive oliguria.
        c. Reduced glomerular or tubular flow (acute renal failure) will reduce urine production.
  vi.   Placing a urinary catheter will allow accurate measurement of urine production.
  vii. Weighing diapers, monitoring bladder size with ultrasound, and weighing the cat are noninvasive but less accurate methods of monitoring urine production.
O. Peritoneal dialysis
  i.   Indications
        a. Anuric renal failure
        b. Oliguric renal failure with hyperkalemia
        c. Oliguric renal failure and fluid overload
        d. Severe clinical uremia (polyuric or oliguric renal failure) unresponsive to fluid therapy
        e. Postrenal uremia resulting from obstruction
        f. Dialyzable toxicities, for example, barbiturates, ethylene glycol
  ii.   Considerations
        a. Requires sedation or anesthesia for placement of peritoneal dialysis catheter
        b. Dialysis catheters can rapidly become occluded. Prior omentectomy is recommended to avoid this (requires general anesthesia and midline celiotomy).
        c. Contraindications
              i.   Peritoneal adhesions
              ii. Compromised peritoneum
                   1. Diaphragmatic hernia
                   2. Recent abdominal surgery (relative)
                   3. Inguinal or abdominal hernias (relative)
              iii. Any condition that may result in increased intra-abdominal pressure
        d. Labor intensive
  iii. Technique
        a. Dialysis catheters

     i.   Percutaneous (short-term)

     ii. Surgically implantable

     iii. Laparoscopic

b. Placement

     i.   Sedation or general anesthesia necessary

     ii. Patient in dorsal recumbency and abdomen shaved

     iii. Patient draped and strict aseptic technique maintained

     iv. Percutaneous trocar technique

        1. Stab incision 3–5 cm lateral to the umbilicus

        2. Catheter tunneled caudally from stab incision before entering abdominal cavity

        3. Catheter threaded off trochar

     v. Surgically placed

        1. Omentectomy via midline celiotomy

        2. End of catheter placed in inguinal region

        3. Catheter to exit abdomen via tunnel 3–5 cm lateral to the umbilicus

     vi. Catheter secured with purse string and Chinese fingertrap.

     vii. Catheters with Dacron cuffs should be used in long-term dialysis patients to avoid the use of suture, which may increase infection rate.

c. Dialysate

     i.   Commercially available products containing various concentrations of dextrose are available.

     ii. "Homemade" using lactated Ringer's solution

     iii. Solutions contain 1.5–4.25% dextrose. Variations in dextrose alter the osmolality of the solution, with the higher concentration being used to remove fluid from the overhydrated patient.

     iv. Some authors recommend the use of heparin (250–1,000 IU/L) in the dialysate for the first few days following catheter placement to help prevent occlusion of the catheter.

     v. Dialysate should be warmed to 38°C to improve permeability of the peritoneum.

     vi. Volume of dialysate instilled should be approximately 10 mL/kg for the initial 24 hours, and gradually increase to 30 mL/kg following this.

d. Dialysis

     i.   Ensure aseptic technique.

     ii. One-third of the calculated dialysate volume should be instilled in the initial 24 hours to prevent high intra-abdominal pressures and dialysate leakage.

     iii. Use a closed Y system to reduce potential for contamination.

     iv. Use "drain first—infuse later" principle to reduce potential for infection.

     v. Instill 10 mL/kg over 10 minutes for the initial 24 hours.

     vi. Gradually increase to 30 mL/kg after the initial 24 hours.

     vii. In the acute setting, dialysate remains in abdomen for approximately 30 minutes (dwell time).

     viii. Dialysate removed under gravity over 20 minutes

     ix. Process repeated every hour until patient clinically improved and serum creatinine and BUN have decreased by one-third.

     x. Do not attempt to reduce the BUN by more than one-third over the initial 24 hours or dialysis disequilibrium syndrome may develop.

     xi. Continue with acute dialysis until BUN has reached 60–100 mg/dL.

     xii. Chronic dialysis with a dwell time of 3–6 hours should then be implemented and rates adjusted accordingly to maintain a BUN of approximately 70 mg/dL.

iv. Concerns

  a. Septic peritonitis

        b. Catheter occlusion

        c. Dialysate leakage

        d. Visceral damage

        e. Electrolyte imbalances

        f. Overhydration

        g. Hypoalbuminemia

P. Hemodialysis

    i. Indications

        a. Anuric renal failure

        b. Oliguric renal failure with hyperkalemia

        c. Oliguric renal failure and fluid overload

        d. Severe clinical uremia (polyuric or oliguric renal failure) unresponsive to fluid therapy

        e. Postrenal uremia resulting from obstruction or rupture to the urinary collecting system

        f. Dialyzable toxicities, for example, barbiturates, ethylene glycol

    ii. Considerations

        a. Limited availability

        b. Expensive

        c. Requires sedation for placement of temporary dialysis catheter or general anesthesia for placement of permanent (tunneled long-term) dialysis catheter

    iii. Complications

        a. Hemorrhage

        b. Catheter-related bloodstream infection

        c. Thrombosis

        d. Dialysis disequilibrium syndrome (too rapid a drop in BUN)

        e. Hypotension while receiving dialysis (due to volume of blood in extracorporeal circuit)

23
UROLOGIC EMERGENCIES: URETER, BLADDER, URETHRA, GN, AND CRF

Annie Malouin

Unique Features
- In cats with urethral obstruction, bradycardia and circulatory collapse might support the presence of severe azotemia, hyperkalemia, and decreased ionized calcium.
- Urine analysis and culture with antimicrobial sensitivity should be performed in the preliminary diagnostic workup of azotemic patients.
- In critically ill cats with renal dysfunction, urine output should be monitored hourly. Also, special attention should be given to match the ins-outs.
- Positive-contrast radiographic studies are useful to diagnose trauma within the urinary tract.
- Parenteral fluid therapy is the most important step in the initial treatment of the uremic cat.

A. Definitions
   a. Azotemia (uremia): the presence of nitrogen-containing compounds in the blood
      i. Prerenal azotemia: due to extrarenal causes that reduce renal blood flow and glomerular filtration
      ii. Renal azotemia: results from loss of functional renal parenchyma
      iii. Post-renal azotemia: caused by reduced renal blood flow caused by increased pressure within the renal collecting system
   b. Isosthenuria: preservation of a constant osmolality of the urine, regardless of changes in osmotic pressure in the blood
   c. Hyposthenuria: excretion of urine of low specific gravity (low osmolality)
   d. Hypersthenuria: excretion of urine of high specific gravity (high osmolality)
   e. Specific gravity of urine: measures of the solute concentration in urine to assess the ability of the renal tubules to concentrate or dilute the glomerular filtrate
   f. Pollakiuria: frequent passage of small amounts of urine
   g. Periuria: urinations in inappropriate locations
   h. Stranguria: slow and painful discharge of urine
   i. Oliguria: reduced urine output
   j. Anuria: complete suppression of urine formation by the kidney
B. Emergency triage assessment
   a. The cat's history might include a recent trauma or a vague malaise that is acute or chronic in duration. The patient's owner might describe more general signs: lethargy to stupor and coma, seizure, anorexia, polydipsia, polyuria, halitosis, vomiting, and diarrhea.

b. More specific signs related to urinary tract abnormalities may also be noted: inappropriate voiding, incontinence, straining to urinate, polyuria, and hematuria.

c. Pet owners often confound straining to urinate for constipation.

d. At presentation to the hospital (on triage), after a brief evaluation of the cat's respiratory and cardiovascular system, the urinary bladder should be palpated as an assessment of its ability to urinate.

e. A cat that presents with a history of inability to urinate and palpation of a large, firm, nonexpressible urinary bladder requires immediate transfer of the animal to the treatment area.

C. Disease conditions

  a. Feline lower urinary tract disease (FLUTD) and feline idiopathic cystitis (FIC)

    i. Definitions

      1. A syndrome of hematuria, dysuria, stranguria, periuria, and/or urethral "plug" formation (with or without urinary obstruction) of undefined etiology

        a. The term *idiopathic* is used because an etiologic diagnosis cannot be found in two-thirds of cats with these signs.

        b. The pathophysiology of FIC is not fully understood and may involve complex interactions between several body systems. Damage to or malfunction of the glycosaminoglycan layer of urothelium and abnormalities in local sensory neurons, sympathetic nervous system, and central nervous system are known to occur in these patients and result in an inappropriate release of inflammatory mediators locally.

    ii. Clinical presentation

      1. Lower urinary tract signs can occur at any age but are unusual in cats less than 1 year of age and most frequent in cats 2–6 years of age. In older cats, neoplasia should be ruled out.

      2. When clinical signs are considered without regard to obstruction, no difference in risk between males and females is observed.

      3. Risk factors include indoor-restricted cats, dry food diet, excessive body weight, decreased activity, multiple-cat household, and Persian cat breeds. The exact nature of these predispositions remains to be determined.

    iii. Diagnostics

      1. Two-thirds of cats with FLUTD signs have FIC, and in approximately 85% of cats with FIC, clinical signs resolve in 2 to 3 days without treatment.

      2. Thus, it is debatable whether any diagnostics should be performed for a young cat in its first presentation of FLUTD signs.

      3. Urinalysis, radiographic studies, and cystoscopy may be necessary to differentiate behavioral disorder from FLUTD and FIC.

      4. Which tests will yield the most benefit for each individual patient must be decided based on the cat's signalment and clinical signs.

        a. Urinalysis may show hematuria, proteinuria, mild sterile pyuria, and crystalluria.

        b. If urine specific gravity is decreased (<1.035 for cats eating solely dry food; <1.025 for cats eating primarily canned foods), a serum biochemical profile and thyroid evaluation should be obtained.

        c. In cats <10 years of age, urine culture is negative 98% of the time.

        d. Urine culture should be performed in all cats:

          i. with recurrent (>2 episodes) FLUTD signs

          ii. older than 10 years old with FLUTD signs

          iii. with a urine specific gravity (USG) <1.030

          iv. that underwent perineal urethrostomy

          v. after a urinary catheter has been placed

      5. A plain abdominal radiograph that includes the entire urinary tract (including urethra) can be a useful to assess for the presence of cystic calculi.

6. Contrast studies of the bladder and urethra in cats with FIC are usually unremarkable, but diffuse or asymmetrical thickening of the bladder wall may be seen.
   a. Contrast studies are especially indicated in elderly cats (> 10 years of age) where FLUTD and FIC are not as likely and the clinical signs persist or keep reoccurring.
   b. A contrast cystogram and urethrogram can be useful to diagnose nonradiopaque calculi and other lesions such as mass lesions, blood clots, and strictures in cats with recurrent episodes.
7. When radiographic findings are negative and a urine culture reveals no growth in cats with no other identifiable abnormalities, the diagnosis of FIC is likely.
8. Ultrasound of the bladder:
   a. May reveal wall thickening that is usually most pronounced cranioventrally. In severe cases, it can become generalized.
   b. Wall thickening somewhat depends on the volume of urine in the bladder. In a nondistended bladder, evaluation of the wall thickness is subjective according to the amount of distension. In a fully distended bladder, normal wall thickening is approximately 1–2 mm.
   c. Diagnostic ultrasound may also help to identify differential diagnosis (e.g., bladder neoplasia, polyps, cystic calculi, etc).
9. Cystoscopy can be performed at referral practices when FLUTD signs fail to resolve after standard therapy in those cats with negative findings from radiography and urine cultures.
   a. Cytoscopy allows visualization of the bladder and urethra, and can exclude less common diseases (small cystic calculi, urachal diverticula, ectopic ureters, and small polyps).
iv. Treatment
1. Many cats improve within 5 days with or without therapy.
2. Subcutaneous fluids (40–60 mL/kg/day) can be given to promote diuresis and dilute urine.
3. Male cats should be watched closely for signs of obstruction.
4. Canned diets can be given to increase water intake.
   a. Easy access to fresh water should be provided at all times.
5. Antibiotics are usually not indicated unless there is a previous history of catheterization and/or severe hemorrhagic cystitis.
6. Metacam is a nonsteroidal anti-inflammatory, specific to COX-2. It can provide analgesia and reduce inflammation and edema; 0.1 mg/kg PO, SC once daily (limit to 4 days use).
7. Amitriptyline is a tricyclic antidepressant that may benefit by stabilizing mast cells and reducing inflammatory changes, and it might relieve stress through mild sedation; 2.5–10 mg once daily in the evening.
8. Phenoxybenzamine is an alpha-adrenergic antagonist that may reduce urethral spasms; 2.5–7.5 mg/cat PO q12h.
9. Diazepam can relax the striated muscle of urethral sphincter and therefore help in the management of urethral spasm; 1–2.5 mg/cat PO q8–12h, or 0.5 mg/kg IV PRN.
v. Prognosis
1. Recurrence rates for FLUTD signs are high. About 50% of cats have a recurrence of clinical signs within 1 year.
b. Urethral obstruction
i. Definitions
1. Urethral plugs made up of a proteinaceous matrix imbedded with struvite crystalline material are the most common causes of obstructions.
   a. Calcium oxalate urethroliths (predominant form of uroliths found in cats), strictures, and neoplasia can also cause obstructions.
   b. Strictures can be secondary to trauma or congenital anatomical abnormalities.
ii. Clinical presentation
1. Male cat with a history of straining to urinate

2. Other signs frequently noted:
   a. Attempting to urinate outside of the litter box
   b. Hematuria
   c. Lethargy
   d. Excessive vocalization as if in pain
   e. Pain on palpation of the abdomen
   f. Loss of appetite and vomiting
3. Owner may mistake cats with urethral obstructions as being constipated, with increased time and effort spent in the litter box.
4. Urethral plugs affect males almost exclusively:
   a. Male cats have a narrow penile urethral lumen and are more at risk to develop a urethral obstruction than are females.
5. Physical examination
   a. Bladder is distended, firm, and nonexpressible with gentle palpation.
      i. Absence of a palpable bladder does not rule out urethral obstruction.
      ii. Seldom, the bladder can rupture because of the severe inflammation and the increased pressure.
      iii. These patients are usually very ill and severely azotemic.
   b. Some cats might have severe cardiovascular compromise, but others are stable.
   c. Dehydration might be present from anorexia and vomiting.
   d. Bradycardia and circulatory collapse might support the presence of hyperkalemia and decreased ionized calcium; therefore, one should monitor an electrocardiogram. See below for a description of ECG changes.
   e. On palpation, the abdomen is often painful.
   f. The tip of the penis might be discolored (dark-red to purple) and swollen, and a urethral plug might be present at its tip.
iii. Diagnostics
   1. In severely ill cats, an extended database (electrolytes, acid-bases, PCV/TS, glucose, and azo-stick) should be completed.
   2. Serum biochemistry, CBC, and urinalysis should be obtained, though it is not necessary to evaluate such results prior to obstruction relief in unstable cats.
   3. Urinalysis may show evidence of inflammation (hematuria, pyuria, proteinuria).
      a. Crystals (struvites or calcium oxalates) may not be present.
      b. Cats with struvite urolithiasis often have a urine pH >6.8 and those with oxalate urolithiasis often have a urine pH <6.5.
      c. USG is often elevated.
   4. Survey abdominal radiographs should be obtained after relief of the obstruction to determine if cystic or renal calculi are present. In cats >8 years old, survey abdominal radiographs should be obtained after relief of the obstruction to determine if cystic or renal calculi are present.
   5. All uroliths and plugs retrieved from a cat should be submitted for quantitative analysis.
      a. This procedure will examine all layers of the urolith and will provide an estimate of the mineral content of each layer.
iv. Treatment
   1. Regardless of the underlying cause, relief of obstructions, reestablishment of urine flow, and correction of fluid, electrolyte, and acid-base imbalances associated with obstruction and postrenal azotemia are the first steps in proper management.
   2. Critically ill cats with urethral obstruction and severe azotemia often have decreased tissue perfusion due to hypovolemia and cardiac dysfunction secondary to metabolic disturbances.

3. An intravenous catheter should be placed and an emergency database (including PCV, TS, dipstick glucose, dipstick BUN, sodium and potassium concentrations, blood gas analysis, and ionized calcium concentration) should be obtained.
4. An ECG should be obtained if a fast, slow, or irregular heart rate is ausculted. Abnormalities cause by hyperkalemia may include
   a. Increased T wave amplitude
   b. Decreased R wave amplitude
   c. ST segment depression
   d. Decreased P wave amplitude
   e. Prolonged PR, QRS, QT
   f. Loss of P wave
   g. Possible ventricular arrhythmias.
5. If severe hyperkalemia is present and causing bradycardia and cardiac electrical conduction disturbances, it should be treated immediately.
   a. Regular insulin, 0.1–0.25 U/kg IV with a 0.25–0.5 g/kg dextrose IV bolus
      i.   IV dextrose should be diluted 1:2 prior administration in a peripheral vein.
      ii. Also, add dextrose to IV maintenance fluids (2.5%–5% concentration) to prevent hypoglycemia.
      iii. Insulin will shift potassium to the intracellular compartment, and its effect lasts 4–6 hours.
   b. A dextrose bolus alone (0.5 g/kg IV) will induce endogenous insulin release in the nondiabetic patient, which translocates potassium intracellularly.
   c. Calcium gluconate 10%, 0.5–1 mL/kg IV slowly over 10 minutes, will rapidly oppose the effect of hyperkalemia on the myocardium, and its effect will last for 10–15 minutes.
      i.   Monitor with ECG. Too-rapid infusion of calcium may manifest on the ECG as prolonged PR intervals, widened QRS complex, shortened QT interval, shortened or absent ST segment, and widened T wave. Bradycardia may progress to complete heart block, asystole, and cardiac arrest. If any of these abnormalities are noted, the calcium infusion should be stopped.
   d. Sodium bicarbonate, 1 mEq/kg IV slowly, will shift potassium to the intracellular compartment, and its effect lasts for up to 2 hours.
      i.   Caution: It may decrease the ionized calcium concentration further, leading to clinical signs of hypocalcemia (tetany, seizures).
   e. Monitor blood gas.
6. If poor tissue perfusion is present (and no obvious physical examination evidence of cardiac disease is present, such as loud heart murmur or gallop rhythm), a bolus of 30 mL/kg/hr of a balanced electrolyte solution should be administered.
   a. After cardiovascular status is improved, parenteral administration of fluid should be continued to promote diuresis (about 3 times maintenance rate), and relief of the urinary obstruction should be attempted.
7. Plugs usually occur at the tip of the penis where the urethra is very narrow, but they can occur anywhere in the urethra.
   a. The tip of the penis should be examined, and if a plug is present it should be dislodged.
8. All items needed to relieve the obstruction should be gathered and ready (fig. 23.1).
   a. An open-end tomcat catheter should primarily be used to relieve the obstruction.
9. Anesthesia is needed to allow proper manipulation of the cat's penis and passage of the urinary catheter (for more in-depth detail, see chap. 5—Guidelines for Anesthesia in Critically Ill Feline Patients and chap. 6—Anesthetic Protocols for Systemically Healthy Cats).
   a. In critically ill cats, this procedure might be well tolerated without sedation.

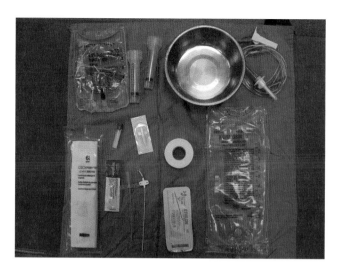

Fig. 23.1. Male urethral catheterization setup:
1. Open-end male cat urethral catheters
2. Sterile lubrication
3. Sterile gloves
4. Red top sample vial for urinalysis
5. White tape
6. 3/0 nylon suture material
7. Sterile bag for urine collection
8. Sterile IV setup for urine collection
9. 10-cc syringes for flushing urinary catheter
10. Sterile saline for flushing urinary catheter
11. Urine collection bowl
12. Catheter adapter

      b. Analgesia should be provided: butorphanol (0.3–0.4 mg/kg), hydromorphone (0.05–0.1 mg/kg), or buprenorphine 8–10 μg/kg).

      c. Then, the combination of ketamine (2.5–5 mg/kg) and diazepam (0.3–0.5 mg/kg), given intravenously to effect, provides adequate sedation for most cats. Ketamine should not be used in patients with cardiac disease, including hyperkalemic cats with EKG abnormalities.

      d. Gas anesthesia with isoflurane administered by facemask or an infusion of propofol (3–5 mg/kg IV) can provide additional sedation and urethral relaxation. These can cause hypotension and the patient's blood pressure should be monitored.

10. The catherization technique should be atraumatic and as gentle as possible.

      a. The severely inflamed urethra and bladder are fragile and can easily rupture.

      b. It is important to follow sterility principles:

         i. Use sterile gloves when placing the catheter.

         ii. Clip the hair from the prepuce and form a small area on the perineum around the prepucial orifice.

         iii. Clean the prepucial orifice with aseptic soap and water.

      c. Small amount of a sterile lubricant gel should be placed at the tip of the tomcat catheter for lubrication.

      d. The prepuce is retracted to extrude the penis and then the penis is pulled caudally to straighten the urethra.

      e. The catheter is inserted into the penis.

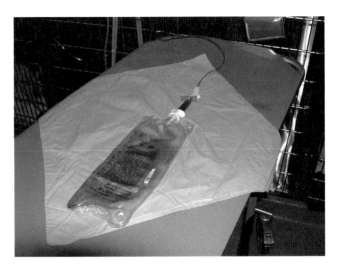

Fig. 23.2. Closed drainage system for urinary catheter.

11. Once the catheter has been inserted into the urethra, it should be advanced gently until resistance is encountered at the site of the urethral plug.
    a. A syringe filled with sterile saline is attached to the urinary catheter and retropulsion with hydraulic forces is performed.
    b. Catheter advancement should be attempted again until it can be introduced in the bladder.
    c. Once the catheter is in the bladder, urine should flow into the catheter.
    d. The bladder can be emptied by aspirating the urine with a syringe attached to the end of the catheter.
    d. Once the bladder is emptied, it should be flushed by inserting about 20 mL of sterile saline through the catheter. This should be done 3–5 times, or until the urine sample is cleared of blood or grit.
    e. An indwelling urinary catheter is then inserted:
        i.   It should be pliable (e.g., red rubber feeding catheter)
        ii. Prior to insertion, the urinary catheter should be measured to assure that the tip of the catheter is about 3 cm past the pelvic inlet.
        iii. The urinary catheter should be attached to a closed drainage system (fig. 23.2).
12. If the urethral plug cannot be dislodged via urethral catheterization, decompressive cystocentesis is recommended.
    a. A small (22- or 23-gauge) butterfly needle inserted into the lateral bladder wall midway between the apex and urethral outflow works well for this procedure and aids in the removal of urine without reinsertion of the needle.
    b. Alternatively, if a longer needle (22-gauge) is necessary, it can be attached to an extension set and urine removed with a syringe in a similar manner.
    c. The bladder should be continuously palpated during the drainage.
    d. Complications are rare but include extravasation of urine into the peritoneal cavity, urinary bladder rupture, or damage to the urinary bladder wall.
13. Urethral catheterization should be attempted again after the cystocentesis.
14. If still unsuccessful at relieving the obstruction, an emergency percutaneous cystostomy tube should be placed until a perineal urethrostomy can be performed.

15. Urine output should be monitored hourly.
    a. Special attention should be given to match the "ins-outs" (see chap. 8—Fluid therapy).
16. Monitor body temperature and provide heat support if needed.
    a. Azotemic animals are often slightly hypothermic.
17. A perineal urethrostomy surgery may be needed to prevent future episodes of urethral obstruction.
    a. This surgery carries some risks or complications such as bacterial UTIs and postoperative strictures.
    b. Clients need to be made aware that this surgery does not correct the underlying problem.
    c. Recurrent uroliths and FIC episodes can still occur.
18. Dietary and environmental changes should be made as needed.
    a. Use of moist rather than dry cat food causes urine dilution and reduces the severity of signs and likelihood of recurrence in cats with idiopathic cystitis.
    b. Struvite uroliths maybe dissolved by feeding a calculolytic diet (Hill's Prescription Diet Feline s/d). Continue diet therapy for 1 month after surveying radiographic evidence of urolith dissolution. Subsequently, feeding magnesium and phosphorus-restricted urine acidifying diets may minimize struvites crystalluria. Several therapeutic foods are available: Hill's Prescription Diet Feline w/d, Hill's Prescription Diet Feline c/d Multicare Feline, and Purina Veterinary Diet UR St/Ox.
    c. Attempts to dissolve calcium oxalate stones have not been successful. For nutritional management of feline oxalate urolithiasis, diets with the highest moisture or protein contents and with moderate amounts of magnesium, phosphorus, or calcium and containing increased dietary sodium (>1%, dry matter basis) are recommended (e.g., Royal Canin Veterinary Diet feline Urinary SO, Hill's Prescription Diet Feline x/d, Hill's Prescription Diet Feline c/d Multicare Feline, and Purina Veterinary Diet UR St/Ox).

v. Prognosis
   1. Prolonged urethral obstruction usually carries more severe morbidity.
   2. Death can occur due to consequences of severe dehydration, hyperkalemia, metabolic acidosis, and hypocalcemia.
      a. Rarely, cats have a ruptured bladder secondary to long-standing urethral obstruction.
      b. Prognosis for survival in these cats is worse.
   3. Almost all cats treated for urethral obstruction at a university referral hospital survived initial treatment and stabilization.
   4. Recurrent obstructions may occur.

c. Urethral tear
   i. History
      1. The history will often lead the clinician to the cause:
         a. Blunt trauma: urethral contusion (HBC)
         b. Laceration/rupture: pelvic (pubic) fractures, penetrating wound (bite wound, gunshot)
         c. Iatrogenic (traumatic catherization)
   ii. Clinical signs
      1. Dysuria, hematuria, pain, swelling, ascites, edematous and swollen hind legs
         a. May or may not be present and voiding may be normal
      2. The hair around perineum should be clipped for better examination of the area: skin discoloration, edema, cellulitis, and fistulous tracts may be present.
   iii. Diagnostics
      1. Perform FAST (focused abdominal sonogram for trauma) to check for abdominal effusion.
      2. Laboratory findings may present dehydration, hypoproteinemia, azotemia, and leukocytosis.
      3. Perform a positive contrast urethrogram to locate the precise site of rupture. Ideally, this procedure should be performed under fluoroscopic guidance to better localize the site of leakage.

iv. Treatment
    1. A balanced crystalloid solution should be administered intravenously to correct electrolyte, acid-base, and perfusion abnormalities.
    2. A small tear in the urethra may not require surgery.
    3. A urinary catheter should be placed and attached to a closed-drainage system.
       a. It should be kept in place for 2–4 weeks, after which a urethrogram should be performed before catheter removal.
    4. Immediate surgical procedure is required for complete urethral tear.
       a. Primary urethroplasty
       b. Temporary cystostomy drainage followed by delayed urethroplasty
d. Bacterial cystitis
  i. History and clinical presentation is usually similar as with FLUTD and FIC.
    1. Bacterial cystitis is rare in cats, but perhaps more common in those with defenses that are compromised due to other diseases or treatments.
    2. Incidence of urinary tract infection rises with age:
       a. Approximately 45% of cats >10 years of age with signs of FLUTD have urinary tract infection
    3. Risk factors for UTIs include:
       a. Urolithiasis
       b. Immunosuppression
       c. Previous indwelling catheterization
       d. Perineal urethrostomy
       e. Tube cystostomies
       f. Diabetes mellitus
       g. Neoplasia
       h. Hyperadrenocorticism
       i. Congenital or acquired anomalies of the lower urinary tract
       j. Chronic renal failure
  ii. Diagnostics
    1. Urinalysis may show signs of inflammation.
       a. Caution should be taken when reporting bacteria from the sediment:
          i. Some cellular breakdown products in the urine can exhibit Brownian motion and look similar to bacteria.
          ii. Bacteria may not be seen, particularly when the USG is low and urine is dilute.
          iii. A urine culture with antimicrobial sensitivity should be performed in all cases.
  iii. Treatment
    1. Subcutaneous fluids (40–60 mL/kg/day) can be given to promote diuresis and dilute urine.
    2. Antimicrobials should be administered based on quantitative urine cultures and sensitivities.
       a. *E. coli* is the most common isolate, but gram-positive cocci such as *Staphylococci* and *Streptococci* account for the next most common isolates.
e. Ureteral obstruction
  i. Definitions
    1. Ureteral obstruction can result from intraluminal and rarely from intramural or extramural causes
       a. Intraluminal obstruction of urine flow can occur as a result of calculi, a blood clot, intramural fibrosis, or a stricture.
       b. Primary ureteral neoplasia has not been reported in cats.
       c. Extramural compression may occur from a retroperitoneal mass, a bladder neoplasm, or from a ligature placed accidentally during surgery.

    d. During ovariohysterectomy, the most common location for inadvertent ureter ligation and/ or transection is near the uterine body and this may result in complete obstruction, with associated hydronephrosis, hydroureter, and eventually permanent renal damage, if not corrected within 7 days.

  ii. Pathophysiology

    1. Obstruction of a ureter can cause ureteral dilatation and progressive distension of the renal pelvis.

    2. As pressure builds up proximal to the site of obstruction, renal blood flow and glomerular filtration decrease, potentially causing permanent renal parenchymal damage.

    3. Chronic renal failure is common at the time of diagnosis of ureteral calculi.

  iii. Clinical presentation and clinical signs

    1. Uroliths tend to develop in middle-aged to older cats, with no sex predilection.

    2. Clinical signs of obstruction may not be apparent unless bilateral obstruction, the contralateral kidney is dysfunctional, or concomitant infection of the urinary tract is present.

    3. Clinical findings are usually nonspecific:

      a. Inappetence

      b. Vomiting

      c. Lethargy

      d. Polyuria

      e. Polydipsia

      f. Hematuria

      g. Lumbar pain

      h. Weight loss

    4. Cats with complete, bilateral obstruction are anuric and may be collapsed at presentation.

      a. Complete, bilateral obstruction that persists for 3 days or longer is fatal without appropriate treatment.

  iv. Diagnostics

    1. Distinction should be made between obstructing and nonobstructing causes of ureteral dilatation.

      a. Pyelonephritis may also cause ureteral dilatation but would not warrant surgery.

      b. Conversely, an obstructing calculus or mass would necessitate early surgical intervention.

    2. A combination of survey radiographs and abdominal ultrasonography is recommended to confirm the diagnosis.

    3. Most ureteral calculi contain calcium oxalate or calcium phosphate and appear radioopaque on radiographs.

      a. However, small calculi, calculi overlying the colonic contents, and radiolucent calculi may be missed on survey radiographs.

    4. Ultrasonography allows limited morphologic assessment of the renal parenchyma and can identify hydronephrosis and hydroureter.

      a. Although ureteral dilatation alone is not a specific sign of obstruction, visualization of focal hydroureter to the level of obstruction can be diagnostic.

      b. Ureteral dilatation usually begins proximally, and as the degree of hydroureter increases, it extends distally.

      c. Ureteral dilatation may not extend to the level of the ureteral obstruction.

      d. Also, in some patients it may be difficult to follow the entire course of the ureter because of its small size and because of interference by other organs.

        i. In these cases, absence or reduced amplitude and duration of ureteral flow at the uretero-vesicular junction can be used as an indirect sign of obstruction.

      e. Ultrasonography may also indicate abnormality in the contralateral kidney (e.g., small size, dilated pelvis), suggestive of preexisting renal parenchymal disease.

5. Additional imaging modalities, such as antegrade pyelography, intravenous urography, nuclear scintigraphy, and computed tomography may be necessary to identify ureteral calculi that are not apparent on survey radiographs and ultrasound images.

   a. Renal scintigraphy allows evaluation of renal function but does not predict what function will be after the obstruction has been relieved.

   b. Excretory urography can identify ureteral dilatation to the point of obstruction and may show a filling defect or stricture if the associated kidney is functional and the patient is not severely compromised.

      i. If renal function is decreased, filtration of the contrast medium will be reduced, which will result in poor opacification of the upper portion of the urinary tract.

      ii. This procedure should not be performed in a dehydrated or severely azotemic cat, as adverse systemic actions to the contrast agent may occur and possibly cause further renal damage.

   c. Percutaneous antegrade pyelography is an accurate diagnostic test for patients in which excretory urography is nondiagnostic, or when concern exists about the adverse effects of systemic contrast administration.

      i. Fluoroscopy or ultrasonography is used to guide needle or catheter placement into the dilated renal pelvis.

      ii. Urine is aspirated from the renal pelvis and submitted for analysis and culture.

      iii. Iodinated contrast material is then injected into the needle or catheter at a volume equal to one-half the aspirated urine volume.

      iv. The flow of contrast is monitored with fluoroscopy or with radiographs taken immediately after contrast injection.

      v. This technique is easily performed and has minimal complications, such as hematuria and leakage of contrast material or urine into the abdomen.

      vi. Fluid diuresis should be performed concurrently to prevent blood clot formation, which may result in obstruction.

6. Laboratory findings include variable elevation of serum creatinine, BUN, and phosphorus.

   a. Factors affecting the degree of azotemia include:

      i. Unilateral or bilateral ureteral obstruction

      ii. The degree of ureteral obstruction

      iii. The degree of impairment of renal function in each kidney

      iv. The degree of prerenal azotemia

   b. Azotemia in cats with unilateral ureteral obstruction indicates reduced renal function in the contralateral kidney or prerenal azotemia.

   c. Some azotemic cats with unilateral blockage may have concurrent infection or a milder degree of ureteral obstruction in the contralateral kidney, which could be caused by undiagnosed ureteral calculi, sediment accumulation, or ureteral stricture.

7. Urine analysis may show crystalluria with amorphous crystals, calcium oxalate crystals, or struvite crystals.

   a. Most uroliths are composed of calcium oxalate and calcium phosphate.

   b. Uroliths should be sent for analysis.

8. Urinary tract infection should be ruled out by obtaining a culture and antimicrobial sensitivity of the specimen.

v. Treatment

   1. Rapid surgical intervention is indicated once the diagnosis has been made because recovery of renal function is inversely related to the duration of obstruction.

      a. The patient should be treated medically until it is stable for definitive surgical correction of the ureteral obstruction.

      b. Fluid, electrolyte, and acid-base balance should be restored.

2. Critically ill cats with ureteral obstruction and acute renal failure often have decreased tissue perfusion due to hypovolemia and cardiac dysfunction secondary to hyperkalemia, acidosis, and dehydration.

3. An intravenous catheter should be placed and an emergency database (including PCV, TS, dipstick glucose, dipstick BUN, sodium and potassium concentrations, blood gas analysis, and ionized calcium concentration) should be obtained.

4. An arterial blood pressure measurement should be obtained.
   a. If the patient blood pressure is decreased (systolic blood pressure <100 mmHg, mean arterial pressure <70 mmHg) and/or if poor tissue perfusion is determined on physical examination:
      i. Administer a bolus of 30 mL/kg/hr of a balance electrolyte solution.

5. An EKG should be obtained if a fast, slow, or irregular heart rate is ausculted.
   a. Hyperkalemia can cause severe cardiac rhythm abnormalities (see above section, "Urethral Obstruction," for a description).

6. If severe hyperkalemia is present and causing bradycardia and cardiac electrical conduction disturbances, it should be treated immediately (see above section, "Urethral Obstruction," for its treatment).

7. After cardiovascular status is improved, parenteral administration of fluid should be continued to promote diuresis (about 3 times maintenance rate). The amount of fluid required for daily maintenance in cats can be calculated using this formula: daily basal water requirement (mL) = (30 × kg) + 70.

8. A urinary catheter should be placed and urine output monitored hourly.

9. Buprenorphine or butorphanol should be administered for pain control.
   a. Pure opioid agonists should be avoided because they may increase ureteral tone, bladder tone, and external sphincter tone, leading to increased difficulty in urination.
   b. Morphine can also cause an increase in antidiuretic hormone release, and thus reduce urine production.
   c. Epidural analgesia may also be given.

10. Furosemide (1–2 mg/kg IV) may be given to promote further diuresis, promoting urine production and passage of the ureteral calculi or blood clot.

11. Amitriptyline can relax urinary tract smooth muscle. Its mechanism of action is by depolarization of the membrane by opening the potassium channels; thus, there is ureteral relaxation and the potential for facilitating stone passage in cats with ureteral calculi. The recommended dosage for amitrityline is 1 mg/kg orally q12–24h.

12. Hemodialysis and emergency placement of nephrostomy catheters can be useful for stabilization of severely uremic patients.
    a. The aim of dialysis is to reduce the degree of azotemia, allow time to determine whether the ureteral calculus will pass on its own, and improve the clinical condition of the cat prior to surgical treatment.
    b. Temporary nephrostomy catheters can be placed in both kidneys in case of bilateral ureteral obstruction.
       i. Placement of temporary nephrostomy catheter diverts urine flow, allows time for physiologic dieresis, and thus preserves renal function.
       ii. It has the additional advantage of allowing a preoperative assessment of remaining renal function in the obstructed kidney.

13. Broad spectrum antibiotherapy should be started if there is any indication of infection on the urine analysis and until results of the urine culture and sensitivity are available. Ampicillin, 20 mg/kg IV q8–12h; amoxicillin-clavulanic acid, 62.5 mg/cat PO q12h; cefazolin 20 mg/kg IV q8–12h; and enrofloxacin, 5 mg/kg IV/SQ/IM/PO q24h.
    a. Any infection should be aggressively treated for 4–8 weeks.

14. During medical management of ureteral calculi, imaging studies should be repeated periodically to evaluate if the calculi have spontaneously passed down the ureter into the bladder.
15. Surgical treatment depends on the cause and duration of obstruction.
    a. If the source of the obstruction is extraluminal, the cause should be removed if possible.
    b. If ureteral calculi are suspected, surgical removal is warranted if there is evidence of partial or complete obstruction of the ureter, or if the calculi are immobile on repeated imaging examinations.
16. Options for surgical treatment of ureteroliths include:
    a. Ureterotomy
    b. Retrograde flushing of calculi into the renal pelvis, followed by pyelolithotomy
    c. Resection of the affected portion of the ureter, followed by primary anastomosis or reimplantation into the bladder
    d. Ureteronephrectomy
17. Complications of ureteral surgery include urine leakage, dehiscence, and stricture formation.
18. Placement of a nephrostomy catheter after surgery may be helpful for diverting urine flow until the ureter heals.
19. Ureteronephrectomy may be required if the ureteral obstruction cannot be corrected, but the contralateral kidney function must be within normal limits.
20. If the obstruction is caused by a urolith, analysis of the stone should be performed, so that dietary and appropriate medical therapy can be initiated.

   vi. Prognosis
1. The longer the obstruction, the less chance of reversibility of renal dysfunction.
2. Medical and surgical treatment of ureteral obstruction can stabilize renal function, although many cats may continue to have impaired renal function.
3. If patency of a completely obstructed ureter is restored within 1 week of obstruction, renal function can return to normal or to its preobstruction function.
4. Irreversible renal damage may occur if complete ureteral obstruction is present for longer than 4 weeks.

  f. Ureteral tear
   i. History
1. Injury to the ureters can occur from:
    a. Blunt or penetrating abdominal injury
    b. Iatrogenically (include complete or partial ligation, transection, kinking, crushing, and devascularization) during abdominal surgery (occurs most commonly as a complication during ovariohysterectomy and resection of a caudal abdominal or pelvic neoplasm) or laparoscopy
    c. Secondary to ureteral obstruction

   ii. Diagnostics
1. Loss of retroperitoneal detail on abdominal radiograph combined with ultrasound findings of free retroperitoneal fluid warrants a suspicion of ureteral rupture, although retroperitoneal hemorrhage can have similar findings.
2. Iatrogenic ureteral injuries are rarely recognized at surgery, and their diagnoses are often a few days after the surgery when the patient becomes clinical.
3. If ureteral injury is suspected during surgery and cannot be confirmed by visual examination, retrograde ureteral catheterization (by cystotomy) can be attempted.
4. Intravenous urography during surgery can also be performed as a single film exposure 10 minutes after injection of the contrast agent to evaluate the integrity of the ureters.

   iii. Treatment

1. Several surgical procedures may be considered, including nephroureterectomy, ureteral anastomosis, ureteral reimplantation, and placement of a ureteral stent with or without nephrostomy drainage.
2. Time of diagnosis, severity, and location of the injury are variables that will guide the surgical treatment.
3. Nephroureterectomy is most often performed in patients with traumatic injury in an effort to eliminate many of the potential complications associated with primary repair procedures.

g. Uroperitoneum
  i. Definition:
    1. Accumulation of urine in the peritoneal cavity following leakage from the kidneys, ureter, bladder, or urethra.
  ii. Clinical presentation
    1. Uroperitoneum commonly results from trauma—either blunt trauma to the abdomen or pelvis, which has created urinary tract injuries, or traumatic catheterization of cats with urethral obstruction and bladder expression.
    2. Less common etiologies include urethral and ureteral tear from obstruction with calculi and bladder rupture from a neoplastic process (lymphoma, transitional cell carcinoma).
  iii. Clinical signs
    1. Anuria and dysuria are the most common historical complaints.
    2. Depressed mentation, dehydration, hypothermia, bradycardia, palpable abdominal fluid wave, and hematuria
    3. Free abdominal fluid may also be identified with a focused abdominal sonogram test.
       a. Abdominocentesis should be performed to obtain a sample of effusion.
  iv. Diagnostics
    1. Definitive diagnosis is supported by finding free urine within the abdominal cavity and with a radiographic contrast study to demonstrate loss of urinary tract integrity, or exploratory surgery to allow direct visualization of the site of urine leakage.
    2. The gross appearance of peritoneal effusion might be misleading in the diagnosis of UP, because it does not always resemble urine.
    3. Free fluid in the abdomen may be identified as urine by
       a. Comparison of the abdominal fluid creatinine and potassium concentration to their concentration in a peripheral blood sample collected at the same time
          i. Large creatinine molecules do not diffuse readily across the peritoneal membrane into the blood, leading to a gradient between creatinine concentration in serum and abdominal fluid.
          ii. A 2:1 ratio of creatinine concentration in the abdominal fluid compared to that in the serum is predictive for uroabdomen.
          iii. A potassium concentration in the abdominal fluid higher than in the serum with a ratio of >1.9:1 is predictive for uroabdomen.
       b. Conversely, the small urea molecules diffuse rapidly across the peritoneal membrane into the blood without allowing a gradient to be established.
          i. A higher BUN in the abdominal fluid than in the serum suggests that the free abdominal fluid is urine, but abdominal fluid with a BUN that is less than or equal to that of serum does not exclude the possibility of the fluid being urine.
    4. Survey radiographs may be suggestive of urinary tract injury but are rarely diagnostic.
       a. They often show a decrease in abdominal detail due peritoneal effusion.
    5. Positive contrast radiographic studies include excretory urography, cystography, and retrograde urethrography.
       a. These methods are very accurate for the diagnosis of urinary tract injuries.
       b. Accuracy depends largely on the amount of contrast medium injected, and false negative results may be from inadequate distension of the bladder with contrast medium.

     c. Excretory urography should not be performed on dehydrated animals because prolonged excretion of dye may cause renal damage.

v. Treatment

   1. Initial stabilization with intravenous fluids should be administered to any traumatized and critically ill patient.

     a. Ventilation support and perfusion support

     b. Electrolyte imbalance and acid-base abnormalities should be treated.

   2. Since uremic patients are at high risk for developing complications during anesthesia, surgical correction of urinary tract leakage should be delayed until metabolic, fluid, and electrolyte disturbances have been corrected.

   3. Severely uremic patients will benefit from peritoneal dialysis, hemoperfusion, or hemodialysis prior to anesthesia and surgery.

   4. The decision between surgical or conservative management is based on the site and the extent of the lesion as well as associated injuries.

     a. Once the patient is stable, surgery should be performed to repair the defect.

   5. A small tear in the bladder and urethra may not require surgery.

     a. A urinary catheter and closed-drainage system can be left in place for 3–10 days.

   6. Conservative therapy

     a. Fluid therapy and drainage of urine from the peritoneal cavity are very important to stabilize the patient.

     b. Effective urine drainage from the peritoneal cavity can be accomplished with an intra-abdominal catheter or with a peritoneal dialysis catheter.

     c. Urethral catheter drainage may be successful in patient with partial urethral tear and small bladder rupture.

     d. The urinary catheter should be kept in place for 2–4 weeks, after which a urethrogram should be performed before catheter removal.

   7. Exploratory surgery should be performed once the patient is stable.

     a. Urine is irritating to the tissues and causes a chemical peritonitis.

     b. The degree of peritonitis may differ depending on duration, amount of urine leakage, and bacterial contamination.

     c. A septic peritonitis may also develop if urinary tract infection was present before urinary tract rupture.

     d. Bacteriologic culture of the peritoneal effusion should be performed and broad-spectrum antibiotic therapy should be initiated. Ampicillin, 20 mg/kg IV q8–12h; amoxicillin-clavulanic acid, 62.5 mg/cat PO q12h; cefazolin 20 mg/kg IV q8–12h; and enrofloxacin, 5 mg/kg IV/SQ/IM/PO q24h.

     e. Bladder rupture at the apex most often results from blunt abdominal trauma.

     f. Defects in the dorsal and ventral aspects of the bladder trigone are more often associated with urethral obstruction and traumatic catheterization.

     g. For detailed instruction on bladder repair, a surgical textbook should be consulted.

vi. Prognosis

   1. Associated injuries caused by trauma are more often responsible for morbidity and mortality.

   2. A delay in diagnostics and treatment may greatly raise the mortality rate.

h. Acute-on-chronic renal failure

i. Pathophysiology

   1. Chronic renal failure (CRF) is common in cats >7 years old.

   2. Possible causes of CRF are:

     a. Sustained systemic hypertension, chronic infection or inflammation, urolithiasis, urine outflow obstruction, polycystic kidney disease or other congenital renal disorder, FIP, and chronic interstitial nephritis (idiopathic).

   b. By the time of diagnosis, the cause(s) of CRF are usually not identifiable or treatable.
3. Cats with loss of two-thirds or more of functional nephrons lose the ability to concentrate urine effectively and are said to have renal insufficiency.
4. Because of the large functional renal reserve and the compensatory hypertrophy of remaining viable nephrons, clinical signs and laboratory data compatible with CRF are not present in most cases until greater than three-fourths or more of functional nephrons have been lost.
5. Serum phosphorus concentration becomes increased with greater than 85% loss of excretory renal function.
6. Once a cat is diagnosed with CRF, regenerative and compensatory nephron changes have had time to occur, yet the presence of azotemia indicates the inadequacy of these compensatory processes.
7. Cats with CRF are polyuric and have a compensatory polydipsia as a result of a decrease in urine-concentrating ability.
8. As long as water intake is adequate and therefore renal blood flow and the glomerular filtration rate (GFR) are maintained, renal failure and severe azotemia can be avoided.
9. Conditions that may produce hypotension, such as dehydration and anesthesia, promote renal hypoperfusion.
   a. These conditions may exacerbate the clinical and laboratory abnormalities of chronic renal insufficiency and failure, perhaps precipitating a uremic crisis: "acute on chronic renal failure."
   b. Further, if dehydration and decreased renal blood flow are severe, additional ischemic renal damage may occur.
   c. Hyperthyroidism can increase the GFR and thereby decrease the serum BUN and creatinine concentration masking underlying renal disease. Treatment of hyperthyroidism may therefore have a negative effect on renal function.
ii. Clinical signs and findings
1. Clinical signs may include anorexia, vomiting, diarrhea, constipation, dehydration, oral ulcerations, and weakness.
2. CRF is usually characterized by polyuria, but affected cats may transiently be oliguric when dehydrated, and permanent oliguria develops during terminal decompensation.
3. Gastrointestinal ulcers and signs of gastroenteritis may occur because uremic toxins stimulate the chemoreceptor trigger zone, increase the production of gastrin, and can produce a uremic vasculitis.
4. Systemic hypertension is seen in 60–75% of cats with CRF.
   a. Glomerular capillary injury, decreased vasodilatory substances, and enhanced renin-angiotensin-aldosterone activation may all lead to hypertension during renal failure.
   b. Indirect blood pressure measurement should be obtained.
   c. Hypertension in cats is defined as a systolic blood pressure >160–170 mmHg.
   d. Fundoscopic evaluation should be performed, since retinal lesions (e.g., edema, hemorrhage, or detachment) are common in cats with hypertension.
5. Cats with CRF should also be evaluated for hyperthyroidism, diabetes mellitus, and cardiac abnormalities.
iii. Diagnostics
1. Initial database should include CBC, biochemistry and acid-base measures, T4, and urinalysis with urine culture.
   a. Blood work findings may include azotemia, metabolic acidosis, hyperphosphatemia, hypokalemia, hypermagnesemia, and nonregenerative anemia.
2. Severe hypokalemia can cause significant muscular weakness, often recognized with neck ventroflexion.

3. Hyperphosphatemia is due to decreased GFR and retained phosphorus, but also decreased activation of vitamin D and decreased calcium absorption.
   a. This may lead to secondary hyperparathyroidism, and therefore a progressive increase in parathyroid hormone occurs to maintain serum calcium concentration.
   b. High levels of parathyroid hormone may cause multiple disorders (e.g., renal osteodystrophy, soft tissue calcification), and it is a significant uremic toxin.
4. Nonregenerative anemia is due to decreased erythropoietin production, gastrointestinal loss due to hemorrhage, and shortened RBC life span.
   a. Platelet function might also be abnormal.
5. Urine analysis can show isostenuria, proteinuria, tubular casts, hematuria, and pyuria.
6. Microalbuminuria detection is marketed for detection of early renal disease:
   a. Detects urine albumin in 2–30 mg/dL range.
   b. Unknown whether it will be specific or predictive as early marker of CRF.
7. Urinary tract infection should be ruled out with a urine culture.
8. Abdominal radiographs can confirm the presence of small kidneys.
9. Renal ultrasonography usually reveals diffusely hyperechoic renal cortices with loss of the normal corticomedullary junction.
   a. The increase in renal echogenicity is caused by fibrous scar tissue replacing the irreversibly damaged nephrons.
10. Radiology and ultrasonography can also help by ruling out potentially treatable causes of CRF like pyelonephritis and renal urolithiasis.
11. Renal biopsy is not routinely performed unless the diagnosis is in question.

iv. Treatment
1. Adequate extracellular fluid volume must be maintained to maximize renal perfusion and assist in excretory function.
2. Parenteral fluid therapy is the most important step in the initial treatment of the uremic cat, and its goals include extracellular fluid volume expansion, correction of electrolyte and acid-base disturbances, and reduction of the magnitude of azotemia.
3. The volume of fluid needed is determined by considering the extent of dehydration and the maintenance and continuing fluid loss of the patient:
   a. Volume replacement (mL) = (body weight [kg]) × (estimated deficit [%]) × 1,000
   b. Fluid deficit should be replaced with a balanced electrolyte solution over 8 hours.
   c. If the cat does not seem dehydrated, 5% of its body weight should be infused over 4 hours to correct subclinical dehydration and promote diuresis.
4. Matching the ins and outs once rehydrated: urine output should be monitored as accurately as possible (weigh diapers, towels, litter, etc.) as well as the fluid administered.
5. Central venous pressures (2–3 mmHg), assessment of body weight, serial measurement of PCV/TS, and frequent pulmonary auscultation can also help gauge the adequacy of fluid therapy and limit possibility of overhydration.
6. Arterial blood pressure should be monitored frequently, and a mean arterial pressure of 80–100 mmHg should be maintained.
7. Once the cat is rehydrated and minimal MAP is maintained, minimal acceptable urine output should be 2 mL/kg/hr.
8. Electrolytes and acid base should be monitored closely, particularly in oliguric, anuric, or severely polyuric patients (see specific treatment for each biochemical abnormality.)
9. Hypokalemia is common, and potassium depletion results from increased urine production along with decreased intake.
   a. Oral supplementation of potassium is preferred over intravenous supplementation, and if at all possible it should be combined with intravenous supplementation during the acute treatment.

    b. Potassium should not be infused intravenously at a rate greater than 0.5 mEq/kg body weight per hour.

    c. Infusion of potassium-containing crystalloid fluids initially may be associated with a decrease in serum potassium concentration as a result of dilution, increased tubular fluid flow in the distal renal tubules, and cellular uptake of potassium.

        i. This effect may be minimized by selecting a fluid that does not contain glucose, administering fluids at an appropriate rate, and beginning oral potassium gluconate (4–8 mEq q24h) as soon as possible.

    d. Clinical improvement usually is observed within 1–3 days.

    e. Chronic treatment involves oral administration of potassium gluconate (2–4 mEq q24h).

    f. Oliguric or anuric cats might be hyperkalemic secondary to decreased excretion and metabolic acidosis.

10. Vomiting can be controlled with the following medications:

    a. Famotidine: 0.25 mg/kg q24h

    b. Ranitidine: 2–4 mg/kg IV q12h

    c. Omeprazole: 0.5–1 mg/kg PO q24h

    d. Odansetron: 0.1 mg/kg PO q12h

    e. Metoclopramide: 1–2 mg/kg/24h added to fluids as a constant rate infusion

11. Hypertension should be treated if systolic pressure exceeds 200 mmHg. The goal of long-term management of hypertension is to maintain a systolic blood pressure below 140–160 mmHg.

    a. Amlodipine besylate, a calcium channel blocker, is an effective antihypertensive agent in cats: 0.625–1.25 mg/cat PO q24h.

12. Proteinuria predicts a worse outcome in cats with CRF. ACE inhibitors decrease proteinuria and increase survival time in cats with proteinuria. A urine protein-to-creatinine >0.4 in cats should prompt intervention: benazepril 0.5–1 mg/kg PO q12–24h, enalapril 0.5 mg/kg PO q12h. Using benazepril is preferable due to decreased renal elimination as compared to enalapril.

13. Iatrogenic blood loss should be minimized.

    a. If severe anemia develops (hematocrit values decline <20% and presence of clinical signs attributable to the anemia), a transfusion of packed RBCs or whole blood is indicated.

    b. The transfusion can be followed by recombinant erythropoietin therapy. There are two different peptides available: epoeitin alfa (Epogen, Procrit) injections: 50–150 U/kg SQ three times weekly, or darbepoetin (Aranesp) 6.25 µg/cat SC weekly, tapering to q2–3 weeks as needed to keep PCV around 30%.

        i. Adequate iron stores are necessary for, and optimal response to, erythropoietin therapy, and iron supplementation is usually required during the initial treatment period. Iron sources: iron dextran 50 mg/cat deep IM injection monthly; ferrous sulfate 50–100 mg/cat PO q24h.

        ii. Hematocrit should be monitored weekly or biweekly until a target hematocrit of approximately 30%.

        iii. Correction of hematocrit to low normal takes approximately 2–8 weeks, depending on the starting hematocrit and dose given.

        iv. Adverse effects related to recombinant erythropoietin therapy may include systemic hypertension, seizures, local reactions at the site of injection, and development of antibodies directed at erythropoietin. Darbepoetin may be less antigenic than the other recombinant EPO therapies.

14. The kidneys are responsible for elimination of many drugs from the body; thus, renal drug clearance is reduced as renal function declines.
    a. Excessive drug accumulation can cause adverse drug reactions and nephrotoxicity; therefore, dose regimens should be adjusted for drugs requiring renal excretion to compensate for decreased organ function.
15. For maintenance therapy, a stepwise therapeutic approach that addresses the progressive complications of renal failure is suggested:
    a. Oral potassium supplementation (see above dosage)
    b. Daily maintenance fluid needs in animal with CRF are higher than those of normal animal because of polyuria.
    c. Dietary management: protein restriction to prevent buildup of nitrogenous wastes and limit diet phosphate content
    d. Phosphorus restriction in conjunction with phosphorus binder (aluminum hydroxide or aluminum carbonate, 30–90 mg/kg q24h divided and administered with meals) to limit phosphorus retention, hyperphosphatemia, renal secondary hyperparathyroidism, and progression of renal disease
    e. Multivitamin supplement is recommended to replace loss of water-soluble vitamins B and C from polyuria.
v. Prognosis
    1. Continued improvement in renal function is a favorable prognostic sign.
    2. CRF is an irreversible and progressive disease.
       a. It is difficult to estimate the extent to which function will return.
       b. Monitoring response to therapy is the only way to monitor the degree of returning function.
    3. With successful renal transplantation, survival times of several years are now expected.
    4. When renal function declines to the point where azotemia/uremia can only be adequately controlled with intravenous fluids and diuresis, the patient's quality of life is usually poor and euthanasia may be an appropriate decision.
i. Acute pyelonephritis
  i. Pathophysiology
      1. Pyelonephritis is a bacterial infection of the upper urinary tract.
      2. Most infections ascend from the lower urinary tract, but hematogenous spread can occur (periodontal disease, bacterial endocarditis, etc).
      3. Acute pyelonephritis can develop from ureteral reflux of bacteria in the urine of animals with lower urinary tract infection.
      4. Other risk factors include urolithiasis, immunosuppression, diabetes mellitus, neoplasia, hyperadrenocorticism, indwelling urinary catheter, and congenital or acquired anomalies of the urinary tract.
      5. Pyelonephritis can result in acute or chronic renal failure.
  ii. Clinical signs
      1. Clinical signs may include fever, anorexia, lethargy, vomiting, dehydration, pain on palpation of the kidneys, and lumbar pain.
  iii. Diagnostics
      1. Laboratory work evaluation
         a. Depending on the extent of renal parenchymal involvement, azotemia, hyperphosphatemia, nonregenerative anemia, and metabolic acidosis may be found.
         b. Common findings on a urine analysis are bacteriuria, pyuria, hematuria, casts (cellular or granular), and low USG.
         c. Urine should be submitted for culture and antimicrobial sensitivity testing.

      i. The most common cause of bacterial pyelonephritis is *E. coli* infection.

      ii. Unfortunately, urinalysis findings may be nonspecific, and urine cultures may be negative in cats with chronic pyelonephritis.

  2. Renal ultrasonography may reveal dilated renal pelvis and proximal ureter, hyperechoic renal pelvis, and changes in the echogenicity of the renal parenchyma.

    a. Renal size may be increased or decreased.

  3. Excretory urography may show dilatation of the renal pelvis, proximal ureter and renal diverticula, decreased uptake of contrast material, or prolonged retention of dye.

    a. A normal study does not rule out pyelonephritis.

  iv. Treatment

    1. Fluid therapy should be administered to restore and maintain hydration.

    2. Antibiotics should be chosen on the basis of culture and sensitivity testing.

      a. Empirically used antibiotics should have a good gram-negative spectrum, good renal penetration (ampicillin, 20 mg/kg IV q8–12h; amoxicillin-clavulanic acid, 62.5 mg/cat PO q12h; cefazolin 20 mg/kg IV q8–12h; and enrofloxacin, 5 mg/kg IV/SQ/IM/PO q24h) and should not be nephrotoxic (e.g., aminoglycosides).

      b. Antibiotic therapy should be continued for 4–8 weeks.

    3. Any predisposing factors (e.g., calculi, obstruction) should be removed.

    4. Urine should be cultured 5–7 days after completing antibiotic therapy.

    5. If infection is still present, antibiotherapy should be continued as indicated by culture and sensitivity for another 6–8 weeks and recultured.

      a. Urine should be cultured every 6–8 weeks until three negative cultures are obtained.

      b. A positive urine culture would require another 6–8-week course of therapy.

    6. If casts are seen in the urine and either acute renal failure or acute-on-chronic renal failure is suspected, the cat should be treated accordingly for this specific condition.

j. Glomerulonephritis (GN)

  i. Pathophysiology

    1. Systemic diseases reported in association with glomerular disorder in cats include bacterial infection (chronic bacterial infections, mycoplasmal polyarthritis), viral infection (feline immunodeficiency virus, feline infectious peritonitis, feline leukemia virus), inflammatory causes (pancreatitis, cholangiohepatitis, chronic progressive polyarthritis, systemic lupus erythematosus, other immune-mediated diseases), neoplasia (leukemia, lymphosarcoma, mastocytosis, other neoplasms), acromegaly, mercury toxicity, familial predisposition, and idiopathic causes.

      a. However, in most reports of GN in cats, no predisposing factors can be found and the disease is classified as idiopathic.

  ii. Clinical presentation

    1. Young adult male cats typically are affected and there is no breed predisposition.

    2. The clinical presentation may fall into two categories:

      a. Classical nephrotic syndrome characterized by subcutaneous edema, ascites, proteinuria, hypercholesterolemia, and hypoalbuminemia without marked azotemia

      b. CRF with azotemia

    3. Signs of thromboembolic disease may be present, such as dyspnea or a decreased or absent peripheral pulse.

    4. Predisposing inflammatory, infectious, or neoplastic process may be found during physical examination.

    5. Blood pressure should be taken, as hypertension is frequent.

    6. Kidney size may be different.

    7. Cats with CRF often have small, firm, irregularly shaped kidneys, whereas those with milder disease often have normal-sized or, occasionally, enlarged kidneys.

iii. Diagnostics
1. Laboratory abnormalities may include proteinuria, hypoalbuminemia, hypercholesterolemia, and nonregenerative anemia.
   a. Azotemia and hyperphosphatemia are not always present.
2. A urine protein–to-creatinine ratio (UPC) greater than 0.5 in a urine sample free of evidence of inflammation and macroscopic hematuria is abnormal and suggestive of significant proteinuria.
3. Hypercoagulability (from loss of antithrombin), thrombocytosis, and hyperfibrinogenemia can be ruled out by thromboelastography.
4. On abdominal radiographs, kidneys may appear normal, small and irregular, or enlarged.
5. Similar changes in shape and size can be seen with sonography.
   a. Increased echogenicity of the cortex and loss of corticomedullary distinction may also be noted.
   b. The renal pelvis may be mildly dilated if polyuria is present or if fluids are being administered.
6. Renal biopsy can provide a definitive diagnosis of glomerular disease.
   a. Membranous nephropathy with IgG and complement deposition are seen histologically.
iv. Treatment
1. The main treatment goals are:
   a. Treatment and elimination of potential underlying diseases
   b. Reduction of proteinuria
   c. Management of uremia and other complications of renal failure
2. Angiotensin-converting enzyme (ACE) inhibitors can significantly reduce proteinuria and delay either the onset or the progression of azotemia. Enalapril 0.5 mg/kg q12–24h or benazepril 0.5–1 mg/kg PO q12–24h. (See comment regarding benazapril versus enalapril above.)
3. If hypertension is still present despite the ACE inhibitor, additional treatment may be needed: Amlodipine besylate, a calcium channel blocker, 0.625–1.25 mg/cat PO q24h.
4. Aspirin is a nonspecific cyclo-oxygenase inhibitor that may be used to reduce glomerular inflammation caused by thromboxane and inhibit platelet aggregation, which may have an added benefit of preventing thromboembolism. Aspirin 25 mg/kg (or ¼ of a 325-mg tablet) PO q48–72h.
5. A diuretic can be given to reduce edema and ascites: Furosemide 2–4 mg/kg q8–24h, Spironolactone 1–2 mg/kg q12–24h.
6. GN associated with immune-mediated disease should be treated with immunosuppressive therapy (prednisolone 2–4 mg/kg q24h).
7. Antiemetics may be use as needed. H_2 blockers are used to manage gastritis: famotidine, ranitidine, cimetidine.
8. Feed a high-quality diet that is restricted in protein and sodium.
9. Fluid therapy regimen
   a. Acute azotemia should be treated with fluid therapy.
   b. Hydration should be corrected with electrolyte-balanced crystalloid solutions.
   c. If edema is present, colloids (hetastarch, dextran 70, plasma, human albumin concentrate) should be administered at a dose of 1–2 mL/kg/day.
   d. Maintenance requirements should be sustained with low-sodium crystalloid solutions (0.45% NaCl with 2.5% dextrose).
10. Cats with azotemia and end-stage renal disease should be treated for CRF.
11. The UPC, urinalysis, body weight, body condition score, and serum albumin and creatinine concentrations should be evaluated monthly or whenever modifications in the therapeutic plan are being made.

v. Prognosis
1. Prognosis is variable.
2. The disease is slowly progressive although remissions are possible.
3. Azotemia, severe proteinuria, systemic hypertension, and marked tubulointerstitial lesions at presentation are the most significant predictors of an unfavorable outcome in most forms of glomerular disease.
4. Cats with end-stage renal disease have the shortest survival times (a few weeks to a few months).
5. Non-azotemic cats presented with the nephrotic syndrome do better and survive several months to several years.

Recommended Reading

Adin CA, Herrgesell EJ, Nyland TG, et al. Antegrade pyelography for suspected ureteral obstruction in cats: 11 cases (1995–2001). J Am Vet Med Assoc, 2003; 222:1576–1581.

Aumann M, Worth LT, Drobatz KJ. Uroperitoneum in cats: 26 cases (1986–1995). J Am Anim Hosp Assoc, 1998; 34:315–324.

Bellah JR. Wound healing in the urinary tract. Semin Vet Med Surg, 1989; 4:294–303.

Buffington CA, Chew DJ, Kendall MS, et al. Clinical evaluation of cats with nonobstructive urinary tract diseases. J Am Vet Med Assoc, 1997; 210(1):46–50.

Cowgill L, James KM, Levy JK, et al. Use of recombinant humans erythropoietin for management of anemia in dogs and cats with renal failure. J Am Vet Med Assoc, 1998; 212(4):521–528.

DiBartola SP, De Morais HA. Disorders of potassium: hypokalemia and hyperkalemia. In DiBartola SP, ed, Fluid Therapy in Small Animal Practice, 3rd ed, pp 91–121. Philadelphia: W.B. Saunders, 2006.

Kirk CA, Ling GV, Franti CE, et al. Evaluation of factors associated with development of calcium oxalate urolithiasis in cats. J Am Vet Med Assoc, 1995; 207(11):1429–1434.

Kyles AE, Hardie AM, Wooden BG, et al. Clinical, clinicopathologic, radiographic and ultrasonographic abnormalities in cats with ureteral calculi: 163 cases (1984–2002). J Am Vet Med Assoc, 2005; 226:932–936.

Kyles AE, Hardie AM, Wooden BG, et al. Management and outcome of cats with ureteral calculi: 153 cases (1984–2002). J Am Vet Med Assoc, 2005; 226:937–944.

Kyles AE, Stone EA, Goodkin J, et al. Diagnosis and surgical management of obstructive ureteral calculi in cats: 11 cases (1993–1996). J Am Vet Med Assoc, 1998; 213:1150–1156.

Lamb CR. Ultrasonography of the ureters. Vet Clin North Am Small Anim Pract, 1998; 28(4):823–848.

Lee JA, Drobatz KJ. The characterization of the clinical characteristics, electrolytes, acid-base and renal parameters in male cats with urethral obstruction. J Vet Emerg Crit Care, 2003; 13(4):227–233.

Lee JA, Drobatz KJ. Historical and physical parameters as predictors of severe hyperkalemia in male cats with urethral obstruction. J Vet Emerg Crit Care, 2006; 16(2):104–111.

Nwadike BS, Wilson LP, Stone EA. Use of bilateral temporary nephrostomy catheters for emergency treatment of bilateral ureter transaction in a cat. J Am Vet Med Assoc, 2000; 217:1862–1865.

Rivers BJ, Walter PA, Polzin DJ. Ultrasonographic-guided, percutaneous antegrade pyelography: technique and clinical application in the dog and cat. J Am Anim Hosp Assoc, 1997; 33(1):61–68.

Weisse C, Aronson LR, Drobatz KJ. Traumatic rupture of the ureter: 10 cases. J Am Anim Hosp Assoc, 2002; 38:188–192.

24
ACUTE INTRINSIC RENAL FAILURE

Cathy Langston

A. Definitions of acute azotemia
  a. Prerenal azotemia is caused by decreased renal perfusion.
      i. Causes include dehydration, hypovolemia, decreased cardiac output, hypotension, and anesthesia.
      ii. Prerenal azotemia is rapidly reversed with correction of the underlying condition.
      iii. Long-standing prerenal azotemia can lead to intrinsic renal failure.
  b. Postrenal azotemia is caused by urinary obstruction or leakage.
      i. Urinary obstruction, which by a combination of neurohumoral events and increased back-pressure in the kidney that opposes filtration, decreases renal clearance.
          1. Azotemia is rapidly reversed by relieving obstruction.
              a. Urethral obstruction
              b. Bilateral ureteral obstruction, or unilateral obstruction with solitary functional kidney
          2. Long-standing obstruction may lead to intrinsic renal failure.
      ii. Urine leakage, which allows filtered substances (i.e., BUN, creatinine, etc.) to be reabsorbed
          1. Azotemia is rapidly reversed by providing drainage of urine, either by drain placement (i.e., peritoneal catheter for uroabdomen) or urinary diversion (i.e., urethral catheter to stent ruptured urethra).
          2. Urine causes inflammatory reaction in tissues
              a. This can lead to sterile peritonitis.
              b. Urine leakage into the abdomen in a patient with a urinary tract infection can lead to a septic peritonitis. This is a surgical emergency.
  c. Intrinsic renal failure is caused by the following factors:
      i. Ischemia
          1. Occurs secondary to poor blood flow to the kidneys
          2. Potential causes include progression of prerenal azotemia, hypotension, hypovolemia, circulatory collapse, excessive renal vasoconstriction, or renal vascular disease (thrombosis, disseminated intravascular coagulation, stenosis)
      ii. Primary renal diseases: pyelonephritis, lymphoma, or other infectious, immune, neoplastic, or degenerative conditions that primarily affect the kidneys
      iii. Nephrotoxins (table 24.1)
          1. Common causes include lily plants, ethylene glycol, and nonsteroidal anti-inflammatory drugs (NSAIDs).
          2. Increased use of NSAID for perioperative pain management may increase incidence of acute renal failure (ARF).

Table 24.1. Substances with nephrotoxic potential.

Classes of Agents	Examples
Antimicrobials	Aminoglycosides, cephalosporins, penicillins, sulfonamides, quinolones, tetracyclines, vancomycin, carbapenems, aztreonam, rifampin, nafcillin
Antiprotozoals	Trimethoprim-sulfamethoxazole, sulfadiazine, thiacetarsamide, pentamidine, dapsone
Antifungals	Amphotericin B
Antivirals	Acyclovir, foscarnet
Chemotherapeutics	Cis- or carboplatin, doxorubicin, azathioprine, methotrexate
Immunosuppressives	Cyclosporine, interleukin (IL) 2
Nonsteroidal anti-inflammatories	All
Angiotensin-converting enzyme inhibitors	All
Diuretics	All
Radiocontrast agents	
Misc. therapeutics	Allopurinol, cimetidine, apomorphine, dextran 40, penicillamine, streptokinase, methoxyflurane, tricyclic antidepressants, lipid lowering agents, calcium antagonists
Heavy metals	Mercury, uranium, lead, bismuth salts, chromium, arsenic, gold, cadmium, thallium, copper, silver, nickel, antimony
Organic compounds	Ethylene glycol, chloroform, pesticides, herbicides, solvents, carbon tetrachloride
Miscellaneous toxins	Gallium nitrate, disphosphonates, mushrooms, grapes, raisins, snake venom, bee venom, lilies, vitamin D_3–containing rodenticides
Endogenous toxins	Hemoglobin, myoglobin

    iv. Systemic diseases: feline infectious peritonitis, pancreatitis, sepsis, systemic inflammatory response syndrome, multiple organ failure, disseminated intravascular coagulation, hemolytic anemia, hyperthermia, heart failure, hyperviscosity

  d. There are four phases of acute kidney injury.

    i. Initiation

      1. When damage occurs, early intervention may prevent progression.

      2. Clinical signs are often not apparent during this phase, which makes intervention difficult.

    ii. Extension: renal hemodynamic alterations, sublethal injury to cell death, intervention may not be successful.

    iii. Maintenance phase: critical amount of irreversible damage has occurred.

    iv. Recovery: regeneration and repair of the renal tissue, lasts weeks to months.

B. Risk factors for development of intrinsic ARF

  a. ARF developing prior to presentation to the veterinarian is generally due to a single cause (i.e., ingestion of nephrotoxin by previously healthy pet).

  b. Combining multiple factors increases the risk of ARF.

    i. Some factors are avoidable. In patients with nonavoidable risk factors, careful attention to minimizing concurrent risk is prudent (see box 24.1).

    ii. Volume depletion is the most significant predisposing factor.

    iii. Risk of aminoglycoside toxicity is increased by prolonged use (>5 days), elevated trough level (>2 μg/mL for gentamicin and tobramycin, >5 μg/mL for amikacin), preexisting renal disease,

---

Box 24.1.   Risk factors of acute renal failure.

Preexisting renal disease
Dehydration and volume depletion
Trauma
Advanced age
Decreased cardiac output
Diabetes mellitus
Fever
Hypotension
Hypoalbuminemia
Sepsis
Electrolyte imbalances
Hyperviscosity syndromes
Liver disease
Concurrent use of potentially nephrotoxic drugs
Dietary protein level
Acidosis

---

dehydration, hypokalemia, hypocalcemia, hypomagnesemia, metabolic acidosis, old age, concurrent nephrotoxic drug administration, diuretics, and antiprostaglandin therapy.

C. Diagnosis
   a. Clinical presentation
      i. Historical findings include recent (generally <1 week) onset of anorexia or polydipsia, lethargy, nausea or vomiting, diarrhea, polyuria or oliguria/anuria, and weakness.
      ii. Cats with exposure to nephrotoxin may present with no other significant historical findings.
         1. Lily ingestion frequently associated with vomiting of leaves or other plant parts.
         2. Acute central nervous system signs may be present early in course of ethylene glycol toxicity.
      iii. Physical examination may reveal some of the following:
         1. Variable degrees of hydration
         2. Generally good body condition
         3. Uremic halitosis or oral ulceration with severe uremia
         4. Renal pain (specific or nonspecific abdominal pain), renal enlargement
         5. Tachycardia or bradycardia
   b. Initial clinical investigation
      i. Hematology and biochemistry findings
         1. Azotemia (elevated BUN, creatinine)
         2. Hyperphosphatemia
         3. Metabolic acidosis
         4. Hypocalcemia
         5. Hypo- or hyperkalemia
         6. Anemia, if concurrent blood loss (i.e., gastrointestinal bleeding) is present
      ii. Urinalysis findings
         1. Isosthenuria or minimally concentrated urine specific gravity (<1.035)
         2. Dipstick findings of proteinuria and glucosuria
         3. Sediment examination

       a. Presence of casts indicates ongoing renal damage. Casts are fragile and may disintegrate if long delay before analysis.

       b. RBCs, WBCs, or bacteria may be present.

       c. Calcium oxalate crystals may indicate ethylene glycol toxicity.

    4. Positive urine culture if pyelonephritis

  iii. Imaging

    1. Radiographs may reveal normal or enlarged kidneys, or nephroliths/ureteroliths.

    2. Abdominal ultrasound may show normal or enlarged kidneys.

       a. Hydronephrosis may indicate obstruction or pyelonephritis. Mild renal pelvic dilation may occur as result of aggressive diuresis.

       b. Dilated ureter may be traced to obstructing stone (frequently difficult to visualize). Mild ureteral dilation extending only minimally past renal pelvis supports inflammation associated with pyelonephritis.

c. Specific diagnostic tests

  i. Rapid ethylene glycol testing may be performed with a commercially available in-house test kit (EGT Test Kit, PRN Pharmacal, Pensacola, FL).

    1. False positive results with propylene glycol (found in etomidate, diazepam, activated charcoal, etc.)

    2. False negative possible with cats due to lower limit of detection of test kit (50 mg/dL)

  ii. Blood concentrations of certain drugs, such as…, are available to determine if toxic concentration is present and to monitor response to therapy

  iii. Renal biopsy may provide specific etiology (e.g., calcium oxalate crystals in renal parenchyma supporting ethylene glycol toxicosis) or show nonspecific changes (e.g., tubular necrosis) consistent with a variety of ischemic or toxic causes.

    1. Risk of bleeding from uremia-induced thrombocytopathy or other complications with percutaneous needle biopsy may limit utilization of renal biopsy.

    2. Renal biopsy may provide prognostic indicators.

d. Differentiating acute from chronic disease

  i. Prognosis differs with acute vs. chronic renal failure.

  ii. Historical findings of long-standing signs (polyuria, polydipsia, partial or complete anorexia, etc.) suggests chronicity.

  iii. Small kidneys, poor body condition suggests chronicity.

  iv. Nonregenerative anemia more common with chronic renal failure.

  v. Enlarged parathyroid glands on cervical ultrasound suggests chronicity.

D. Therapy of acute renal failure

a. Medical management

  i. Fluid balance

    1. Careful management of fluid balance is the most effective therapy of ARF.

    2. Regulation of the volume and type of fluid administered is necessary.

       a. Volume of intravenous fluid

         i. Rehydration

           1. Body weight (in kg) × estimated % dehydration = fluid deficit in L

           2. Administered over 2–4 hours to rapidly reverse any ongoing renal damage from poor perfusion, and to rapidly assess urine output

           3. Administered over longer time frame if cardiovascular compromise prohibits rapid fluid administration

         ii. Maintenance fluid therapy

           1. 66 mL/kg/day presumes normal urine output and no excessive losses (i.e., vomiting, diarrhea).

           2. Urine output in a cat with ARF may be high, low, or normal.

   3. Cats with ARF may be unable to excrete this fluid volume and have "relative oliguria."
   4. Cats with ARF may have polyuria and require rates of administration exceeding maintenance volumes to avoid dehydration.
iii. Fluid therapy to promote diuresis
   1. In cats with the ability to increase urine output in response to a fluid challenge, administration of a volume of fluid exceeding "maintenance" can improve excretion of some uremic toxins.
   2. Volume is varied based on clinical situation and clinician preferences, but generally ranges from 2.5–6% of body weight per day, in addition to maintenance fluid administration rate.
   3. 60 mL/kg/day = 6% of body weight (i.e., twice the maintenance fluid rate is equivalent to a maintenance rate plus a 6% "push" for diuresis)
iv. "Ins-and-outs" method
   1. It is used when urine output varies from normal, usually below normal, but it is useful for polyuric cats also.
   2. Should only be used after rehydration is complete (not appropriate if a patient is still dehydrated or hypovolemic)
   3. There are three components of volume calculation.
      a. Insensible loss (fluid lost via respiration and normal stool) = 22 mL/kg/day
      b. Urine volume replacement calculated by actual measurement (see below for measuring techniques)
      c. Ongoing losses (i.e., vomiting, diarrhea, body cavity drainage) generally estimated
   4. If no fluid pump available, calculate daily insensible fluid needs and divide by administration interval (i.e., if adjusting fluid rate 4 times a day, divide daily fluid need by 4). Add to this volume the amount of urine produced in previous 6 hours, and add a volume estimate of other losses.
   5. If a fluid pump is available, calculate daily insensible fluid needs and divide by 24 to get hourly rate. Add to this the hourly volume of urine output over the previous monitoring interval, plus an estimate of ongoing losses.
   6. Sample calculations without fluid pump: 4.5-kg cat × 22 mL/kg/day = 100 mL/day, ÷4 = 25 mL per 6 hours; 30 mL urine output over previous 6 hours; vomiting about 3 times a day (~8 mL each time) = 6 mL over 6 hours: 25 + 30 + 6 mL = 61 mL to administer over next 6 hours
   7. Sample calculations with fluid pump: 4.5 kg × 22 mL/kg/day = 100 mL/day, ÷24 = 4 mL/hr; 30 mL urine output over previous 6 hours ÷ 6 = 5 mL/hr; vomiting about 3 times a day (~8 mL each time) = 1 mL/hr: 4 + 5 + 1 = 10 mL/hr
b. Type of IV fluid to administer
   i. Balanced polyionic (i.e., lactated Ringer's solution [LRS], Plasmalyte, Normosol) appropriate in most situations
   ii. 0.9% NaCl contains no potassium; suitable choice for hyperkalemic patient
   iii. Lower sodium fluid more appropriate after rehydration (i.e., 0.45% NaCl with 2.5% dextrose, ½-strength LRS with 2.5% dextrose).
   iv. 5% dextrose in water (D5W) rarely appropriate as sole fluid choice, but may be combined with LRS or 0.9% saline to make ½- or ¾-strength sodium solutions (25 mL LRS + 25 mL D5W = 50 mL ½-strength LRS + 2.5% dextrose).
   v. Colloidal solution (i.e., Hetastarch, 6% Dextran) may be appropriate if hypoalbuminemia present. Generally administered at 20 mL/kg/day (which may replace insensible loss if using ins-and-outs method).

      c. Other fluids included in fluid balance calculations: medications, transfusions, and nutrition.

   3. Urine output and other fluid loss should be monitored.

      a. Monitoring fluid loss

         i. Monitoring urine volume

            1. Indwelling urinary catheter with closed collection system

            2. Weigh dry litter, subtract weight from wet litter: $1\,g = 1\,mL$

            3. Weigh diaper pads, subtract weight of dry diaper: $1\,g = 1\,mL$

        ii. Losses from vomiting, diarrhea—usually estimated

        iii. Other losses

            1. Body cavity drainage (ascites, pleural effusion)

            2. Nasogastric tube suctioning

      b. Inadequate urine production

         i. Oliguria is defined as $<1\,mL/kg/hr$.

         ii. Anuria is defined as essentially no urine.

        iii. Prior to starting diuretic therapy, ensure the cat is adequately hydrated and has sufficient blood pressure to perfuse kidneys (mean arterial pressure >60–$80\,mmHg$, Doppler systolic pressure >80–$100\,mmHg$).

        iv. Diuretics that may be used include:

            1. Mannitol: 0.25–$0.5\,g/kg$ IV over 20 minutes, followed by constant rate infusion (CRI) of 1–$2\,mg/kg/min$ IV if successful at inducing urine production

               a. Contraindicated in face of dehydration or volume overload

               b. Doses in excess of $4\,g/kg$ may cause ARF

            2. Furosemide: 2–$6\,mg/kg$ IV, followed by 2–$6\,mg/kg$ q6h or 0.25–$1.0\,mg/kg/hr$ CRI

               a. No evidence that furosemide improves outcome

               b. Electrolyte abnormalities possible if brisk diuresis ensues; monitor electrolytes at least twice daily

  ii. Treatment of uremic signs

      1. Gastrointestinal manifestations—nausea, vomiting

         a. Inhibitors of gastric acid secretion

            i. Famotidine 0.25–$0.5\,mg/kg$ SC, PO SID (do not give IV in cats).

            ii. Ranitidine 0.5–$2.5\,mg/kg$ IV, IM, SC, PO SID

            iii. Cimetidine 5–$10\,mg/kg$ IV, IM, PO BID

            iv. Omeprazole $0.7\,mg/kg$ PO SID

         b. Antiemetics

            i. Metoclopramide 0.2–$0.4\,mg/kg$ SC QID or 0.01–$0.02\,mg/kg/hr$ IV as CRI

            ii. Chlorpromazine 0.2–$0.5\,mg/kg$ IM, SC TID–QID

            iii. Ondansetron $0.1\,mg/kg$ PO BID–TID, 0.1–$0.3\,mg/kg$ IV BID–TID

            iv. Dolasetron $0.5\,mg/kg$ PO, SC, IV SID

         c. Motility modifiers:

            i. Cisapride 0.1–$0.5\,mg/kg$ PO BID–TID

            ii. Metoclopramide (see dose above)

            iii. Ranitidine (see dose above)

         d. Gastric protectants—if evidence of GI ulceration (hematemesis, melena, increased BUN-to-creatinine ratio, panhypoproteniemia with acute anemia): sucralfate $0.25\,g/cat$ PO TID)

      2. Hyperkalemia

         a. It causes bradycardia, small or absent p waves, tall tented T waves, and wide and bizarre QRS complex.

         b. Treatment of hyperkalemia involves translocation of potassium into cells until urine flow can be reestablished or dialysis instituted (see table 24.2).

Table 24.2. Drugs to treat hyperkalemia.

Drugs	Doses	Routes	Onsets of Actions	Indications	Comments
10% calcium gluconate	0.5–1 mL/kg	IV over 10 minutes	Immediate	Immediately life-threatening arrhythmia	Must monitor EKG during administration; does not decrease [K]
Regular insulin	0.25 u/kg	IV	30 minutes	Moderate to severe hyperkalemia	Must give dextrose to avoid hypoglycemia
Dextrose (with insulin)	1–2 gm per unit insulin	IV as bolus, and IV over next 6–8 hours	30 minutes		Give initial IV dose as bolus and continue as IV infusion
Dextrose (without insulin)	0.25–0.5 g/kg	IV as bolus	30 minutes	Mild to moderate hyperkalemia	
Sodium bicarbonate	1–2 mEq/kg	IV over 10–20 minutes	30 minutes	Mild to severe hyperkalemia	Contraindicated if PCO_2 elevated; may cause hypernatremia or paradoxic CNS acidosis

      i.   10% calcium gluconate
          1. 0.5–1 mL/kg IV over 10 minutes
          2. Effective immediately
          3. Cardioprotective but does not decrease potassium concentration
          4. Requires concurrent electrocardiographic monitoring
     ii. Regular insulin (0.25 U/kg IV) and dextrose (1–2 g/U insulin IV, then 1–2 g/U IV over next 4–6 hours) requires 30 minutes to onset of action.
   iii. Dextrose alone at a dose of 0.25–0.5 g/kg can be administered to stimulate endogenous insulin release from the pancreas.
   iv. Sodium bicarbonate (1–2 mEq/kg IV over 10–20 minutes) is contraindicated if PCO_2 is elevated, and it may cause hypernatremia or paradoxic CNS acidosis.
3. Metabolic acidosis
   a. Treat if pH <7.1.
   b. One half of the calculated sodium bicarbonate dose (body weight [kg] × 0.3 × [desired bicarbonate – measured bicarbonate]) is administered over 20–30 minutes and the rest over the next 2–4 hours.
   c. Hypernatremia is a possible complication, and bicarbonate is contraindicated if PCO_2 is elevated.
4. Hypertension
   a. Goal is to decrease systolic pressure to <180 mmHg (as measured by Doppler or oscillometric techniques), but avoid precipitous decrease.
   b. Antihypertensive drugs to consider:
      i. Amlodipine (0.625 mg PO SID) response may be seen within 24–48 hours. Can be administered rectally if vomiting

      ii. ACE inhibitors: generally avoided in ARF

      iii. Hydralazine (2.5 mg/cat PO or SC once): reserved for unmanageable or severe hypertension.

         1. Blood pressure must be monitored closely after administration.

         2. Onset in 15 minutes (SQ) to 1 hour (PO)

  5. Anemia

    a. Anemia may occur due to GI bleeding, repeated blood sampling, or dilution associated with volume overload.

    b. Administer blood transfusion if clinical signs of anemia. Packed RBC preferred to whole blood if volume overloaded and/or oliguric.

      i. Clinical signs of anemia include tachycardia, heart murmur, weakness, dull mentation, anorexia, and so on.

      ii. Clinical signs of anemia overlap with signs of ARF.

      iii. There is no absolute degree of anemia to dictate transfusion.

         1. More liberal criteria if anemia acutely develops

    c. More stringent criteria if chronic

    d. Recombinant erythropoietin products generally not indicated in ARF due to long onset to effect (weeks).

  6. Coagulation abnormalities

    a. Uremia induces a platelet function defect.

    b. Buccal mucosal bleeding time is prolonged; coagulation profile is normal.

    c. No effective treatment is available other than controlling uremia.

  7. Pancreatitis

    a. Common occurrence in cats with ARF

    b. No known effective treatment strategies—antiemetics, pain management, and early nutritional support (parenteral if vomiting not controlled, feeding tube if anorexic but not vomiting) are commonly used by author.

iii. Specific treatments

  1. Pyelonephritis

    a. Gram negative bacteria are the most common causes.

    b. Antibiotics to consider include the following:

      i. Fluoroquinolones have good spectrum and renal tissue penetration.

         1. Enrofloxacin 5 mg/kg IV SID

         2. Do not exceed 5 mg/kg due to potential for acute blindness

      ii. Ampicillin, amoxicillin, amoxicillin-clavulanic acid, or cephalosporins may be effective.

         1. Ampicillin/amoxicillin 15–22 mg/kg IV TID

         2. Clavamox 10–20 mg/kg IV BID

      iii. Trimethoprim-sulfa drugs are effective against *E. coli* and gram positive bacteria.

         1. Sulfonamides do not reach effective intrarenal concentrations.

         2. Only the trimethoprim component is effective.

         3. Dose 30 mg/kg PO BID

      iv. Aminoglycosides are a last resort due to the potential for nephrotoxicity.

    c. Treat for at least 4–6 weeks.

      i. Culture urine 3–7 days after completing antibiotic therapy.

      ii. If negative culture, repeat in one month.

      iii. If positive culture, treat for additional 4 weeks with appropriate antibiotic.

  2. Nephrotoxicity

    a. Ethylene glycol

      i. Treatment should be started within 8 hours of ingestion.

Box 24.2.   Ethanol treatment for ethylene glycol toxicosis.
1. Dilute ethanol to 20% solution (200 mg/mL) in 0.9% saline (e.g., 26.6 mL of 75% ethanol plus 73.4 mL 0.9% saline).
2. Day 1: Give 5 mL/kg IV at hours 0, 6, 12, 18, and 24.
3. Day 2: Give 5 mL/kg IV at hours 8, 16, and 24.
4. Day 3: Give 5 mL/kg IV at hour 8 (last treatment).
5. Monitor level of consciousness during treatment. Cat should be visibly sedate but not comatose.

---

      ii. 4-methylpyrazole is not effective in cats at standard doses. A higher dose of 125 mg/kg IV once followed by 31.25 mg/kg at 24, 48, and 72 hours after the initial dose can be used.
        1. Although no azotemia developed in experimental cats, oxalate crystals in the urine indicated there was some ethylene glycol metabolism.
        2. Side effect is mild sedation.
      iii. 20% ethanol is given at 5 mL/kg q6h for 5 treatments, then q8h for 4 treatments (see box 24.2).
   b. NSAID
      i. Misoprostol (PGE analogue)—1–3 µg/kg PO TID–QID
  3. Ureterolithiasis
   a. Surgical removal after medical stabilization is associated with 91% survival rates at 1 year.
   b. Some ureteroliths can pass into bladder over time (days to months).
 iv. Nutritional support (see chap. 9—Nutritional Support for the Critically Ill Feline Patient)
  1. Early institution of nutritional support improves prognosis in humans. ARF is a highly catabolic disease.
  2. If vomiting prohibits enteral feeding, total or partial parenteral nutrition may be utilized.
  3. Once vomiting is controlled, a feeding tube is placed if the patient remains inappetant.
  4. A moderately protein-restricted diet (such as used for CRF) is appropriate in most situations; higher protein intake may be needed with greater catabolic stress.
  5. Oral phosphate binders can be added when enteral feeding is started.
   a. Aluminum hydroxide, 30–90 mg/kg/day, divided and given with meals
   b. Calcium acetate, 60–90 mg/kg/day, divided and given with meals
 b. Renal replacement therapies
  i. Hemodialysis and continuous renal replacement therapy
   1. Removes uremic toxins by diffusion from bloodstream through dialyzer outside the body
   2. Exogenous toxins that are readily removed by dialysis include ethylene glycol, methanol, salicylate, lithium, ethanol, phenobarbital, acetaminophen, aminoglycosides, and tricyclic antidepressants.
   3. Requires referral to university or specialty private practice
  ii. Peritoneal dialysis
   1. Removes uremic toxins by diffusion from peritoneal membrane into dialysate infused into abdomen, then drained
   2. Necessary supplies are readily available, but is time consuming
   3. Common complications include catheter occlusion and peritonitis.
  iii. Renal transplantation
   1. Not suitable as emergency procedure
   2. If cat stabilized (medically or with hemodialysis) but renal function does not recover, transplantation can be considered.

E. Monitoring
    a. Frequency of monitoring depends on severity of disease.
    b. Check hydration status at least BID, namely, skin turgor, mucus membrane tackiness, body weight, urine output, blood pressure, PCV, total solids, and central venous pressure.
    c. Acid-base and electrolyte determinations are done multiple times daily if severe abnormalities exist.
    d. BUN and creatinine are measured SID–QOD.
F. Prognosis
    a. Potential outcomes include death, euthanasia, stabilization with permanent chronic renal failure, or functional recovery.
    b. Overall mortality is about 40–50%, and 50% of survivors have subsequent CRF, although there are differences in survival associated with etiology.
        i. Ischemia: 75% survival
        ii. Nephrotoxins: 20–50% survival
        iii. Infectious/other: 50–100% survival
    c. Polyuria has a better outcome than oliguria or anuria.

Recommended Reading

Cowgill LD, Francey T. Acute uremia. In Ettinger SJ, Feldman EC, eds, Textbook of Veterinary Internal Medicine, 6th ed. Philadelphia: Elsevier Saunders, 2005.

Elliott DA, Cowgill LD. Acute renal failure. In Bonagura JD, ed, Current Veterinary Therapy XIII Small Animal Practice. Philadelphia: W.B. Saunders, 2000.

Grauer GF. Prevention of hospital-acquired acute renal failure. Vet Forum, Jan 1999; pp. 46–54.

Langston CE. Renal emergencies. In Ettinger SJ, Feldman EC, eds, Textbook of Veterinary Internal Medicine, 6th ed, p 447. St. Louis: Elsevier Saunders, 2005.

25
GENERAL APPROACH AND OVERVIEW OF THE NEUROLOGIC CAT

Daniel J. Fletcher

Unique Features
- Neurologic exam in the cat can be challenging and should be done as efficiently as possible, in discrete segments with pauses between if necessary.
- Conscious proprioception is generally better evaluated in the cat using tactile placing rather than the paw-placement test.
- Cats are more sensitive to the neurologic effects of pyrethrins and pyrethroids than most other species. Even exposure to products specifically labeled for cats can lead to tremors and seizures.
- Idiopathic epilepsy is uncommon in the cat compared to the dog; therefore, cats presenting acutely with seizures should be fully evaluated for other extracranial and intracranial causes of seizures.

A. Feline neurologic emergencies
  a. The initial approach to the acutely neurologic cat is identical to that of any critically ill cat. Initial triage and primary assessment should proceed as with any other emergent feline patient (see chap. 1—Approach to the Critically Ill Cat). Once life-threatening extra–central nervous system (CNS) abnormalities have been identified and addressed, a complete secondary CNS assessment should be done.
  b. Secondary CNS assessment
    i. Mentation
      1. Normal—alert and appropriately responsive to the environment
      2. Depressed—alert and aware, but not appropriately responsive to environmental stimuli
      3. Obtunded—unconscious, but arousable with nonnoxious stimuli, such as loud noises, light, or gentle manipulation
      4. Stuporous—unconscious and arousable only with painful stimulation
      5. Comatose—unconscious and nonarousable, even with the application of noxious stimuli
    ii. Ambulation
      1. Determine the ability of the patient to ambulate. Stressed cats often will not walk. If the cat is responsive, place on the floor in an enclosed room and encourage to move.
      2. If the cat is ambulatory, thoroughly assess the gait.
        a. Evaluate each limb for strength and appropriate movement.
          i. Paresis—decreased voluntary motor function
          ii. Paralysis/plegia—absent voluntary motor function

       iii. The brainstem (red nucleus) is the most important center for walking in cats.
         1. Forebrain lesions rarely cause paresis or paralysis.
         2. Brainstem or spinal cord lesions commonly cause paresis or paralysis.
    b. Look for evidence of crossing over or incoordination in the thoracic and/or pelvic limbs
       i. Ataxia—uncoordinated motor function
       ii. Usually due to disease affecting the following:
         1. Cerebellum
         2. Vestibular system
         3. Spinal cord
    c. Note exaggerated movements (hypermetria) or truncated movements (hypometria)
       i. Most commonly seen with cerebellar disease
       ii. Can be seen with head movements, resulting in overshooting of movements followed by correction (intention tremors)
    d. If the patient collapses in the thoracic or pelvic limbs, note the side to which the patient is falling.
    e. Look for evidence of circling behavior.
       i. Circling is a sign of intracranial disease.
       ii. Direction is generally toward the affected side of the brain.
      iii. Size of circles can help localize lesion
        1. Tight circles—vestibular disease
        2. Wide circles, wall-hugging—forebrain disease
 iii. Posture
   1. Vestibular disease
     a. Unilateral—head tilt, leaning to one side
     b. Bilateral—wide-based stance
   2. Decerebrate (opisthotonus; fig. 25.1)
     a. Rigid extension of thoracic and pelvic limbs
     b. Rigid neck extension
     c. Severe brainstem disease
   3. Decerebellate
     a. Rigid extension of thoracic limbs
     b. Relaxed pelvic limbs
     c. Cerebellar disease

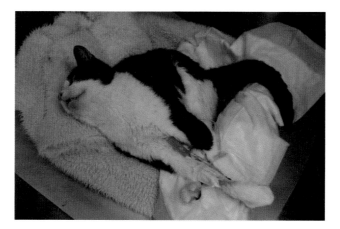

Fig. 25.1. Cat with decerebrate posture. Note extension of all four limbs. (Photo courtesy of Curtis W. Dewey.)

    4. Schiff-Scherrington
      a. Rigid extension of thoracic limbs and neck when in lateral recumbency
      b. T3-L3 myelopathy
    5. Cervical ventroflexion (without neck pain)
      a. Neuromuscular disease (weakness)
      b. Metabolic diseases such as hypokalemia
    6. Postural reactions should be evaluated in all four limbs.
      a. Tactile placing and hopping are often easier to evaluate in the cat than the paw-position test.
      b. The complete ascending sensory pathways from the limbs, up the spinal cord, through the brainstem and thalamus, to sensorimotor cortex as well as the descending pathways through the spinal cord to the effector muscles must be intact. Lesions in any of these pathways will lead to deficits.
  iv. Cranial nerves
    1. A thorough cranial nerve exam is essential for accurate neurolocalization of intracranial disease.
    2. Clinical signs associated with specific cranial nerves include
      I.   Olfactory
                i. Limited clinical usefulness
                ii. Loss of smell
      II.   Optic
                i. Loss of vision
                ii. Loss of pupillary light reflex
      III.   Oculomotor
                i. Eye movement abnormalities (loss of function of dorsal, ventral, and medial recti resulting in ventrolateral strabismus)
                ii. Loss of pupillary light reflex
      IV.   Trochlear
                i. Rotary strabismus due to paralysis of the dorsal oblique muscle
      V.   Trigeminal
                i. Loss of palpebral reflex
                ii. Loss of facial sensation
                iii. Temporal and/or masseter muscle atrophy
                iv. Sunken eye due to paralysis of pterygoid muscle
      VI.   Abducens
                i. Loss of globe retraction due to paralysis of retractor bulbi muscle
                ii. Medial strabismus due to paralysis of lateral rectus muscle
      VII.   Facial
                i. Facial and lip droop (fig. 25.2)
                ii. Loss of palpebral reflex and menace response but still retains vision. Can sometimes see just third eyelid movement when cat attempts to blink if abducens function still intact.
                iii. Keratoconjunctivits sicca
      VIII.   Vestibulocochlear
                i. Ataxia, head tilt, nystagmus, strabismus
                ii. Circling and leaning behaviors
                iii. Deafness
                iv. Vomiting
     IX/X/XI. Glossopharyngeal, vagus, spinal accessory
                i. Loss of gag reflex

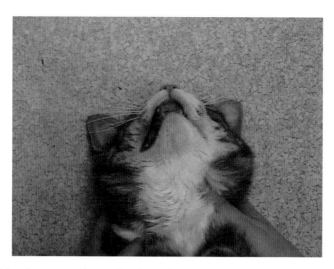

Fig. 25.2. Cat with lip droop secondary to facial paralysis. (Photo courtesy of Curtis W. Dewey.)

           ii. Dysphagia
           iii. Laryngeal paralysis
           iv. Megaesophagus
      XII.   Hypoglossal
           i. Dysphagia
           ii. Deviation of tongue
           iii. Unilateral atrophy of tongue
    3. VII and the sympathetic trunk pass through the middle ear. Otitis media/interna can cause a combination of signs
      a. Vestibular
      b. Facial/lip droop, facial sensation deficits
      c. Horner's syndrome (fig. 25.3)
        i. Ptosis
        ii. Miosis
        iii. Enophthalmus
    4. V, VII, and VIII arise from the area of the cerebello-pontine angle. Brainstem lesions affecting this area can cause signs associated with all three cranial nerves.
  v. Spinal reflexes
    1. Spinal reflexes are useful for localization of spinal cord lesions as well as peripheral neuropathies.
    2. Absence of spinal reflexes is a lower motor neuron sign, indicating spinal cord damage to the cervical intumescence in the case of thoracic limb deficits (C6–T2 spinal cord segments) or the lumbar intumescence with pelvic limb deficits (L4–S3).
    3. Absence or deficits of individual reflexes can further localize a spinal cord lesion.
  c. Specific neurologic emergencies
    i. Disorders of posture and ambulation
      1. Flaccid paralysis/paresis (lower motor neuron signs)
        a. Flaccid paralysis may be due to diseases affecting the muscle, neuromuscular junction, peripheral nerves, or spinal cord. The most consistent finding is loss or decrease of

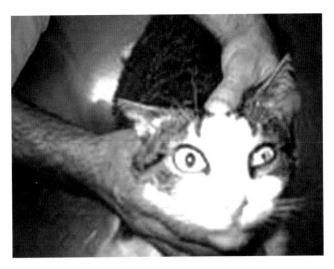

Fig. 25.3. Cat with Horner's syndrome in the left eye. (Photo courtesy of Curtis W. Dewey.)

voluntary motor function and muscle tone with a concurrent loss of segmental reflexes in the affected limb or limbs.
  b. Myopathies and neuromuscular junction disease are uncommon in cats, but there are several described congenital diseases that can cause flaccid paralysis.
    i.   Burmese cats: hypokalemic myopathy
    ii. Norwegian forest cats: glycogen storage disease
    iii. Devon Rex: congenital myopathy
    iv. Congenital muscle and neuromuscular junction disorders without breed predilection also occur.
      1. Congenital myotonia
      2. Hypertrophic feline muscular dystrophy
      3. Laminin alpha-2 deficiency
      4. Myasthenia gravis (most common in Siamese cats)
    v.   Acquired myasthenia gravis has also been reported in cats, although less commonly than dogs. Abyssinian cats may be predisposed.
  c. Peripheral neuropathies are commonly due to systemic disease or metabolic disturbances.
    i.   Diabetes mellitus: diabetic polyneuropathy, commonly affecting the tibial nerve, results in a characteristic plantigrade stance.
    ii. Hyperlipemia
    iii. Brachial plexus avulsion secondary to trauma results in lower motor neuron signs to a single thoracic limb. Ipsilateral loss of the cutaneous trunci reflex and Horner's syndrome may also be present.
  d. Spinal cord disease of the cervical (C6–T2) or lumbar (L4–S3) intumescence can also cause flaccid paralysis. Differential diagnoses include intervertebral disk disease, neoplasia (commonly lymphoma), infectious disease (FIP, cryptococcus), thromboembolic disease, and trauma.
2. Spastic paralysis/paresis (upper motor neuron signs)
  a. Spastic paralysis or paresis is characterized by loss or decrease of voluntary motor function in the affected limb or limbs with preservation of normal or increased segmental reflexes. It is due to spinal cord disease cranial to the affected limbs or brain disease.

   b. Damage to descending motor and ascending sensory pathways causes the signs, which affect only the pelvic limbs (T3–L3 myelopathy) or both the thoracic and pelvic limbs (C1–C6 myelopathy).
   c. Differential diagnoses are the same for those noted for spinal cord disease causing flaccid paralysis above.
3. Incoordination/ataxia
   a. Sensory ataxia
      i. Sensory ataxia is associated with loss of proprioception in the thoracic and pelvic limbs (C1–C6 myelopathy) or only the pelvic limbs (T3–L3 myelopathy).
      ii. This type of ataxia is also often associated with paresis.
      iii. It is caused by spinal cord disease, and differential diagnoses are the same for those described above for flaccid paralysis due to spinal cord dysfunction.
   b. Vestibular ataxia
      i. Peripheral
         1. Damage to the vestibular apparatus of the inner ear or the cranial nerve VIII can lead to vestibular ataxia.
         2. In addition to ataxia, head tilt toward the side of the lesion and nystagmus with the fast phase away from the side of the lesion are common. Nystagmus should not be positional but may be of any type (rotary, horizontal, or vertical). Tight circling or falling to the side of the lesion are also common.
         3. No paresis, proprioceptive deficits, or alterations in mentation are present.
         4. The sympathetic trunk runs through the middle ear, making Horner's syndrome a possible finding (miosis, ptosis, and enophthalmos ipsilateral to the lesion).
         5. Ventral strabismus may be present ipsilateral to the lesion with extension of the neck. This may also be present with central vestibular disease (see below).
         6. Common causes include otitis media/interna, neoplasia, nasopharyngeal polyps, trauma (including overly aggressive ear flushing), and ototoxic drugs (aminoglycosides, metronidazole).
         7. A full otoscopic exam may provide evidence of disease, but imaging of the skull (radiographs or CT) is often required to identify disease affecting the bullae.
      ii. Central
         1. Damage to the vestibular nuclei in the brainstem leads to central vestibular signs.
         2. Proprioceptive deficits or paresis ipsilateral to the lesion, combined with head tilt (toward the side of the lesion) and/or nystagmus (fast phase away from the side of the lesion) are diagnostic for central vestibular disease.
         3. Nystagmus may be positional with central vestibular disease and is more commonly rotary or vertical than in peripheral vestibular disease. Tight circling or falling to the side of the lesion are also common.
         4. Other cranial nerve deficits may accompany the vestibular signs with central vestibular disease.
         5. Mental dullness, obtundation, stupor, or coma may be present due to the close proximity of the reticular activating system.
         6. Ventral strabismus may be present ipsilateral to the lesion with extension of the neck. This may also be present with peripheral vestibular disease (see above).
         7. Common causes include neoplasia, trauma, infection (e.g., FIP), parasitic disease (e.g., Cuterebra), toxins (lead, hexachlorophene), thromboembolic disease, or storage diseases.
      iii. Paradoxical central
         1. The presence of head tilt or nystagmus in the opposite direction to other localizing signs such as paresis or proprioceptive deficits is indicative of paradoxical vestibular disease.

2. This is caused by lesions of the flocculonodular lobes of the cerebellum or the caudal cerebellar peduncles.

3. Lesion localization is ipsilateral to the proprioceptive signs or paresis.

4. Causes are the same as those for central vestibular disease described above.

   iv. Bilateral

1. Cats with bilateral vestibular disease usually do not have head tilts or nystagmus.

2. A side-to-side swaying of the head is often noted (this can be subtle, so look closely).

3. A characteristic wide-based stance is often present.

4. Can look disoriented, reluctant to move, and vocalize without side-to-side head movements

  c. Cerebellar ataxia

    i. Cerebellar ataxia is commonly associated with hypermetria, truncal ataxia, intention tremors (especially of the head), and a wide-based stance.

    ii. Menace response is often decreased to absent in cats with diffuse cerebellar disease.

    iii. Motor and sensory tracts are not affected; therefore, no proprioceptive deficits or paresis are present.

    iv. Acute cerebellar damage can be associated with decerebellate posture (see above). Hyperreflexia may also be present. Animals that survive the acute stage often develop the other signs of cerebellar disease described above.

    v. Common causes include neoplasia, infection (e.g., FIP), cerebellar abiotrophy, storage diseases, and toxins (lead, organophosphates).

ii. Disorders of mentation

1. Altered mentation

  a. Patients that are alert and responsive but are exhibiting abnormal mentation or behaviors most commonly have diseases affecting the prosencephalon.

  b. Cranial nerve, proprioceptive, or motor deficits can help localize focal disease, with deficits occurring contralateral to the affected hemisphere. Animals with prosencephalic disease often walk in wide circles in the direction of the lesion.

  c. Disinhibition due to frontal lobe disease may lead to compulsive stereotypic pacing and head pressing.

  d. Potential causes of altered mentation may be divided into extracranial and intracranial diseases.

    i. Extracranial

1. Hepatic encephalopathy

2. Uremic encephalopathy (see chap. 23—Urologic Emergencies: Ureter, Bladder, Urethra, GN, and CRF and chap. 24—Acute Intrinsic Renal Failure)

3. Toxins such as early ethylene glycol ingestion, antidepressants, sedatives, illicit drugs, heavy metals, and other neuroactive substances

4. Other metabolic disturbances such as hypoglycemia or extreme changes in sodium concentration

    ii. Intracranial causes include neoplasia, infection (e.g., FIP, toxoplasmosis, cryptococcus), congenital brain diseases, thiamine deficiency leading to polioencephalomalacia, and head trauma.

  e. Diagnostics include ruling out major extracranial causes (complete blood count, serum chemistry analysis, resting blood ammonia, serum osmolality, toxicology screen, blood pressure), followed by intracranial causes (toxoplasmosis titer, retinal examination, brain imaging such as MRI, and cerebrospinal fluid analysis).

2. Obtundation, stupor, or coma

  a. Patients that are unconscious either have diffuse cerebral disease or damage to the rostral brainstem (containing the reticular activating system).

   b. Localization of the lesion may be possible based on neurologic examination.
      i.   Deficits in motor function (hemiparesis or tetraparesis) are commonly noted, contralateral to the lesion with cerebral disease, ipsilateral to the lesion with brainstem disease.
      ii. Vision is commonly absent with diffuse cerebral disease but present with rostral brainstem lesions.
      iii. Pupil size and pupillary light response are normal with diffuse cerebral disease, but pupils are often unresponsive with rostral brainstem lesions.
      iv. Eye movements are generally normal with diffuse cerebral disease, but patients will not follow moving objects due to loss of vision. Ventrolateral strabismus ipsilateral to the lesion, and decreased physiologic nystagmus is common with rostral brainstem lesions.
   c. Likely causes of stupor or coma vary depending on the presence of lateralizing signs.
      i.   Lateralizing signs present: neoplasia, trauma causing focal hemorrhage, and thromboembolic disease
      ii. Lateralizing signs not present: congenital malformations, extracranial causes (see "Altered mentation" above), thiamine deficiency, encephalitis (infectious or noninfectious), toxins, or trauma leading to cerebral edema.
iii. Neurotrauma
   1. Head trauma
      a. Etiology
         i.   The most common causes of head injuries in cats include crush injuries, penetrating wounds, vehicular injury, fall from height, and purposeful harm.
         ii. Many cats present with head trauma of unknown cause.
      b. Pathophysiology
         i.   Primary injury
            1. Primary injury is the direct result of the traumatic event, and includes cerebral contusion, hematoma, laceration, axonal injury, and skull fracture.
            2. With the exception of extra-axial hemorrhage causing a space occupying lesion and unstable skull fracture, primary injury is not amenable to treatment.
         ii. Secondary injury
            1. Secondary injury is the result of a series of biochemical processes that ultimately lead to neuronal cell death.
            2. These processes include the following:
               a. Excitotoxicity due to release of neurotransmitters such as glutamate.
               b. Intracellular accumulation of sodium and calcium, leading to cellular edema.
               c. Ischemia-reperfusion injury and production of reactive oxygen species.
               d. Release of inflammatory mediators via the arachidonic acid pathway.
               e. Migration and activation of inflammatory cells such as neutrophils and monocytes.
               f. Activation of platelets and the coagulation cascade leading to microvascular thrombosis and compromise of local perfusion
            3. The end result of these processes is perpetuation of neuronal cell death and development of cerebral edema.
         iii. Because the brain is contained within the rigid skull, once compensatory mechanisms are exhausted, cerebral edema can eventually lead to increases in intracranial pressure (ICP).
            1. Cerebral oxygen and nutrient delivery is dependent on adequate cerebral perfusion pressure (CPP).
            2. CPP is defined as the difference between mean arterial blood pressure (MAP) and ICP.
               a. CPP = MAP – ICP

When ICP increases, CPP decreases, and cerebral ischemia results.
c. Treatment
   i. Extracranial stabilization
      1. Perfusion
         a. Because CPP is dependent on MAP, hypotension cannot be tolerated in patients with head injury.
         b. Aggressive fluid therapy should be used to maintain normotension.
         c. Isotonic crystalloids
            i. 15–20 mL/kg bolus over 15–20 minutes
            ii. Repeat as necessary to maintain normotension (mean blood pressure 80–100 mmHg).
         d. Synthetic colloids (hetastarch)
            i. 5 mL/kg bolus over 15–20 minutes.
            ii. Repeat as necessary to maintain normotension.
            iii. Suggested maximum daily dose of hetastarch is 20 mL/kg. This is due to an acquired decreased ability to coagulate when this dose is exceeded, although specific studies in cats have not been performed.
            iv. Do not use in dehydrated patients.
         e. Blood products
            i. Use packed red blood cells or fresh whole blood for anemic patients.
            ii. Hemoglobin concentration is the major determinant of oxygen carrying capacity.
            iii. Consider fresh frozen plasma (10–15 mL/kg) in patients with coagulopathy.
      2. Oxygenation
         a. Maintain SpO_2 >95%.
         b. All patients should receive oxygen supplementation during initial stabilization.
            i. Flow by mask
            ii. Nasal cannulae (avoid inducing sneezing as this can increase ICP)
            iii. Nasal catheters (avoid inducing sneezing)
            iv. Oxygen cage
            v. Oxygen tent
      3. Ventilation
         a. Elevations in CO_2 lead to cerebral vasodilation, pooling of blood within the calvarium, and potentially, increases in ICP.
         b. Altered mentation and/or airway obstruction due to trauma can cause hypoventilation in patients with head trauma.
         c. If patients cannot maintain normocapnea ($PaCO_2$ of 35–45 mmHg, $PvCO_2$ of 40–50 mmHg), they should be mechanically ventilated.
      4. Avoid compression of the jugular veins (holding off jugular for blood draw, bending of the neck, etc.)
   ii. Intracranial stabilization
      1. Osmotic therapy
         a. Mannitol
            i. There are multiple proposed mechanisms of actions by which mannitol decreases ICP, including reflex vasoconstriction of brain vasculature via decreasing blood viscosity, reduction of cerebrospinal fluid production, scavenging free-radical species, and osmotically drawing extravascular edema fluid into the intravascular space.
            ii. Administer intravenously over 10–20 minutes at a dosage of 0.5–1.5 g/kg. A recent human clinical trial supports the use of higher doses of mannitol

(1.4 g/kg) rather than lower doses (0.7 g/kg) in patients with severe brain injury.

    iii. Serum osmolality and electrolytes should be measured with repeated mannitol use; osmolality should be maintained at or below 320 mOsm/L to reduce the risk of renal failure due to renal vasoconstriction (see chap. 24).

    iv. Because of mannitol's diuretic properties, volume status should be closely monitored (either by measuring urine output via a urinary catheter or weighing diaper pads or closely monitoring body weight), and crystalloid and/or colloid therapy should be adjusted to address any volume deficits (see chap. 24).

  b. Hypertonic saline

    i. Hypertonic saline (7%) is a hyperosmotic solution that may be used as an alternative to mannitol in patients with head injury.

    ii. Administer intravenously at a dose of 2–3 mL/kg over 15–20 minutes.

    iii. Other beneficial effects include improved hemodynamic status via volume expansion and positive inotropic effects, as well as beneficial vasoregulatory and immunomodulatory effects.

    iv. Monitor serum sodium concentrations to avoid hypernatremia.

2. Glucocorticoids

  a. High dose methylprednisolone sodium succinate (MPSS) and prednisolone sodium succinate have been recommended as neuroprotective agents after head injury. However, a recent, large human clinical trial demonstrated worse outcome in patients with head trauma treated with MPSS compared with controls. The use of these high-dose protocols is no longer recommended.

  b. Dexamethasone and prednisone have been shown to be effective for treating vasogenic edema associated with intracranial neoplasia but have not been shown to be beneficial when treating patients with cytotoxic edema due to head trauma.

  c. It is the author's opinion that corticosteroids should not be used in patients with head trauma.

3. Facilitation of venous drainage

  a. Elevation of the head by 15–30 degrees reduces cerebral blood volume by increasing venous drainage, decreasing ICP, and increasing CPP without changes in cerebral oxygenation.

  b. A slant board should be used to prevent occlusion of the jugular veins. Higher elevations may cause a detrimental decrease in CPP.

4. Decompressive craniectomy

  a. Indications for surgery after head trauma include presence of extra-axial hemorrhage causing compression of the brain (diagnosed by CT or MRI), open skull fractures, depressed skull fractures (with associated neurologic impairment), and retrieval of potentially contaminated bone fragments or foreign material lodged in brain parenchyma.

  b. Surgical intervention should be considered in head-traumatized cats that are deteriorating neurologically despite aggressive medical therapy.

  d. Prognosis

    i. The overall prognosis for victims of severe head trauma is considered guarded to poor.

    ii. The Modified Glasgow Coma Scale scoring system, adapted from a human coma scale, has been shown in one retrospective study to predict survival to 48 hours in dogs with head injury. Its prognostic value has not been evaluated in cats, but it is a useful quantitative scale to evaluate severity of neurologic injury and to monitor progression.

iii. Presence and persistence of hyperglycemia have been shown to be prognostic indicators in people with head trauma. However, in a veterinary study including cats with head trauma, admission hyperglycemia was associated with severity of injury but not with outcome.

iv. There is a tremendous recuperative ability in cats, especially younger animals, and prognosis can be difficult to predict at admission. It is the author's clinical experience that many cats with severe neurologic deficits at admission can show remarkable improvement in the first 24–48 hours postinjury.

2. Spinal cord trauma

  a. Etiology

    i. The most common causes of spinal trauma in cats include motor vehicle accidents, animal-animal interactions, falls from heights, and crush injuries.

    ii. Spontaneous intervertebral disk herniation is rare in cats but can occur.

  b. Pathophysiology

    i. Primary injury

      1. Primary injury is the direct result of the traumatic event and includes spinal luxation and vertebral fracture, traumatic intervertebral disk herniation, spinal cord contusion, and extra-axial hemorrhage.

      2. Surgical and medical therapies can help correct or mitigate the impact of primary spinal injuries.

    ii. Secondary injury

      1. Secondary injury results from activation of a number of biochemical pathways that ultimately lead to continued neuronal damage or death.

      2. These processes include the following:

        a. Excitotoxicity due to release of neurotransmitters such as glutamate.

        b. Intracellular accumulation of sodium and calcium, leading to cellular edema.

        c. Ischemia-reperfusion injury and production of reactive oxygen species.

        d. Release of inflammatory mediators via the arachidonic acid pathway.

        e. Migration and activation of inflammatory cells such as neutrophils and monocytes.

        f. Activation of platelets and the coagulation cascade leading to microvascular thrombosis and compromise of local perfusion.

  c. Diagnostics

    i. Spinal radiographs are indicated in all cats with spinal trauma but have been shown to have low sensitivity for fracture (72%) or spinal luxation (77.5%) in dogs. No data are available in cats, but given their generally smaller size, it is unlikely the sensitivity is higher. Patients should be immobilized by taping them to a back board before sedation and radiographs to reduce the risk of further spinal cord trauma during manipulation, and ventrodorsal views should be obtained using a horizontal beam technique.

    ii. Advanced imaging techniques such as myelography, CT, or MRI are often required to definitively diagnose spinal injuries. All of these modalities require anesthesia, and care should be taken to immobilize patients to prevent further trauma to the spinal cord.

  d. Treatment

    i. Extra-CNS stabilization

      1. Recognition and treatment of concurrent life-threatening injuries in the spinal trauma patient is of paramount importance. Aggressive therapy to maintain perfusion, oxygenation, and ventilation must be instituted as soon as possible.

      2. See "Extracranial stabilization" in the Head Trauma section above for specific therapeutic recommendations.

    ii. Primary injury treatment

1. Spinal luxation and vertebral fracture
   a. Surgical management: Surgical options for stabilization and internal fixation include the use of bone plates, screws, Steinmann pins, and polymethylmethacrylate (PMMA) cement. Surgical management often results in accelerated stabilization of the spine and more rapid return to function, but it is expensive, may result in worsening of spinal cord injury during anesthesia and surgical manipulation, and carries the risk of implant failure or complications, such as infection and implant fracture.
   b. Nonsurgical management: External coaptation and strict cage rest for 6–8 weeks are the basic principles of nonsurgical management. Fiberglass, thermoplastics, plaster, metal rods, or other materials can be fashioned to conform to the patient's body shape. The entire spine must be immobilized and the splint held in place using bandage material. Soiled bandages must be replaced immediately. Nonsurgical management requires intensive nursing care, longer recovery periods, and a greater likelihood of persistent neurologic deficits.
2. Traumatic intervertebral disk herniation
   a. Surgical and nonsurgical management are options for these types of injuries.
   b. In general, surgical management is recommended when voluntary motor function is absent or severely decreased, or if clinical signs are progressing in spite of conservative treatment.
   c. Conservative management consists of strict cage rest for 6–8 weeks.
3. Spinal cord contusion
   a. There are no direct therapies for spinal cord contusion.
iii. Secondary injury treatment
1. Maintenance of perfusion, oxygenation, and ventilation are of paramount importance in reducing secondary injury in the patient with traumatic spinal cord injury. See "Extracranial stabilization" in the Head Trauma section above for specific recommendations.
2. Methylprednisolone sodium succinate (MPSS) has been extensively studied as a therapy to address secondary injury. The free-radical scavenging effects are likely the most important for providing neuroprotection.
   a. Although the anti-inflammatory effects of other common corticosteroids (e.g., dexamethasone, prednisone) are likely to reduce the discomfort associated with spinal trauma, they are unlikely to have any significant neuroprotective effect.
   b. There have been no placebo-controlled trials evaluating the efficacy of MPSS in veterinary patients with spinal cord injury. It is well known that high-dose corticosteroids can have significant side effects in cats, including immunosuppression, decreased renal blood flow, and gastrointestinal effects, although anecdotally, cats appear to be more resistant to these side effects compared with dogs.
   c. Given the clinical and experimental evidence, MPSS at an initial dose of 30 mg/kg followed by a constant rate infusion (CRI) of 5.4 mg/kg/hr or repeated boluses of 15 mg/kg every 6 hours for 24–48 hours may be considered as neuroprotective therapy in patients with spinal cord injury. However, given the potential side effects and the lack of clinical trials in cats demonstrating efficacy, it is the author's opinion that the risks of this treatment outweigh the potential benefits. There is no clinical or experimental evidence of a neuroprotective effect of other corticosteroids, such as dexamethasone or prednisone, but these drugs may be useful at an anti-inflammatory dose (initially 1–2 mg/kg/day prednisone, 0.15–0.3 mg/kg/day dexamethasone, tapering over 1–2 weeks) to reduce discomfort associated with the injury.

   3. Polyethylene glycol (PEG) is a polymer that has been shown to repair defects in damaged nerve fibers. In addition, PEG seals damaged cells and reduces the release of cytotoxic substances leading to secondary injury. A clinical trial of intravenous PEG (two doses, 2 mL/kg of a 30% solution intravenously 4–6 hours apart) in dogs with acute intervertebral disk herniation within 72 hours of injury showed that treated dogs had improved outcomes compared with historical controls. Although no data are available in cats, PEG may provide a promising new therapy for acute spinal trauma.

iv. Seizures
   1. Pathophysiology
      a. Seizures are initiated by a high-frequency burst of action potentials within a hypersynchronized population of neurons. Individual neurons within the population experience a sequence of events including the following:
         i. A burst of action potentials (700–1,000 per second) mediated by an influx of calcium and sodium
         ii. A sustained depolarization
         iii. Rapid repolarization and hyperpolarization mediated by GABA receptors, which promote either chloride influx or potassium efflux.
      b. Many areas of the brain, including the subcortical nuclei, thalamus, cerebrum, and brainstem, can participate in seizure genesis and propogation.
      c. This population of hypersynchronized neurons then overcomes normal physiologic surround inhibition, allowing propagation of the seizure into surrounding areas as well as distant areas of the brain via long-distance pathways (e.g., the corpus callosum).
   2. Classification
      a. Generalized seizures: Generalized seizures (also called tonic-clonic seizures or grand mal seizures) are associated with a loss of consciousness and symmetrical effects on the brain. These events can manifest in a number of ways, including paddling or tonic-clonic movement of all limbs or generalized rigidity.
      b. Focal/partial seizures: Focal seizures (also called partial seizures) are initiated by abnormal activity in a circumscribed region of the brain. Clinical signs are related to the area of the brain affected and are often lateralized. Patients remain conscious during partial seizures, but changes in behavior and mentation may occur. Simple partial seizures (also called partial motor seizures) result in abnormal, often rhythmic contraction of a single muscle group, such as facial muscles or muscles of a single limb. Complex partial seizures (also called psychomotor seizures) are characterized by abnormal, quasi-purposeful behaviors. Quasi-purposeful behaviors are normal behaviors that are repeated inappropriately or exhibited at inappropriate times. Behaviors such as fly-biting, fear, or aggression are typical of quasi-purposeful behaviors. Simple or complex partial seizures may progress to generalized seizures.
      c. Cluster seizures: There are various definitions of cluster seizures in the literature, but the most widely accepted is two or more separate seizures in a 24-hour period. In order to be considered separate, the animal should return to normal mentation and neurologic status between the seizures.
      d. Status epilepticus: Patients who continue to have seizure activity for more than 5 minutes, or who have repeated seizures without returning to normal neurologic status between epiosodes are considered to be in status epilepticus. Patients presenting with cluster seizures or status epilepticus are at high risk of developing systemic sequelae, including hyperthermia, disseminated intravascular coagulation, systemic inflammatory response syndrome, and multiple organ failure. In addition, there is a risk of permanent brain damage and expansion of the seizure focus in the brain.

3. Etiology
   a. Extracranial diseases: Metabolic disturbances and systemic disease can lead to alterations in the electrophysiology of the brain, causing paroxysmal neuronal discharges and seizures. In general, these types of diseases are likely to cause widespread disturbances affecting both hemispheres. Therefore, generalized seizures are more common than focal seizures. Endogenous toxins accumulating due to hepatic or renal disease can lead to seizures. Metabolic disturbances, such as hypoglycemia, hyperlipidemia, hypernatremia or hyponatremia, and hypocalcemia, as well as endocrine diseases such as hypothyroidism and diabetes mellitus (hyperosmolar nonketotic) can also lead to seizures. Many toxicoses, including early ethylene glycol intoxication, bromethalin, pyrethrins, theobromine, caffeine, cocaine, lead, or organophosphate poisoning may also result in seizures.
   b. Intracranial diseases: There are many, primary intracranial causes of seizures. A classification scheme, such as DAMNIT-V, can be helpful for organizing this large list.
      i.   Degenerative: storage diseases
      ii.   Anomalous: hydrocephalus, lissencephaly
      iii. Metabolic: see "Extracranial diseases" above
      iv.   Neoplastic: primary brain tumors as well as metastatic disease
      v.   Nutritional: thiamine deficiency in cats fed exclusively fish diets
      vi.   Infectious: viral (FIP, FeLV), bacterial, fungal (cryptococcus), protozoal (toxoplasma)
      vii. Idiopathic: epilepsy
      viii. Trauma: head trauma
      ix.   Toxin: see "Extracranial diseases" above
      x.   Vascular: thromboembolic disease, intracranial hemorrhage
4. Treatment
   a. Individual, infrequent, and short-duration seizures may not require therapy, but severe, acute seizures are life-threatening emergencies, and aggressive therapy is warranted. Cluster seizures and status epilepticus are the two most life-threatening types of seizures. In addition to direct neuronal damage, systemic sequelae of severe seizures include traumatic injury to other parts of the body, hyperthermia leading to disseminated intravascular coagulation, aspiration pneumonia, and noncardiogenic pulmonary edema.
   b. Anticonvulsant therapy
      i.   Benzodiazepines: Intravenous diazepam (0.5–1.0 mg/kg) or midazolam (0.066–0.22 mg/kg) should be considered first-line therapy for patients with severe, acute seizures. These drugs are GABA agonists, leading to hyperpolarization of neurons and cessation of seizure activity. For patients in whom intravenous access is not readily available, diazepam at a dose of 1–2 mg/kg is rapidly absorbed intrarectally. If the patient responds to benzodiazepine therapy but rapidly recrudesces, an intravenous CRI is a good option. Diazepam at 0.5–2.0 mg/kg/hr is often effective. Diazepam administered undiluted via a peripheral vessel can cause vasculitis; use of a central line or dilution in intravenous fluids is recommended. Diazepam may be mixed with 0.9% saline or 5% dextrose in water. Avoid mixing with lactated Ringer's solution as the calcium will precipitate the diazepam. Plastic will adsorb diazepam and may make the actual CRI dose of diazepam unpredictable.
      ii. In addition, injectable benzodiazepines are light sensitive, so infusion lines should be wrapped.
      iii. Barbiturates: For patients refractory to benzodiazepine therapy, barbiturates (Pentobarbital, Phenobarbital) can sometimes be effective. Pentobarbital (2–15 mg/kg IV) can effectively terminate the physical manifestations of seizure activity within

several minutes, but it is not generally considered to be an effective anticonvulsant and is unlikely to stop seizure activity in the brain. Phenobarbital is an effective anticonvulsant (2–6 mg/kg IV) but can take 15–20 minutes to have an effect. If an effect is not noted within 15–30 minutes, the dose may be repeated to raise blood levels to the therapeutic range more rapidly (to a maximum loading dose of 16 mg/kg within the first 24 hours), but care must be taken to avoid overdose.

   iv. Propofol: Propofol is a rapidly acting injectible anesthestic that is a centrally acting GABA agonist. It may be administered via slow IV injection at a dose of 1–6 mg/kg and has been shown to be effective for stopping seizure activity (cluster seizures and status epilepticus) in human and veterinary medicine. If the initial bolus dose is effective but seizures recur, a CRI at 0.1–0.6 mg/kg/min may be instituted. Apnea and cardiovascular depression are important side effects to consider, and it is the author's opinion that any animal receiving a propofol infusion should be intubated to protect the airway, and ventilation should be closely monitored to avoid the sequelae of hypoventilation. In addition, propofol has been associated with transient seizure activity on induction and discontinuation of infusion in people. Additionally, propofol may be associated with increased Heinz body formation in cats, but recent studies suggest that these are not clinically significant.

   v. Levetiracetam (Keppra): Levetiracetam is a piracetam anticonvulsant that has shown efficacy for treatment of seizures in people and experimental animals. The mechanism of action of this drug is not known. It has a high bioavailability and is excreted unchanged in the urine without any significant hepatic metabolism, suggesting that it may be safer than benzodiazepines or barbiturates for treatment of seizures in patients with hepatic disease. There are no published doses for cats, but anecdotal reports have noted seizure control with 20 mg/kg intravenous boluses q8hr. It has no sedative side effects, making it easier to evaluate neurologic status in treated patients. Although the use of this drug for severe, acute seizures has not yet been described in the veterinary literature, a recent report showed significant improvement in seizure control in epileptic cats with the use of the oral formulation of this drug as an adjunct to phenobarbital therapy. It may prove to be a useful addition to the anticonvulsant armamentarium for cats and is available in an intravenous formulation (UCB Pharmaceuticals, Inc., Smyma, GA, USA).

  c. Once seizures are controlled, aggressive supportive care targeted at the cerebral and systemic sequelae of seizures should be undertaken.

   i. Fluid therapy with or without the addition of pressors should be instituted to aggressively treat perfusion deficits and maintain a mean blood pressure of 80 mmHg.

   ii. Ventilation should be closely monitored with blood gas analysis, and normocapnea maintained with intubation and ventilation if required.

   iii. Oxygenation should be maintained using supplemental oxygen therapy.

   iv. Hyperosmolar therapy (mannitol at 0.5–1.5 g/kg over 15–20 minutes or 7% hypertonic saline at 2 mL/kg over 15–20 minutes) should be considered for all patients with evidence of increased intracranial pressure, such as cranial nerve deficits, abnormal mentation, or hypertension and bradycardia (Cushing's reflex).

    1. Cushing's reflex occurs as result of increased intracranial pressure resulting in brain ischemia. The physiologic response to this is a release of catecholamines causing increased blood pressure and reflex bradycardia. It is a sign of clinically significant increased intracranial pressure and requires aggressive therapy.

   v. Body temperature should be monitored and active cooling instituted in all patients with body temperatures greater than 105°F.

 v. CNS toxins (see chap. 39)

1. Many toxins have the potential to induce neurologic signs in cats, but few have specific antidotes. Therefore, general decontamination procedures are recommended in all cats with suspected neurotoxin ingestion.
   a. Emesis induction: If the patient has been exposed within 4–6 hours and is not currently exhibiting altered mentation, emesis may be induced with oral hydrogen peroxide administration (1–5 mL/kg PO) or intravenous xylazine (0.44 mg/kg).
   b. Gastric lavage: In patients with neurologic signs or in which emesis induction is otherwise contraindicated, anesthesia, intubation, and gastric lavage are recommended.
   c. Activated charcoal: After emesis induction or gastric lavage, activated charcoal administration is recommended, either PO or via stomach tube. Administration should be repeated q6h when toxins undergoing enterohepatic recirculation are ingested. Activated charcoal with a cathartic (such as sorbitol) may be administered once, but only cathartic-free formulations should be repeatedly administered.
2. Specific toxins
   a. Bromethalin
      i. Bromethalin is a newer rodenticide that exerts its toxic effects via uncoupling of oxidative phosphorylation, resulting in ATP depletion, inactivation of sodium-potassium ATPases, and development of cerebral edema.
      ii. Common clinical signs of acute intoxications include seizure, coma, and death. Chronic exposure to lower doses can lead to pelvic limb paresis and altered mentation.
      iii. There is no specific antidote for Bromethalin intoxication. Decontamination protocols (as described above) and supportive care for seizures and cerebral edema are recommended.
      iv. Bromethalin undergoes enterohepatic recirculation. Repeated doses of activated charcoal for 24–48 hours are recommended.
      v. Prognosis is poor once signs have developed.
   b. Pyrethrins and pyrethroids
      i. Exposure most commonly occurs after administration of over-the-counter topical flea and tick products in cats. Because some cats are extremely sensitive to these compounds, even products specifically labeled for cats have been known to cause clinical signs when used at the recommended dose. Ingestion during grooming rather than transdermal absorption is most likely the cause of toxicosis.
      ii. Pyrethrins are the naturally occurring forms of these compounds (derived from chrysanthemum flowers), and pyrethroids are synthetic analogs.
      iii. These compounds prolong the opening of sodium channels in neural tissue by inhibition of GABA, resulting in prolonged membrane depolarization. This leads to muscle tremors, seizures, and ataxia, as well as hypersalivation, anorexia, and vomiting.
      iv. Treatment
         1. Gastric decontamination is risky in symptomatic patients and is unlikely to be effective.
         2. Bathing should be done as soon as possible to remove any remaining compound from the skin and to decrease additional transdermal or oral absorption.
         3. Medical therapy is targeted at stopping tremors or seizures.
            a. Methcarbamol (50–150 mg/kg slow IV to effect) is the treatment of choice for muscle tremors. It can be repeated as needed, but the total dose should not exceed 330 mg/kg/day, although the author has rarely exceeded this dose in severe or persistent cases.
            b. Barbiturates (such as phenobarbital) or general anesthesia with propofol or inhalants may rarely be required to stop seizures.

    4. Patients are commonly hyperthermic on presentation and should be cooled if body temperature is greater than 105°F. Hypothermia commonly develops after tremors or seizures are controlled and the cat is bathed; therefore, close monitoring of temperature and thermal support are important aspects of management.

    5. Most cats recover within 24 hours, but some may remain clinically affected for 48–72 hours.

c. Organophosphates and carbamates

    i. These insecticides are acetylcholinesterase inhibitors that lead to increased concentrations of actylcholine at somatic, sympathetic, and parasympathetic preganglionic synapses.

    ii. Clinical signs can vary depending on the type or types of receptors stimulated.

        1. Muscarinic: The most common clinical signs are a result of parasympathetic stimulation and include salivation, lacrimation, urination, and defecation (SLUD).

        2. Nicotinic: Tremors and muscle fasciculations can develop secondary to stimulation of nicotinic receptors.

        3. Central cholinergic: Stimulation of central cholinergic receptors results in seizures.

    iii. Treatment

        1. Gastrointestinal decontamination should be instituted if exposure is sufficiently acute and there are no contraindcations.

        2. Anticholinergic therapy (atropine 0.1–0.2 mg/kg, ¼ IV, the remainder SQ) if muscarinc signs are present.

        3. Pralidoxime chloride (2-PAM) results in the release of the toxin from acetylhcholinesterase and will treat nicotinic and muscarinic effects. The drug is administered IM at 20 mg/kg BID. Because carbamates spontaneously dissociate from acetylcholinesterase, 2-PAM should not be used to treat carbamate intoxication.

d. Lead

    i. Lead exerts its toxic effects via multiple enzyme systems, binding to ligands nonspecifically via sulfhydryl groups. This produces a variety of cellular effects, including interference with cellular metabolism, damage to heme production, and endothelial damage. It is present in many household items, including paint produced prior to 1950, curtain sinkers, pottery, roofing materials, and many other substances.

    ii. Neurologic signs include blindness, seizures, ataxia, altered mentation, coma, or tremors. Other clinical signs include mild anemia, vomiting, diarrhea, and megaesophagus.

    iii. Diagnosis is definitively determined via blood lead level determination. Consult your diagnostic laboratory to determine the appropriate sample for lead level determination. Other suggestive findings include increased nucleated red blood cells and red blood cell basophilic stippling.

    iv. Treatment includes gastrointestinal decontamination for acute exposures as described above, chelation therapy, and symptomatic treatment.

        1. Chelation may be accomplished with any of the following:

            a. Calcium EDTA: 25 mg/kg SQ q6h for 5 days. The 100 mg/mL solution should be diluted with 0.9% NaCl to a 10 mg/mL solution.

            b. D-Penicillamine: Should be considered after Calcium EDTA therapy if lead levels remain elevated. Give 125 mg PO q12h for 5 days.

            c. Succimer: 10 mg/kg PO q8h for 10 days is the published dose for dogs. No dose has been published for cats.

        2. Seizures should be controlled and supportive care administered. See "Seizures" above for specific recommendations.

   3. Methocarbamol may be used to treat tremors at a dose of 15–44 mg/kg PO or IV, not to exceed a total dose of 330 mg/kg/day.
e. Metronidazole
   i. When administered at a dose of greater than 30 mg/kg/day, metronidazole can lead to neurologic signs, including central vestibular signs, cerebellar ataxia, seizures, blindness, and abnormal mentation. The pathophysiology of this toxicosis is not known, but similar histopathologic lesions affecting the reticular system have been found in cats, dogs, and rats after metronidazole overdose.
   ii. Diagnosis is based on history and compatible clinical signs.
   iii. Treatment consists of discontinuation of metronidazole therapy and supportive care. Fluid therapy and antiemetics are indicated for patients with significant vomiting and/or nausea. Diazepam at a dose of 0.5 mg/kg IV q8h for 3 days can reverse many of the clinical signs associated with this toxicosis. Note that the use of oral diazepam in cats has been associated with rare but catastrophic hepatic necrosis, and is not recommended. Prognosis is good, and most animals recover within 1–3 weeks.

26
NEUROLOGIC EMERGENCIES: BRAIN

Jessica M. Snyder

Unique Features

1. Potassium bromide may be associated with a respiratory syndrome similar to feline asthma in approximately 40% of cats treated with the medication. This is generally reversible when the medication is discontinued.
2. Diazepam can cause a fatal, irreversible hepatic necrosis in cats when administered orally.
3. Rectally administered valium is not reliably absorbed in cats.
4. Hepatic encephalopathy due to hepatic lipidosis is a more common metabolic cause of severe prosencephalic disease in cats than portosystemic shunting, and should be considered in any icteric or historically inappetent cat. Cats with hepatic encephalopathy often display ptyalism as a clinical sign.
5. Thiamine deficiency is uncommon in cats but should be suspected in a neurological cat on an all-raw fish diet or with a history of prolonged anorexia.
6. Permethrin toxicity is a common cause of severe generalized tremoring in cats. This can occur after some dog flea products are applied to cats.
7. Idiopathic vestibular disease occurs in cats of all ages.
8. Granulomatous meningoencephalomyelitis is an extraordinarily rare cause of intracranial disease in cats, as opposed to dogs.
9. Siamese cats and other oriental breeds normally will have a pendular nystagmus.
10. Seizure activity and other clinical signs of forebrain disease are more commonly seen in cats with Metronidazole toxicosis, in addition to symptoms of central vestibular disease.
11. Ketamine anesthesia, especially in Persian cats, has been associated with cerebellar disease.
12. Prolonged hepatic metabolism makes several third-line anticonvulsant drugs unsuitable for use in cats, including Primidone, Phenytoin, and Valproic acid.
13. Idiopathic epilepsy is less common in the cat than the dog. Diagnostic testing should be pursued to rule out an identifiable underlying cause regardless of age.
14. Cerebellar hypoplasia, caused by in utero panleukopenia infection (feline parvovirus), is a common cause of nonprogressive cerebellar dysfunction in kittens.

A. General approach to the critically ill cat
   a. The brain can be subdivided broadly into four major anatomic and functional regions that cause distinct clinical syndromes: prosencephalon, diencephalon; midbrain/pons/medulla; and cerebellum.
B. Prosencephalon: Emergency manifestations of prosencephalic disease include seizure, stupor/coma, and tremors.

a. Seizure
  i. Seizure management
    1. Initial stabilization
      a. Evaluate for airway patency, breathing, and circulation.
      b. Administer diazepam (0.5–1 mg/kg IV). Venous access should be obtained. If venous access cannot be obtained, diazepam may be provided per rectum (dosing at 1–2 mg/kg can be attempted, but some report that absorption is unreliable in cats as opposed to dogs).
    2. Diazepam should not be used in cases of chlorpyrifos exposure as it may worsen the signs of acute toxicity.
    3. A blood glucose, serum calcium, BUN, and TP/PCV should be assessed immediately.
      a. 10% calcium gluconate (5–15 mg/kg IV over 10–15 minutes) may be administered to the hypocalcemic cat.
      b. 50% dextrose (1–2 mL/kg IV diluted with sterile water or 0.9% sodium chloride) may be administered to the hypoglycemic cat.
        i. If hypoglycemia is the cause, expect cessation of seizures within 1 minute of administration.
    4. Intravenous diazepam may be given up to three times to control acute seizures.
      a. A diazepam constant rate infusion (CRI) may be started at 0.5–2.0 mg/kg/hr if seizure activity quickly recurs.
        i. Diazepam may be mixed with 0.9% saline or 5% dextrose in water. Avoid mixing with lactated Ringer's solution as the calcium will precipitate the diazepam.
        ii. Plastic will adsorb diazepam and may make the actual CRI dose of diazepam unpredictable.
      b. If diazepam is not effective in controlling the seizures, then propofol (bolus of 1–4 mg/kg followed by 0.01–0.25 mg/kg/min CRI) or another anesthetic drug (i.e., volatile anesthetic agent such as isoflurane) should be used.
    5. Any icteric or historically inappetent cat (in which hepatic encephalopathy is suspected) should be treated with lactulose enemas (dose of 1 mL/kg per rectum); oral dose of 1 mL/5 kg PO q8h may be used in stable, aware patients.
    6. If the cat has had recurrent seizures, it may be phenobarbital loaded. Intravenous phenobarbital takes 20 minutes to obtain blood levels following administration (therefore, phenobarbital is not immediately effective for control of ongoing seizure). A loading dose of phenobarbital is approximately 15 mg/kg. This may be given as a single slow intravenous push, or it may be divided into four 4 mg/kg doses, administered every 30 minutes to 4 hours, depending on the frequency of seizure.
      a. If cat is severely sedated or comatose prior to next dose, then withhold dose.
      b. Adequacy of ventilation and airway protection should be monitored in any cat that has received multiple doses of anticonvulsants and is heavily sedated. If gag reflex is absent, an endotracheal tube should be placed to protect the airway.
    7. After the seizure is stopped, rectal temperature should be measured. Appropriate cooling measures should be undertaken if the cat is extremely hyperthermic (e.g., >105°F). Intravenous fluids may be administered.
    8. If the cat is in status epilepticus (see 8a below), and in any cat with severe seizures and obtundation, nystagmus, unresponsive pupils, bradycardia and hypertension, or anisocoria, a dose of mannitol (0.5–1 g/kg over 15–20 minutes IV) may decrease cerebral edema. Limit treatment to three doses in a 24-hour period. Furosemide administration at 2 mg/kg intravenously prior to mannitol infusion may provide synergistic effect in reducing intracranial pressure and also prevent the mild increase in intracranial pressure that occurs when mannitol is first administered. The cat should be hydrated prior to the administration of mannitol and fluid therapy continued to avoid hypotension or dehydration secondary to mannitol administration.

Table 26.1. Causes of seizure in the cat (bold denotes common cause).

Degenerative	Lysosomal storage disease; leukodystrophies
Anomalous	Lissencephaly; intracranial intra-arachnoid cyst; hydrocephalus; hydranencephaly; exencephaly; meningoencephalocoeles
Metabolic	**Hepatic encephalopathy**; uremic encephalopathy; hypoglycemia (**insulin overdose**, insulinoma); hypocalcemia; acid-base disturbances (respiratory acidosis most common), polycythemia
Neoplastic	**Meningioma**; **lymphosarcoma**; pituitary tumor; other primary or metastatic brain tumor
Nutritional	Thiamine deficiency
Infectious	**Feline infectious peritonitis**; other viral; rabies; *Cryptococcus neoformans*; other fungal disease; bacterial; *Toxoplasma gondii*; parasitic (Cuterebra larvae myiasis)
Idiopathic	Idiopathic epilepsy reportedly uncommon in cats in the U.S.; eosinophilic
Toxin	Veterinary drugs (recent ketamine anesthesia); lead; organophosphates; ethylene glycol; metronidazole
Trauma	**Common**
Vascular	Feline ischemic encephalopathy; hypertensive encephalopathy

      a. Status epilepticus can be defined as a seizure that lasts >5 minutes continuously or multiple seizures lasting less than this without complete neurologic recovery between seizures.

    9. Blood pressure (systolic of 90 mmHg) and oxygenation (Hb saturation of >95% if possible) should be monitored and maintained in any cat with suspected increased intracranial pressure.

  ii. Causes of seizure in the cat (table 26.1)

  iii. Emergency diagnostic workup for the seizuring cat

    1. CBC/Chemistry/UA/T4; FeLV/FIV test (if status unknown)

    2. Bile acids/NH$_3$ in cases of possible hepatic encephalopathy

    3. Thoracic +/– abdominal radiographs if indicated

    4. Blood pressure measurement

      a. Hypertension

        i. Hypertensive encephalopathy can be an underlying cause of seizures.

        ii. Hypertension can occur secondary to increased intracranial pressure (Cushing's reflex; see chap. 25—General Approach and Overview of the Neurologic Cat).

    5. Fundoscopic evaluation

  iv. Further therapy

    1. Anticonvulsant of choice: phenobarbital at 2 mg/kg PO BID.

    2. Potassium bromide may be associated with a respiratory syndrome identical to feline asthma in 40% of cats (see chap. 13—Parenchymal Disease).

    3. Oral diazepam may cause irreversible and fatal hepatic necrosis, although this is relatively rare.

    4. Drugs to avoid: phenytoin, primidone, valproic acid due to the prolonged half life in cats and potential for hepatotoxicity and other side effects (extreme sedation with phenytoin and hyperactivity and alopecia with valproic acid).

    5. Other anticonvulsants may be used: Levetiracetam (Keppra) (20–25 mg/kg PO or IV q8–12h) or Zonisamide 5–10 mg/kg PO q24h. Keppra seems to be tolerated better by cats and is not metabolized by the liver.

    6. Hepatic encephalopathy or liver disease (see chap. 21—Management of Specific Gastrointestinal Conditions for more details).

         a. Lactulose

         b. Antibiotic therapy to decrease gastrointestinal bacterial load

            i. Neomycin

            ii. Amoxicillin 22 mg/kg PO q12h or Ampicillin 22 mg/kg IV q12h

            iii. Metronidazole 7.5 mg/kg PO or IV q12h

     7. Blood pressure support as appropriate (see chap. 8—Fluid Therapy)

         a. Blood pressure support is indicated when the doppler is <90 or the mean arterial pressure is <60–80 mmHg after adequate fluid replacement.

            i. Dopamine 5–15 µg/kg/min

            ii. Norepinephrine 0.1–3 µg/kg/min

            iii. Dobutamine should not be used as an initial theraputic agent due to reports of seizure activity secondary to dobutamine CRI.

     8. Thiamine deficiency: thiamine (vitamin B1) at 20–100 mg/cat IM or SQ q12–24h, begin oral supplementation when stable.

         a. Thiamine deficiency is rare in cats but is seen in cats receiving purely overly cooked diets or pure raw fish diets or cats with prolonged anorexia.

         b. Clinical signs are a result of polioencephalomalacia of the brain gray matter and include ataxia, seizures, and pupillary dilatation due to oculomotor nerve paralysis. A characteristic sign is ventroflexion of the neck when the cat is lowered head first to the ground. Clinical signs should improve within 24 hours of administration of thiamine.

b. Stupor/coma: Global lesions of the cerebrum or of the ascending reticular activating system may cause stupor or coma.

    i. Causes of stupor/coma: see table 26.1

    ii. Management of stupor/coma

        1. Manage airway, breathing, circulation, and provide oxygen support.

          a. $PaCO_2$ <30 mmHg reduces cerebral blood flow and cerebral edema.

            i. Goal: $PaCO_2$ 35–40 mmHg

          b. Maintain PaO_2 at 100 mmHg in cats (pulse oximetry SaO_2 >95% mmHg if arterial blood gas not available).

        2. Keep head at 30-degree elevation and avoid compressing jugular veins and angling the neck.

        3. Body temperature should be maintained between 99° and 102°F.

        4. Maintain PCV between 20% and 40% ideally.

        5. Monitor electrolytes—magnesium maintains cellular enzymatic reactions and mitochondrial stability in the injured brain.

        6. Good nursing care is essential.

          a. Monitor and maintain normal body temperature (hypothermia is a common problem).

          b. Turn cat from one side to the next or place sternal every 2–4 hours.

          c. Express urinary bladder as needed to prevent overdistention.

          d. Keep cat dry and prevent soiling.

          e. Keep eyes lubricated with artificial tear ointment if blink reflex is affected.

          f. Keep tongue moist if unable to retract tongue.

        7. Mannitol if indicated (0.5–1 g/kg over 15–20 minutes IV).

        8. Nutritional support when appropriate.

    iii. Head trauma patients with stupor/coma should be treated to reduce the effects of the secondary injury (continued hemorrhage and edema). (For more details, see chap. 25—General Approach and Overview of the Neurologic Cat.)

        1. Maintain blood pressure of a doppler >90 mmHg or a mean arterial pressure of >60–80 mmHg. Hetastarch may be administered to cats at a dose of 5 mL/kg over 5–10 minutes. Hypertonic saline (7% NaCl) may also be used at a dose of 2–3 mL/kg over 15–20 minutes, although there is some concern that this treatment may disrupt the blood brain barrier.

2. All other treatments should be similar to the treatment of cats with stupor or coma above.
  iv. Emergency diagnostic workup (see seizure section above). Tests that may be used to confirm brain death include BAER testing (brainstem auditory-evoked response testing) and electroencephalography.
c. Tremors
  i. Causes of generalized twitching in the cat: A thorough history should be taken including possible exposure to toxins or administration of topical flea control (particularly products that contain permethrins).
     1. Prosencephalic disease (table 26.1)
     2. Metabolic: hypernatremia, hypocalcemia, hypomagnesemia, uremia, hepatic encephalopathy.
     3. Toxin: permethrin products (common), hexachlorophene, heavy metals, organophosphates, chlorinated hydrocarbons, mycotoxins, poisonous plants, strychnine, metaldehyde, bromethalin
     4. Cerebellar disease
     5. Primary disorders of the muscles, nerves, or neuromuscular junction
  ii. Management of tremors
     1. Decontamination in case of intoxication
        a. For recent oral exposures, may induce emesis and then administer activated charcoal. This should not be done in impaired animals or those who have ingested a CNS stimulant (see chap. 39—Toxicological Emergencies).
        b. In cases of dermal exposure, the cat should be bathed.
     2. Diazepam at 0.2–0.5 mg/kg IV may help control tremors.
     3. Methocarbamol: Administer 44 mg/kg IV as slow push (may repeat); do not exceed 330 mg/kg/day.
        a. This is particularly effective and is the drug of choice to treat permethrin-induced tremors in cats.
C. Diencephalon: comprises the thalamus and hypothalamus
  a. Signs of diencephalic disease
     i. Abnormal temperature regulation (hypothermia, hyperthermia)
     ii. Abnormal urine concentrating ability (central diabetes insipidus)
     iii. Electrolyte derangements (hypernatremia, hyponatremia)
     iv. Blind eye(s) with dilated, unresponsive pupil(s)
     v. Vestibular disease
     vi. Endocrine dysfunction including diabetes insipidus, acromegaly, hypothyroidism, and hyperadrenocorticism (all uncommon in cats)
     vii. Abnormal eating patterns
     viii. Nonspecific pain (uncommon)
     ix. Stupor/coma
  b. Causes of diencephalic disease: see table 26.1
  c. Emergency management of diencephalic disease
     i. Hypernatremia: Hypernatremia in cats can lead to the shrinkage of brain parenchymal cells and should be corrected by administration of fluids hypoosmolar to the patient.
        1. The water deficit (L) can be calculated as $0.6 \times$ lean BW (kg) $\times$ patient's Na^+/normal $Na^+ - 1$.
           a. This calculation should be used as an initial guide, but response varies from cat to cat. Therefore, initial calculation should be made and rate administered for 1–2 hours, and then sodium concentration should be evaluated. Adjustments of fluid infusion rate can be made empirically as sodium concentration changes.
        2. Chronic hypernatremia should be corrected over 48–72 hours.
           a. Serum sodium should not be decreased faster than 0.5 mEq/hr.

b. If the hypernatremia is corrected too rapidly, it can lead to intracellular swelling within the brain parenchymal cells.

ii. Hyponatremia: Hyponatremia in cats can result in swelling of brain parenchymal cells with subsequent brain edema and should be corrected by administration of sodium-containing fluids such as normal, or in rare, acute, severe cases, hypertonic saline.

1. The sodium deficit (mEq/L) can be calculated as $0.6 \times$ lean BW (kg) $\times$ (normal Na^+ – patient's Na^+).

2. Chronic hyponatremia should also be corrected over 48–72 hours.

a. Serum sodium should not be increased faster than 0.5 mEq/hour.

b. If the hyponatremia is corrected too rapidly, it can lead to intracellular dehydration within the brain parenchymal cells.

c. Initial fluid therapy should be instituted using 0.9% sodium chloride, and the sodium measured closely (every 1–2 hours for the first 6–12 hours).

d. If the sodium is increasing too quickly, addition of a lower sodium fluid is indicated.

e. Ideally, serum sodium concentration should not be increased greater than 0.5 mmol/L/hr.

iii. Temperature regulation

1. Temperature can vary depending upon if the thermoregulatory center is specifically affected or not. Temperature should be monitored closely in cats with severely altered mentation and should be maintained between 99° and 102°F.

iv. Mannitol if indicated (0.5–1 g/kg over 15–20 minutes IV).

v. Appropriate intravenous fluid therapy

1. Maintenance fluid therapy is indicated for patients that have normal electrolytes but are not eating/drinking and do not have ongoing losses (vomiting, diarrhea, fever; see chap. 8).

D. Midbrain/pons/medulla: the portion of the brainstem not including the diencephalon, which is anatomically and functionally distinct from the remainder of the brainstem

a. Emergency manifestations of disease include vestibular disease and stupor/coma.

b. Vestibular disease: signs include head tilt, nystagmus, strabismus, and a vestibular ataxia.

i. Peripheral versus central vestibular disease (table 26.2)

ii. Causes of central vestibular disease are similar to those for seizure (see table 26.1), although metabolic causes are less likely.

iii. Peripheral vestibular disease is caused by a lesion of CN VIII and may be seen in conjunction with CN VII dysfunction or a Horner's syndrome. Causes of peripheral vestibular disease:

1. Congenital: Siamese, Burmese, and Tonkinese kittens

2. Neoplastic: involving temporal bone or middle ear

3. Idiopathic: cats of all ages. Stabilization of clinical signs should occur within 72 hours and recovery in 2–4 weeks. No other cranial nerve deficits should be present.

Table 26.2. Distinguishing peripheral from central vestibular disease.

Clinical signs	Peripheral Vestibular Disease	Central Vestibular Disease
Mentation	Alert +/− disoriented	+/− dull, stupor, coma
Other cranial nerve deficits	+/− cranial nerve 7 dysfunction	+/− cranial nerve 5, 6, 7, 9–11 dysfunction
Proprioceptive deficits	None	Possible
Nystagmus	Horizontal, rotary; fast phase away from side of head tilt	Horizontal, rotary, vertical; fast phase toward or away from side of head tilt
Horner's syndrome	common	rare
Vestibular ataxia	Mild to severe	Mild to severe
Degree of head tilt	Mild to severe	Mild to severe

      4. Infectious: bacterial otitis media/interna most common (*Staphylococcus*, *Streptococcus*, and *Pseudomonas* spp.)

      5. Inflammatory: feline nasopharyngeal polyps (cats often <2–5 years of age); may also see clinical signs of otitis or upper respiratory signs

      6. Trauma

      7. Toxin: aminoglycoside antibiotics; loop diuretics; propylene glycol, chlorhexidine, and cetrimide; five-lined skink (SW US); some antineoplastics (cisplatin); heavy metals (arsenic, lead, mercury)

    iv. Emergency management of the acutely vestibular cat

      1. Lubricate eyes in cases of facial nerve paralysis.

      2. Protect animal from self-trauma.

      3. Antihistamines (diphenhydramine, meclizine) may decrease severity of head tilt, nystagmus, and nausea.

        a. Diphenhydramine 2–4 mg/kg PO, IM q8h

        b. Meclizine 6.25 mg/5 kg PO q24h

      4. Antibiotic therapy in cases of suspected otitis interna/media

        a. First-generation cephalosporins

          i. Cefazolin 10–30 mg/kg IV or IM q8h

          ii. Cephalexin 22 mg/kg PO q8h

          iii. Cefadroxil 22 mg/kg PO q8–12h

        b. Clavamox 62.5 mg/cat PO q12 or Baytril 5 mg/kg PO, IV q24h, although this has been associated with renal degeneration and blindness in some cats.

      5. Mannitol if indicated (0.5–1 gram/kg over 15–20 min. IV).

    v. Emergency diagnostic workup (p = peripheral vestibular disease; c = central vestibular disease)

      1. CBC/Chemistry/UA +/– thoracic radiographs (p, c)

      2. Otoscopic examination (p, c)

      3. Noninvasive blood pressure measurement (c)

      4. +/– Skull radiographs (p)

E. Cerebellum

  a. Signs of cerebellar disease include tremor of the head and limbs (may worsen with purposeful activity), nystagmus, decreased menace response, opsithotonus, and dysmetria.

  b. Causes of cerebellar disease

    i. Generally similar to causes of prosencephalic disease (see table 26.1); in addition, consider cerebellar abiotrophies, cerebellar hypoplasia (common), and toxins (ivermectin, lead, hexachlorophene, organophosphates, plants, and ketamine anesthesia [especially in Persian cats]).

  c. Emergency management and diagnostic workup: see "Vestibular disease" above.

27
NEUROLOGIC EMERGENCIES: SPINAL CORD

Jessica M. Snyder

Unique Features

1. A history of rabies vaccination or possible exposure should always be obtained in the cat that presents with unexplained paralysis.
2. Clinically significant intervertebral disk disease is uncommon in cats as opposed to dogs, and the lumbar spine is most often affected. Clinically significant cervical disk disease in cats is extremely uncommon.
3. Lymphoma is the most common neoplasm to affect the spinal cord in cats, and it most often involves the thoracic and lumbosacral spine. Lymphoma may be diagnosed on cerebrospinal fluid analysis in up to one-third of the cases.
4. Fibrocartilaginous embolic myelopathy does occur in (most often middle-aged to older) cats and involves the thoracic and lumbar intumescences more frequently.
5. Feline infectious peritonitis is the most common infectious disease to affect the spinal cord of cats, although intracranial signs often are seen as well.
6. When a spinal, metabolic, or vascular cause of paraparesis or tetraparesis cannot be identified in cats, the possibility of intracranial disease should be investigated.

A. General approach: Spinal cord injuries can generally be assigned to one of four neuroanatomic locations within the spinal cord based on the neurological examination findings (see table 27.1).
B. **L4-S3 myelopathy:** The approach to the L4-S3 myelopathy is illustrated in figure 27.1. Diffuse lower motor neuron disease or orthopedic disease should be suspected in the cat with decreased reflexes or a short-strided gait in both the pelvic and thoracic limbs. With an L4-S3 myelopathy, only the pelvic limbs are affected.
   a. With S1-S3 disease, tail tone and rectal tone may be decreased, and the perineal reflex may be absent. Sacrococcygeal dysgenesis is an inherited condition in Manx cats that may be associated with lower motor neuron signs of the pelvic limbs, urinary bladder, and anus, generally in a young cat (see figs. 27.2, 27.3, and 27.4).
   b. With disease of the L3-5 lumbar spine, the patellar (femoral nerve) reflex may be decreased to absent and the sciatic nerve reflexes present. With disease of the L6-S3 spine, the patellar reflex may be increased (pseudohyperreflexia) and the sciatic nerve reflexes depressed (see Special Section).
   c. Differential diagnoses for the cat with L4-S3 myelopathy (see table 27.2).
   d. Emergency diagnostic workup:
      i. Palpate femoral pulses.
      ii. CBC, chemistry, UA; FeLV/FIV if status unknown

Table 27.1. Clinical signs of spinal cord disease by spinal cord segment.

	C1-5	C6-T2	T3-L3	L4-S3
Pelvic limb tone	Normal to ↑	Normal to ↑	Normal to ↑	Normal to ↓
Pelvic limb reflexes	Normal to ↑	Normal to ↑	Normal to ↑	Normal to ↓
Thoracic limb tone	Normal to ↑	Normal to ↓	+/– increased (Schiff-Sherrington)	+/–increased (Schiff-Sherrington)
Thoracic limb reflexes	Normal to ↑	Normal to ↓	Normal	Normal
Paraparesis/plegia	Yes	Yes	Yes	Yes
Tetraparesis/plegia	Yes	Yes	No	No
Proprioceptive deficits	+/– all limbs	+/– all limbs	+/– pelvic limbs	+/– pelvic limbs
Spinal pain	+/– cervical	+/– cervical	+/– thoracic	+/– lumbar
Anal and tail tone	Present	Present	Present	+/–↓
Bladder	+/– large, firm, and difficult to express	+/– large, firm, and difficult to express	+/– large, firm, and difficult to express	+/– large, flaccid, and easy to express
Horner's syndrome	Possible, ipsilateral	Possible, ipsilateral	No	No

Note: C = cervical spinal cord segment; T = thoracic spinal cord segment; L = lumbar spinal cord segment.

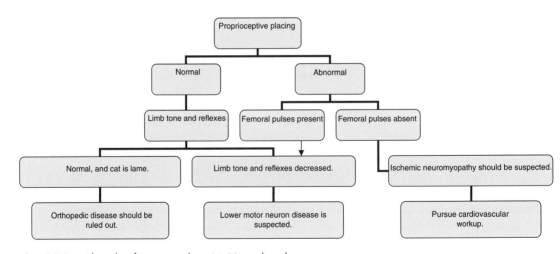

Fig. 27.1. Algorithm for approaching L4-S3 myelopathy.

    iii. Survey spinal radiographs (two-view ideal) if any suspected history of trauma; use caution positioning the cat until vertebral fracture/luxation is ruled out.

  e. Emergency therapeutic plan:

    i. Bladder expression

    ii. If history of trauma is unknown, minimize movement/manipulation of lumbar spine; if a fracture is identified or suspected, the cat may be immobilized by taping to a backboard.

    iii. High-dose methylprednisolone sodium succinate (SoluMedrol) treatment for acute spinal trauma:

      1. This treatment is controversial, and efficacy has not been proven in controlled clinical trials in small animals. The protocol in human medicine consists of an initial slow intravenous

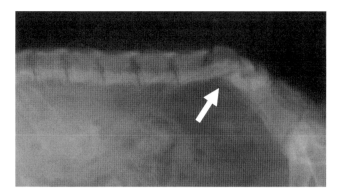

Fig. 27.2. Lateral radiograph of the lumbar spine in an 11-week-old Manx cat. Note the vertebral incongruity and deformity of L6 and L7 (arrow). There are absent sacral and coccygeal vertebrae.

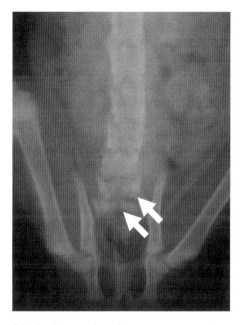

Fig. 27.3. Ventrodorsal view of the lumbar spine in the same cat. Note the incomplete fusion of the L6 and L7 vertebrae (arrows), which suggests spina bifida in this cat.

injection of 30 mg/kg SoluMedrol, followed by a constant rate infusion of 5.4 mg/kg/hr for the next 23 hours. A modified protocol has been proposed for use in veterinary medicine. This involves an initial bolus of 30 mg/kg IV with subsequent doses of 15 mg/kg administered at 2 and 6 hours. Results from human clinical trials suggest that treatment may be deleterious if administered >8 hours following the trauma.

2. Potential side effects include hyperglycemia, and SoluMedrol should not be administered to a hyperglycemic patient. Gastrointestinal ulceration has been reported in dogs receiving the high-dose SoluMedrol protocol.

iv. Surgical decompression and stabilization is recommended in cases of moderately to severely displaced vertebral fracture/luxation, in patients with severe neurological dysfunction (non-ambulatory paraparesis) and deteriorating neurological status. Advanced imaging (myelography,

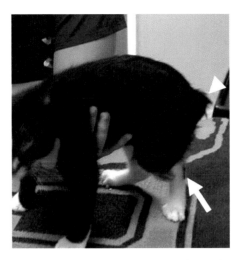

Fig. 27.4. Eleven-week-old Manx cat in a characteristic posture in the hind end. The cat is tucked under in the hind end, dropped in the hocks (arrow), and it bunny hops. The tail is absent (arrowhead).

Table 27.2. Differential diagnosis for spinal disease in the cat (common causes presented in bold type).

Degenerative	Clinically significant intervertebral disk disease (L4-5 most common site); storage diseases
Anomalous	Spinal arachnoid cyst; syringomyelia or hydromyelia; sacrocaudal dysgenesis (Manx cats); multiple cartilaginous exostoses
Neoplasia	**Lymphosarcoma** (most common in cats 2–8 years old); vertebral neoplasms (most common >8 years old); peripheral nerve sheath tumors; metastatic neoplasms
Nutritional	Metabolic osteodystrophy
Infectious	**Feline infectious peritonitis**; *Cryptococcus neoformans* (other fungal such as coccidiodomycosis reported, but less likely); *Toxoplasma gondii*; bacterial (including discospondylitis); *Sarcocystis neurona*; FeLV associated myelopathy; feline polioencephalomyelitis
Trauma	Vertebral fracture or luxation (L2-3 and L4-5 most common sites); subdural hematoma; traumatic intervertebral disk herniation; fracture/luxation of the sacrococcygeal region due to traction injury; traumatic feline ischemic myelopathy (due to vasospasm or thrombosis of lumbar arteries supplying the spinal cord)
Vascular	Fibrocartilaginous embolic myelopathy

       computed tomography, or magnetic resonance imaging) is indicated when possible to rule out spinal cord compression, including traumatic intervertebral disk herniation in the absence of obvious spinal fracture.

v.   Nonsurgical management can be attempted in cats with less severe neurological dysfunction, in cats with no evidence of spinal instability or spinal cord compression, or in cases with financial constraints. Some authors suggest that the prognosis is similar for cats with exogenous spinal trauma treated surgically and nonsurgically, although study sizes are small. Cats do not tolerate external support bandages or casts as readily as dogs, although this treatment has been reported. Conservative therapy should involve 4–6 weeks of cage rest with or without an attempt at external coaptation.

vi.   In one study of cats with thoracic and lumbar spinal cord injuries due to external trauma, the survival rate was 50%. The presence or absence of deep pain was the most important prognostic indicator, with no cat with paraplegia and loss of deep pain perception surviving. Cats with intact pain perception made a complete or functional recovery in 15/22 cases (68%).

vii. For cases with no history or radiograph evidence of trauma, the cat should be kept cage confined. Antibiotics (Clindamycin at 10–15 mg/kg BID) and/or corticosteroids (Prednisone at 1 mg/kg BID) may be used in case of infectious or inflammatory spinal cord disease if the clinical signs are severe. Treatment with Prednisone prior to diagnostic testing may interfere with diagnosis of neoplastic (lymphoma) or inflammatory disease and may worsen infectious disease. The paralyzed, systemically stable cat with no radiographic abnormalities should be referred for advanced imaging as soon as possible.

C. **T3-L3 myelopathy**
   a. Clinical signs: see table 27.1.
   b. There may be focal loss of the cutaneous trunci reflex.
   c. Schiff-Sherrington posture is caused by a severe (although not irreversible) lesion of the thoracolumbar spine and is characterized by increased tone in the thoracic limbs due to a lack of ascending inhibition. This posture should not be confused with a lesion in the cranial cervical spine; postural reactions should be normal in the thoracic limbs in a cat with Schiff-Sherrington posture and decreased in a cat with a C1-C5 myelopathy.
   d. Differential diagnoses: see table 27.2.
   e. Emergency diagnostic workup: see "B. L4-S3 myelopathy: d. Emergency diagnostic workup."
   f. Emergency therapeutic plan: see B.e.

D. **C6-T2 myelopathy**
   a. Clinical signs: see table 27.1.
   b. The cat, if ambulatory, may walk with a short-strided gait in the thoracic limbs and a long-strided, ataxic gait in the pelvic limbs.
   c. The cutaneous trunci response may be absent on the ipsilateral side in case of a lesion affecting the lateral thoracic nerve where it exits the spinal cord at T1-T3.
   d. Respiratory difficulty may occur in severe cases, characterized by an "abdominal" breathing pattern.
   e. Differential diagnoses: see table 27.2.
   f. Emergency diagnostic workup: see B.d.
      i. Perform a blood gas with CO_2 (to assess adequacy of ventilation) in the cat with cervical spinal disease and increased respiratory effort or decreased thoracic wall excursions.
   g. Emergency therapeutic plan: see B.e.
      i. Ventilation may be required in cases of severe respiratory compromise.
         1. $PaCO_2$ >50 mmHg on arterial blood gas
         2. $PvCO_2$ >60–70 mmHg on venous blood gas (as long as perfusion is good)
         3. Significant respiratory distress

E. **C1-C5 myelopathy**
   a. Clinical signs of a C1-C5 myelopathy: see table 27.1.
   b. With very high cervical disease, the postural ability in the thoracic limbs may be worse than that in the pelvic limbs.
   c. With markedly increased muscle tone, the segmental spinal reflexes may paradoxically appear diminished.
   d. May see respiratory difficulty with poor chest excursions and diaphragmatic movements.
   e. Differential diagnoses: see table 27.2.
      i. Additionally, atlanto-axial instability occasionally occurs in cats, and feline hypervitaminosis A (in cats fed exclusively liver diets) can be associated with exostoses of cervical and thoracic vertebrae. Diagnosis is based on serum vitamin A concentration.
   f. Emergency diagnostic plan: see B.d.
   g. Emergency therapeutic plan: see B.e.

Special Section: Performing the Feline Neurological Examination

General attitude: Is the cat depressed, dull, stuporous (responsive to noxious stimuli), or comatose (unresponsive even to noxious stimuli)? Is the cat mentally appropriate? Does the cat seem disoriented?

Posture: Is there a head tilt or a body curve, which may suggest vestibular disease? Is there a head turn, which may suggest forebrain disease? Is there ventroflexion of the neck or a plantigrade stance, which may suggest neuromuscular disease? Does the cat show decerebrate rigidity (extension of all limbs, with or without opisthotonus), decerebellate rigidity (opisthotonus, forelimb extension, and hind limb flexion), or Schiff-Sherrington posture (see fig. 27.3)?

Gait: Observe the animal's gait, if possible. Cats will infrequently walk on a leash. Ideally, take the cat into a small examination room with the door closed. Many cats will refuse to ambulate in an unfamiliar environment. Luring them with food or with their open cat carrier may help in some instances. Note any tendency to circle. Ataxia (an uncoordinated gait) can be classified as a **proprioceptive (spinal) ataxia**, characterized by a long-strided, ataxic gait with crossing, interference, and floating of the limbs; a **vestibular ataxia**, characterized by tilting, leaning, veering, and circling in tight circles; or a **cerebellar ataxia**, characterized by head bobbing, hypermetria or dysmetria, and a truncal sway. Note any lameness, which may suggest orthopedic or lower motor neuron disease (see fig. 27.1).

Cranial Nerve Examination

Menace response (cranial nerve 2 afferent, cranial nerve 7 efferent). Covering one eye, make a menacing gesture in front of the open eye. Be careful not to touch the whiskers, and do not move the hand forcefully enough to direct air movement toward the eye. Some cats will be anxious in the hospital and reluctant to completely close the eye. If there is doubt about the patient's vision, cotton balls can be thrown in front of the cat, to observe for visual tracking. Kittens younger than 8–12 weeks normally may lack a menace response.

Pupillary light response (cranial nerve 2 afferent, cranial nerve 3 efferent). Observe the pupils for any disparity in size or shape. Shine a bright light into one pupil, and observe for constriction of both pupils. Repeat with opposite eye. Some cats will be anxious in the hospital and will have dilated pupils that respond poorly to light. Performing the test in a dark room may enhance the pupil's response to bright light.

Facial sensation and movement (cranial nerve 5 afferent, cranial nerve 7 efferent). Tickle the nares and the upper and lower lips with a closed hemostat, and observe for moving the head away from the stimulus and retracting the lip.

Palpebral blink (cranial nerve 5 afferent, cranial nerve 7 efferent). Touch the medial canthus of the eye with a finger or closed hemostat. The appropriate response is to close the eyelid completely.

Nystagmus (cranial nerve 8). Observe for pathologic nystagmus at rest and in both lateral recumbencies and dorsal recumbency.

Strabismus (cranial nerves 3, 4, 6). Observe the globe for deviation in any direction, and then elicit physiological nystagmus by moving the head from side to side. A positional ventrolateral strabismus may be present in an animal with a head tilt, and reflects disease of cranial nerve 8.

Gag response Not routinely performed in cats. The mouth should be opened if possible during the examination, and the tongue should be inspected for atrophy (cranial nerve 12).

Proprioceptive Testing

All limbs: Knuckle the paw so that the animal is standing on the dorsum of the paw (fig. 27.5). Observe for correcting paw placement. Many normal cats will not allow you to put the paw on the ground in an abnormal position (fig. 27.6).

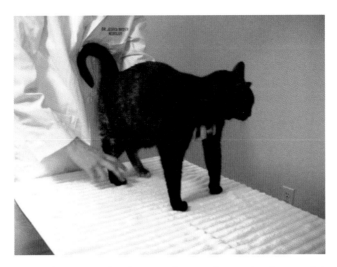

Fig. 27.5.   Preparing to turn the paw so that the animal is standing on the dorsum of the paw.

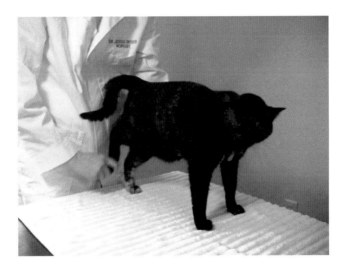

Fig. 27.6.   Many normal cats will not allow you to put the paw on the ground in an abnormal position.

Postural reactions: Holding the cat under the abdomen, walk the cat forward on the thoracic limbs only. Then hold the cat up to a table, allowing the limbs to hit the edge of the table. The normal cat should lift the legs to stand on the table. Now, holding the cat under the axillary regions, walk the cat backwards on the pelvic limbs (fig. 27.7).

Segmental Spinal Reflex and Limb Examination

Pelvic limbs: Note the tone in the pelvic limbs and tail.

Quadriceps (Femoral nerve): Percuss the patellar tendon with the straight edge of a pleximeter, and observe for extension of the stifle (fig. 27.8).

Withdrawal (sciatic nerve): Pinch the toe and observe for flexion of the hock, stifle, and hip (fig. 27.9). The lateral aspect of the foot is innervated by the sciatic nerve. The medial digit is innervated by the femoral

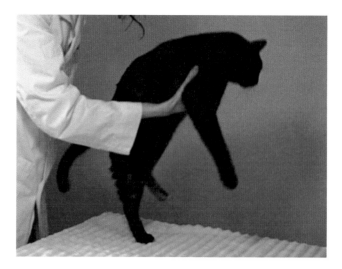

Fig. 27.7. Walking the cat backward on the pelvic limbs.

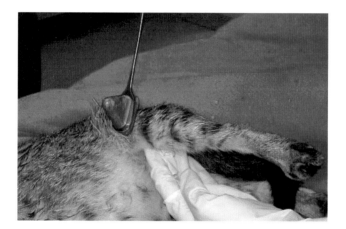

Fig. 27.8. Observing for extension of the stifle.

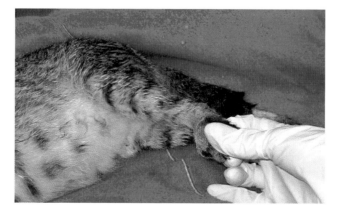

Fig. 27.9. Observing for flexion of the hock, stifle, and hip.

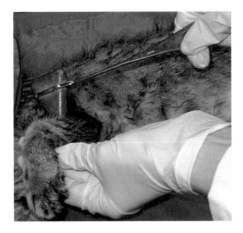

Fig. 27.10. Observing for extension of the carpus.

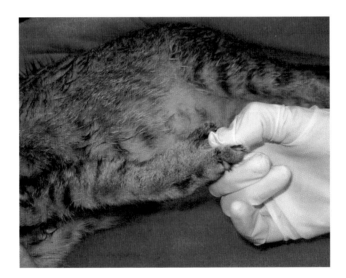

Fig. 27.11. Observing for flexion of the carpus, elbow, and shoulder.

nerve, so in some cases of femoral nerve disease, pinching the medial digit will not elicit withdrawal of the limb.

Perineal reflex (perineal and pudendal nerves): Lightly stroke the perineum lateral to the anus. The anal sphincter should contract and the tail flex.

Thoracic limbs: Note the tone in the thoracic limbs.

Extensor carpi radialis (radial nerve): Percuss the extensor carpi radialis muscle on the dorsal aspect of the antebrachium with the pointed end of the pleximeter (fig. 27.10). Observe for extension of the carpus.

Withdrawal (musculocutaneous, axillary, median, ulnar, and radial nerves): Pinch the toe, and observe for flexion of the carpus, elbow, and shoulder (fig. 27.11).

Cutaneous trunci response: Can be elicited in some cats by pinching the skin lateral to the thoracolumbar spine with hemostats. This reflex is considered unreliable in cats.

Hyperpathia: Palpate the spine for pain by firmly pressing on the dorsal spinous processes of the thoracic and lumbar spine. Move the head and neck in a full range of motion.

Recommended Reading

General

Dewey CW. Disorders of the cauda equina. In Dewey CW, ed, A Practical Guide to Canine and Feline Neurology, pp 337–355. Ames: Iowa State Press, 2003.

Dewey CW. Myelopathies: disorders of the spinal cord. In Dewey CW, ed, A Practical Guide to Canine and Feline Neurology, pp 277–336. Ames: Iowa State Press, 2003.

LeCouteur RA. Proceedings of the ESFM Feline Congress, Stockholm, September 2002. Spinal cord disorders. J Feline Med Surg, 2003; 5:121–131.

Marioni-Henry K, Vite CH, Newton AL, et al. Prevalence of diseases of the spinal cord of cats. J Vet Intern Med, 2004; 18:851–858.

Spinal Cord Trauma

Anderson A, Coughlan AR. Sacral fractures in dogs and cats: a classification scheme and review of 51 cases. J Small Anim Pract, 1997; 38:404–409.

Bagley RS. Spinal fracture or luxation. Vet Clin N Am Small Anim Pract, 2000; 30:133–153.

Bagley RS, Harrington ML, Silver GM, et al. Exogenous spinal trauma: clinical assessment and initial management. Comp Contin Educ Pract Vet, 1999; 21:1138–1143.

Bracken MB, Collins WF, Freeman DF, et al. Efficacy of methylprednisolone in acute spinal cord injury. J Am Med Assoc, 1984; 251:45–52.

Bracken MB, Holford TR. Neurological and functional status 1 year after acute spinal cord injury: estimates of functional recovery in National Acute Spinal Cord Injury Study II from results modeled in National Acute Spinal Cord Injury Study III. J Neurosurg, 2002; 96:259–266.

Bracken MB, Shepard MJ, Collins WF, et al. A randomized, controlled trial of methylprednisolone or naloxone in the treatment of acute spinal cord injury. New Engl J Med, 1990; 322:1405–1411.

Bracken MB, Shepard MJ, Holford TR, et al. Administration of methylprednisolone for 24 or 48 hours or tirilazad mesylate for 48 hours in the treatment of acute spinal cord injury. J Am Med Assoc, 1997; 277:1597–1604.

Braughler JM, Hall ED. Lactate and pyruvate metabolism in injured cat spinal cord before and after a single large intravenous dose of methylprednisolone. J Neurosurg, 1983; 59:256–261.

Grasmueck S, Steffen F. Survival rates and outcomes in cats with thoracic and lumbar spinal cord injuries due to external trauma. J Small Anim Pract, 2004; 45:284–288.

Kraus KH. Medical management of acute spinal cord disesase. In Bonagura, JD, ed, Kirk's Current Veterinary Therapy XIII, pp 186–190. Philadelphia: W.B. Saunders, 2000.

Kuntz CA. Sacral fractures and sacrococcygeal injuries in dogs and cats. In Bonagura, JD, ed, Kirk's Current Veterinary Therapy XIII, pp 1023–1026. Philadelphia: W.B. Saunders, 2000.

Olby N. Current concepts in the management of acute spinal cord injury. J Vet Intern Med, 1999; 13:399–407.

Voss K, Montavon PM. Tension band stabilization of fractures and luxations of the thoracolumbar vertebrae in dogs and cats: 38 cases (1993–2002). J Am Vet Med Assoc, 2004; 225(1):78–83.

Congenital Disease

Bagley RS, Silver GM, Kippenes H, et al. Syringomyelia and hydromyelia in dogs and cats. Comp Contin Educ Vet Pract, 2000; 22:471–478.

Bone DL, Wilson RD. Primary syringomyelia in a kitten. J Am Vet Med Assoc, 1982; 181:928–929.

Crawley AC, Muntz FH, Haskins ME, et al. Prevalence of Mucopolysaccharidosis type VI mutations in Siamese Cats. J Vet Intern Med, 2003; 17:495–498.

Galloway AM, Curtis NC, Sommerland SF, et al. Correlative imaging findings in seven dogs and one cat with spinal arachnoid cysts. Vet Rad Ultrasound, 1999; 40:445–452.

Haskins ME, Bingel SA, Northington JW. Spinal cord compression and hindlimb paresis in cats with Mucopolysaccharidosis VI. J Am Vet Med Assoc, 1983; 182:983–985.

Plummer SB, Bunch SE, Khoo LH, et al. Tethered spinal cord and an intradural lipoma associated with meningocele in a Manx-type cat. J Am Vet Med Assoc, 1993; 203:1159–1161.

Vignoli M, Rossi F, Sarli G. Spinal subarachnoid cyst in a cat. Vet Rad Ultrasound, 1999; 40:116–119.

Watson AG. Congenital occipitoatlantoaxial malformation in a cat. Compend Contin Educ Prac Vet, 1985; 7:245–252.

Wilson JW. Spina bifida in the dog and cat. Compend Contin Educ Prac Vet, 1982; 4:626–632, 636–637.

Degenerative/Nutritional

Goldman AL. Hypervitaminosis A in a cat. J Am Vet Med Assoc, 1992; 200:1970–1972.

Mesfin GM, Kusewitt D, Parker A. Degenerative myelopathy in a cat. J Am Vet Med Assoc, 1980; 176:62–64.

Polizopoulou ZS, Kazakos G, Patsikas MN, et al. Hypervitaminosis A in the cat: a case report and review of the literature. J Feline Med Surg, 2005; 7:363–368.

Intervertebral Disk Disease

Knipe MF, Vernau KM, Hornof WJ, et al. Intervertebral disk extrusion in six cats. J Feline Med Surg, 2001; 3:161–168.

Lu D, Lamb CR, Wesselingh K, et al. Acute intervertebral disc extrusion in a cat: clinical and MRI findings. J Feline Med Surg, 2002; 4:65–68.

McConnell JF, Garosi LS. Intramedullary intervertebral disk extrusion in a cat. Vet Rad Ultrasound, 2004; 45:327–330.

Muñana KR, Olby NJ, Sharp NH, et al. Intervertebral disk disease in 10 cats. J Am Anim Hosp Assoc, 2001; 37:384–389.

Rayward RM. Feline intervertebral disk disease: a review of the literature. Vet Comp Orthop Traumatol 2002; 15:137–144.

Fibrocartilaginous Embolic Myelopathy

Abramson CJ, Platt SR, Stedman NL. Tetraparesis in a cat with fibrocartilaginous emboli. J Am Anim Hosp Assoc, 2002; 38:153–156.

MacKay AD, Rusbridge C, Sparkes AH, et al. MRI characteristics of suspected acute spinal cord infarction in two cats, and a review of the literature. J Feline Med Surg, 2005; 7:101–107.

Mikszewski JS, Van Winkle TJ, Troxel MT. Fibrocartilaginous embolic myelopathy in five cats. J Am Anim Hosp Assoc, 2006; 42:226–233.

Scott HW, O'Leary MT. Fibrocartilaginous embolism in a cat. J Small Anim Pract, 1996; 37:228–231.

Turner PV, Percy DH, Allyson K. Fibrocartilaginous embolic myelopathy in a cat. Can Vet J, 1995; 36:712–713.

Spinal Neoplasia

Irving G, McMillan MC. Flouroscopically guided percutaneous fine-needle aspiration biopsy of thoraco-lumbar spinal lesions in cats. Prog Vet Neurol, 1990; 1:473–475.

Lane SB, Kornegay JN, Duncan JR, et al. Feline spinal lymphosarcoma: a retrospective evaluation of 23 cats. J Vet Intern Med, 1994; 8:99–104.

Levy MS, Mauldin G, Kapatkin AS, et al. Non-lymphoid vertebral canal tumors in cats: 11 cases (1987–1995). J Am Vet Med Assoc, 1997; 210:663–664.

Noonan M, Kline KL, Meleo K. Lymphoma of the central nervous system: a retrospective study of 18 cats. Compend Contin Educ Pract Vet, 1997; 19:497–503.

O'Brien D. Osteosarcoma of the vertebra causing compression of the thoracic spinal cord in a cat. J Am Anim Hosp Assoc, 1980; 16:497–499.

Okada M, Kitagawa M, Shibuya H, et al. Malignant peripheral nerve sheath tumor arising from the spinal canal in a cat. J Vet Med Sci, 2007; 69:683–686.

Spodnick GJ, Berg J, Moore FM, et al. Spinal lymphoma in cats: 21 cases (1976–1989). J Am Vet Med Assoc, 1992; 200:373–376.

Stigen O, Ytrehus B, Eggertdottir AV. Spinal cord astrocytoma in a cat. J Small Anim Pract, 2001; 42:306–310.

Sumner J, Simpson DJ. Surgical management of a recurrent spinal meningioma in a cat. Aust Vet J, 2007; 85:276–280.

Infectious Myelopathies

Addie DD, Jarett O. Feline coronavirus infection. In Greene CE, ed, Infectious Diseases of the Dog and Cat, 2nd ed, pp 58–69. Philadelphia: W.B. Saunders, 1998.

Carmichael KP, Bienzle D, McDonnell JJ. Feline leukemia virus-associated myelopathy in cats. Vet Pathol, 39; 536–545.

Dubey JP, Benson J, Larson MA. Clinical sarcocystis neurona encephalomyelitis in a domestic cat following routine surgery. Veterinary Parasitology, 2003; 112:261–267.

Dubey JP, Lappin MR. Toxoplasmosis and neosporosis. In Greene CE, ed, Infectious diseases of the dog and cat, 2nd ed, pp 493–509. Philadelphia: W.B. Saunders, 1998.

Foureman P, Longshore R, Plummer S. Spinal cord granuloma due to *Coccidioides immitis* in a cat. J Vet Intern Med, 2005; 19:373–376.

Heidel JR, Dubey JP, Blythe LL, et al. Myelitis in a cat infected with *Toxoplasma gondii* and feline immu-nodeficiency virus. J Am Vet Med Assoc, 1990; 196:316–318.

Kline KL, Joseph RJ, Averill DR. Feline infectious peritonitis with neurologic involvement: clinical and pathologic findings in 24 cats. J Am Anim Hosp Assoc, 1994; 30:111–118.

Kornegay JN. Multiple neurologic deficits: inflammatory diseases. Probl Vet Med, 1991; 3:426–439.

Legendre AM, Whitenack DL. Feline infectious peritonitis with spinal cord involvement in two cats. J Am Vet Med Assoc, 1975; 167:31–32.

Malik R, Latter M, Love DN. Bacterial discospondylitis in a cat. J Small Anim Pract, 1990; 31:404.

Norsworthy GD. Discospondylitis as a cause of posterior paresis. Feline Pract, 1979; 9:39.

Packer RA, Coates JR, Cook CR, et al. Sublumbar abscess and diskospondylitis in a cat. Vet Radiol Ultrasound, 2005; 46:396–399.

Singh M, Foster DJ, Child G, et al. Inflammatory cerebrospinal fluid analysis in cats: clinical diagnosis and outcome. J Feline Med Surg, 2005; 7:77–93.

Vinayak A, Kerwin SC, Pool RR. Treatment of thoracolumbar spinal cord compression associated with *Histoplasma capsulatum* infection in a cat. J Am Vet Med Assoc, 2007; 230:1018–1023.

Watson E, Roberts RE. Discospondylitis in a cat. Vet Radiol Ultrasound, 1993; 34:397–398.

28
NEUROLOGIC EMERGENCIES: PERIPHERAL

Jessica M. Snyder

Unique Features

1. Ventroflexion is a common clinical sign in cats with neuromuscular disease and is most commonly associated with hypokalemia, myasthenia gravis, hyperthyroidism, and thiamine deficiency.
2. Megaesophagus and regurgitation are less common in cats with acquired myasthenia gravis than in dogs.
3. The prognosis for cats with myasthenia gravis is better than that for dogs, and the one year mortality rate for cats is 15%.
4. Diabetes mellitus should always be ruled out in the cat that presents with a plantigrade stance.
5. Cats are more sensitive to acetylcholinesterase inhibitors, and immunosuppression with prednisone is often the most effective therapy in feline myasthenia.

A. General approach
   a. Broadly, the peripheral nervous system can be subdivided into three major neuroanatomic locations: muscle, peripheral nerve, and neuromuscular junction. Clinical signs of peripheral nervous system disease are generally similar for these three divisions (see box 28.1).
B. Muscle
   a. Inflammatory myopathies
      i. Infectious (see table 28.1)
         1. Toxoplasmosis: generally cats >3 months of age
            a. Clinical signs: related to CNS, respiratory, and gastrointestinal signs; myopathic signs include muscle weakness and possible muscle pain.
            b. Diagnosis
               i. Serum IgM titer >1:64.
               ii. A fourfold increase in the serum IgG titer is indicative of a recent or active infection.
            c. Treatment: Clindamycin 10 mg/kg TID +/− trimethoprim-sulfadiazine 10–15 mg/kg PO q12h pyrimethamine 0.25–1.0 mg/kg PO q8–12h.
      ii. Immune-mediated (see table 28.1)
   b. Noninflammatory myopathies
      i. Metabolic (see table 28.1)
         1. Hypokalemic myopathy: total potassium depletion caused by decreased potassium intake, increased excretion secondary to chronic renal failure, polyuria/polydipsia secondary to

351

> **Box 28.1.** Clinical signs of peripheral nervous system disease.
> • Short-strided, choppy gait
> • Muscle weakness
> • Ventroflexion of the neck
> • Regurgitation (megaesophagus) and/or dyspnea
> • Muscle atrophy (rarely hypertrophy with primary muscle disorders)
> • Hypotonia and/or hyporeflexia
> • Fecal and urinary incontinence

Table 28.1. Causes of myopathy and neuropathy in cats.

	Myopathies	**Neuropathies**
Inflammatory: Infectious	*Toxoplasma gondii*; Clostridial myositis; Feline immunodeficiency virus	Feline leukemia virus (may see in association with urinary incontinence); feline immunodeficiency virus (generally subclinical); mycobacterial neuritis
Inflammatory: Immune mediated	Feline idiopathic polymyositis; systemic lupus erythematosus; paraneoplastic; toxin (penicillamine, cimetidine, trimethoprim-sulfa)	Paraneoplastic; chronic inflammatory demyelinating polyneuropathy; toxin (Salinomycin; Acrylamide; Pyrethrins/pyrethroid)
Congenital	Feline muscular dystrophy; myotonia congenita; hereditary myopathy of Devon Rex cats; defects of glycogen metabolism	
Metabolic	Hypokalemic myopathy; glucocorticoid myopathy; hyperthyroid myopathy; hypoadrenocorticism-associated myopathy; hypokalemic periodic paralysis	Diabetic neuropathy; hyperthyroid neuropathy; primary hyperlipoproteinemia

hyperthyroidism, diabetes mellitus, hyperaldosteronism (often accompanied with hypertension, and hypomagnesemia.

2. The most life-threatening concern for severe hypokalemia is respiratory muscle weakness resulting in hypoventilation and even respiratory arrest. This usually does not occur until potassium is <2.0–2.5 mmol/L. Mechanical ventilation will be required in these cases until normal potassium concentration is restored and respiratory muscle weakness is resolved.
   a. Laboratory abnormalities: CK elevated 10–30 times normal; serum potassium concentration <3.5 mEq/L; serum BUN and creatinine may be elevated with with renal disease.
   b. Treatment:
      i. In the stable animal, begin supplementation with potassium gluconate at 2–4 mEq PO BID until signs resolve and then maintain at 2–4 mEq PO per day.
      ii. In more severe cases, intravenous potassium chloride may be used at a dose not to exceed 0.5 mEq/kg/hr.
3. Congenital (see table 28.1)
   1. Most congenital feline myopathies manifest by 12–18 months of age.
C. Nerve
   a. Polyneuropathies

     i. Chronic (see table 28.1)

        1. Diabetic neuropathy: Classic clinical signs include a pelvic limb distal polyneuropathy with a plantigrade stance; strict glycemic control reverses the clinical signs of this neuropathy in some cats.

        2. Hyperthyroid neuropathy: Clinical signs include muscle tremors and ventroflexion of the neck; weakness typically results from the myopathic effects of disease and usually reverses with control of the hyperthyroidism.

     ii. Acute onset of flaccid tetraparesis: uncommon in cat; differential diagnoses include fulminant myasthenia gravis, black widow spider (preceded by muscle spasticity and pain progressing to flaccid tetraparesis) and coral snake envenomation, organophosphate and salinomycin toxicity, and myopathies (see above); tick paralysis and polyradiculoneuritis reported in cats but very uncommon.

  b. Mononeuropathies (see table 28.1)

     i. Peripheral nerve sheath tumors: uncommon; lymphoma, sarcoma, and carcinomas may also affect the peripheral nerve.

     ii. Trauma: Trauma can cause either temporary signs resulting from a localized conduction block in the nerve or more severe permanent signs if complete transection of the axons occurs. Treatment consists of stabilizing other systemic injuries and tincture of time. The rate of axonal regrowth is 1–4 mm/day. The time period expected for return of function of most traumatic peripheral nerve injuries is within 6 months. Beyond this time, it is unlikely that there will be return of function. The most important prognostic indicator is presence of deep pain sensation.

        1. Brachial plexus avulsion: ventral nerve roots more often affected; may see ipsilateral Horner's syndrome (a partial Horner's syndrome with miosis of the pupil should not be confused with intracranial trauma); may also see loss of the ipsilateral cutaneous trunci reflex; cats with cranial avulsions (less common than caudal plexus avulsions) may still be able to fix the elbow and bear weight on the limb.

           a. Treatment for this injury includes physical therapy (passive range of motion exercises and massage, to prevent muscle contracture) and protecting the limb from self-mutilation and from dragging on the ground. If there is no improvement within 4–6 months, it is not likely that there will be return of function, and amputation may be necessary. The prognosis for return to function is guarded.

        2. Pelvic limb: Approximately 10% of pelvic fractures in cats are associated with peripheral nerve injury (generally of the sciatic nerve); sciatic nerve injury may also be seen with intramuscular injections, bites, and lacerations of the caudal thigh; cats with sciatic nerve injuries are able to bear weight on the limb, but they walk with a plantigrade stance.

           a. Therapy for this condition includes surgical correction of pelvic fractures and tincture of time. Sciatic nerve paralysis may be treated with talocrural joint fusion and muscle transfer.

     iii. Vascular: ischemic neuromyopathy; most affected cats have hypertrophic cardiomyopathy and emboli lodge in the aortic trifurcation (brachial artery occlusion has also been reported); suspect if there are poor peripheral pulses, swollen and painful limb muscles, and cyanotic food pads. The prognosis for this condition is guarded, with a median survival of 117 days and recurrence in 25% of cats (see chap. 16—Management of Thromboembolic Disease Secondary to Heart Disease).

D. Neuromuscular junction

  a. Myasthenia gravis: rare in cats

     i. Acquired and congenital forms are possible; the acquired form involves production of antibodies against acetylcholine receptors in the postsynaptic membrane. Acquired myasthenia gravis is most commonly noted in Abyssinian cats. Myasthenia gravis may also be associated with methimazole administration in hyperthyroid cats (extremely rare; <0.5% of cats receiving methimazole) and the clinical signs can be reversible when methimazole treatment is discontinued.

ii. Clinical signs
  1. Appendicular muscle weakness (85% of cats)
  2. Regurgitation or vomiting (60%)
  3. Ventroflexion of the neck (20%)
  4. Decreased palpebral reflex (60%)
iii. Diagnostic testing
  1. Thoracic radiographs
    a. Cranial mediastinal mass present in 15% of cases.
    b. Megaesophagus in 35–40% of cases.
  2. Administration of edrophonium chloride (0.1 mg/kg IV not to exceed 0.5 mg/cat IV following pretreatment with atropine [0.02–0.04 mg/kg atropine subcutaneously 15 minutes prior to edrophonium administration]) may result in improvement in muscle strength.
  3. Serum Ach-receptor antibody titer >0.3 nM/L.
iv. Treatment: pyridostigmine (0.25 mg/kg/day) and corticosteroids (0.25–2 mg/kg/day prednisone PO).
b. Toxins
  i. Organophosphate and carbamate toxicity
    1. Clinical signs: tachycardia; tremors; muscle weakness; respiratory paralysis; salivation; lacrimation and bronchial hypersecretion; vomiting; urination; diarrhea; and possible seizures and coma.
    2. Treatment
      a. Pralidoxime chloride (2-PAM, 20–50 mg/kg diluted in 10% glucose solution and administered slowly IV) if animal showing nicotinic signs (muscle stiffness, muscle fasiculations, tremors, weakness, flaccid paralysis).
        i. 2-PAM is contraindicated in cases of carbamate intoxication.
        ii. Prior to administration, atropine should be administered at a dose of 0.1 mg/kg IV, followed by a dose of 0.3 mg/kg IM.
      b. Diazepam (0.5 mg/kg IV) may be administered to control seizure activity.
      c. Severe intoxication may require continuous electrocardiographic monitoring, oxygen therapy, potentially mechanical ventilation, and correction of metabolic acidosis.
  ii. Tick paralysis: in cats, occurs only in Australia.
  iii. Elapid neurotoxins; envenomation by black widow spider; toad poisoning; algal blooms (see chap. 40)
  iv. Drug-induced neuromuscular blockade; aminoglycoside antibiotics; streptomycin, gentamicin; antiarrhythmic agents; phenothiazines; methoxyflurane; magnesium
E. Autonomic nervous system/miscellaneous conditions
  a. Dysautonomia: rare in the United States in cats; cause undetermined but most likely is a result of changes in the autonomic ganglia affecting both sympathetic and parasympathetic nervous systems; poor prognosis.
    i. Clinical signs: may develop over a few hours to several weeks and include anorexia, obtundation, gastrointestinal stasis, dry mucous membranes, constipation, urinary bladder atony, reduced tear production, regurgitation or vomiting, protrusion of the nictating membranes, mydriasis, and bradycardia
    ii. Diagnostic testing
      1. Response to one drop of 0.1% pilocarpine in the eye
        a. There should be no change in normal cats. Denervation hypersensitivity in cats with dysautonomia results in miosis and retraction of the third eyelid.

2. One drop of 0.25% physostigmine in the eye
   a. Rapid miosis will occur in the normal cat and no response will occur in the cat with dysautonomia.
3. Plasma catecholamine assay
   a. May be decreased in cats with dysautonomia, but these are not commonly measured.
iii. Treatment: primarily symptomatic and supportive
   1. Promote gastrointestinal motility
      a. Cisapride 2.5–5.0 mg/cat PO q8–12h
      b. Metoclopramide 0.2–0.4 mg/kg IM, IV, PO 30 minutes prior to feeding
   2. Decrease urinary retention
      a. Bethanecol 2.5 mg/cat PO q8–12h (monitor for bradycardia/cardiac arrhythmias)
   3. Stimulate lacrimation
      a. Pilocarpine 1% one drop OU q6h
   4. General supportive care
      a. Express bladder, colon care
      b. Physical therapy
      c. Maintain feeding and hydration
b. Megaesophagus: uncommon in cats. Prognosis is fair to guarded.
   i. Causes: idiopathic (43% of cats), myasthenia gravis, mediastinal mass, vascular ring anomalies and other congenital disease, dysautonomia, esophageal stricture, and lead toxicosis.
   ii. Treatment:
      1. Treat underlying cause. It is rare that megaesophagus resolves once it develops.
      2. Supportive care
         a. Sucralfate 0.25 g/cat PO BID–TID to reduce esophagitis secondary to regurgitation
         b. H$_2$ antagonists (famotidine at 0.5 mg/kg SID–BID or ranitidine at 2.5–3.5 mg/kg BID). Used to decrease stomach pH, which may help reduce esophageal irritation in dogs with reflux esophagitis.
         c. Metoclopramide 0.2–0.4 mg/kg as a prokinetic to promote gastrointestinal motility. Of questionable benefit with megaesophagus.
         d. Feed from elevated position (gruel/liquid diet) and encourage to remain in upright position for 10–15 minutes after feeding.
c. Tetanus: rare in cats, but generalized and localized forms of disease have been reported in cats.
   i. Clinical signs: seen within 21 days (usually 5–10 days) of wound contamination and may progress to generalized contraction and rigidity of appendicular and facial muscles, then recumbency with extension of all four limbs and opisthotonus. Respiratory depression and paralysis may occur in generalized cases, and mechanical ventilation may be required.
   ii. Treatment
      1. Wound debridement
      2. Antibiotics such as penicillin G (20,000–80,000 IU/kg IV or IM TID), metronidazole (10 mg/kg IV BID–TID), or clindamycin (3–10 mg/kg IV BID–TID)
      3. Administration of antitoxin (100–1,000 IU/kg IV) after pretreatment with diphenhydramine 1 mg/kg IM +/– dexamethasone 0.1–0.2 mg/kg IV. Corticosteroids are indicated if a hypersensitivity reaction to antitoxin is suspected.
      4. Sedation if needed (intravenous diazepam 0.5 mg/kg IV PRN, phenobarbital 1–3 mg/kg IV BID, acepromazine 0.02–0.1 mg/kg IV, IM, SC PRN (caution as acepromazine can cause hypotension)
      5. Minimize stimulation (keep cat in a quiet, dimly lit area).
      6. Nursing care
d. Urinary system dysfunction: Failure to completely empty the bladder can be attributed to failure of detrusor contractile function, anatomic or functional urethral obstruction, or both. Anatomic

obstructive disorders are more common and should always be ruled out, especially if no other neurologic deficits are present.

i. An upper motor neuron bladder is large, firm, and difficult to express. The urethral sphincter tone may be increased. This type of bladder is seen with spinal lesions cranial to L5-7.

1. Diagnostic evaluation: See chapter 27 for diagnostic approach to spinal cord disease. Additionally, consider CBC, serum chemistry, urinalysis and urine culture, and imaging of the urinary tract (survey or contrast radiography or ultrasonography). Urodynamic studies (cystometrogram, urethral pressure profiles) may add additional information.

2. Therapeutic plan

a. Address primary neurologic, metabolic, or obstructive disease.

b. Prevent urinary bladder from becoming overdistended. Place indwelling urinary catheter to empty bladder and to keep bladder small, or intermittently catheterize or manually express bladder.

c. Treat urinary tract infection, if present. Monitor for development of urinary tract infection.

d. Decrease urethral resistance with diazepam (0.2–0.5 mg/kg IV prior to expression) or phenoxybenzamine (1.25–5 mg/cat PO SID–BID). Blood pressure should be monitored in the animal receiving phenoxybenzamine, and the effects may not be seen for 2–3 days. This drug should be used with caution in cases of cardiac disease, renal disease, or diabetes mellitus. Oral diazepam may be used in cats, but owners should be cautioned of the risk of hepatic necrosis.

ii. A lower motor neuron bladder is flaccid, distended, and easily expressed. This type of bladder is seen with spinal lesions caudal to L5-L7, with peripheral neuropathies, and with autonomic dysfunction (dysautonomia). Bladder atony may also result from chronic distention secondary to urinary retention (seen in cats that are stressed, painful, or receiving anticholinergic agents, opioids, or tricyclic antidepressants, or post urethral obstruction).

1. Diagnostic evaluation: See diagnostic approach to upper motor neuron bladder above.

2. Therapeutic plan: See therapeutic plan for upper motor neuron bladder above.

a. Consider Bethanecol at 1.5–5 mg per cat PO TID. Bethanecol is contraindicated in cases of gastrointestinal or urinary obstruction. Bethanecol may increase urethral resistance in some cases, and should be administered with phenoxybenzamine (1.25–5 mg/cat PO q12–24h) or diazepam (0.1–0.5 mg/kg PO q12–24h, risk of hepatotoxicity in some cats) if this occurs.

b. Other agents used less frequently to increase bladder contraction include:

i. Metoclopramide 0.2–0.4 mg/kg IM, PO, SC q6h

ii. Cisapride 0.1–1 mg/kg PO q8–12h

1. Cisapride is no longer commercially available; must be obtained through a compounding pharmacy.

29
HEMATOLOGIC EMERGENCIES: BLEEDING

Susan G. Hackner

Unique Features
— Primary thrombocytopenia is uncommon in cats. The majority of cats with thrombocytopenia have an underlying disease. Most common are viral (FeLV, FIP), neoplasia, and hepatobiliary disease.
— DIC in cats is characterized by microvascular thrombosis. Overt hemorrhage is unusual. When it occurs, it is a late-stage event, always preceded by thrombosis.

---

1. General
   a. Bleeding disorders may be due to disorders of primary or secondary hemostasis, or both.
      i. Primary hemostatic disorders result from either thrombocytopenia, platelet dysfunction (thrombopathia), or rarely, from vasculopathies.
      ii. Secondary hemostatic disorders (coagulopathies) result from low concentration or activity of coagulation factors.
      iii. Mixed hemostatic disorders occur when primary and secondary disorders coexist, such as in disseminated intravascular coagulation (DIC).
   b. Spontaneous bleeding disorders are uncommon in cats, but subclinical hemostatic abnormalities are relatively common, particularly in cats with underlying disease, such as neoplasia, viral disease, or hepatopathy.
   c. The vast majority of bleeding disorders in cats are acquired.
   d. Bleeding disorders should always be considered life-threatening. Even the stable patient can decompensate rapidly due to massive bleeding, or bleeding into a vital organ.
2. Presenting signs
   a. Clinical signs are extremely variable and depend on the site, extent, and duration of hemorrhage, as well as the presence of any underlying disorder.
   b. Clinical status can range from stable to extremely compromised.
   c. The patient with a bleeding disorder may demonstrate:
      i. Abnormal hemostatic testing, in the absence of any evidence of bleeding.
      ii. Bleeding that is evident to the owner (e.g., epistaxis)
      iii. Apparently unrelated symptoms due to bleeding (such as blindness due to hyphema)
      iv. Compromised hemodynamics and/or organ function as a result of acute hemorrhage:
         1. If acute, substantial blood loss has occurred, signs of hypoperfusion predominate.
         2. Hemorrhage into the brain, spinal cord, myocardium, or lungs can result in acute organ compromise without significant anemia or shock.

   1. Primary survey
   2. Establish vascular access.
   3. Collect pretreatment blood samples:
       -   minimum database (MDB)
       -   blood smear
       -   EDTA plasma (for later CBC, reticulocyte count, platelet count, blood typing, immune
           testing, PCR, etc.)
       -   serum (for later chemistry profile, serologic testing, etc.)
       -   citrated plasma (for later coagulation testing)
   4. Initiate therapy to stabilize the patient:
       -   support of airway and/or breathing, if indicated
       -   control of hemorrhage, if present
       -   fluid therapy, as needed to maintain adequate perfusion
       -   blood transfusion, if sufficient compromise exists due to massive hemorrhage or
           anemic crisis
   5. Secondary survey
       -   complete history
       -   thorough physical examination
       -   MDB interpretation
   6. Formulate problem list and differentials
   7. Formulate plan, and write orders, for ongoing supportive care and monitoring
   8. Diagnostic workup
   9. Specific therapy

Fig. 29.1.   Approach to the emergent bleeding patient.

      v.   Signs related to anemia from subacute or chronic hemorrhage
           1. If bleeding has been gradual, and there has been sufficient time for compensatory fluid shifts,
              the patient is weak and lethargic, but hemodynamically stable. Mucus membranes are pale,
              and a flow murmur may be evident.
           2. Severe anemia that overwhelms compensatory mechanisms results in an anemic crisis. The
              patient is depressed or moribund, with pallor, tachypnea, tachycardia, and bounding pulses.
   3. Initial stabilization and monitoring
      a. The patient in crisis requires rapid intervention, with an initial goal of stabilizing life-threatening
         emergencies (fig. 29.1).
      b. A primary survey is performed to determine if a life-threatening situation exists. (see chap. 1—Approach
         to the Critically Ill Cat). Hypovolemic shock, an anemic crisis, and pulmonary or brain hemorrhage
         constitute life-threatening situations in the bleeding patient.
      c. Venous access should be established without delay, by placement of a peripheral catheter.
      d. Blood is collected from the catheter immediately following placement, for a minimum database,
         including a PCV and total solids (TS).
      e. Additional blood samples should be collected prior to initiating therapy, to avoid treatment-induced
         changes in laboratory parameters. These should include:
         i.   blood smear
         ii. serum sample
         iii. EDTA-plasma sample
         iv. citrated-plasma sample(s) (preferably two)
      f. Initial therapy is aimed at stabilizing the patient while diagnostic testing continues. It includes:
         i.   Control of hemorrhage, where possible
         ii. Blood volume replacement, if the patient is hypoperfused. In hemorrhagic shock, hypoperfusion
              constitutes the most life-threatening problem. Initial therapy, therefore, is aimed at correcting
              perfusion via aggressive fluid therapy (crystalloid +/– colloid) until blood is available. There is no

justification to withhold fluid therapy in the anemic patient. Hypoperfusion will only serve to exacerbate the tissue hypoxia.

  iii. Blood transfusion, if anemic crisis or massive hemorrhage

g. Secondary survey. Once stabilization is initiated, attention should be focused on the rapid establishment of a diagnosis. This begins with a thorough history and physical examination. This allows generation of an initial problem list and differentials, and formulation of a diagnostic plan.

h. Ongoing care and monitoring. Pending diagnosis and institution of specific therapy, a plan should be formulated, and orders written, for supportive care and monitoring (see chap. 1—Approach to the Critically Ill Cat).

  i. Absolute cage rest should be prescribed and enforced.

  ii. Avoid unnecessary surgical or medical procedures that could exacerbate bleeding.

  iii. Subcutaneous injections should be avoided where possible.

  iv. Venipuncture should only be performed when required for platelet enumeration. Venipuncture sites should be held off with manual pressure for 5 minutes.

  v. Jugular veins should never be used for venipuncture in the coagulopathic patient as bleeding from this site can be difficult, if not impossible, to control.

  vi. An intravenous sampling catheter can usually be safely placed in the femoral vein and used to collect all other blood samples.

  vii. The patient should be closely monitored for evidence of ongoing or recurrent hemorrhage. This includes, at a minimum:

    1. Perfusion status, mucous membrane color, pulse rate, and quality
    2. General attitude
    3. Respiratory rate and effort
    4. Neurologic status
    5. Temperature
    6. PCV/TS
    7. Blood pressure

4. Clinical assessment

a. General: The clinical assessment of the bleeding patient includes a history, physical examination, and a few selected screening laboratory tests. The information gleaned from these should answer three initial questions that will narrow the list of differentials and guide a systematic and efficient diagnostic workup:

  i. Is the bleeding due to local factors, or does the patient have a generalized bleeding disorder?

  ii. If a systemic bleeding disorder does exist, what is the nature of the defect (primary or secondary hemostasis)?

  iii. Is the defect congenital or acquired?

b. History

  i. The history should aim to determine whether bleeding is due to local factors or to a systemic bleeding disorder, and to try to narrow down the possible etiologies.

  ii. The signalment of the patient may be informative. Inherited disorders are generally apparent within the first 6 months of life. Some milder forms, however, may not be diagnosed until surgery, trauma, or concurrent disease precipitate bleeding.

  iii. Questions should ascertain:

    1. If there is bleeding in multiple sites that may indicate a systemic bleeding disorder
    2. If there is a history of repeated bleeding episodes that may indicate an inherited or longstanding disorder
    3. Whether bleeding occurred spontaneously or was precipitated by injury or surgery. Some disorders (e.g., thrombocytopenia) produce spontaneous bleeding, whereas milder forms of these diseases and other conditions (e.g., hemophilia) more commonly require some form of trauma or surgery to make the impairment clinically apparent.

Table 29.1. Clinical features helpful in differentiating primary and secondary hemostatic disorders.

Disorders of Primary Hemostasis	Disorders of Secondary Hemostasis
Petechiae common	Petechiae rare
Hematomas rare	Hematomas common
Bleeding often involves mucous membranes	Bleeding into muscles and joints common
Bleeding usually at multiple sites	Bleeding frequently localized
Prolonged bleeding from cuts or venipuncture	Bleeding may be delayed at onset, or stop and start again

4. The response to previous trauma. This may enable the clinician to date the onset of the disorder. A patient who has tolerated surgery is unlikely to have an inherited bleeding disorder.

5. Previous or current illnesses. Some systemic diseases can compromise hemostasis and precipitate clinical bleeding, particularly in a patient with an already compromised hemostatic mechanism.

6. Past and present medications. Numerous drugs have been associated with thrombocytopenia (e.g., methimazole), thrombopathias, and coagulopathies (e.g., phenobarbital).

7. Home environment and exposure to other cats, to elucidate the potential of infectious disease

8. Environmental and behavioral history, to determine potential exposure to toxins, trauma, or insect vectors

9. Medical history of family members, where available

c. Physical examination

  i. A thorough physical examination should focus particular attention on the following:

  1. The distribution and extent of current hemorrhage

     a. This requires careful examination of all body systems, including the skin, mucous membranes, eyes, and joints, as well as the urine and feces. The ear pinna is a common site of petechiation in the cat.

     b. The presence of hemorrhage in more than one site suggests a bleeding disorder.

     c. The nature of the hemorrhage helps to characterize the defect (table 29.1).

        i. Defects of primary hemostasis are characterized by petechiation or ecchymosis, as well as spontaneous bleeding from mucosal surfaces, including epistaxis, gingival bleeding, hyphema, hematuria, and melena.

        ii. Defects of secondary hemostasis are usually characterized by single or multiple hematomas and bleeding into subcutaneous tissue, body cavities, muscles, or joints.

        iii. Some acquired disorders, such as DIC, defy this classification because multiple hemostatic defects are present.

  2. Evidence of any systemic disease that may impair hemostasis. These include: neoplasia, viral disease, and hepatopathy.

  3. Evidence of immune-mediated disease (e.g., cutaneous or mucocutaneous lesions, arthropathy, chorioretinitis)

d. Screening laboratory tests (table 29.2)

  i. The screening laboratory tests globally evaluate aspects of primary and secondary hemostasis.

  ii. These tests need to be performed carefully and interpreted in the light of clinical findings, with their limitations in mind.

  iii. The usual screening panel includes platelet enumeration, prothrombin time (PT), partial thromboplastin time (PTT), and fibrin split products (FSPs) or D-dimers. In the emergency setting, platelet enumeration, PT, and PTT (or an activated clotting time, ACT) are generally sufficient to allow characterization and to guide further testing.

Table 29.2. Screening laboratory tests of hemostasis.

Screening Test	Component(s) Evaluated	Reference Values
Primary hemostasis		
Platelet enumeration	Platelet numbers	$200–600 \times 10^3/\mu L$
Platelet estimation[a]	Platelet numbers	11–25/hpf
BMBT[a]	Platelet numbers and function, vascular integrity	1.4–3.2 min.
Secondary hemostasis		
Activated clotting time (ACT)[a]	Intrinsic and common pathways: factors XII, XI, IX, VIII, X, V, II, and fibrinogen	50–75 sec.
Prothrombin time (PT)[b]	Extrinsic and common pathways: factors III, VII, X, V, II and fibrinogen	9–12 sec.[c]
Partial thromboplastin time (PTT)[b]	As with ACT, but more sensitive	15–21 sec.[c]
Fibrinolysis		
Fibrin split products (FSPs)[b]	Products of fibrinolysis	$<10 \mu g/mL$
D-dimers[b]	Products of fibrinolysis, specific for lysis of cross-linked fibrin	<250 mg/dL

a. In-house test.
b. In-house testing option(s) available.
c. Reference values are laboratory- and technique-dependent. Normal values for patient-side coagulometers are provided by the manufacturer.

iv. General principles
1. Blood samples should be collected prior to the initiation of any therapy.
2. Hemostatic tests make high demands on sampling techniques. Improper technique or handling leads to false results.
3. For platelet enumeration, EDTA blood is required. Most of the other hemostatic tests are performed on citrated blood or plasma. Citrated tubes contain sufficient volume of citrate solution such that the ratio of citrate to blood is 1:9. Should there be deviations in this ratio, false test results are obtained. This ratio, however, is valid for animals with a physiologic hematocrit. It can be adjusted via controlled underfilling for patients with a markedly decreased hematocrit.
4. Blood collection should be performed without, or after brief (<30-second), venous congestion. Puncture should be quick and atraumatic. Puncture of the same vein should not be repeated within 30 minutes. Venipuncture of the jugular veins should be avoided in the patient with a bleeding tendency, as bleeding from this site can be extremely difficult to control.
5. Collected blood should be rapidly and thoroughly mixed with the anticoagulant via careful inversion and rotation.

v. Platelet enumeration (platelet count)
1. The platelet count detects quantitative platelet disorders. A count should be performed in all patients with a suspected bleeding disorder.
2. Feline platelets tend to clump rapidly, placing high demand on rapid and atraumatic sampling. Even with excellent technique, however, clumping can occur. Decreased counts, therefore, should always be verified via blood smear examination.
3. In cats, there is considerable overlap between erythrocyte and platelet volumes, resulting in erroneous results from automated cell counters. Feline platelets should therefore be enumerated manually (via hemocytometer).

vi. Platelet estimation (via blood smear)
1. Blood smear examination allows for rapid estimation of platelet numbers.
2. This is essential in the emergency setting where manual enumeration is often not feasible and automated counts are frequently inaccurate.
3. Accurate assessment is highly dependent on the quality of the smear and systematic, careful evaluation.
4. Feline platelets clump readily. It is therefore extremely important to assess the feathered edge of the smear for platelet clumps. If large clumps are present, platelet numbers are likely adequate and counts from this sample will be erroneously low.
5. In a well-distributed smear without platelet clumps, approximately 11–25 platelets per oil immersion or high-power field (1,000×) is considered normal. In such a field, each platelet represents a count of approximately 15,000/μL.
6. Large platelets (macroplatelets or "shift" platelets) generally indicate megakaryocytic hyperplasia and a regenerative response but may also be seen with viral diseases and myelodysplastic syndromes.

vii. Buccal mucosal bleeding time (BMBT)
1. The BMBT reflects in vivo primary hemostasis. It is prolonged with thrombocytopenia, thrombopathia, or vascular anomalies.
2. It is indicated in patients with a suspected primary hemostatic defect when the platelet count is adequate. The test is unnecessary in the thrombocytopenic patient.
3. Cats usually require light sedation. The patient is restrained in lateral recumbency. A strip of gauze is tied around the maxilla to fold up the upper lip tightly enough to cause moderate mucosal engorgement. In cats, there may not be sufficient space to accommodate this, and the lip must be held manually. A two-blade, spring-loaded device (Simplate II, Organon Teknika Corporation, Jessup, MD) is used to make two 1-mm-deep incisions in the mucosa of the upper lip. The incisions should be made at a site devoid of visible vessels and inclined so that the blood flows toward the mouth. Shed blood is carefully blotted with filter paper, taking extreme care not to disturb the incisions. The BMBT is the time from incision to cessation of bleeding (fig. 29.2).
4. Normal BMBT in the cat is less than 3.2 minutes.

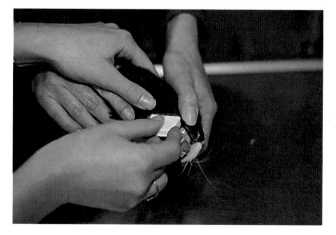

Fig. 29.2. Performance of a buccal mucosal bleeding test. A spring-loaded device is used to make two 1-mm incisions in the upper lip.

viii. Activated clotting time (ACT)
1. The ACT is a simple in-office screening test for the intrinsic and common coagulation pathways (fig. 29.3).
2. In the traditional ACT, blood (2 mL) is drawn into a prewarmed (37°C) commercial tube containing diatomaceous earth, which serves as a chemical activator. (The first few drops of blood are discarded because of the possible presence of tissue factor.) The sample is mixed by inversion and then placed into a 37°C heat block or water bath for 50 seconds. It is inverted every 10 seconds, observed for clot formation, and replaced. The ACT is the time interval to first clot formation (table 29.2).
3. A patient-side coagulometer (SCA 2000, Synbiotics, San Diego, CA) allows automated ACT testing. Given that this coagulometer also enables PT and PTT testing, which are more sensitive, the use of the ACT in this situation is hard to justify.
4. The ACT test is relatively insensitive. A single coagulation factor must be decreased to less than 10% of normal before ACT prolongation occurs.
5. ACT prolongation may be due to:
   a. Severe anomaly/anomalies of the intrinsic and/or common coagulation pathways
   b. Severe thrombocytopenia (<10,000 platelets/µL)
   c. Some thrombopathias
   d. Hypofibrinogenemia
ix. Partial thromboplastin time (PTT)
1. The PTT tests the intrinsic and common pathways (fig. 29.3). Only factors VII and XIII are not evaluated.
2. This test is more sensitive than the ACT and is not affected by primary hemostatic disorders.

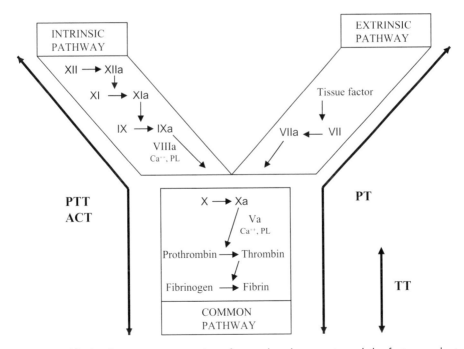

Fig. 29.3. A simplified, schematic representation of secondary hemostasis and the factors evaluated by the screening laboratory tests. PT = prothrombin time; PTT = partial thromboplastin time; ACT = activated clotting time; Ca = calcium; PL = platelet phospholipid.

      3. In general, at least one factor must be decreased to below 25–30% of normal concentration before prolongation occurs.

      4. A patient-side coagulometer (SCA 2000, Synbiotics, San Diego, CA) is an attractive alternative to conventional laboratory PTT determination in the emergency setting.

          a. While the methodology enables testing of either nonanticoagulated blood or citrated whole blood, the latter is preferable with respect to sensitivity and specificity.

          b. Using citrated whole blood, reported sensitivity in dogs is 100%, with a specificity of approximately 83%. As such, it is an excellent screening test for defects of the intrinsic and common pathways. False positives, however, do occur.

          c. A prolonged PTT on the SCA should be validated via conventional laboratory testing. In the author's experience, marked prolongations are usually clinically significant; mild prolongations should be interpreted with caution.

   x. Prothrombin time (PT)

      1. The PT tests the extrinsic and the common pathways (fig. 29.3). It is the principal test of the extrinsic pathway.

      2. Because of the short half-life of factor VII, the PT is very sensitive to vitamin K deficiency or antagonism. It is less sensitive to heparin than is the PTT.

      3. The patient-side coagulometer is a relatively accurate methodology for PT testing.

          a. Using citrated whole blood, reported sensitivity and specificity in dogs are approximately 86% and 96%, respectively. That is, some defects of the extrinsic system will not be detected, and false positives occur.

          b. In the author's experience, this instrument is reliable in detecting clinically significant disorders of the extrinsic pathway that result in hemorrhage. Mild defects, however, may not be detected, and mild prolongations should be interpreted with caution.

          c. Results that do not correlate with clinical findings should be verified via conventional laboratory testing.

   xi. Thrombin time (TT)

      1. The TT assesses the conversion of fibrinogen to fibrin (the common pathway) and bypasses all other steps (fig. 29.3).

      2. The TT may be prolonged by hypofibrinogenemia (<100 mg/dL), by dysfibrinogenemia, or by substances that inhibit thrombin (heparin, FSPs).

   xii. Fibrin split products (FSPs)

      1. FSPs are generated with fibrinolysis.

      2. Elevated FSP concentrations commonly occur in DIC but are not universally present, nor specific for the syndrome. Increased concentrations can also occur in hepatic disease (due to enhanced fibrinolysis and reduced clearance). False elevations may occur in patients on heparin therapy, or those with dysfibrinogenemia.

      3. Commercial latex agglutination kits (Thrombo-Wellcotest, Wellcome Reagents, Beckenham, England) constitute a rapid, semi-quantitative method for FSP determination (table 29.2).

   xiii. D-dimers

      1. D-dimers are unique FSPs that are formed when cross-linked fibrin is lysed by plasmin.

      2. In contrast to FSPs, D-dimers are specific for active coagulation and fibrinolysis.

      3. The half-life of D-dimers is short. As such, they are only useful for detection of recent or ongoing fibrinolysis.

      4. D-dimers are a relatively sensitive test for DIC, and likely superior to traditional FSP assays. However, they are neither universal nor specific for DIC. Elevated concentrations have been demonstrated in dogs with thromboembolism, intracavitary hemorrhage, neoplasia, hepatic disease, renal failure, cardiac failure, and following surgical procedures. Less is known about the significance of D-dimers in feline patients.

5. As with FSPs, D-dimers should be considered an ancillary diagnostic test, with the diagnosis of DIC relying on the appropriate constellation of clinical findings and abnormal results of hemostatic testing.

6. The traditional laboratory assay of D-dimers is the ELISA test. An in-office latex bead agglutination test (Accuclot D-dimer, Sigma) has been shown to compare favorably in dogs but remains to be fully evaluated in cats.

5. Diagnostic approach
   a. Bleeding disorders are classified as disorders of primary or secondary hemostasis (figs. 29.4 and 29.5). Since etiologies are distinct, this classification is an essential early step in the diagnostic workup. Distinction is generally possible from the history and physical examination.
   b. If a disorder of primary hemostasis is suspected (fig. 29.6):
      i. Platelet enumeration/estimation is the first step. It is extremely important that sampling is performed correctly and that a smear is evaluated to assess for platelet clumping, thus avoiding erroneous interpretation (see above).
      ii. If the platelet count is sufficiently low to explain spontaneous bleeding (<40,000/μL), then workup for thrombocytopenia should follow (see below—Specific conditions: Thrombocytopenia).
      iii. If the platelet count does not explain bleeding, assess tests for secondary hemostasis.
          1. If the platelet count is normal and PT and/or PTT (or ACT) is prolonged, then a disorder of secondary hemostasis should be pursued.
          2. If the platelet count is mildly or moderately decreased and PT and/or PTT (or ACT) is prolonged, then there is either a combined defect or a disorder of secondary hemostasis with consumptive thrombocytopenia due to bleeding.
          3. If platelet counts and tests for secondary hemostasis are normal, a BMBT should be performed to assess in vivo primary hemostasis.
   c. If a disorder of secondary hemostasis is suspected (fig. 29.7):
      i. Review the history regarding the possibility of an inherited disorder.
      ii. Assess PT and PTT.
          1. If PT is prolonged and PTT is normal, there is a disorder in the extrinsic pathway (factor VII). This could be caused by early anticoagulant rodenticide toxicity, warfarin therapy, an inherited factor VII deficiency, or (occasionally) early hepatic failure or biliary obstruction. Following collection of samples, plasma transfusion and vitamin K can be administered if needed (see below, 6.c. Acquired vitamin K deficiency).
          2. If PTT is prolonged and PT is normal, there is a disorder(s) in the intrinsic pathway. This is seen with DIC, heparin therapy, hepatic failure (less commonly), or an inherited coagulopathy. Evaluation of D-dimers or FSPs, platelet count, viral serology, and hepatic function should follow.
          3. If both PT and PTT are prolonged, there are multiple disorders or there is a disorder in the common pathway.
             a. Evaluate for DIC (clinical evidence, D-dimers or FSPs, platelet enumeration). If findings are compatible, search for underlying disorder (neoplasia, viral, etc).
             b. Evaluate for hepatopathy.
             c. Consider anticoagulant rodenticide intoxication or other cause of vitamin K deficiency.
             d. Consider a circulating anticoagulant. If no compatible drug history, verify the presence of an anticoagulant by mixing patient plasma and normal plasma at ratio of 1:1 and repeating the tests. The absence of an anticoagulant will result in normalization of testing.
             e. If above are negative, or deemed extremely unlikely, consider an inherited disorder and submit samples for specific factor assays.
                i. Comparative Coagulation Section. Animal Health Diagnostic Center. College of Veterinary Medicine, Cornell University. (607) 253-3900. www.diaglab.vet.cornell.edu/coag/

Thrombocytopenia
Decreased production (megakaryocytic hypoplasia):
Pure megakaryocytic hypoplasia
Immune-mediated megakaryocytic hypoplasia
Vaccination (panleukopenia virus)
Infectious (FeLV, FIV)
Panhypoplasia
Aplastic pancytopenia
Infectious: FeLV, FIP, FIV, chronic ehrlichiosis, parvovirus, endotoxemia/septicemia
Drug-associated: chemotherapeutic agents, griseofulvin, sulfadiazine, methimazole, albendazole
Myelophthisis
Myelofibrosis
Hematopoietic neoplasia
Dysthrombopoiesis
Myelodysplastic syndromes (MDS)
Increased destruction:
Immune-mediated (ITP)
Primary idiopathic
Secondary
Drugs (methimazole, propylthiouracil, cephalosporins, penicillin, oxytetracycline, phenobarbital)
Viral (FeLV, FIP)
Neoplasia
Rickettsial disease (ehrlichiosis, hemobartonellosis)
Bacterial infection
Infectious
Viral: FeLV, FIV, FIP, parvovirus
Rickettsial: Hemobartonellosis, ehrlichiosis
Protozoal: cytauxzoonosis
Bacterial: bacteremia, sepsis, leptospirosis, salmonellosis
Fungal: histoplasmosis, disseminated candidiasis
Consumption/sequestration:
Disseminated intravascular coagulation
Sepsis
Vasculitis
Hepatic disease
Profound, acute hemorrhage
Microangiopathy (hemangiosarcoma, splenic disease)
Thrombopathia
Acquired:
Hepatic disease
Myeloproliferative disorders
Dysproteinemia (myeloma)
Uremia
Drugs (calcium channel blockers, dextran, hetastarch, propanalol, cephalosporins, sulfonamides, aminophylline, isoproteranol)
Inherited:
Von Willebrand's disease
Type I (Himalayan)
Type III (domestic shorthair, domestic longhair)
Chediak-Higashi syndrome (Persian cats)
Vascular Disorders
Vasculitis (FIP)
Hyperadrenocorticism

Fig. 29.4. Causes of primary hemostatic disorders in cats.

Acquired:
Disseminated intravascular coagulation
Hepatopathy
Vitamin K deficiency/antagonism
       Anticoagulant rodenticide intoxication
       Hepatic disease, extrahepatic biliary obstruction
       Pancreatic insufficiency
       Phenobarbital
Circulating anticoagulants
Hornet venom

Inherited factor deficiencies:
I:	Hypo/dysfibrinogenemia (domestic shorthair, domestic longhair)
VII:	Hypoproconvertinemia (domestic shorthair)
VIII:	Hemophilia A (Abyssinian, domestic shorthair, domestic longhair, Havana brown, Himalayan, Siamese)
IX:	Hemophilia B (British shorthair, domestic shorthair, domestic longhair, Siamese)
X:	Stuart Prower trait (domestic shorthair)
XII:	Hageman factor deficiency (domestic shorthair, domestic longhair, Siamese)
Other:	Vitamin K-dependent factors (Devon rex)

Fig. 29.5.   Causes of secondary hemostatic disorders in cats.

     f. Plasma transfusion can be given if necessary. Because this can interfere with future hemostatic testing, however, samples for laboratory testing should be collected prior to transfusion. Vitamin K therapy should be initiated if there is concern for deficiency/ antagonism.

  iii. If only ACT testing is available:

    1. If ACT is prolonged:

      a. Consider DIC, hepatic failure, vitamin K deficiency/antagonism, circulating anticoagulant, or an inherited coagulopathy. Consider the possibility of erroneous prolongation due to severe thrombocytopenia or thrombopathia.

      b. Evaluate a blood smear for platelet estimation.

      c. Evaluate hepatic values.

      d. Submit samples for PT, PTT, D-dimers (or FSP) testing, prior to any therapy. Save additional plasma.

      e. Initiate therapy, if required, with fresh frozen plasma. If rodenticide intoxication or hepatic failure is considered possible, vitamin K therapy should be initiated. For long-acting rodenticide intoxication, vitamin K is administered at 3–5 mg/kg/day SC, IM, or PO; for short-acting rodenticides, and other vitamin K deficiencies, doses of 1–2 mg/kg/day SC, IM, PO are considered adequate. High doses (>5 mg/kg) can result in Heinz body anemia.

    2. If ACT is normal:

      a. Consider the possibility of a primary hemostatic disorder. Evaluate blood smear for platelet estimation.

      b. Consider the insensitivity of the ACT, and the possibility of a subtle disorder. Submit samples for PT, PTT, D-dimers (or FSP) testing, prior to any therapy. Save additional plasma.

6. Specific conditions

  a. Thrombocytopenia

    i. General

      1. Thrombocytopenia can be due to decreased platelet production, destruction, consumption, or sequestration (fig. 29.4).

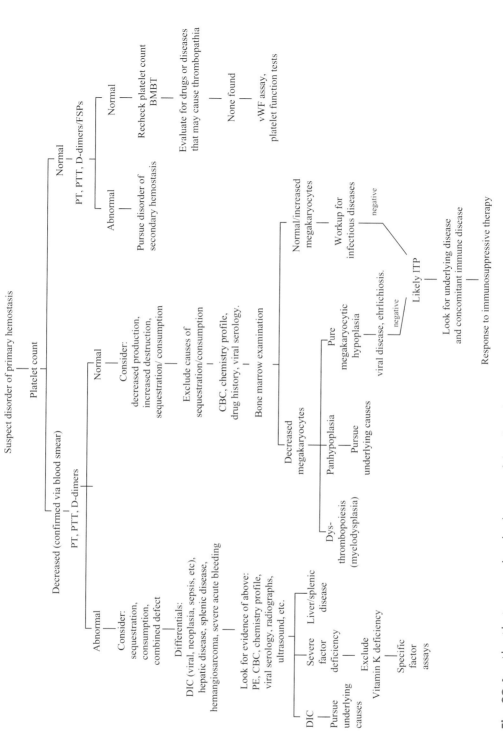

Fig. 29.6. Algorithmic approach to the diagnosis of disorders of primary hemostasis. PT = prothrombin time; PTT = partial thromboplastin time; FSPs = fibrin split products; DIC = disseminated intravascular coagulation; BMBT = buccal mucosal bleeding time; ITP = immune-mediated thrombocytopenia; vWf = von Willebrand factor.

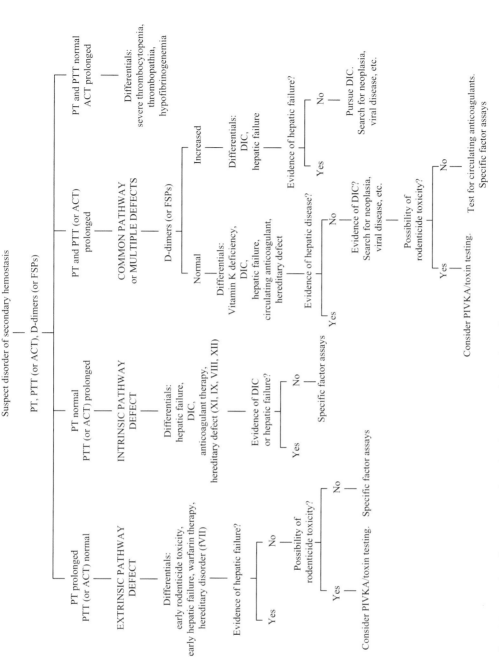

Fig. 29.7. Algorithmic approach to the diagnosis of disorders of secondary hemostasis. PT = prothrombin time; PTT = partial thromboplastin time; FSPs = fibrin split products; ACT = activated clotting time; DIC = disseminated intravascular coagulation; PIVKA = test for proteins induced by vitamin K absence or antagonism.

2. Most thrombocytopenic patients do not bleed overtly. Rather, they are presented for lethargy, weakness, or clinical signs related to the underlying disease. Thrombocytopenia is often first identified on blood work.

3. Spontaneous bleeding generally does not occur until platelet counts are below approximately 40,000/μL, unless another concomitant bleeding disorder exists. Many patients will tolerate lower counts without evidence of hemorrhage.

4. CBC may show evidence of other cytopenias (nonregenerative anemia, leukopenia). This suggests marrow panhypoplasia and is an absolute indication for bone marrow examination.

5. Primary idiopathic thrombocytopenia is relatively uncommon in cats (estimated at less than 2%). The majority of cats with thrombocytopenia have underlying disease. Most common are viral disease (approx. 30%) and neoplasia (approx. 20%). It is imperative, therefore, that a finding of thrombocytopenia prompts a thorough workup for underlying disorder(s).

6. The drug history should be carefully appraised for any drug(s) that may be associated with thrombocytopenia, and the potential for infectious disease thoroughly investigated (fig. 29.4).

7. The secondary hemostatic mechanisms should be evaluated in all thrombocytopenic patients, to evaluate for DIC or other combined defects.

8. If the cause of thrombocytopenia is not obvious (e.g., compatible drug history), bone marrow examination is indicated to evaluate platelet production. This is important in feline patients because primary thrombocytopenia is uncommon, and intramarrow disorders are common.
   a. Both a bone marrow aspirate and a core biopsy should be collected.
      i. Bone marrow aspirate cytology allows rapid interpretation of megakaryocyte numbers and evaluation of cellular morphology. At least three good quality smears must be evaluated.
      ii. Histopathology (via core biopsy) allows more accurate evaluation of cellularity, proportions, maturation sequences, and other marrow components.
      iii. Bone marrow aspirate samples should be tested for FeLV (via IFA) where blood serology is negative.
   b. Samples can be collected from the proximal humerus, iliac crest, or femur. Where thrombocytopenia is severe, it may be prudent to select a site with less covering muscle mass (e.g., the proximal humerus).
   c. A current blood smear and CBC results should accompany the submission of bone marrow samples.
   d. Thrombocytopenia is not a contraindication to bone marrow sampling. In fact, it is frequently the only means of establishing a diagnosis and prognosis. If the patient is actively bleeding, blood transfusion may be administered prior to sampling (CBC, however, should be collected beforehand).

ii. Megakaryocytic hypoplasia
   1. Decreased platelet production can result from the following:
      a. Conditions that affect only the platelet precursors (pure megakaryocytic hypoplasia)
      b. Conditions that can affect multiple marrow progenitor cells (panhypoplasia)
      c. Dysthrombopoiesis, where platelet maturation is abnormal (fig. 29.4).
   2. Suspicion or confirmation of hypoplasia should prompt revision of the drug and vaccination history, and testing for infectious diseases.
   3. Intramarrow conditions (aplastic pancytopenia, myelodysplastic syndromes, myelophthisis, myelofibrosis, and hematopoietic neoplasia are diagnosed via marrow histopathology (see chap. 30).
   4. Immune-mediated megakaryocytic hypoplasia can present a diagnostic dilemma, which is usually resolved by exclusion of other causes of hypoplasia, and evaluation of the response to immunosuppressive therapy (see below).

5. Treatment
   a. General principles apply.
   b. Specific therapy of intramarrow disorders and infectious diseases is addressed in chapter 30.
iii. Consumptive or sequestration thrombocytopenia
   1. As a general rule, most causes of consumptive thrombocytopenia lead to a mild or moderate decrease in circulating platelet numbers. DIC and sepsis are exceptions and may occasionally result in profound thrombocytopenia. In such cases, however, thrombocytopenia is usually associated with concomitant anomalies in secondary hemostatic testing.
   2. Causes (fig. 29.4) can usually be identified or excluded based on clinical findings. Bone marrow examination is seldom necessary. When performed, megakaryocyte numbers are normal or increased.
   3. Treatment is directed to the underlying cause. If this is reversed, platelet numbers normalize within days.
iv. Immune-mediated thrombocytopenia (ITP)
   1. Primary ITP is uncommon in the cat. ITP is usually secondary to viral disease, drugs, or neoplasia (especially lymphoid; fig. 29.4). It is rarely associated with other systemic immune-mediated diseases (e.g., systemic lupus erythematosus).
   2. Diagnosis is difficult and is based largely on exclusion of other causes of thrombocytopenia. A clue to possible ITP is a profound thrombocytopenia (<20,000/μL) in the absence of other cytopenias.
   3. Bone marrow examination usually reveals a profound megakaryocytosis; less commonly, megakaryocyte numbers are within normal limits. Immune-mediated megakaryocytic hypo-plasia also occurs (see above).
   4. The drug history should be carefully reviewed (fig. 29.4.). Drug-induced ITP usually occurs at least 7–10 days following initiation of the drug, or at least 3 days after its reintroduction (second exposure).
   5. Suspicion of ITP should prompt a thorough search for underlying disease. In addition to a CBC, serum biochemical analysis, and urinalysis, diagnostic testing should include thoracic radiology, abdominal ultrasonography, and testing for viral and other infection.
   6. Treatment (table 29.3)
      a. The goals of therapy are to arrest bleeding, to replace losses as needed, to halt ongoing platelet destruction, and to treat the underlying disorder.
      b. Blood losses can be replaced via the transfusion of whole blood or packed RBCs and plasma. Provision of platelets, however, can only be achieved via fresh whole blood transfusion. This is indicated with severe, active hemorrhage.
      c. Treatment of the underlying disorder is essential to a sustained beneficial response. Where drug-induced thrombocytopenia is suspected, all drugs the patient is receiving should be discontinued.
      d. Immunosuppressive therapy
         i. Immunosuppressive therapy should be initiated with prednisolone at 1–2 mg/kg PO q12h. If parenteral therapy is preferable, dexamethasone can be substituted, at 0.1–0.25 mg/kg SC or IV q12h.
         ii. Response to glucocorticoid therapy is generally seen in 2–7 days.
         iii. Patients should be hospitalized until platelet counts are above 50,000/μL and bleeding has ceased. Thereafter, platelet counts should be regularly monitored. When these are within reference range, prednisolone dose is decreased by approximately 25%. The dose is then decreased gradually (every 4 weeks) over 3–6 months, with close monitoring of platelet counts.
         iv. Relapses of thrombocytopenia with decreases of the prednisolone dose are unpredictable and not uncommon. If relapse occurs, the dose should be increased temporarily

Table 29.3. Drug table.

Drugs	Classes	Primary Mechanism(s)	Adverse Effects	Contraindications or Precautions	Doses and Routes
Cyclosporine A	Immunosuppressant Calcineurin inhibitor	Inhibits early T-cell activation, T-helper cells, and the production and release of certain cytokines (interleukin-2).	Inappetance generally occurs only with high plasma levels (>1,000 ng/mL). Nephrotoxicity and hepatoxocity only reported with severe overdose (plasma levels >3,000 ng/mL). Hirsutism reported. May increase susceptibility to infection.	1. Bioavailability is reduced by food. Should be administered on an empty stomach (1 hour before or 2 hours after a meal). 2. Bioavailability is variable, and different forms of the drug are not bioequivalent. Trough plasma levels should be measured if response is inadequate, or overdose suspected. 3. Cyclosporine can increase plasma levels of digoxin. Some drugs can increase cyclosporine levels (ketoconazole, metoclopramide, calcium channel blockers). Some drugs can decrease cyclosporine levels (trimethoprim/sulfa, phenobarbital, omeprazole).	4–6 mg/kg PO or IV q12h (Doses are for Neoral or Atopica.) Goal: trough plasma level of 250–500 ng/mL.
Dexamethasone	Glucocorticoid	Numerous systemic mechanisms. Immunomodulating effects include decreasing T-lymphocytes, inhibition of phagocyte migration, inhibition of chemotactic factors, cytokines, and complement.	Occasional polyphagia, polyuria, polydipsia. Can precipitate diabetes mellitus. Muscle and joint weakness with prolonged use. Iatrogenic hyperadrenocorticism is rare.	1. Use in the diabetic patient is likely to increase insulin requirements. 2. Patients on corticosteroids should not receive live virus vaccination.	0.11–0.25 mg/kg IV or SC q12h initially; then taper or switch to prednisolone.

Drug	Class	Action/Mechanism	Adverse effects	Precautions/Contraindications	Dosage
Heparin sodium	Anticoagulant	Enhances activity of antithrombin, thus inactivating thrombin and factors IX, X, XI, and XII.	Excessive bleeding possible with large doses.	1. Contraindicated in patients with thrombocytopenia that is not related to DIC or thromboembolism. 2. Contraindicated in patients with bleeding that is not due to DIC. 3. Use with caution in patients on concurrent anticoagulant or antiplatelet therapy.	See text.
Prednisolone	Glucocorticoid	Numerous systemic mechanisms. Immunomodulating effects include decreasing T-lymphocytes, inhibition of phagocyte migration, inhibition of chemotactic factors, cytokines, and complement.	Occasional polyphagia, polyuria, polydipsia. Can precipitate diabetes mellitus. Muscle and joint weakness with prolonged use. Iatrogenic hyperadrenocorticism is rare.	1. Use in the diabetic patient is likely to increase insulin requirements. 2. Patients on corticosteroids should not receive live virus vaccination.	1–2 mg/kg PO, SC q12h initially; then taper according to response.
Vincristine	Vinca alkaloid	Binds tubulin in mitotic spindle, preventing cell division during metaphase. Immunosuppression. Mechanisms of promoting thrombocyte release are unclear.	Inappetence, constipation, diarrhea. Myelosuppression (mild). Peripheral neuropathy. Profound tissue irritation and necrosis with extravasation.	1. Must be given strictly IV. 2. Use with caution in patients with leukopenia, infection, preexisting neuromuscular disease, or hepatic disease.	0.025 mg/kg, or 0.5 mg/m² once weekly, strictly IV.
Vitamin K1	Fat-soluble vitamin		Heinz body anemia can result from high doses (>5 mg/kg).	1. PO absorption enhanced by feeding a fatty meal. 2. PO absorption adversely affected by biliary obstruction and malassimilation disorders.	Long-acting rodenticides: 3–5 mg/kg/day SC, IM, PO. Short-acting rodenticides and other vitamin K deficiencies: 1–2 mg/kg/day SC, IM, PO.

(until counts rebound) and another immunosuppressive agent added to the therapeutic regimen.

    1. Cyclosporine is the drug of choice for adjunctive immunosuppression. Target trough plasma cyclosporine levels are 400–600 ng/mL. Monitoring of levels, however, is generally recommended only where response is inadequate, or where adverse responses occur.

    2. Responses have also been reported to weekly vincristine therapy (0.025 mg/kg strict IV, once weekly).

    3. Experience with mycophenolate and intravenous immunoglobulins in cats is extremely limited. As such, it is impossible to give evidence-based recommendations for their use.

    4. Azathioprine should not be used in cats due to the lack of metabolizing enzyme in this species and the resultant high incidence of severe myelosuppression.

  v. Infectious thrombocytopenia

    1. Infectious diseases that can cause thrombocytopenia are listed in figure 29.4.

    2. The mechanisms by which these diseases result in thrombocytopenia are often multifactorial and incompletely understood. They include DIC, vasculitis, splenic platelet sequestration, decreased thrombopoiesis, and/or immune mediated.

    3. The history and clinical signs may be suggestive of an infectious etiology. Geographic location and travel history can also be informative.

    4. Depending on the etiologic agent, definitive diagnosis may depend on organism identification or culture, serologic testing, or PCR amplification of DNA.

    5. Specific diagnostic testing, and treatment, is addressed elsewhere.

b. Thrombopathia

  i. Vascular disorders are a relatively uncommon cause of bleeding in the cat. In the patient with a primary hemostatic disorder and normal platelet numbers, a platelet function defect is likely. A prolonged BMBT in such a patient confirms thrombopathia.

  ii. Diseases known to precipitate platelet dysfunction should be excluded and the drug history appraised (fig. 29.4). If no obvious cause of acquired thrombopathia can be found, a hereditary disorder is suspected.

  iii. Von Willebrand disease (vWD) is rare in cats. Isolated cats with types I and III have been reported. Assay can be performed by specialized laboratories.

  iv. The patient with a suspected non-vWD hereditary thrombopathia should be referred to a tertiary referral institution for specific platelet function testing.

c. Acquired vitamin K deficiency

  i. Vitamin K deficiency or antagonism results in failure to activate vitamin K-dependent factors (factors II, VII, IX, and X), resulting in a secondary hemostatic disorder.

  ii. Causes:

    1. Anticoagulant rodenticide intoxication. This is uncommon in cats. Clinical signs generally occur 2–3 days postingestion.

    2. Severe hepatic disease, or extrahepatic biliary obstruction

    3. Pancreatic insufficiency

    4. Phenobarbital therapy. This has been associated with dose-dependent decreases in the activities of factors II and VII.

  iii. Diagnosis

    1. Prolongation of the PT occurs first, but by the time hemorrhage is evident, the PT, PTT, and ACT are usually all prolonged.

    2. FSP, D-dimer, and fibrinogen concentrations are generally normal.

    3. The platelet count is usually normal but may be decreased due to hemorrhage-related consumption.

4. The cat should be evaluated for hepatobiliary disease and the drug history appraised.

5. Toxicological testing for specific rodenticides or for proteins induced by vitamin K antagonism (PIVKA) is not usually helpful in the emergency situation but may serve to confirm an uncertain diagnosis.

    iv. Treatment

        1. Initial therapy

           a. General

             i. General therapeutic and monitoring principles apply.

             ii. Hemorrhagic shock should be managed via appropriate fluid therapy +/− blood transfusion.

             iii. Oxygen supplementation may be indicated in cats with respiratory compromise due to pulmonary or pleural space hemorrhage.

           b. Vitamin K is essential to management.

             i. Initiate vitamin K therapy subcutaneously, using a small-gauge needle. For long-acting rodenticide intoxication, vitamin K is administered at 3–5 mg/kg/day; for short-acting rodenticides and other vitamin K deficiencies, doses of 1–2 mg/kg/day are considered adequate.

             ii. The intravenous route should be avoided, due to the potential for anaphylaxis.

           c. Plasma

             i. Response to vitamin K commonly takes up to 12 hours. Emergency needs for clotting factors can be met only by plasma transfusion.

             ii. Plasma transfusion should be should be administered at 5–10 mL/kg and repeated every 6 hours for the first 12–18 hours (due to the short half-life of transfused factors).

             iii. Whole blood transfusion (fresh or stored) is indicated when severe anemia is present.

        2. Ongoing therapy

           a. The cause of the deficiency must be reversed where appropriate (e.g., treatment of hepatobiliary disease).

           b. After 24 hours, if the patient is not vomiting, vitamin K1 therapy is administered orally.

           c. Therapy should be maintained until the toxin has been metabolized, or the underlying disease sufficiently resolved.

             i. With rodenticide intoxication, the duration of therapy depends on the type of rodenticide. If the anticoagulant is known to be warfarin, 10–14 days of therapy is usually sufficient. If the anticoagulant is unknown or a second-generation rodenticide, oral vitamin K1 should be continued for at least 3–4 weeks.

           d. Evaluate the PT 48–72 hours after cessation of therapy. If it is prolonged, therapy should be reinstituted for an additional 2 weeks, and the PT again reevaluated after discontinuation.

  d. Hepatic disease

    i. Hepatobiliary disease is one of the more common bleeding disorders in cats, resulting in abnormal results of hemostatic testing. Spontaneous hemorrhage, however, is relatively infrequent. Bleeding generally occurs following surgical or medical procedures. This underlies the importance of routine hemostatic testing in cats with hepatobiliary disease.

    ii. Severe disease can result in one or more of the following: decreased production of coagulation factors, interference with hepatic vitamin K recycling, decreased vitamin K absorption (biliary obstruction), quantitative and/or qualitative platelet disorders, excessive fibrinolysis, and reduced clearance of FSPs.

    iii. Diagnosis

        1. In very acute cases, only PT elevation may occur. Thereafter, both PT and PTT elevations are usually noted.

2. Mild to moderate thrombocytopenia may occur.

3. FSPs and D-dimers may be elevated.

4. Antithrombin and fibrinogen concentrations may be reduced.

5. Differentiation from DIC is sometimes impossible based on coagulation testing alone, and depends on clinical findings, serum chemistries, and liver function testing.

iv. Treatment

1. Bleeding tendencies must be corrected before pursuing hepatic biopsy or other invasive procedures.

2. Plasma transfusion can temporarily offset factor deficiencies.

3. Vitamin K1 may be beneficial in some patients. Efficacy should be ascertained by repeating coagulation testing at least 12 hours after initiating therapy.

e. Disseminated intravascular coagulation (DIC)

i. DIC is an acquired syndrome, characterized by the excessive activation and loss of regulation of coagulation, with subsequent microvascular thrombosis.

ii. Aberrant expression of tissue factor (by neoplastic cells or cytokine-stimulated monocytes) initiates excessive coagulation. This is sustained and amplified by the consumption of coagulation inhibitors (antithrombin, protein C). In systemic inflammatory response syndromes (SIRS), a self-perpetuating cycle occurs, whereby inflammatory mediators activate coagulation and activated coagulation factors promote inflammation.

iii. DIC is always secondary to inciting illness. Most common in the cat are neoplasia (lymphoma and others), pancreatitis, and sepsis. Other reported causes include severe hepatic disease, trauma, heatstroke, viral infection (FIP), SIRS, and tissue necrosis. Secondary factors, such as vascular stasis, acidosis, and hypoxia, exacerbate the systemic response and promote DIC.

iv. DIC is a dynamic process. Initially, a compensated or "non-overt" hypercoagulable phase occurs, in which procoagulant activity is counterbalanced by the natural inhibitors of coagulation. With continued activation, however, inhibitors become overwhelmed, and uncompensated or "overt" DIC results, with widespread microvascular thrombosis. In a subset of patients, platelets and coagulation factors are consumed, leading to hypocoagulation and bleeding.

v. The hemorrhagic phase of DIC is a late-stage event, always preceded by thrombosis. It is uncommon in cats, occurring in <20% of feline DIC patients.

vi. Mortality is very high and is usually the result of microvascular thrombosis and organ failure.

vii. Clinical signs

1. DIC can be subclinical, mild or severe, and acute or chronic.

2. Overt DIC usually manifests as failure of one or more organs. Spontaneous bleeding is uncommon. When it occurs, it may be suggestive of a primary hemostatic disorder, a secondary hemostatic disorder, or both.

viii. Diagnosis

1. Diagnosis is generally challenging, owing to the variability in clinical manifestations, the difficulty in detecting thrombosis, and the lack of pathognomonic laboratory tests. Diagnosis of DIC requires careful consideration of both the clinical and laboratory findings.

2. Diagnosis depends on the following:

a. Identification of an inciting cause (see above).

b. Laboratory testing. There is no single test or combination of tests that serves as a gold standard for DIC diagnosis. Findings are extremely variable.

i. Thrombocytopenia is frequently, but not universally, present. Relative changes may be undetected unless a recent platelet count is available for comparison.

ii. The PTT is usually prolonged; less commonly, the PT.

iii. Elevated FSP concentrations are highly suggestive but nonspecific. D-dimers appear to be very sensitive in cats and likely superior to FSP assays. They are also nonspecific.

      iv. Antithrombin behaves as an acute phase reactant in cats and is inconsistently decreased with DIC.

      v. Scizocytosis is consistent with DIC, but schizocytes are not invariably present and may occur with other conditions.

      vi. Thromboelastography shows promise to identify both hyper- and hypocoagulability.

  ix. Treatment

    1. Identification and correction of the underlying cause. This is paramount, and should be accomplished as rapidly as is possible.

    2. Further management should focus on preventing or reversing factors that may exacerbate the DIC. This includes optimization of perfusion via appropriate fluid therapy, correction of acid-base and electrolyte disorders, supplemental oxygen therapy where indicated, maintenance of adequate renal perfusion, and the prevention of secondary sepsis.

    3. Plasma transfusion remains controversial but has theoretic merit. It provides antithrombin and replaces depleted coagulation factors. Moreover, there may be additional indications for plasma administration relating to the underlying disease (e.g., sepsis, SIRS, pancreatitis).

    4. Heparin therapy (table 29.3) has no proven efficacy in human patients and remains to be evaluated in cats. It is therefore impossible to give evidence-based recommendations for its use. Dosing regimens are uncertain, and most published doses are anecdotal. These have included 50–200 iu/kg SC q8h for mild cases, and 300–700 iu/kg SC q8h for moderate and severe cases. Monitoring of the cat on heparin therapy is difficult, as PTT does not appear to be well correlated with plasma heparin concentrations in this species.

f. Inherited coagulopathies

    i. In contrast with dogs, cats with heritable disorders seldom bleed spontaneously. They are frequently discovered when excessive bleeding occurs following surgery or trauma.

    ii. Inherited coagulopathies are rare in the cat (fig. 29.5).

      1. Factor XII (Hageman factor) deficiency is the most common, resulting in prolongation of the PTT; but it does not result in a bleeding disorder unless other hemostatic abnormalities develop. Coexistence of factor XII deficiency and hemophilia has been reported in domestic shorthair cats.

      2. Hemophilia A and B are recessive sex-linked traits, thus manifesting in males.

    iii. An inherited coagulopathy should be suspected, particularly in younger cats, if PT and/or PTT are prolonged in the absence of other abnormal testing and if acquired secondary hemostatic defects have been ruled out. A history of prior or recurrent bleeding is highly suggestive.

    iv. Definitive diagnosis requires specific factor assays, performed by specialized laboratories.

    v. Treatment

      1. Treatment adheres to general principles of bleeding control.

      2. If bleeding is severe or unrelenting, factors should be provided via plasma transfusion.

Recommended Reading

Bick RL. Disseminated intravascular coagulation: current concepts of etiology, pathophysiology, diagnosis, and treatment. Hemat Oncol Clin North Am, 2003; 17(1):149–176.

Catalfamo JL, Dodds WJ. Thrombopathias. In Feldman BF, Zinkl JG, Jain NC, eds, Schalm's Veterinary Hematology, 5th ed, pp 1042–1050. Philadelphia: Lippincott Williams & Wilkins, 2000.

Dodds WJ. Other hereditary coagulopathies. In Feldman BF, Zinkl JG, Jain NC, eds, Schalm's Veterinary Hematology, 5th ed, pp 1030–1036. Philadelphia: Lippincott Williams & Wilkins, 2000.

Estrin ME, et al. Disseminated intravascular coagulation in cats. J Vet Int Med, 2006; 20(6):1334–1339.

Grindem CB. Infectious and immune-mediated thrombocytopenia. In Bonagura JD, ed, Kirk's Current Therapy XIII, pp 438–442. Philadelphia: W.B. Saunders, 2003.

Jordan HL, et al. Thrombocytopenia in cats: a retrospective study of 41 cases. J Vet Int Med, 1993; 7(5):261–265.

Peterson JL, et al. Hemostatic disorders in cats: a retrospective study and review of the literature. J Vet Int Med, 1995; 9(5):298–303.

Stokol T, Brooks M. Diagnosis of DIC in cats: is it time to go back to the basics? (Editorial). J Vet Int Med, 2006; 20(6):1289–1290.

Tseng LW, et al. Evaluation of a point-of-care coagulation analyzer for measurement of prothrombin time, activated partial thromboplastin time, and activated clotting time in dogs. Am J Vet Res, 2001; 62(9):1455–1460.

Weiss DJ. Platelet production defects. In Feldman BF, Zinkl JG, Jain NC, eds, Schalm's Veterinary Hematology, 5th ed, pp 469–471. Philadelphia: Lippincott Williams & Wilkins, 2000.

Zimmerman KL. Drug-induced thrombocytopenias. In Feldman BF, Zinkl JG, Jain NC, eds, Schalm's Veterinary Hematology, 5th ed, pp 472–477. Philadelphia: Lippincott Williams & Wilkins, 2000.

30
HEMATOLOGIC EMERGENCIES: ANEMIA

Susan G. Hackner

Unique Features
— Immune-mediated hemolytic anemia is a less common cause of anemia in cats than in dogs. When it does occur, it is usually secondary to viral disease, parasitic infection, or antithyroid medication.
— Feline hemoglobin is extremely sensitive to oxidant denaturation. Heinz bodies occur in association with many conditions and do not necessarily correspond to hemolytic anemia in the cat. Heinz bodies, therefore, should be interpreted in the light of other clinical findings.
— Iron deficiency may be difficult to recognize in cats. Automated cell counters may not count microcytes, MCHC is usually normal, and microcytic hypochromia is difficult to appreciate on blood smear evaluation. Diagnosis rests on identification of an underlying cause and measurement of serum iron parameters. Red cell distribution width may be helpful.
— Nonregenerative anemias are common in cats. Examination of the bone marrow is essential in the diagnostic workup of any patient with nonregenerative anemia. This is best achieved via both cytology (aspirate) and histopathology (core biopsy).
— Feline leukemia virus (FeLV) is commonly associated with anemia in cats. Mechanisms include: immune-mediated, secondary infection (hemobartonellosis), anemia of inflammatory disease, and intramarrow disorders (pure red cell aplasia, myelodysplasia, myelofibrosis, hematopoietic neoplasia, and aplastic anemia). As such, serologic testing is mandatory in anemic cats. Treatment should focus on the mechanism of the anemia.

A. General
    a. Anemia is defined as a decrease in the red blood cell mass, occurring due to decreased production, increased destruction (hemolysis), or loss (hemorrhage) of red blood cells.
    b. The consequences of anemia are tissue hypoxia and, ultimately, death.
B. Presenting signs
    a. Anemic cats are usually presented for progressive weakness, lethargy, and inappetence, which may culminate in collapse.
    b. The duration of signs ranges from peracute to chronic.
    c. Pallor is the hallmark sign and should be differentiated from pallor associated with hypoperfusion, by determination of perfusion parameters (heart rate, pulse quality, blood pressure) and the packed cell volume (PCV; see chap. 3—Shock).
    d. Other clinical manifestations may include bounding pulses, a gallop rhythm, and a systolic flow murmur. Signs of an underlying disease may also be evident.

1. Primary survey
2. Establish vascular access
3. Collect pretreatment blood samples:
   - minimum database
   - blood smear
   - EDTA plasma (for later CBC, reticulocyte count, platelet count, blood typing, immune testing, PCR, etc.)
   - serum (for later chemistry profile, serologic testing, etc.)
   - citrated plasma, if bleeding suspected/possible (for later coagulation testing)
   - in-saline agglutination test, if hemolysis suspected/possible
4. Initiate therapy to stabilize the patient:
   - support of airway and/or breathing, if indicated
   - control of hemorrhage, if present
   - fluid therapy, as needed to maintain adequate perfusion
   - blood transfusion, if indicated
5. Secondary survey
   - complete history
   - thorough physical examination
   - MDB interpretation
6. Formulate problem list and differentials
7. Formulate plan, and write orders, for ongoing supportive care and monitoring
8. Diagnostic workup
9. Specific therapy

Fig. 30.1. Approach to the emergent anemic patient.

    e. Patients in an anemic crisis are moribund or extremely depressed, with marked pallor, tachypnea, tachycardia, and bounding pulses. If the anemia is due to severe blood loss, signs of hypoperfusion predominate.

C. Initial stabilization and monitoring

    a. The patient in crisis requires rapid intervention, with an initial goal of stabilizing life-threatening emergencies (fig. 30.1).

    b. The primary survey of the emergent patient is the rapid assessment of vital organ systems to determine whether a life-threatening situation exists (see chap. 1—Approach to the Critically Ill Cat). In the anemic patient, an anemic crisis or hemorrhagic shock constitutes life-threatening emergencies.

    c. Venous access should be established without delay, by placement of a peripheral catheter, ideally the largest bore possible, in case aggressive fluid therapy is warranted.

    d. Blood is collected from the catheter immediately following placement, for a minimum database including a PCV and total solids (TS).

    e. Additional blood samples should be collected prior to initiating therapy, to prevent treatment-induced changes in parameters. These should include:

      i. Blood smear
      ii. In-saline agglutination test
      iii. EDTA-plasma sample
      iv. Serum sample
      v. Citrated plasma sample

    f. Initial therapy should be instituted without delay. This is aimed to stabilize the patient while diagnostic testing continues. It includes:

       i. Control of hemorrhage, where applicable

      ii. Blood transfusion if the cat is in an anemic crisis

     iii. Blood volume replacement, where hypoperfusion is present (see chap. 3—Shock and chap. 8—Fluid Therapy).

     iv. The severely anemic cat can be remarkably fragile and decompensate rapidly with stress. It is important that stress is minimized, therefore, and nonessential procedures delayed until the patient is stabilized.

    g. Following initial stabilization, attention should be directed to the establishment of a diagnosis. The secondary survey includes a thorough history and physical examination, and interpretation of the minimum data base. This allows generation of an initial problem list and formulation of a diagnostic plan.

    h. Ongoing care and monitoring:

       i. Pending diagnosis and institution of specific therapy, a plan should be formulated, and orders written, for supportive care and monitoring (see chap. 1—Approach to the Critically Ill Cat).

      ii. The patient should be kept quiet and unstressed.

     iii. Nonessential procedures are avoided until a bleeding disorder has been ruled out.

     iv. Monitor closely for evidence of worsening anemia and decompensation. This includes, at a minimum:

         1. attitude and mental status

         2. respiratory rate and effort

         3. perfusion status

         4. mucous membrane color

         5. temperature

         6. PCV/TS

         7. blood pressure

D. Clinical assessment

    a. History

       i. The signalment of the patient may be informative. Young animals are more likely to have congenital disease or blood loss due to parasites, whereas older animals are at greater risk for malignancies.

      ii. The owner should be questioned on the following:

         1. The duration and progression of clinical signs. This may allow one to date the onset of disease. Determination of chronicity is useful in formulating differential diagnoses. (For example, the cat with a chronic progressive clinical course is unlikely to have suffered an acute toxic insult.) It also allows one to predict whether there has been sufficient time (2–4 days) for a regenerative response.

         2. The degree of functional compromise

         3. The presence of any other signs not directly related to the anemia (e.g., vomiting or dyspnea)

         4. Whether anorexia is present and, if so, its duration. This is always relevant in the cat where hepatic lipidosis can complicate other diseases (and resulting icterus may be misinterpreted as being directly related to the anemia).

         5. Diet, travel, and home environment (indoor/outdoor), which may elucidate the potential for trauma, toxin exposure, or infectious disease

         6. Present and past illnesses

         7. Any history of past or current bleeding—melena, hematuria, epistaxis, etc.

         8. Vaccines and medications, which may predispose to immune-mediated disease or marrow suppression.

         9. History of viral serologic testing for FeLV/FIV and exposure to other cats.

10. The medical history of other household cats. If other cats have similar signs, environmental (toxin), genetic (if the other cats are related), or infectious causes should be considered. The viral status of other household cats may be informative.
  b. Physical examination. A thorough examination should focus particular attention on the following:
    i. A thorough search for evidence of hemorrhage: evaluation of the body cavities, examination of the skin, mucous membranes and joints, rectal and fundic examinations
    ii. The presence of icterus, which may be due to hemolysis or hepatobiliary disease
    iii. The presence of splenomegaly, which could be consistent with hemolysis, neoplasia, infectious disease, or extramedullary hematopoiesis
    iv. Any evidence of neoplasia, infectious disease, or immune-mediated disease
  c. Diagnostic tests
    i. Complete blood count (CBC)
      1. The CBC is part of the laboratory database in any ill patient and is essential in the anemic patient.
      2. The total erythrocyte count (RBC) and hemoglobin concentration (Hb) confirm the presence and severity of anemia. Discrepancies between these values and the PCV may occur in several situations:
        a. Heinz bodies may increase erythrocyte fragility, causing lysis, thus lowering the PCV and increasing the Hb.
        b. Microcytic erythroctes can result in a lower PCV and Hb relative to the RBC.
        c. Laboratory error
      3. The erythrocyte indices, mean corpuscular volume (MCV), and mean corpuscular hemoglobin concentration (MCHC), may be useful but should never be considered pathognomonic. Four patterns can be recognized:
        a. Microcytic anemia usually indicates iron deficiency.
        b. Normocytic, normochromic anemia is generally suggestive of a nonregenerative response but should always be verified via reticulocyte count.
        c. Macrocytic, hypochromic anemia usually indicates a regenerative response but should always be verified via reticulocte count.
        d. Macrocytic, normochromic anemia may also occur with regeneration. In the cat without regeneration, however, it may be suggestive of FeLV or myelodysplasia. Macrocytosis can also be an artifact in day-old samples. Vitamin B12 or folic acid deficiency are rare causes of macrocytosis.
      4. The total white cell count (WBC) and differential counts are informative. Leukocytosis suggests infection, inflammation, or neoplasia. Leukopenia may be indicative of an intramarrow disorder.
      5. Automated platelet counts are not reliably accurate for cat blood.
    ii. Blood smear
      1. Blood smear examination is invaluable in the evaluation of the anemic patient.
      2. Accurate assessment is highly dependent on the quality of the smear and systematic, careful evaluation.
      3. Erythrocyte morphology may indicate an etiology (table 30.1), for example, toxic damage (Heinz bodies, eccentrocytes), physical damage (schizocytes), or erythrocyte parasites (*Mycoplasma, Babesia, Cytauxzoon*; see below). Microcytosis and spherocytosis are generally not recognizable in cats.
      4. It is important to realize that regeneration cannot be accurately assessed on blood smear examination in cats. Due to the different forms of reticulocytes in this species (see below), the absence of identifiable reticulocytes does not exclude regeneration. Conversely, evidence of any degree of reticulocytosis on blood smear examination in a cat indicates an acute and profound regenerative response.

Table 30.1. Erythrocyte morphologic changes that may be observable on blood smear examination.

Abnormality	Associated Disorder(s)
Acanthocytosis	Chronic liver disease
Eccentrocytosis	Onion toxicity
Echinocytes	Crenation artifact
Heinz bodies	Oxidative red cell injury
Hypochromia	Iron deficiency
Macrocytosis	Active regeneration, myelodysplasia, FeLV infection, hypernatremia, artifact
Nucleated red blood cells	Active regeneration, splenic disease, postsplenectomy, lead toxicity, systemic stress, some intramarrow disorders
Parasitic inclusions	*Hemobartonella, Babesia, Cytauxzoon*
Scizocytosis	Microangiopathy

5. Smear examination also allows assessment of other cell lines. The clinician should evaluate platelet numbers and morphology (see Bleeding Disorders). Leukocyte assessment is informative with regard to white cell numbers and proportions and may indicate the presence of a left shift, neoplastic changes, or parasites (*Ehrlichia* morulae). Approximately 18–51 leukocytes per ×10 objective field is considered normal.

iii. Reticulocyte count

1. A reticulocyte count should be performed in all anemic patients, providing the only accurate assessment of the regenerative response.

2. The clinician should be aware of the species peculiarities in the cat regarding reticulocyte counts.

   a. Automated counts are not accurate in cats. Counts should be performed manually via vital staining that allows visualization of ribosomes. A few drops of EDTA-anticoagulated blood are mixed with an equal volume of 0.5% new methylene blue in physiological saline. The solution is allowed to incubate for 10–20 minutes, remixed, and a thin smear made. A thousand red blood cells are counted, and the percentage of reticulocytes recorded.

   b. The cat has two types of reticulocytes: aggregate reticulocytes, in which the organelles are coalesced into aggregates, and punctate reticulocytes, in which the organelles are present as small particles. Aggregate reticulocytes are released from the marrow and mature into punctate forms within 12 hours. The latter mature to erythrocytes over 10–12 days. Aggregate forms therefore indicate active regeneration, whereas punctate forms indicate recent, cumulative regeneration. Because punctate forms are not recognizable on routine staining, the degree of regeneration may be underestimated in cats. If both forms are counted and not distinguished, active regeneration may be overestimated (fig. 30.2).

3. The degree of reticulocytosis must be interpreted relative to the degree of anemia, by calculation of the absolute reticulocyte count (numbers/μL of blood) or a corrected reticulocyte count (percentage; fig. 30.3). An increase in either of these parameters provides the best evidence for a regenerative response. An absolute count of >50,000 aggregate reticulocytes/μL, or a corrected reticulocyte count of >0.5% is considered regenerative (table 30.2).

4. Aggregate reticulocytes generally appear in the circulation within 48 hours of hemorrhage or hemolysis, peak by 4–6 days, and then decline. Punctate reticulocytes, on the other hand, persist for up to 2 weeks following insult.

iv. In-saline agglutination test

1. This evaluation for autoagglutination is indicated in all anemic patients, except those with obvious hemorrhage. It is particularly indicated in the patient with confirmed or suspected hemolysis.

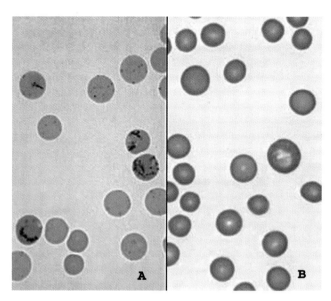

Fig. 30.2. Blood smears from a cat with regenerative anemia. A: New methylene blue staining, demonstrating both punctate and aggregate reticulocyte forms. B: Diff-Quik staining, in which only aggregate reticulocytes are identifiable as large, basophilic erythrocytes (courtesy of Dr. Elizabeth Spangler, Oregon State University).

$$\text{Absolute reticulocyte count (reticulocytes/}\mu L):$$
$$= \frac{\% \text{ reticulocytes} \times RBC/\mu L}{100}$$

$$\text{Corrected reticulocyte count (\%):}$$
$$\text{observed reticulocyte \%} \times \frac{PCV \text{ of the patient}}{37}$$

Fig. 30.3. Calculation of the reticulocyte response.

Table 30.2. Grading of the reticulocyte response in cats.

| Reticulocytosis | Corrected (%) | Absolute | |
		Aggregate/µL	Punctate/µL
Mild	0.5–2	>50,000	>500,000
Moderate	2–4	>100,000	>1,000,000
Marked	>4	>200,000	>1,500,000

2. The test is performed by mixing a drop of blood with an equal or greater volume of saline on a glass slide. Macroagglutination can be visualized grossly but is present in only a small percentage of cases. Microscopic evaluation of a fresh wet mount should always be performed. This will allow detection of microagglutination and differentiation from rouleau formation. Agglutination appears as "grapelike" accumulations of erythrocyte, whereas rouleau formations are more linear, resembling stacks of coins.

      3. Convincing agglutination is evidence of immune-mediated hemolytic anemia (IMHA) but is not universally present. A diagnosis of IMHA should not be excluded based on a negative agglutination test.

  v. Bone marrow evaluation

    1. Indications for bone marrow examination

      a. Nonregenerative anemia of greater than 2–4 days' duration

      b. Thrombocytopenia without evidence of a consumptive disorder

      c. Pancytopenia

      d. To investigate for, or stage, certain neoplastic conditions (e.g., myeloma, lymphoma)

      e. To assess for Feline Leukemia virus (FeLV) infection, when blood serology is negative

    2. Both a bone marrow aspirate and a core biopsy should be collected in cats.

      a. Samples can be collected from the humerus, ilial crest, or femur.

      b. Bone marrow aspirate cytology allows rapid impressions of cellularity and evaluation of cell morphology.

      c. Histopathology (via core biopsy) allows more accurate evaluation of cell numbers, proportions, maturation sequences, and other marrow components. This is important in cats, where myeloid dysplasia, aplasia, and myelophthisis are relatively common.

      d. Aspirate samples should be tested for FeLV (via IFA) if blood serology is negative.

    3. A current CBC and blood smear should accompany submission of marrow samples.

E. Diagnostic approach

  a. Causes of anemia are classified by mechanism: decreased erythropoiesis, hemolysis, or hemorrhage (fig. 30.4). Determination of the mechanism is an essential process in the diagnostic workup.

  b. The essential first step is to determine whether the anemia is regenerative or nonregenerative.

    i. The only reliable indication of regeneration in the cat is via manual reticulocyte count (see above). Nucleated red blood cells are not a reliable indicator, as they may be present in numerous conditions in spite of a quiescent marrow.

    ii. The presence of regeneration indicates either hemolysis or hemorrhage.

    iii. In general, a nonregenerative anemia indicates decreased erythropoiesis. There are, however, three important exceptions (table 30.3):

      1. Acute hemorrhage or hemolysis of less than 2–4 days' duration, as there has been insufficient time for reticulocytosis

      2. Concomitant disease that precludes an appropriate bone marrow response, for example, renal failure

      3. IMHA, where the immune response is targeted to the red cell precursors

    iv. Therefore, if the anemia is regenerative, the next step is to determine if it is due to hemolysis or hemorrhage. If the anemia is nonregenerative, decreased erythropoiesis should not be assumed.

  c. Hemolysis vs. hemorrhage. Blood loss is not always obvious, so a careful search must be made for evidence of hemorrhage. Several clinical clues may assist in differentiating hemolysis from hemorrhage (table 30.4).

  d. Other factors that should be considered:

    i. The severity of anemia (table 30.5). Some anemias (e.g., anemia of inflammatory disease) are characteristically mild or moderate and would be excluded from consideration in a severe anemia.

    ii. The progression of disease. Anemias of decreased erythropoiesis tend to have a chronic progression (weeks to months), corresponding to erythrocyte life span. Hemolytic and hemorrhagic anemias may be more acute (days to weeks). There are, however, exceptions (e.g., chronic hemorrhage, acute hematopoietic neoplasia).

    iii. The magnitude of clinical signs relative to the PCV. Animals with an acute onset of hemolysis or hemorrhage will develop clinical signs at a higher PCV than animals with a gradual onset of anemia due to decreased erythropoiesis.

Hemolysis
Antibody mediated
Immune-mediated hemolytic anemia
Primary/idiopathic
Secondary
Viral (FeLV, FIV, FIP)
Bacterial (various acute and chronic infections)
Protozoal (hemobartonellosis, ehrlichiosis, babesiosis)
Drugs (methimazole, propylthiouracil)
Neoplasia
Neonatal isoerythrolysis
Transfusion reaction
Oxidative damage
Food
Onions, propylene glycol (semi-moist foods), some fish-based diets
Drugs
Acetaminophen, phenacetin, phenazopyridine, methylene blue, DL-methionine, propofol
Diseases
Diabetes/diabetic ketoacidosis, hyperthyroidism, neoplasia (lymphoma), hepatic disease, renal disease, others
Toxins
Zinc
Naphthalene
Infectious
Hemobartonellosis
Babesiosis
Cytauxzoonosis
Microangiopathic
Disseminated intravascular coagulation
Near-drowning (fresh water)
Heat stroke, severe burns
Neoplasia
Splenic disease, hepatic disease, vasculitis
Congenital
Pyruvate kinase deficiency (Abyssinian, Somali, domestic shorthair)
Porphyria (Siamese, domestic shorthair)
Increased osmotic fragility (Abyssinian, Somali)
Poikilocytosis (domestic shorthair)
Methemoglobin reductase deficiency (domestic shorthair)
Miscellaneous
Hypophosphatemia
Hemorrhage
Trauma/surgery
Bleeding disorders
Ectoparasites
Gastrointestinal (endoparasites, ulceration, neoplasia)
Neoplasia (hemangiosarcoma, others)

Fig. 30.4. Causes of anemia in cats.

Decreased or ineffective erythropoiesis
Extramarrow disease
Anemia of inflammatory disease
Iron deficiency (severe)
Renal failure
Endocrine/metabolic disorders
hypothyroidism, hypoadrenocorticism, panhypopituitarism
Starvation–inadequate protein intake
Intramarrow disease
Pure red cell aplasia
Aplastic pancytopenia (aplastic anemia)
Infectious: FeLV, FIV, chronic ehrlichiosis, parvovirus, endotoxemia/septicemia
Drug associated: chemotherapy, griseofulvin, albendazole, sulfadiazene
Myelodysplastic syndromes
Myelophthisis
Myelofibrosis
Hematopoietic neoplasia
Infectious
Feline leukemia virus
Feline immunodeficiency virus
Ehrlichiosis
Parvovirus
Endotoxemia

Fig. 30.4. *Continued.*

Table 30.3. Mechanisms of regenerative versus nonregenerative anemia.

Regenerative Anemia	Nonregenerative Anemia
• Hemolysis • Hemorrhage	• Decreased or ineffective erythropoiesis • Acute hemolysis or hemorrhage <2–4 days • Hemolysis or hemorrhage with concurrent disease precluding regeneration • Immune-mediated destruction of erythrocyte precursors

Table 30.4. Clinical features helpful in differentiating hemorrhage from hemolysis.

Clinical Features	Hemorrhage	Hemolysis
Evidence of bleeding	Common	Rare
Serum protein	Low to normal	Normal to high
Hemoglobinemia/uria	No	May be present if intravascular hemolysis
Icterus	No, unless concurrent or underlying hepatobiliary disease	Common, but not invariably present
Splenomegaly	No, unless concurrent or underlying disease, or extramedullary hematopoiesis	Common, but not invariably present

Table 30.5. Guidelines for classification of the severity of anemia.

Severity of Anemia	PCV/Hematocrit (%)
Mild	20–26
Moderate	14–19
Severe	10–13
Very severe	<10

    1. Severe signs, relative to the degree of anemia, indicate either an acute anemia or that another process is contributing to the symptomatology.

    2. Mild signs, relative to the degree of anemia, generally reflect a chronic process, usually either decreased erythropoiesis or chronic blood loss.

F. Specific conditions

  a. Hemolytic anemia

    i. Immune-mediated hemolytic anemia (IMHA)

      1. Hemolysis is usually extravascular but may be intravascular.

      2. IMHA can be primary (idiopathic) or secondary to tick-borne disease (hemobartonellosis, babesiosis), viral infection (FeLV, FIV), various acute/chronic bacterial infections, drugs (methimazole, propylthiouracil), or neoplasia (especially lymphosarcoma).

      3. IMHA may be accompanied by other immune-mediated processes (such as immune-mediated thrombocytopenia). Rarely, it is a component of a systemic immune-mediated disease.

      4. Clinical signs

        a. The onset of signs is usually acute or subacute.

        b. Signs of anemia usually predominate. Splenomegaly is common, as is icterus and fever. Signs of an underlying disease may be evident.

      5. Diagnosis

        a. Diagnosis requires elimination of other causes of hemolysis and demonstration of immune-mediated erythrocyte injury.

        b. The anemia is usually regenerative. Up to one-third of cats with IMHA, however, have reticulocytopenia.

        c. Neutrophilia is not uncommon. Thrombocytopenia may occur.

        d. Autoagglutination is convincing evidence of IMHA but is not always present.

        e. A positive direct Coombs' test supports the diagnosis but should be interpreted with caution. False positives have been reported with FeLV and FIP infections, hemobartonellosis, neoplasia, and some chronic bacterial infections. Conversely, a negative test does not rule out IMHA.

        f. Spherocytosis cannot be identified in cats, owing to the small size and lack of central pallor of normal feline erythrocytes.

        g. If agglutination and Coombs' tests are negative, a saline fragility test helps to document erythrocyte injury. This is performed by some university laboratories.

        h. If the anemia is nonregenerative, bone marrow examination is indicated. This may reveal erythrophagocytosis, a maturation block at one stage of erythroid development, or pure red cell aplasia. Diagnosis of IMHA in these cases can be difficult, and response to therapy provides important diagnostic information.

        i. A diagnosis, or suspicion, of IMHA should prompt a thorough search for underlying causes. In addition to a CBC, biochemical profile, and urinalysis, testing should include radiology and/or ultrasound, viral serology (FeLV, FIV), and testing for hemobartonellosis (smear examination, polymerase chain reaction) and other parasites.

      6. Treatment

a. General treatment principles apply. The guidelines for blood transfusion are no different from those for other forms of anemia.

b. Management of any underlying cause. In the absence of an identifiable underlying cause, treatment for hemobartonellosis should be instituted.

c. Immunosuppression

   i. Glucocorticoids are the backbone of immunosuppressive therapy and should be initiated without delay, following diagnosis and evaluation for underlying neoplasia.

     1. Therapy is initiated with prednisolone (1–2 mg/kg PO, SC q12h). If a parenteral route is preferable, dexamethasone may be substituted (0.11–0.20 mg/kg IV or SC q12h).

     2. Most patients with regenerative IMHA show a response to glucocorticoid therapy within 5–7 days. Response is considerably slower in patients with nonregenerative forms.

     3. Corticosteroids are continued at the initial dosage until the hematocrit increases, usually a minimum of 3–4 weeks. They are then gradually tapered (by 50% every 3–4 weeks) according to response.

   ii. Adjunctive immunosuppressive therapy

     1. Indications

       a. Intravascular hemolysis

       b. Autoagglutination

       c. Severe hyperbilirubinemia

       d. Unrelenting aggressive hemolysis

       e. Delayed or incomplete response to corticosteroids

       f. Unacceptable adverse effects to corticosteroids

       g. Relapse with weaning of corticosteroids

     2. Cyclosporine is the most appealing option for adjunctive immunosuppressive therapy in cats, as it is rapid acting and well tolerated. Cyclosporine (Neoral or Atopica) is dosed at 4–6 mg/kg PO or IV q12h. As bioavailability is reduced by food, the drug should be administered on an empty stomach (1 hour before or 2 hours after a meal). Adverse effects are rare and generally occur only with overdose (inappetance, hepatotoxicity, nephrotoxicity). Determination of trough plasma levels are generally recommended only for patients that do not respond appropriately, or where overdose is suspected. Samples are collected 12 hours after dosing, just prior to the next dose. The recommended therapeutic range is a trough cyclosporine concentration of 250–500 ng/mL.

     3. Vincristine (0.025 mg/kg, or 0.5 mg/m², once weekly, strictly IV) is an alternative if cyclosporine therapy is not feasible, or if the patient fails appropriate cyclosporine therapy. The drug must be administered strictly IV as profound tissue irritation and necrosis occur with extravascation. Potential adverse effects include inappetance, constipation, diarrhea, myelosuppression (mild), and peripheral neuropathy.

     4. Splenectomy may be considered in patients that do not respond to aggressive immunosuppressive therapy, or that have intractable drug-induced side effects. There is little or no published data to support this practice in cats, but there are anecdotal reports of success. Prior to splenectomy, it is important to rule out tick-borne disease and ascertain marrow activity (via marrow examination).

     5. Azathioprine should not be used in cats because of the potential for development of fatal toxicity.

 ii. Hemolytic transfusion reactions

   1. Isoantibodies, directed against erythrocyte antigens, result in acute or delayed hemolytic transfusion reactions.

2. Isoantibodies occur naturally in cats, necessitating blood typing of both the donor and recipient prior to transfusion.

iii. Neonatal isoerythrolysis

1. Occurs in type A or type AB neonates of type B queens. Strong maternal anti-A alloantibodies are transferred via colostrum, resulting in lysis of the neonate's erythrocytes. This can occur even in primiparous queens.

2. Clinical signs

   a. Kittens are born healthy; signs develop within hours to days.

   b. Peracute death may occur in the first day of life in the absence of clinical signs. More commonly, kittens stop nursing and fail to thrive. Signs include hemoglobinuria, anemia, +/– icterus.

   c. Kittens that are subclinical, or survive the acute disease, may develop tail tip necrosis and/or a positive Coombs' test.

3. Treatment

   a. Kittens should be removed from the queen for the first 2–3 days of life. During this time, they can be fed a milk replacer or be foster nursed by a type A queen.

   b. Severely anemic kittens require blood transfusions. In the first 3 days of life: washed type B blood. Thereafter: type A blood. Blood is washed by centrifugation, removal of the plasma supernatant, and reconstitution with normal saline. This washing procedure is generally repeated twice.

iv. Hemobartonellosis (feline infectious anemia)

1. Caused by the epicellular erythrocyte organism, *Mycoplasma hemofelis* (previously named *Hemobartonella felis*) and the less pathogenic *Mycoplasma hemominutum*.

2. Infection appears to occur via bloodsucking ectoparasites and, possibly, bite wounds. Newborns may become infected from the queen. Iatrogenic infection can occur via blood transfusion.

3. The organism is opportunistic; it is usually associated with other underlying disease. Approximately 50% of cats with hemobartonellosis are FeLV positive.

4. Parasitemia is cyclic and can last for weeks to months.

5. Parasitized erythrocytes lose deformability and elicit an immune response, resulting in phagocytosis. Hemolysis is usually extravascular.

6. Clinical signs

   a. Depend on the degree of anemia, the stage of infection, and the immune status of the patient

   b. Anemia can be gradual or precipitous.

   c. Icterus is rare. Splenomegaly is common. Cyclic fevers can occur during periods of parasitemia.

7. Diagnosis

   a. Hemobartonellosis should be considered in any cat with anemia of any duration, particularly if hemolysis is suspected. It should also be evaluated for in cats with IMHA or FeLV infection.

   b. Anemia is usually regenerative but can be nonregenerative if there is a coexisting disorder that results in chronic inflammation.

   c. Diagnosis is confirmed by organism identification on blood smear.

      i. Samples should be collected prior to therapy.

      ii. Since parasitemia is cyclic, a negative test does not rule out the disease. Smear examination should be repeated daily.

      iii. Fresh blood must be used, as the organisms are epicellular and can be dislodged in EDTA.

      iv. The smear should be well fixed prior to staining, to avoid organism dislodgement.

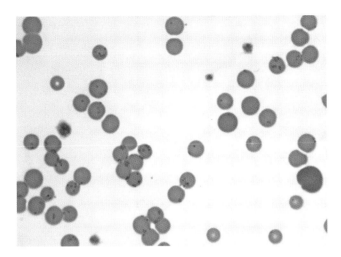

Fig. 30.5. *Mycoplasma hemofelis* organisms on feline erythrocytes (Diff-Quik; courtesy of Dr. Raquel Walton, University of Pennsylvania).

      v. Any Romanowsky-type stain can be used (e.g., Diff-Quik, Wright's-Giemsa). New methylene blue staining is not appropriate as organisms can be confused with other inclusions.

      vi. Organisms appear as blue-staining ring, rod, or coccoid forms on the surface of erythrocytes (fig. 30.5).

    d. Polymerase chain reaction (PCR) tests to detect mycoplasma-DNA are reliable. However, a positive test may indicate a carrier state or infection with *Mycoplasma hemominutum* and is not necessarily associated with hemolytic anemia.

    e. In-saline agglutination and Coombs' tests may be positive, due to the role of immune-mediated erythrocytic destruction in this disease.

    f. Testing for associated conditions (including FeLV) is imperative.

8. Treatment

    a. Antibiotic therapy for 21 days:

      i. Doxycycline (5 mg/kg PO or IV twice daily) is the drug of choice. Tetracycline (12–25 mg/kg PO q8–12h) is an alternative. Due to the risk of esophagitis with oral doxycycline administration, the drug should be delivered as a dilute suspension. The most common adverse effects are GI irritation (inappetance and vomiting). These tend to be less severe with tetracycline and can be reduced by administration with food. Dental staining can occur in young animals. IV doxycycline must be diluted and administered slowly via continuous rate infusion. Rapid injection can result in hypotension, collapse, and vomiting.

      ii. Enrofloxacin (5 mg/kg PO, SC, or IV q24h) may be used when tetracyclines are not tolerated. Efficacy, however, is not established. The most common adverse effects are GI intolerance (inappetance, vomiting, diarrhea). These may be reduced by administration with a meal. Ocular toxicity has been reported at high doses (15 mg/kg). Enrofloxacin can cause cartilaginous damage when administered to young, growing animals.

      iii. A doxycycline/tetracycline and enrofloxacin drug combination may be helpful in refractory infections.

    b. Corticosteroids (e.g., prednisolone 1–2 mg/kg PO q12h) are prescribed for the first 7 days.

      c. Supportive care and blood transfusion (packed RBC) as indicated.

      d. Parasitemia typically resolves rapidly following institution of appropriate antibiotic therapy, and a clinical response is generally seen within days.

      e. Antibiotics do not entirely clear the infection; treated cats remain carriers. Relapses, however, are uncommon.

  v. Babesiosis

    1. *Babesia* species that infect cats include *B. felis*, *B. cati*, *B. herpailuri*, and *B. pantherae*.

    2. Disease is reported in cats in Africa, South America, and southern Asia.

    3. Organisms are intracellular in the erythrocyte, resulting in intra- and extravascular hemolysis.

    4. Clinical signs

      a. Cats usually have a chronic anemia, which may be severe.

      b. Fever and icterus are rare.

      c. Diarrhea and splenomegaly are common.

    5. Diagnosis

      a. Babesiosis should be a differential diagnosis in cats with a compatible travel history and with a chronic regenerative hemolytic anemia.

      b. Definitive diagnosis depends on demonstration of the organism within erythrocytes or positive serologic testing.

        i. Parasitemia may be low in chronically infected cats, making organism identification difficult. Yield can be improved by:

          1. Smear preparation from capillary blood collected from the ear tip or nail bed.

          2. Examination of erythrocytes in the feathered edges of multiple blood smears.

        ii. Organisms are intra-erythrocytic and basophilic. *B. felis* and *B.cati* appear as small, single, or paired annular bodies; *B. herpailuri* appear as large piriform bodies.

    6. Specific treatment

      a. Primaquine phosphate (0.5 mg/kg IM or SC once) is effective. Extreme caution must be exercised with dosing as the therapeutic index is low (lethal dose is 1.0 mg/kg). Adverse effects include myelosuppression, hemolysis, and methemoglobinemia.

      b. The need for immunosuppressive therapy is unclear. Short-term use should be considered if anemia persists following antiprotozoal therapy.

  vi. Cytauxzoonosis

    1. An uncommon disease, caused by *Cytauxzoon felis*, affecting cats in the midwestern and southern United States.

    2. Wildcats appear to be the reservoir, with ticks serving as vectors.

    3. Merozoites infect erythrocytes, leading to severe intravascular hemolysis.

    4. Clinical signs

      a. Anemia, fever, icterus, pigmenturia, dyspnea. Organ dysfunction, particularly pulmonary, is common. DIC may occur.

      b. The disease is rapidly progressive, generally leading to death within a week.

    5. Diagnosis

      a. Should be considered a differential diagnosis in the cat that has access to tick-infested wooded areas, becomes depressed, febrile, anemic, and possibly icteric

      b. Diagnosis is confirmed by organism identification on Romanowsky-stained blood smear. Infection is usually low (1–2 piroplasms in <5% of erythrocytes). Organisms appear as basophilic cocci, rings with eccentric nuclei (signet ring), or oblong rings with bipolar nuclei (safety pin; fig. 30.6).

      c. The tissue phase of the organism may be demonstrated on aspirates or impression smears of bone marrow, spleen, liver, or lymph node (fig. 30.7).

      d. Serologic tests are not commercially available.

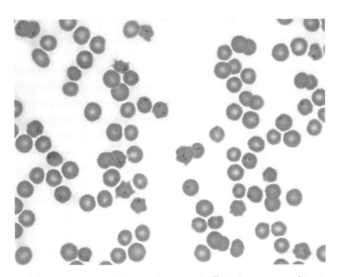

Fig. 30.6. *Cytauxzoon felis* organisms on feline erythrocytes (Diff-Quik; courtesy of Dr. Raquel Walton, University of Pennsylvania).

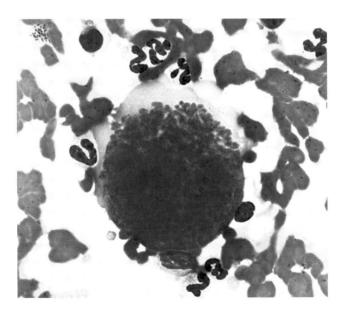

Fig. 30.7. Bone marrow aspirate of a cat with cytauxzoonosis (Diff-Quik; courtesy of Dr. Raquel Walton, University of Pennsylvania).

      6. Treatment
         a. Therapy with a diamidine, either diminazene aceturate (2 mg/kg IM once) or imidocarb (5 mg/kg IM q 14 days), may be attempted, together with supportive therapy. These drugs are of variable efficacy and are associated with significant morbidity (see table 29.3).
         b. Mortality is extremely high, even with therapy.
   vii. Heinz body anemia

1. Heinz bodies are aggregates of precipitated hemoglobin, attached to the internal surfaces of RBC membranes. They result from oxidative damage of globin sulfhydryl groups.
2. In normal, healthy cats, Heinz bodies should not be present in more than 5% of erythrocytes. Increased numbers occur readily in numerous situations because feline hemoglobin is very susceptible to denaturation by oxidants, and the spleen is inefficient in Heinz body removal.
3. The presence of increased Heinz bodies, even in high concentrations, is not necessarily associated with anemia.
4. Hemolysis, when it occurs, is primarily extravascular. Intravascular hemolysis is less common.
5. Causes of Heinz bodies:
    a. Drug induced. Oxidant drugs are likely to cause an acute anemia due to the rapid rate of formation.
    b. Diet induced. Anemia is not always present. When it occurs, it is generally mild or moderate. An exception is onion toxicity, which can cause significant anemia. Onions can be ingested in raw, cooked, dehydrated, or powdered forms. The latter is common in baby food.
    c. Disease associated. Numerous diseases can result in significant Heinz body formation. Most notable is diabetic ketoacidosis, which can result in up to 80% Heinz bodies. A mild to moderate anemia generally occurs but is seldom acute.
6. Severe drug-induced Heinz body anemia may also be associated with methemoglobinemia.
    a. Methemoglobin is formed when the heme moiety of hemoglobin is oxidized to the ferric form.
    b. Exposure to oxidant drugs can result in significant methemoglobinemia, with or without anemia. Methemoglobin is unable to bind oxygen, resulting in hypoxemia.
    c. Clinical signs of methemoglobinemia: Cyanosis is evident when concentrations reach 10% of total hemoglobin, but serious clinical signs are not usually appreciated until a concentration of 40%. These include lethargy, dyspnea, and exercise intolerance, and can progress to stupor, coma, and death. Cats with acetaminophen toxicity also exhibit facial swelling.
7. Diagnosis of Heinz body anemia
    a. Anemia is usually regenerative and ranges from subclinical to severe.
    b. The clinical history should elucidate the potential for drug- or diet-associated oxidants and concurrent diseases.
    c. Heinz bodies are confirmed by blood smear examination (fig. 30.8).
        i. They can be easily missed with routine staining, where they appear as pale inclusions within erythrocytes, or as bulges from the surface.
        ii. They are readily visualized as dark, refractile inclusions in new methylene blue "wet" preparations. Rapid evaluation can be achieved by placing a drop of new methylene blue on a dried blood smear and covering it with a coverslip.
        iii. The presence of eccentrocytes (fig. 30.9), erythrocytes in which the hemoglobin is concentrated on one side of the cell, is suggestive of oxidant injury.
        iv. A high percentage of Heinz bodies does not necessarily correspond to significant hemolytic anemia in the cat. Conversely, drug-induced Heinz bodies can result in a severe life-threatening anemia. It is important, therefore, that the number of Heinz bodies be interpreted in the light of other clinical findings: severity of anemia, history, and exclusion of other causes of anemia.
    d. In cases of severe drug-induced hemolytic anemia, the patient should be evaluated for methemoglobinemia:
        i. A simple spot test can detect clinically important methemoglobinemia. If a tube of blood, or a drop of blood on filter paper, remains brown after exposure to air,

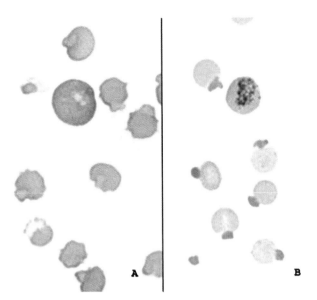

Fig. 30.8. Heinz bodies. A: Diff-Quik stained blood smear, showing Heinz bodies evident as pale bulges from the erythrocyte surface. B: New methylene blue staining of a blood smear from the same cat. Heinz bodies are evident as dark blue inclusions on the periphery of the erythrocytes (courtesy of Dr. Elizabeth Spangler, Oregon State University).

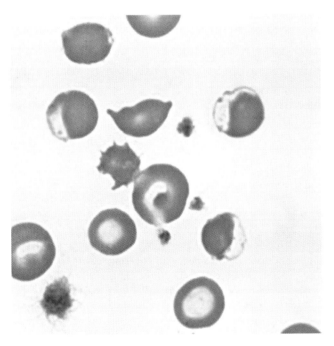

Fig. 30.9. Eccentrocytes, characterized by the eccentric distribution of hemoglobin within the erythrocyte (Diff-Quik; courtesy of Dr. Elizabeth Spangler, Oregon State University).

compared to a control sample that turns red, methemoglobin concentration exceeds 10%.

    ii. Accurate quantification can be performed by commercial laboratories.

  8. Treatment

    a. The oxidant source should be removed where possible.

    b. Supportive therapy, including blood transfusion (packed red cells), as indicated.

    c. If severe intravascular hemolysis is present, intravenous fluid therapy should be administered to ameliorate the risk of hemoglobinuria-induced nephrosis.

    d. The hematocrit or PCV should be closely monitored because the nadir is not generally reached until several days after oxidant exposure.

    e. Following oxidant removal/withdrawal, Heinz bodies disappear gradually over 1–4 weeks.

viii. Methemoglobinemia:

  1. Oxygen supplementation is of limited benefit, as the methemoglobin cannot bind oxygen.

  2. Routine decontamination should be attempted after a known or suspected ingestion.

  3. Mild to moderate methemoglobinemia does not require specific therapy to reduce the methemoglobin content. If the oxidant source is eliminated, erythrocytes can reduce the methemoglobin within 24 hours.

  4. Ascorbic acid (30 mg/kg PO q6h) should be administered to assist in the reduction of methemoglobin to hemoglobin.

  5. Severe methemoglobinemia can be corrected via a single administration of Methylene blue. However, the drug has the potential to actually cause Heinz bodies and exacerbate anemia. It is considered contraindicated in cats by some clinicians. It should only be used with extreme caution, and only when absolutely necessary. Methylene blue is given at 1.0–1.5 mg/kg via slow IV injection, once only. A dramatic response should be seen 30 minutes after administration.

  6. In cats with acetaminophen toxicity, N-acetylcysteine should be administered. This provides an alternate substrate for one of the active metabolites of acetaminophen. Moreover, it provides cysteine, to restore glutathione synthesis. A loading dose of 140 mg/kg is given IV in D5W, or PO, followed by 70 mg/kg PO q6–8h for 3–7 days.

ix. Zinc toxicity

  1. Less common in cats compared with dogs due to their more discriminating eating habits. They are unlikely to ingest pennies, zinc nuts, or bolts. Toxicity, however, can occur via ingestion of topical protectants.

  2. Toxic concentrations of zinc result in severe intravascular hemolysis and gastrointestinal irritation. Acute renal failure can result from massive hemoglobinuria.

  3. Diagnosis

    a. Zinc toxicity should be considered in the patient with acute hemolytic anemia without autoagglutination or morphological abnormalities on blood smear.

    b. Hemoglobinemia and hemoglobinuria are common.

    c. Reticulocytosis may or may not be present, depending on the duration of hemolysis.

    d. A tentative diagnosis is based on a history of exposure, the presence of intravascular hemolysis, and the exclusion of other causes of such.

    e. Metal-dense foreign objects can sometimes be seen radiographically, but their absence should not exclude a diagnosis.

    f. Definitive diagnosis requires the presence of convincing clinical signs or an elevated blood zinc concentration. Samples should be submitted in special trace mineral tubes to avoid contamination from rubber stoppers and erroneous results. Due to the high mortality associated with this condition, these cases are serious emergencies and treatment should not be delayed pending results.

4. Treatment
   a. If a foreign body is present, it should be removed (via endoscopy or laparotomy) following stabilization of the patient.
   b. Appropriate fluid therapy, based on perfusion parameters and renal function.
   c. Packed red blood cells should be transfused as necessary.
   d. H_2-receptor antagonists are recommended to decrease leaching of zinc from the source (e.g., famotidine 0.5 mg/kg PO, SC, or dilute IV, q12–24h).
   e. Chelation therapy with calcium ethylenediamine tetra-acetic acid (CaEDTA) should be initiated at 25 mg/kg, as a 1% solution in 5% dextrose water, SC q6h. This is achieved by diluting 1 mL EDTA (200 mg/mL) with 19 mL 5% dextrose water. The resulting solution administered at 2.5 mL/kg. EDTA is nephrotoxic. It is contraindicated in patients with anuria and should be used with caution in patients with renal failure or on concurrent therapy with potentially nephrotoxic drugs. The duration of chelator therapy remains unclear, as serum zinc concentrations may take 2–21 days to decline following removal or elimination of the toxin. The decision should be based on normalization of the serum zinc concentration.
   f. The prognosis for complete recovery is good with timely and aggressive intervention.

x. Microangiopathic anemia
   1. Numerous conditions can cause physical damage to erythrocytes, resulting in fragmentation and hemolysis.
   2. Microangiopathic hemolysis is usually mild and subclinical. Signs of the underlying disease predominate.
   3. Diagnosis is based on the following:
      a. Identification of an underlying trigger condition
      b. Identification of schizocytes on blood smear examination. These erythrocyte fragments appear as small, misshapen, often helmet-shaped or triangular structures (fig. 30.10). They are significant when present but are not specific for microangiopathy.
      c. Elimination of other causes of anemia
   4. Treatment

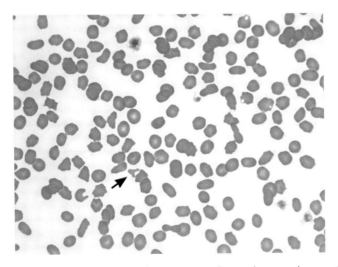

Fig. 30.10. Schizocytes (arrow) are indicative of microangiopathic erythrocytic damage (Diff-Quik; courtesy of Dr. Raquel Walton, University of Pennsylvania).

a. Besides supportive care, treatment is directed at the underlying disease.

b. Prognosis is guarded to poor unless the underlying condition is corrected.

  xi. Hypophosphatemia

    1. Patients are rarely presented for hypophosphatemic anemia. Hypophosphatemia generally occurs in hospitalized patients, resulting in anemia and increased morbidity.

    2. Causes

      a. Diabetes mellitus, diabetic ketoacidosis

      b. Hepatic lipidosis

      c. Starvation-refeeding syndrome (enteral or parenteral)

      d. Phosphate-binding antacids (rare)

    3. Phosphorus concentrations can drop precipitously in ketoacidotic patients following insulin therapy and in patients with lipidosis or prolonged starvation following refeeding.

    4. Decreased serum phosphorus is generally evident 24 hours after initiation of therapy but may continue to decline thereafter.

    5. Depletion of ATP results in erythrocytic damage and intravascular hemolysis. It can also result in myopathy and neurologic dysfunction.

    6. Clinical signs

      a. Acute hemolytic anemia: weakness, pallor, sometimes icterus and/or hemoglobinuria

      b. Neuromuscular signs: weakness, disorientation, ataxia, convulsions

    7. Diagnosis

      a. Hypophosphatemia should be suspected if acute anemia (or acute worsening of anemia) occurs in the ketoacidotic patient following initiation of therapy or in the patient with lipidosis or starvation following refeeding.

      b. Hemoglobinemia is usually evident; less commonly, gross hemoglobinuria.

      c. Diagnosis is confirmed via serum phosphorus determination (<2.0 mg/dL). This can underestimate the phosphate depletion and may be erroneously higher due to hemoglobinemia and hyperbilirubinemia.

    8. Treatment

      a. Intravenous supplementation, as potassium phosphate or sodium phosphate, at 0.03–0.06 mM/kg/hr, infused over 6 hours. This is best achieved by diluting the dose with a small volume of normal saline or balanced electrolyte solution, and administering via syringe pump. Alternatively, the dose can be added to the patient's usual crystalloid fluids. Serum phosphorus concentration should be reassessed following infusion, and the infusion repeated as necessary.

      b. Oral supplementation is sufficient when hypophosphatemia is mild and subclinical, where further decline is not anticipated, and if the patient is eating and not vomiting. This is achieved via milk or commercial phosphate products (0.5–2.0 mM/kg/day).

    9. Prevention. The clinician should predict clinical situations in which hypophosphatemia is likely to occur. In such patients:

      a. Serum phosphorus should be measured prior to therapy. Borderline or low-normal concentrations should prompt IV phosphate supplementation.

      b. Serum phosphorus should be measured 24 hours after initiation of therapy in patients at risk. Hypophosphatemia, or a significant decline, are indications for supplementation.

      c. Close monitoring of PCV and mucous membranes, and observation of plasma for hemoglobinemia

b. Hemorrhagic anemia

  i. Acute blood loss

    1. Acute blood loss reduces both the RBC mass and the circulating volume.

2. Blood loss constituting less than 20% of the blood volume is generally well tolerated. When loss exceeds 20%, cardiovascular effects are evident. Initial compensatory responses attempt to maintain perfusion to vital organs (see chap. 3). These include tachycardia and peripheral vasoconstriction (resulting in pallor and a prolonged capillary refill time). As loss exceeds 30–40%, cardiac output and blood pressure decrease, resulting in hypoperfusion, shock and, ultimately, death.

3. If blood loss is rapid, cardiovascular collapse can occur before any changes in PCV and TP. If loss is gradual, fluid shifts occur into the vascular compartment to maintain vascular volume, resulting in decreased PCV and TP. In the absence of fluid therapy, these shifts, and the associated drop in PCV, are gradual (2–3 days). The PCV, therefore, can underestimate the extent of hemorrhage.

4. Marrow response to anemia takes several days, so the initial anemia is nonregenerative. Aggregate reticulocytosis is evident by 2–4 days.

5. Diagnosis:
   a. Acute, external hemorrhage is usually obvious. The extent and severity should be assessed via evaluation of perfusion parameters.
   b. Internal hemorrhage should be considered in any patient with hypoperfusion and/or acute anemia. Potential sites of significant blood loss include the gastrointestinal tract, abdominal cavity, thoracic cavity, retroperitoneal space, and musculofascial planes. The clinician should be aware that melena may not be evident for several days following GI hemorrhage.

6. Treatment
   a. Four main goals in management
      i. Intravascular volume replacement (fluid therapy)
      ii. Control of hemorrhage
      iii. Provision of red cells (transfusion)
      iv. Treatment of the underlying disorder
   b. With acute, substantial blood loss, the effects of hypoperfusion are more critical than those of a reduced red cell mass. Initial treatment, therefore, must be directed toward intravascular volume expansion and reestablishment of adequate perfusion. There is no rationale to withhold fluid therapy in these patients; hypoperfusion will only serve to exacerbate the tissue hypoxia. Fluid choice (crystalloid/colloid) and administration rate depend on the severity and rapidity of hemorrhage, the clinical status of the patient, and whether other concomitant injuries are present (see chap. 3—Shock and chap. 8—Fluid Therapy).
   c. The transfusion trigger may be difficult to determine, because the PCV and TP do not accurately reflect the extent of loss until intravascular volume is normalized. Moreover, hypoperfusion contributes to the hypoxia. Transfusion, therefore, should be based on the status of the patient, not the PCV.
   d. After control of hemorrhage, red cell mass generally returns to normal over 1–2 weeks (unless transfusion[s] has been given). Iron supplementation is not required.

ii. Chronic blood loss—iron deficiency anemia
   1. With chronic internal blood loss, iron is recycled, and an iron deficiency does not occur. The anemia is regenerative, the magnitude depending on the extent of blood loss and of marrow response.
   2. Chronic external blood loss results in iron loss and eventual deficiency. Iron deficiency leads to excessive cell division of erythroid precursors and the production of smaller erythrocytes (microcytosis).
   3. In contrast to humans, iron deficiency anemia is usually regenerative. In the most advanced stages, a nonregenerative anemia may occur.

4. Young, nursing kittens are particularly susceptible to iron deficiency from any type of blood loss, as stores are low and milk contains little iron.
5. Causes of external loss
   a. Gastrointestinal loss (most common): parasitism, ulcers, neoplasia, malabsorption
   b. Hematuria
   c. Severe flea infestation, in kittens or very small cats
   d. Overzealous and repeated phlebotomies, particularly in small cats
6. Clinical signs
   a. Anemia is generally insidious occurring over weeks and allowing remarkable adaptation.
   b. Pica is a classical manifestation, exhibited by the eating of cat litter or dirt.
   c. Signs relating to the primary disorder may be evident. Melena, however, is often intermittent or occult.
7. Diagnosis
   a. CBC
      i. MCV is generally normal initially. If deficiency persists, microcytic cells constitute a significant portion of the RBC population, and MCV decreases.
         1. Some electronic counters may not count microcytic cells, resulting in a spuriously normal or increased MCV. (An erythrocyte histogram will provide evidence that this has occurred.)
         2. A decreased MCV may not be evident in the neonate as the MCV is normally higher at birth.
         3. Marked microcytosis is almost pathognomonic for iron deficiency. Mild microcytosis may be seen with other conditions, for example, anemia of inflammatory disease, portosystemic shunt.
      ii. A decreased MCHC is rarely present in cats.
      iii. Red cell distribution width (RDW) may be high, reflecting the presence of microcytes together with normal erythrocytes.
      iv. Thrombocytosis can occur.
   b. Reticulocyte count: Absolute reticulocytosis generally occurs. As the magnitude of depletion increases, reticulocytosis decreases.
   c. Hypochromia is usually not evident on blood smear examination in cats.
   d. Bone marrow is characterized by mild to moderate erythroid hypoplasia. Evaluation for stainable iron is of limited value in the cat, as normal cats store only small amounts of iron in the marrow.
   e. Iron parameters
      i. Serum iron concentrations are low, but this can occur in other disorders.
      ii. Total iron binding capacity (TIBC) is usually normal or slightly increased; transferrin saturation is decreased.
      iii. Serum ferritin concentration is usually low. Since ferritin is an acute phase protein, however, concentrations may increase in inflammatory conditions.
      iv. Iron parameters are affected by transfusions, iron supplements, and corticosteroid administration.
   f. Investigation of underlying disease. This should include evaluation for intestinal and urinary sources of blood loss. Since melena may not be grossly apparent, testing for fecal occult blood may be necessary.
8. Treatment
   a. Correction of the underlying cause
   b. Supportive care
   c. Blood transfusion, if anemia is severe and the patient sufficiently compromised, or if surgery is to be performed

    d. Iron supplementation
        i. Oral supplementation (ferrous sulfate (50–100 mg PO q24h) is preferable. Gastrointestinal intolerance is the primary adverse effect. Division of the daily dosage may ameliorate this effect, but dosage reduction may be necessary in some patients. Supplementation should be continued beyond correction of hematocrit and erythrocyte parameters, to replenish iron stores. This may take several months. Oral iron should be avoided in neonates during the first week of life, due to potential for liver injury.
        ii. Injectable iron dextran (10 mg/kg IM q 3–4 weeks) may be used if oral therapy is ineffective or results in adverse effects, if the patient is uncooperative, or if the owner is unwilling to give oral preparations. Injections, however, are painful and irritating.
        iii. Blood transfusion is an excellent source of iron, but use should be restricted to severely anemic patients.
  c. Decreased and ineffective erythropoiesis
    i. Extramarrow disorders
     1. Anemia of inflammatory disease (AID)
       a. AID (formerly known as anemia of chronic disease) is a nonregenerative anemia that often accompanies inflammatory and neoplastic disorders.
       b. Pathogenesis may include mediators that inhibit erythropoiesis, decreased serum iron, a blunted erythropoietin response, and decreased erythrocyte life span.
       c. Clinical signs vary depending on the underlying disorder. Presenting complaints are seldom directly related to the anemia, but anemia may be contributory.
       d. Diagnosis:
         i. CBC and reticulocyte count
          1. Mild or moderate, nonregenerative anemia
          2. MCV is usually in the low end of the reference range but may be mildly decreased.
          3. MCHC and RDW are normal.
         ii. Serum iron and TIBC are normal or decreased. Serum ferritin is normal or increased.
       e. Treatment: The anemia is reversible with effective treatment of the underlying disorder.
     2. Iron-deficiency anemia
       a. Severe iron deficiency can result in nonregenerative anemia and marrow hypoplasia (see above).
     3. Anemia of renal failure
       a. Nonregenerative anemia is relatively common in cats with renal failure, especially chronic and severe failure. It is usually mild to moderate but can be severe.
       b. The pathophysiology is complex and may include erythropoietin (EPO) deficiency, presence of circulating toxins that suppress erythropoiesis or reduce RBC life span, AID, gastrointestinal ulceration, and/or thrombopathia. EPO appears to play less of a role in the pathogenesis of anemia in cats compared to dogs. Cats with renal failure may have a normal or only modestly decreased EPO concentration.
       c. Diagnosis:
         i. A nonregenerative anemia in a patient with significant renal failure is suggestive.
         ii. Other causes of anemia should be excluded, particularly if the degree of anemia is disproportionate to the magnitude and duration of renal failure.
         iii. Measurement of plasma EPO concentration is useful to determine pathogenesis and predict potential response to EPO therapy.
       d. Treatment
         i. Management of the renal disease and uremia.
         ii. Blood transfusion if the anemia is severe and the patient has associated compromise.
         iii. EPO therapy (using human recombinant EPO) can result in the development of antibodies after several weeks of use. Therefore, it is only indicated if the patient has

clinical signs related to the anemia or is significantly affected (PCV < 20%). EPO therapy is initiated 100 units three times weekly until the target hematocrit is reached. It is then reduced to twice weekly. The lowest possible maintenance dose should be used. Treatment should not be initiated in patients with hypertension or iron deficiency until these problems have been corrected. Blood pressure and serum iron should be monitored during therapy. If refractory anemia occurs despite therapy and a normal serum iron concentration, EPO therapy should be withheld and bone marrow evaluated. Erythroid hypoplasia suggests the development of autoantibodies, necessitating cessation of EPO therapy and support via blood transfusion.

    iv. Other therapeutic strategies should be directed toward factors that may be contributing to the anemia, including gastrointestinal ulcers and reduced nutrient intake.

ii. Intramarrow disorders

  1. General

    a. Result in nonregenerative anemia. With the exception of pure red cell aplasia, variable degrees of neutropenia and thrombocytopenia may occur.

    b. Taking a history usually reveals a chronic, progressive course. Acute hematopoietic neoplasia is an exception.

    c. General clinical signs include lethargy, inappetance, and weight loss. Other signs may be present relating to the cytopenia: weakness and pallor with anemia, infections and fever with neutropenia, and bleeding with thrombocytopenia. Splenomegaly may occur due to extramedullary hematopoiesis or neoplastic infiltration.

    d. Intramarrow disorders should be suspected in the patient with the following:

      i. A nonregenerative anemia together with another cytopenia(s)

      ii. A nonregenerative anemia and a history of exposure to viral disease or potentially myelosuppressive drugs

      iii. A nonregenerative anemia of more than 3–5 days' duration, in which other causes have been eliminated

    e. Diagnosis and differentiation depends on bone marrow examination (cytology and histopathology). A current CBC and blood smear should accompany sample submission.

    f. Cats with intramarrow disorders should be evaluated for viral disease, neoplasia, and immune-mediated disease. If FeLV blood serology is negative, IFA should be performed on marrow aspirate samples.

    g. General treatment principles:

      i. Supportive care includes fluid and electrolyte therapy to maintain adequate hydration and electrolyte balance and nursing care to ensure comfort.

      ii. Blood transfusion, if indicated

      iii. Broad spectrum antibiotics, if significant neutropenia (<2,500/µL) exists. Examples include amoxicillin/clavulanate (15–22 mg/kg PO q12h) and enrofloxacin (5 mg/kg PO, SC, dilute IV q24h).

      iv. Nutritional support. Many of these cats are chronically inappetant and malnutritioned, requiring appetite stimulants or enteral nutrition (see chap. 9—Nutritional Support for the Critically Ill Feline Patient).

  2. Pure red cell aplasia (PRCA)

    a. A severe nonregenerative anemia associated with depletion of erythroid precursor cells in the bone marrow

    b. Secondary PRCA occurs in cats with FeLV infection. Primary PRCA is likely immune mediated.

    c. Diagnosis:

      i. CBC reveals a severe anemia; white cell and platelet counts are within normal limits.

      ii. Confirmed via bone marrow examination: Erythrocyte precursors are often virtually absent; myeloid and megakaryocytic elements are preserved.

      iii. Viral serology should be performed as well as Coombs' testing.

    d. Specific treatment

      i. Primary PRCA: Generally responds to immunosuppressive therapy within 3–4 weeks (see IMHA—Treatment).

      ii. Secondary PRCA: No specific therapy for the anemia. Immunosuppressive and interferon therapy can be attempted (see below: FeLV).

3. Aplastic anemia (Aplastic pancytopenia)

    a. Characterized by pancytopenia of blood and panhypoplasia of bone marrow with marrow space replaced by adipose tissue.

    b. Acute and chronic forms are seen

      i. Acute. Clinical signs develop within 2 weeks of marrow injury. Neutropenia develops 5–6 days after the insult, followed by thrombocytopenia at 8–10 days. Anemia is generally mild or absent.

      ii. Chronic. Clinical signs develop over weeks or months. Signs of severe anemia usually predominate. Neutropenia and thrombocytopenia are often of insufficient magnitude to result in infection and/or hemorrhage.

    c. Causes:

      i. Infectious. Parvovirus and endotoxemia/septicemia result in acute aplastic anemias. Chronic ehrlichiosis results in chronic aplastic anemia. Uncommonly, FeLV and FIV may cause a chronic aplastic anemia.

      ii. Drug-induced. Chemotherapeutic drugs, griseofulvin, sulfadiazine, and albendazole can cause acute aplastic anemia.

      iii. Idiopathic cases are rare in cats.

    d. Diagnosis

      i. Careful history taking should elucidate possible exposure to drugs or infectious agents.

      ii. Pancytopenia with a nonregenerative anemia

      iii. Diagnosis is confirmed on bone marrow evaluation. Hemic tissue occupies less than 25% of the marrow space, with the remainder replaced by adipose tissue.

      iv. In the absence of a compatible drug history, testing for infectious causes is indicated.

    e. Specific treatment

      i. Acute: Withdrawal of offending drug, or treatment of the underlying disease. Severe leukopenia (neutrophil count <1,500/µL) can be managed with granulocyte colony stimulating factor (G-CSF, filgrastim) at 5 µg/kg SC q24h. This is administered as pulse therapy for 3–5 days until the neutrophil count increases above 3,000/µL.

      ii. Chronic: Specific treatment is not reported for animals. Bone marrow transplantation is limited by a lack of compatible donors and high incidence of rejection. Management of severe cytopenias may be attempted via hematopoietic growth factor therapy (EPO, G-CSF).

    f. Prognosis

      i. Acute aplastic anemias tend to be reversible after elimination of the initiating cause and with adequate supportive care.

      ii. Chronic aplastic anemias are less amenable to therapy. However, with supportive care, recovery can occur weeks to months after diagnosis.

4. Myelodysplastic syndromes (MDS)

    a. MDSs are a group of hematopoietic stem cell disorders, characterized by ineffective hematopoiesis and evidence of disturbed maturation in blood and bone marrow.

b. MDSs are heterogenous with respect to clinical signs and laboratory abnormalities.
c. MDS can evolve into acute myeloid leukemia (AML). Even in the absence of neoplasia, MDSs are lethal in many cases due to the severe cytopenias.
d. FeLV is the probable cause for MDS in most cats. Other potentially mutagenic events include exposure to chemotherapeutic agents, radiation, or certain chemicals.
e. Diagnosis:
   i. CBC findings are variable. Multiple cytopenias are common, but decreased mature cell numbers in one or two lines may be accompanied by normal or increased numbers of other cells.
      1. A nonregenerative anemia is present in almost all patients and is often severe. Macrocytosis is usually present. Nucleated red blood cells may be profoundly increased.
      2. The majority of patients have thrombocytopenia; few have thrombocytosis. Abnormal platelets may be evident on blood smear evaluation.
      3. Neutropenia and monocytopenia are common, but profound leukocytosis may also occur. Immature and dysplastic eosinophils are relatively common. Circulating myeloid blast cells generally represent less than 10% of white cells.
   ii. Bone marrow examination by an experienced hematopathologist is essential to diagnose and classify MDS.
   iii. The diagnosis can be difficult in patients that lack convincing evidence of multilineage dyspoiesis or excess blast cells. In such cases, benign or potentially reversible disorders should be excluded. These include nutritional deficiencies (folate, cobalamin), drugs (vincristine, chloramphenicol), and immune-mediated ineffective erythropoiesis.
f. Treatment
   i. Administration of hematopoietic growth factors (EPO, G-CSF) can alleviate the effects of cytopenias.
   ii. The benefits of corticosteroid therapy in these patients is uncertain but may be attempted.
   iii. Low-dose cytosine arabanicide has been reported to be effective in a small number of cases.
   iv. Adjunctive therapy with interferon may be of some benefit in patients with FeLV-associated MDS.
g. Prognosis is guarded. Survival times generally range from days to months. Progression to AML is unpredictable. Cats with mild to moderate cytopenias and low blast counts can live for months to years with therapy.

5. Myelophthisis
   a. Characterized by the replacement of bone marrow with nonmarrow elements. These can be neoplastic cells, infectious granulomas, or fibrous tissue.
   b. Anemia usually normocytic, normochromic. Nucleated red blood cells are frequently increased. Marked anisocytosis and poikilocytosis are also common. Immature white cells and immature, abnormal megathrombocytes may be evident.
   c. Diagnosis depends on demonstration of inappropriate invading cells on bone marrow histopathology.
   d. Specific treatment and prognosis depend on the type of invading cell. Prognosis is generally poor.

6. Myelofibrosis
   a. Characterized by an increase in bone marrow collagen and extracellular matrix. A pivotal role for megakaryocytes in the pathogenesis has been demonstrated in several species.
   b. Myelofibrosis is a reactive process associated with various diseases. In cats, the most common underlying diseases are MDS and AML. Other causes include infectious diseases, radiation, drugs, and immune-mediated nonregenerative anemias.

    c. Diagnosis:
       i. CBC reveals variable cytopenias. Thrombocytosis is not uncommon.
      ii. Bone marrow histopathology confirms a diagnosis and may indicate an underlying disease.
     iii. Further workup should include investigation of drug history, infectious diseases, and immune-mediated diseases.
    d. Specific therapy
       i. Myelofibrosis can resolve with correction of the underlying disease. As such, diagnosis and treatment of such is paramount.
      ii. Adjunctive therapy with hematopoietic growth factors may be beneficial.
  7. Hematopoietic neoplasia
    a. Characterized by replacement of normal hemic tissue with abnormal clonal proliferation
    b. Acute and chronic myeloproliferative and lymphoproliferative disorders are recognized in cats.
    c. Viral infection (FeLV or FIV) is commonly associated.
    d. Diagnosis
       i. The history should provide clues as to chronicity.
      ii. Nonspecific bone pain can occur.
     iii. Variable cytopenias occur. Neoplastic cells in the peripheral blood occur frequently but not universally.
     iv. Infiltration of other hematopoietic tissues (spleen, liver, lymph nodes, central nervous tissue) is common. Sampling of these sites may reveal neoplasia.
      v. Marrow examination serves to confirm a diagnosis and may suggest cell type. Flow cytometry or immunocytochemical staining is necessary for accurate classification.
     vi. Viral serology should be performed.
    e. Specific treatment and prognosis
       i. Chemotherapy options depend on the tumor type and the status of the patient. Therapy may offer some prolongation of life and improved quality, but responses are generally palliative and not curative.
iii. Infectious
  1. Feline leukemia virus (FeLV)
    a. At least 50% of cats with FeLV infection are anemic. Possible mechanisms include:
       i. Anemia of inflammatory disease related to FeLV-associated disease(s).
      ii. Intramarrow disorders: pure red cell aplasia, MDS, myelofibrosis, hematopoietic neoplasia, or aplastic anemia.
     iii. Hemolysis associated with secondary infection (hemobartonellosis) or immune-mediated mechanisms.
    b. The type of anemia reflects the pathologic process. If anemia is caused by an intramarrow disorder or AID, it is usually normocytic normochromic and nonregenerative. Where anemia results from hemolysis, a regenerative macrocytic anemia generally occurs. Some cats defy these patterns in that they demonstrate a macrocytic normochromic nonregenerative anemia.
    c. Clinical signs may reflect anemia, other cytopenias, and/or other FeLV-associated diseases.
    d. Diagnosis
       i. FeLV infection should be suspected and tested for in any anemic cat without obvious cause.
      ii. Diagnosis of FeLV is confirmed via ELISA or IFA testing for viral antigens. If testing of blood samples is negative, marrow aspirate samples should be tested via IFA.
    e. Treatment
       i. Treatment should focus on the mechanism for the anemia, be it immune mediated, parasitic, or intramarrow.

ii. Adjunctive interferon (IFN) therapy. Beneficial results have been reported using oral recombinant human IFN-alpha (Roferon, Hoffman Laroche; Intron A, Schering-Plough) or injectable recombinant feline IFN-omega (Virbagen omega, Virbac). Oral rh-IFN is dosed at 30 u per cat daily, on a 7-day-on, 7-day-off cycle. The IFN is provided in a concentrated form and is diluted as follows: The entire contents of a 3-million-unit vial are diluted in 1 liter of sterile normal saline to yield a 3,000 u/mL solution. This is then divided into 10-mL aliquots in plastic tubes and frozen. Such aliquots are stable for years. When needed, an aliquot is thawed and diluted in 1 liter of saline to yield a 30 u/mL solution. This final solution is stable for 3–6 months if refrigerated. Injectible feline-IFN-omega is dosed at 10^6 u/kg SC daily for 5 consecutive days, on days 0, 14, and 60.

f. Prognosis is variable and depends on the pathogenesis of the anemia and the presence of other FeLV-associated disorders. If the cause of the anemia is reversible or manageable, many of these cats can enjoy a good quality of life for an extended period. The contagious nature of the disease and the consequential risk to other cats, however, should be addressed with the owner.

2. Feline immunodeficiency virus (FIV)
   a. Anemia occurs frequently in FIV-infected cats (18–36%). This is likely related to AID rather than a direct result of infection.
   b. Other CBC findings may include neutropenia, lymphopenia, lymphocytosis, monocytosis, and thrombocytopenia.
   c. Diagnosis is confirmed by demonstration of FIV antibodies via ELISA, IFA, or Western Blot assays.

3. Ehrlichiosis
   a. Ehrlichiosis in cats has been recognized with increasing frequency worldwide. There appear to be two forms: one caused by *Ehrlichia canis*, with inclusions in neutrophils, and another caused by *Anaplasma (Ehrlichia) phagocytophilum*, with inclusions in mononuclear cells.
   b. Clinical signs are variable. Anorexia, lethargy, weight loss, pallor, fever, hyperesthesia or joint pain, lymphadenopathy, splenomegaly, and/or dyspnea are most common.
   c. Laboratory findings
      i. A nonregenerative, normocytic, normochromic anemia is usually present. Leukopenia, leukocytosis, or thrombocytopenia can occur. Less commonly, anemia is regenerative.
      ii. Hyperglobulinemia is not uncommon. This is usually a polyclonal gammopathy, although a monoclonal gammopathy is also described.
      iii. Antinuclear antibody testing is frequently positive.
      iv. Bone marrow changes include hypoplasia and dysplasia.
   d. Diagnosis
      i. Demonstration of intracytoplasmic inclusions in neutrophils or monocytes may be possible in acute cases. But these are inconsistent findings, making this an insensitive method of diagnosis.
      ii. Serologic testing (IFA) for antibodies is available, but false negatives and positives occur.
      iii. PCR testing is specific and confirms a diagnosis, but false negatives occur, particularly in patients that have received antibiotic therapy.
      iv. Ehrlichiosis should be a differential diagnosis in the cat with nonregenerative anemia due to hypoplasia or dysplasia, or in the cat with immune-mediated disease. A tentative diagnosis is based on a combination of clinical and laboratory findings consistent with the disease, exclusion of other causes, positive serologic testing, and response to therapy. A positive PCR test or demonstration of morulae confirms the diagnosis.

e. Treatment
   i. Doxycycline, for 3–4 weeks
   ii. Clinical response is generally good. Complete eradication of the organism may be difficult, however, particularly in patients on concurrent immunosuppressive therapy.

Recommend Reading

Blue JT. Myelodysplastic syndromes and myelofibrosis. In Feldman BF, Zinkl JG, Jain NC, eds, Schalm's Veterinary Hematology, 5th ed, pp 682–688. Philadelphia: Lippincott Williams & Wilkins, 2000.

Feldman BF. Nonregenerative anemia. In Ettinger SJ, Feldman EC, eds, Textbook of Veterinary Internal Medicine, 6th ed, pp 1908–1917. St. Louis: Elsevier Saunders, 2005.

Giger U. Regenerative anemias caused by blood loss or hemolysis. In Ettinger SJ, Feldman EC, eds, Textbook of Veterinary Internal Medicine, 6th ed, pp 1886–1907. St. Louis: Elsevier Saunders, 2005.

Harvey JW. Methemoglobinemia and Heinz body hemolytic anemia. In Bonagura JD, ed, Kirk's Current Therapy XII, pp 443–446. Philadelphia: W.B. Saunders, 1995.

McSherry LJ. Techniques for bone marrow aspiration and biopsy. In Ettinger SJ, Feldman EC, eds, Textbook of Veterinary Internal Medicine, 6th ed, pp 285–288. St. Louis: Elsevier Saunders, 2005.

Tvedten H, Scott M, Boon GD. Interpretation of cytograms and histograms of erythrocytes, leukocytes, and platelets. In Bonagura JD, ed, Kirk's Current Therapy XII, pp 381–390. Philadelphia: W.B. Saunders, 2002.

Tvedten H, Weiss DJ. Classification and laboratory evaluation of anemia. In Feldman BF, Zinkl JG, Jain NC, eds, Schalm's Veterinary Hematology, 5th ed, pp 143–150. Philadelphia: Lippincott Williams & Wilkins, 2000.

31
MANAGEMENT OF SPECIFIC ENDOCRINE AND METABOLIC DISEASES: DIABETES

Tara K. Trotman

Unique Features

- A small number of cats develop "transient" diabetes mellitus, in which hyperglycemia and glucosuria resolve sometime during the course of treatment, and therapy is no longer required. This "resolution" of diabetes mellitus can be temporary or permanent.
- Cats can tolerate higher blood glucose levels than dogs without showing overt clinical signs.
- Cats may have a strong catecholamine response to stress, leading to a stress hyperglycemia, which must be differentiated from diabetes mellitus.
- Because cats are obligate carnivores, gluconeogenesis is ongoing. Therefore, nutritional recommendations are to feed a diet high in protein content, with limited carbohydrates.
- May be able to regulate feline diabetes mellitus with oral hypoglycemic agents such as glipizide.

I. Diabetes mellitus
   A. Background
      a. Diabetes mellitus is defined as persistent fasting hyperglycemia and glucosuria.
      b. Historically, two types of diabetes mellitus exist.
         i. Type 1—also known as insulin-dependent diabetes mellitus, associated with an absolute deficiency of insulin
         ii. Type 2—also known as non-insulin-dependent diabetes mellitus, associated with a relative insulin deficiency or insulin resistance
      c. While most commonly thought to be insulin-dependent diabetics, felines have been reported to have non-insulin-dependent diabetes mellitus, and some will respond to dietary management and/or oral hypoglycemics, without the need for exogenous insulin administration.
      d. "Transient" diabetes mellitus: see Unique Features box.
   B. Pathophysiology
      a. Diabetes mellitus occurs secondary to an absolute or relative deficiency of insulin secretion from the pancreas. Lack of insulin leads to an inability of tissues to utilize glucose as a source of nutrients, and an increase in hepatic glycogenolysis and gluconeogenesis. This leads to hyperglycemia in the blood circulation, which leads to glucosuria when the feline renal threshold of approximately 280 mg/dL is exceeded.

b. Glucosuria causes an osmotic diuresis leading to the classic clinical sign of polyuria, which is followed by a compensatory polydipsia.

c. A decrease in the utilization of nutrients by the peripheral tissues leads to weight loss.

d. Glucose typically inhibits the satiety center to decrease hunger, but because a lack of insulin reduces the ability for glucose to enter the satiety center, polyphagia ensues.

e. Cats can tolerate higher blood glucose levels than dogs without showing overt clinical signs.

C. Signalment, history, clinical signs, and physical examination

a. Older cats (greater than 6 years, with a mean of 10 years) are diagnosed most frequently, but cats of any age may be affected.

b. Neutered male cats tend to be overrepresented.

c. A history of polyuria, polydipsia, polyphagia, and weight loss is typical, although owners may also report lethargy, decreased grooming activity, or an unkempt hair coat. These signs are not diagnostic for diabetes mellitus, as other feline diseases such as hyperthyroidism can cause similar signs.

d. Owners may report hind limb weakness, due to a plantigrade posture.

e. Findings on physical examination can vary, but unless concurrent disease is present, or diabetic complications such as diabetic ketoacidosis have occurred, many cats are in good or even obese body condition, and no classic examination findings are seen.

D. Diagnosis

a. Persistent fasting hyperglycemia with glucosuria is necessary for diagnosis.

b. Because cats have a strong catecholamine response to stress, which leads to stress-induced hyperglycemia, it is extremely important to document glucosuria, as well as an appropriate history. Rarely, cats may have glucosuria secondary to stress-induced hyperglycemia. If in doubt, further testing to establish a diagnosis may include repeated blood and urine glucose measurements, allowing the owner to check for glucosuria at home in a nonstressful environment, or measurement of a fructosamine.

i. Fructosamines are proteins that have been glycated, and they typically measure the glucose concentration for the prior 3 weeks.

ii. Normal reference ranges for fructosamine are laboratory dependent. Typically, the higher the fructosamine concentration, the higher the average blood glucose concentration for the preceding 3 weeks.

E. Treatment of the uncomplicated feline diabetic patient

a. Diet therapy

i. Obesity is a common finding in diabetic cats and may cause reversible insulin resistance. Therefore, obese diabetic cats may become better regulated if weight management practices are undertaken.

ii. Historically, nutrition recommendations for diabetic cats have relied on feeding a diet high in fiber, which has been shown in studies of cats and dogs to improve glycemic control because of its ability to inhibit or slow intestinal glucose absorption.

iii. Newer information suggests that feeding diabetic cats a high-protein, low-carbohydrate diet may be more effective in improving glycemic control in cats.

1. The pathophysiologic reason for this is that cats are carnivores, and as such they use amino acids and fat, rather than carbohydrates, as their energy source. Thus, dietary carbohydrates may lead to higher postprandial glucose concentrations.

2. Current feeding recommendations for cats with diabetes mellitus are to feed a diet with a high protein level, limited carbohydrates, and a fixed amount of fat. Diets such as Purina DM (Nestle Purina Pet Care Company, St. Louis, MO), Hills M/D, or kitten foods with this type of content, are suggested.

3. These diets may not be ideal for cats with preexisting renal disease because of the high protein content.

b. Oral hypoglycemic
   i. Many oral hypoglycemic agents exist, with a variety of goals including improvement of insulin secretion, suppression of hepatic glucose production, decrease in insulin resistance, or a reduction of glucose absorption via the GI tract.
   ii. Little evidence exists in feline medicine for the use of such agents; however, they may be successful in regulating diabetes mellitus in a small portion of cats. These agents are not thought to have any benefit in dogs with diabetes mellitus.
   iii. The most commonly used oral hypoglycemic agent in feline diabetes mellitus is glipizide.
      1. Glipizide is a sulfonylurea, which acts by increasing insulin secretion from pancreatic beta cells.
         a. Glipizide is recommended for use in cats with mild to moderate hyperglycemia that are clinically stable.
         b. Start at 2.5 mg PO BID for 2 weeks.
         c. If patient is still hyperglycemic and no adverse side effects are noted, possibly increase to 5 mg PO BID.
         d. If blood glucose remains above 300–400 mg/dL after 1–2 months, treatment is discontinued and subcutaneous insulin injections should be started.
      2. Adverse side effects of glipizide include hypoglycemia, GI intolerance, and/or hepatic toxicity/icterus.
c. Insulin administration
   i. It is very important that owners are made aware upfront that diabetes mellitus is most often a disease that requires lifetime therapy with twice daily subcutaneous injections.
   ii. There are many insulin types being used for the treatment of feline diabetes mellitus. The uncomplicated diabetic cat is typically administered an intermediate or long-acting insulin subcutaneously, at 0.5 units/kg BID. Some insulin types, such as glargine or PZI, may be effective when administered once daily.
   iii. See box 31.1.
   iv. Most stable newly diagnosed diabetic cats can be treated as outpatients.
   v. Owner instructions must be clear so as to ensure the insulin is being handled and administered properly.
   vi. Insulin must be stored at constant temperature, avoiding major fluctuations.
   vii. Prior to use, the bottle must be mixed. *Never shake the insulin bottle.* Mix the contents by gently rolling the bottle between two hands.
   viii. Injections are administered subcutaneously, with proper technique demonstrated to the owner. They can practice using 0.9% saline if needed. Owners should be told that if they are unsure if the dose was administered properly, they should *not* repeat the dose. They should wait until the next injection before administering insulin again, and give the regular dose at that time.
   ix. The pet should always be fed prior to insulin administration to ensure adequate intake. If the pet does not eat, half the dose should be administered. If the pet misses a second meal, the veterinarian should be contacted immediately.
   x. It is important to inform owners of the risks of hypoglycemia and hyperglycemia.
d. After starting insulin therapy, the pet should be seen back for a 12–24 hour blood glucose curve in 7–10 days. This curve requires blood glucose checks every 2 hours. This is very important. *Dose adjustments should never be made based on one spot blood glucose.* A 12-hour curve, along with report on resolution of clinical signs, should be monitored regularly.
e. Fructosamine, as mentioned previously, can be used to monitor glycemic control in fractious animals. Veterinarians should be aware that they can be difficult to interpret at times, especially if the animal is receiving excess insulin, leading to the somogyi effect, which then could lead to a high fructosamine despite excess insulin dose.

Box 31.1. Insulin therapy for newly diagnosed diabetic cat.

1. Humulin NPH
   a. Intermediate-acting insulin
   b. Duration of action ≤ 12 hours
   c. Onset of action: 4–6 hours
   d. Administration: 0.5 units/kg, subcutaneously, BID
2. Glargine
   a. Long-acting insulin
   b. "Peakless" insulin in humans, although this has not proven true in felines
   c. Its activity is dependent on the acidity of the solution, and therefore, glargine cannot be diluted.
   d. Duration of action 23 +/– 0.9 hours (Rand, Marshall 2006)
   e. Reports differ as to the best dosing regimen.
      i. May start anywhere from 0.25 units/kg to 0.5 units/kg SID-BID subcutaneously
   f. Studies suggest that some cats may go into remission with use of this insulin type; therefore, cats in which this type of insulin is used must be monitored closely for signs of hypoglycemia (weakness, lethargy, disorientation, ataxia, seizures).
3. While other insulins such as PZI and vetsulin may be used to treat newly diagnosed diabetic patients, the author has found that therapy with NPH or glargine insulin leads to more consistent results and diabetic stabilization.

II. Diabetic ketoacidosis (DKA)
   A. Pathophysiology
      a. DKA is a serious, life-threatening complication of diabetes mellitus characterized by formation of ketone bodies, which may lead to severe metabolic acidosis and electrolyte derangements.
      b. Ketone bodies are generated when the body perceives a deficiency of glucose; they are utilized as an energy source by many tissues of the body.
      c. The ketone bodies present in the body during a DKA episode are acetoacetate, β-hydroxybutyrate, and acetone.
      d. Insulin is a potent inhibitor of lipolysis and fatty acid oxidation. A lack of insulin leads to increased lipolysis, which causes an increase in free fatty acids, promoting the formation of ketones.
      e. Feline patients are typically in one of two categories when they present with a DKA episode.
         i. Newly diagnosed, untreated diabetic patient that has not received insulin previously. Insulin deficiency leads to ketone formation.
         ii. A second category of feline patients is already receiving insulin at the time of DKA diagnosis. These patients often have concurrent disease, leading to overproduction of counterregulatory hormones and a relative insulin deficiency secondary to insulin resistance. Therefore, DKA ensues despite the presence of insulin in circulation.
   B. History and physical examination
      a. In the previously undiagnosed diabetic cat, clinical signs of diabetes may have been present but were subtle and went unnoticed by the owner. The ongoing lack of insulin therapy then leads to the development of ketone formation, which leads to progressive systemic signs such as anorexia, lethargy, and vomiting as the metabolic acidosis develops.
      b. In the cat being treated with insulin, systemic signs such as anorexia, lethargy, and vomiting also may occur, along with signs related to the presence and severity of a concurrent disease (e.g., renal failure, heart disease, infection, neoplasia).
      c. Physical examination can vary as well but often reveals dehydration, depression, weakness, acetone odor of the breath, and tachypnea.

C. Diagnosis
   a. The diagnosis of DKA requires the diagnosis of diabetes mellitus (persistent fasting hyperglycemia along with glucosuria), as well as ketonuria or ketonemia and metabolic acidosis.
      i. The most common technique used for detecting ketonuria or ketonemia involves the use of nitroprusside reagent (used in most urine dipstick tests). This agent readily detects acetone and acetoacetate in the urine or serum, but β-hydroxybutyrate may not be detected via this method. Because β-hydroxybutyrate may be present in higher concentrations than the other ketone bodies, the severity of ketonemia and ketonuria may be underestimated if additional methods are not used for its detection.
         1. Adding one drop of hydrogen peroxide to the dipstick may aid in detection of β-hydroxybutyrate.
   b. CBC/ chemistry screen
      i. Elevated total solids and hematocrit secondary to dehydration
      ii. Elevation of white blood cells due to inflammation and/or infection
      iii. Liver enzyme elevations
      iv. Hyperbilirubinemia
      v. Azotemia
      vi. Acidosis
      vii. Severe electrolyte shifts
         1. Hyponatremia
         2. Hypokalemia
         3. Hypophosphatemia
         4. Hypomagnesemia
   c. Urinalysis
      i. May show pyuria or bacteriuria if an infection is present.
      ii. A sterile cystocentesis sample should always be obtained and analyzed to rule out a urinary tract infection.
      iii. A culture should always be done in the diabetic cat to rule out an infection, as bacteria or white blood cells may not be present in the urine despite an infectious process.
   d. Imaging may reveal disease within the thorax (thoracic radiographs—heart failure, neoplasia, pneumonia), or abdomen (abdominal radiographs and/or ultrasound—pancreatitis, pyometra, neoplasia, hepatic lipidosis).
D. Therapy of the feline DKA patient
   a. Due to severe fluid and electrolyte shifts, these patients are often critical and require intensive management for stabilization.
   b. Fluid therapy
      i. After obtaining intravenous access (preferably central venous access if possible), fluid therapy should be started immediately. Choice of fluids depends on the presence of electrolyte abnormalities; however, rate may be calculated by determining the percent dehydration, ongoing and insensible losses, and amount needed for maintenance.
      ii. If the patient is hypovolemic and/or hypotensive, more aggressive therapy with fluid may be indicated (see chap. 3—Shock).
   c. Insulin administration
      i. Fluid therapy should be administered for at least 4–6 hours before insulin therapy is started, in order to better hydrate the patient and evaluate electrolyte status. Blood glucose will often decline significantly with fluid therapy alone. Once the patient is more stable and the hydration status has improved, insulin therapy can be started.
      ii. Recheck measurements of potassium and phosphorus levels should be done prior to initiating insulin therapy and supplementation provided if necessary, as these levels will decrease with insulin treatment. A short-acting insulin with rapid onset of action, such as regular insulin,

Box 31.2. Continuous rate infusion of insulin for the diabetic ketoacidotic feline patient.
1. Place 1.1 units/kg of regular insulin into 240 mL of 0.9% NaCl.
2. Run approximately 50 mL of this through the primary venoset line so that insulin adheres to the inner portions of the tubing.
3. Blood glucose measurements should be made every 2 hours.
    a. A catheter should be placed that can be used for sampling, and minimal amount of blood should be drawn to limit the potential for iatrogenic anemia.
4. The following is only a guideline—rates and concentrations may need to be adjusted based on an individual's response to therapy.

Blood Glucose	Rate of Insulin CRI	Dextrose [conc]
>350 g/dL	10 mL/hr	0%
250–350 g/dL	7 mL/hr	0%
200–250 g/dL	5 mL/hr	0%
150–200 g/dL	3 mL/hr	0%
100–150 g/dL	1 mL/hr	2.5%
<100 g/dL	0 mL/hr	5%

5. Care should be taken to avoid fluid overload. Any additives (i.e., potassium, phosphorus, magnesium, etc.) should be placed in a separate fluid line and given at a different rate that can be adjusted as needed (see chap. 8—Fluid Therapy).

      should be used. Methods for its use have been described elsewhere but typically involve either intermittent intramuscular injections or continuous rate intravenous infusion (see box 31.2).

   iii. Gradual decline of the blood glucose level is ideal, as rapid changes in blood glucose concentration can lead to rapid fluid and electrolyte shifts that can be life-threatening in extreme cases.

   iv. The goal of treatment is to allow the body to start utilizing glucose and thus to stop ketone formation. Therefore, once blood glucose levels fall below a certain level (usually around 100 mg/dL), dextrose should be added to the fluids to increase the blood glucose level so that insulin can continue to be administered.
     1. The only way to stop the body from continuing to make ketones is to allow it to utilize glucose by providing insulin.
     2. Blood glucose levels should be maintained at a relatively consistent level (i.e., 150 mg/dL to 250 mg/dL).

   v. Insulin therapy is continued as an intramuscular or intravenous dosing until the patient begins to eat regularly, at which point the insulin can be switched to a longer acting, subcutaneous dosing schedule (see above).

  d. Electrolytes
   i. Potassium
     1. These patients are invariably depleted of their total body potassium, even if the blood potassium levels are normal at presentation. Once insulin administration begins, potassium is pushed into the cells and serum potassium levels may drop dramatically. Aggressive supplementation may be required. Potassium administration should not be given at a rate higher than 0.5 mEq/kg/hr. If rates at or above that should become necessary, intensive monitoring with continuous ECG and frequent blood sampling must be provided.
     a. Some cats with DKA require higher rates of potassium than 0.5 mEq/kg/hr (Kmax).

      b. If potassium concentration remains below 3.5 mEq/L despite potassium supplementation at Kmax, potassium constant rate infusion can be increased in increments of 0.25 mEq/kg/hr.

      c. At rates above Kmax, heart rate should be monitored regularly, and a continuous ECG used if possible. If arrhythmias occur, potassium infusion should be discontinued and potassium checked immediately.

  ii. Phosphorus

    1. Similar to potassium, these patients are often depleted of their total phosphorus stores, and once insulin administration is begun, phosphorus is pushed into cells. If levels reach below 1.5 mg/dL, clinical signs such as hemolysis, lethargy, and neurologic changes such as seizures and weakness due to decreased 2,3-DPG concentration may occur. Phosphorus supplementation should be provided as needed.

      a. P supplementation can be given as potassium phosphate (potassium 4.4 mEq/mL, phosphate 3 mM/mL) at 0.03–0.12 mM phosphate/kg/hour, but K administration must be taken into account.

        i. Recheck potassium and phosphorus within 6 hours of instituting supplementation, then every 6–8 hours.

  iii. Magnesium

    1. Magnesium levels may drop also. Hypomagnesemia may cause hypokalemia to be refractory to supplementation. If potassium remains low despite appropriate supplementation, magnesium should be evaluated.

    2. Magnesium can be administered at a rate of 1 mEq/kg/24 hours. Magnesium should be checked at least once every 24 hours.

  e. Acidosis

    i. It is rare that bicarbonate administration is required in these patients because acidosis typically responds to fluid therapy and resolution of ketones.

    ii. Bicarbonate therapy may be necessary if pH < 7.1 despite adequate fluid resuscitation and institution of insulin therapy. The following formula may be used to calculate the bicarbonate deficit:

      1. $NaHCO_3$ (mL) = 0.3 × body weight (kg) × base deficit

      2. The patient should be given ¼ to ⅓ of this amount slowly (over 1–2 hours), and then the acidosis should be reassessed.

      3. Contraindications to use of sodium bicarbonate administration include hypernatremia and/or respiratory compromise, which could lead to hypercarbia.

  f. Concurrent diseases

    i. Common concurrent diseases may include pancreatitis, hepatic lipidosis, pyelonephritis, neoplasia, and cholangitis. A thorough workup should always be performed to look for underlying diseases, and the concurrent disease must be addressed as well. Tests should include at least the following:

      1. Complete blood count

      2. Chemistry screen

      3. Urinalysis

      4. Urine culture and sensitivity

      5. Thyroid testing, T4

      6. Chest radiographs

      7. Abdominal radiographs and/or abdominal ultrasound

      8. Additional tests may be performed depending on the results of initial evaluation.

  g. Nutrition

    i. Depending on the severity of the disease, as well as the concurrent disorder, these patients may require supplemental enteral (nasoesophageal-, esophagostomy-, gastrostomy-, jejunostomy-tube placement) nutrition, or possibly administration of total parenteral nutrition (see chap. 9—Nutritional Support for the Critically Ill Feline Patient).

E. Follow–up

    a. Once stable, these patients may be sent home with an appropriate dose of insulin and reevaluated as discussed in the chapter on diabetes mellitus.

    b. An appropriate dose to send these patients home with is usually 0.5 units/kg of an intermediate or long-acting insulin.

       i. Exceptions to this are:

         1. Patient is extraordinarily sensitive to insulin therapy in the hospital, and the veterinarian is concerned this may be a transient diabetic (i.e., resolving pancreatitis with newly diagnosed diabetes). This patient may be sent home with a lower dose of insulin, such as 0.25 units/kg BID subcutaneously.

         2. Patient is extraordinarily resistant to insulin while in the hospital and has a known reason to be insulin resistant (acromegaly, neoplasia, pyelonephritis, hyperadrenocorticim). This patient may require a higher dose of insulin.

         3. No matter what dose the patient is sent home with, the owners must always be aware of possible complications from hypo- or hyperglycemia.

III. Hyperglycemic, hyperosmolar syndrome

  A. Definition

    a. In humans, this syndrome is characterized by a patient with a blood glucose greater than 600 mg/dL, osmolality over 350 mOsm/kg, severe dehydration, and a lack of serum or urine ketones.

    b. While the syndrome is less well defined in cats, one study defines it as occurring in cats with blood glucose greater than 600 mg/dL, osmolality over 350 mOsm/kg, and negative urine ketones.

    c. This syndrome is reportedly seen most commonly in older cats that are long-standing diabetics and have been receiving insulin. It is thought that the presence of insulin may prevent the development of ketosis but allow for profound dehydration and development of hyperosmolarity.

    d. Common reported clinical signs include polyuria, polydipsia, and lethargy, and many cats are found to have neurologic (stupor, obtundation, coma, seizures) and respiratory signs (dyspnea and/or tachypnea due to pleural effusion from cardiac failure or neoplasia, pulmonary edema, or asthma).

    e. Concurrent diseases are commonly found in this population of cats and include diseases found in many older cats. Such diseases include renal failure, respiratory disease, infection, heart disease, neoplasia, and gastrointestinal disease.

    f. Most cats present with profound dehydration, azotemia, and acidosis.

    g. The survival rate for these cats is typically low, with one study reporting a mortality rate of 64.7%. No variables evaluated in this study were associated with a better or worse chance for survival. It is possible that given the severity of clinical signs with which these animals present, and the common finding of concurrent disease such as renal failure and infection, these animals were euthanized early in the course of treatment.

  B. Diagnosis

    a. Because many patients will present with neurologic signs such as obtundation, twitching, seizures, or disorientation, it is important to differentiate between HHS and hypoglycemia.

    b. These patients will have a profound hyperglycemia, hyperosmolality, and glucosuria.

    c. Renal values and full electrolyte panel should be evaluated upon presentation and will help to calculate serum osmolality if an osmometer is not available.

    d. Serum osmolality = $2(Na + K) + (BUN/2.8) + (glucose/18)$. Reference range: 292–308 mosm/L.

    e. Urinalysis, hematrocrit, and total solids may help differentiate between renal and prerenal azotemia, since these patients are often profoundly dehydrated.

    f. Additional testing should include complete blood count, serum chemistry, urinalysis and urine culture, thyroid level, and serum osmolality. Other testing may include radiography, abdominal ultrasound, and echocardiography as indicated.

Box 31.3.   Step-by-step diagnostics and therapy for feline diabetic ketoacidotic patients.

1. Diagnostics
   a. Extended database
      i.   Blood glucose
      ii.   Serum and/or urine ketones
      iii.   PCV
      iv.   Total solids
      v.   pH, HCO_3^-, base deficit
      vi.   Sodium, chloride
      vii.   Potassium
      viii. Phosphorus
      ix.   Magnesium
   b. Blood pressure
   c. Complete blood count
   d. Chemistry screen
   e. Urinalysis
   f. Urine culture
   g. T4
   h. Chest and abdominal imaging
   i. Miscellaneous testing such as fPLI
2. Therapeutics
   a. Obtain intravenous access, preferably central venous access.
   b. Begin fluid therapy.
      i.   May require fluid boluses to stabilize patient—see chap. 3—Shock and chap. 8—Fluid Therapy.
      ii. Once hemodynamically stable, begin replacement and maintenance fluid therapy.
      iii. Continue to monitor electrolyte, blood glucose, and blood pressure closely.
   c. Start insulin continuous rate infusion—usually after at least 4–6 hours of replacement fluids have been administered.
      i. See box 31.2 for further details.
      ii. Blood glucose should be checked every 2 hours.
   d. Once insulin therapy has started, expect further shifts in electrolytes such as potassium, magnesium, and phosphorus. Check these levels at least every 8–12 hours. Most cats will need supplementation of one or more of these electrolytes to prevent complications.
   e. If underlying infection such as urinary tract infection is suspected, antibiotics should be started after obtaining a sterile urine sample for culture.
   f. If protracted vomiting occurs, antiemetics should be administered.
   g. Gastrointestinal protectants such as famotidine may be used to limit acid secretion in the stomach.
   h. Treat underlying diseases as indicated.

C. Differential diagnosis
   a. Hyperosmolar, hyperglycemic syndrome must be differentiated from other diabetic emergencies such as insulin overdose, and hypoglycemia, and diabetic ketoacidosis. It should be remembered that the urine dipstick does not measure β-hydroxybutyrate. While it is unlikely that a patient would have diabetic ketoacidosis only due to production of this ketone body, it is possible.
   b. Other causes of neurologic abnormalities should be considered, including renal failure, hepatoencephalopathy, primary neurologic disease, metabolic derangements such as hypokalemia or hypocalcemia, and toxicity (ethylene glycol, etc.).

D. Treatment

   a. Treatment protocol follows that of DKA; however, rehydration must be performed more slowly to prevent cerebral edema and worsening of neurologic signs.

   b. It is very important to allow the glucose concentration to be slowly corrected as well to prevent rapid fluid and electrolyte shifts that could lead to cerebral edema. The rate of decline of serum glucose should not exceed 75–100 mg/dL/hr.

   c. Sodium concentrations should be monitored closely as well, and the serum sodium concentration should not decline (or rise) more rapidly than 10–12 meEq in a 24-hour period.

   d. As with DKA patients, potassium, phosphorus, and magnesium concentrations should be monitored closely to prevent extreme reductions in their total body levels.

   e. The absolute goal of therapy is to allow for gradual rehydration and gradual correction of the serum glucose levels, leading to correction of the hyperosmolar state. Underlying diseases need to be treated as well.

Recommended Reading

Feldman EC, Nelson RW. Canine and Feline Endocrinology and Reproduction, 3rd ed. Elsevier Science, 2004.

Greco DS. Diagnosis of diabetes mellitus in cats and dogs. In Behrend EN, Kemppainen RJ, eds, The Veterinary Clinics of North America Small Animal Practice: Endocrinology, pp 845–853. Philadelphia: W.B. Saunders, 2001.

Koenig A, Drobatz KJ, Beale AB, King LG. Hyperglycemic, hyperosmolar syndrome in feline diabetics: 17 cases (1995–2001). J Vet Emerg Crit Care, 2004; 14(1):30–40.

Rand J, Marshall R. Feline diabetes mellitus: which insulin do I choose and how do I adjust the dose? ACVIM Proceedings, June 2006.

Rand JS, Martin GJ. Management of feline diabetes mellitus. In Behrend EN, Kemppainen RJ, eds, The Veterinary Clinics of North America Small Animal Practice: Endocrinology, pp 881–913. Philadelphia: W.B. Saunders, 2001.

32
MANAGEMENT OF SPECIFIC ENDOCRINE AND METABOLIC DISEASES: OTHER

Cynthia R. Ward

Unique Features
- Cats with thyroid storm present with acute manifestations of thyroid hormone excess and should be aggressively treated to minimize mortality.
- The most common cause for a low Na:K ratio in the cat is cavitary effusion and not hypoadrenocorticism; cortisol sampling times for ACTH-stimulation testing in the cat using the IV protocol are at 0, 60, and 90 minutes.
- Hyperaldosteronism in the cat is a rare endocrinopathy that results in severe hypokalemia and hypertension.
- Medical treatment for hyperadrenocorticism in cats using trilostane has been successful.

I. Thyroid storm
   A. Thyroid storm is an acute thyrotoxic manifestation of hyperthyroidism in cats and can be a significant cause of mortality.
   B. Etiology
      1. Rapid increases in free thyroid hormone
      2. Increased cellular sensitivity to the hormone
      3. Increased activity of the sympathetic nervous system
   C. Precipitating events that may be linked to the development of thyroid storm
      1. Surgery
      2. Nonthyroidal illness
      3. Vigorous palpation of the thyroid gland
      4. Sudden withdrawal of antithyroid medication
      5. Administration of iodine-containing agents, such as radioiodine or potassium iodide
      6. Trauma
   D. Clinical presentation
      1. Signalment—middle- to older-aged cats, no breed/sex predilection
      2. Cardiovascular
         a. Congestive heart failure
         b. Cardiac arrhythmias
         c. Cardiac murmurs
         d. Gallop sounds
         e. Thromboemboli

   3. Neurologic
      a. Hyperactivity
      b. Hyperesthesia
      c. Ataxia/paresis
      d. Altered mentation
      e. Seizure
      f. Coma
   4. Muscular
      a. Severe muscle atrophy
      b. Generalized weakness
      c. Neck ventroflexion
   5. Gastrointestinal-hepatic dysfunction
      a. Diarrhea
      b. Vomiting
      c. Unexplained hyperbilirubinemia
   6. Acute respiratory distress
   7. Hypovolemia
   8. Hypertension
   9. Hyperthermia
E. Clinical pathology abnormalities
   1. CBC
      a. Mild erythrocytosis
      b. Macrocytosis
      c. Mature neutrophilia, lymphopenia, eosinopenia (stress leukogram)
   2. Chemistry
      a. Mild hyperglycemia
      b. Elevated liver enzymes (ALT, SAP, LDH, AST)
      c. Hyperbilirubinemia
      d. Mild-severe hypokalemia
   3. Lack of urine concentrating ability
   4. Elevated serum T4 or elevated serum T4 and fT4
F. Diagnosis
   1. Newly or previously diagnosed hyperthyroidism
   2. Clinical signs as listed above
   3. Presence of clinical abnormalities in three or more separate organ systems may indicate impending thyroid storm.
G. Treatment (table 32.1)
   1. Treatment of nonthyroidal illness or other precipitating cause
   2. Inhibition of hyperactive thyroid gland tissue
      a. Methimazole 2.5–5 mg BID
         i. Oral
         ii. Transdermal—in PLO gel
         iii. Rectal—dissolve crushed tablet in warm water
      b. Iodine preparations
         i. Prevents release of preformed thyroid hormone in thyroid gland
         ii. Give methimazole 1 hour before administration of these compounds to prevent new hormone synthesis.
         iii. Iopanoic acid 100–150 mg PO q24h
         iv. Potassium iodate 25 mg q8h
   3. Inhibition of peripheral thyroid hormone effects

Table 32.1. Medications used in managing feline endocrine diseases.

Medications	Usages	Doses	Comments
Methimazole	Blocks thyroid hormone production	2.5–5 mg q12h, orally, transdermally, rectally	Immune-mediated side effects
Iopanoic acid	Blocks peripheral T4 to T3 conversion	100–150 mg PO q24h	
Potassium iodate	Blocks thyroid hormone release	25 mg q8h PO	
Atenolol	Beta-blockade	1–3 mg/kg PO q12–24h	
Propanolol	Beta-blockade, inhibits T4 to T3 peripheral conversion	0.02 mg/kg slow IV 2.5–5 mg PO q8–12h	
Esmolol	Short acting Beta-blockade	Load: 200–500 µg/kg IV over 1 min 25–200 µg/kg/min CRI	
Dexamethasone	Weak inhibitor of peripheral T4 to T3 conversion	0.1 mg/kg q12–24h	
	Glucocorticoid replacement	0.0.02–0.04 mg/kg IV q24h	
	Adrenal Axis testing	0.1 mg/kg IV	10x canine dose
Amlodipine	Antihypertensive	0.625–1.25 mg PO or rectally q12–24h	
Enalapril or benazepril	Antihypertensive	0.25–0.5 mg/kg q12–24h	
Nitroprusside	Antihypertensive	0.5–5 µg/kg/min as a CRI	
Potassium gluconate	Potassium replacement	0.5 mEq/kg PO q24h	
Potassium chloride	Potassium replacement	0.1–0.5 mEq/kg/hr IV	
B complex vitamins	Support	2–4 mL/L of IV fluids	
Unfractionated heparin	Anticoagulation	200–400 U/kg SQ q8h	
Cortrosyn	Adrenal axis testing	125 mg IV or IM	Postinjection sampling times differ depending on route of delivery
ACTH gel	Adrenal axis testing	2.2 U/kg IM	Obtain at reliable compounding pharmacies. May not be standardized strength
Prednisone	Glucocorticoid replacement	0.2–0.4 mg/kg PO q24h	
Methylprednisolone acetate	Glucocorticoid replacement	5–10 mg SQ, IM once per month	May cause diabetes mellitus
Desoxycorticosterone pivalate (DOCP)	Mineralocorticoid replacement	2.2 U/kg IM q25–28 days	
Fludrocortisone acetate (Florinef)	Mineralocorticoid replacement	0.1 mg PO q24h	
Spironolactone	Blockage of aldosterone	2–3 mg/kg PO q12h	
Trilostane	Medical treatment of hyperadrenocorticism	5 mg/kg PO q24h	

a. B-blockade
    i. Atenolol 1–3 mg/kg PO q12–24h
    ii. Propanolol
        a. May also have weak activity to inhibit T4 to T3 peripheral conversion

          b. 0.02 mg/kg slow IV, may repeat up to four times

          c. 2.5–5 mg PO q8–12h

        iii. Esmolol

          a. Load at 200–500 μg/kg IV over 1 min

          b. 25–200 μg/kg/min CRI

    b. Dexamethasone

      i. Inhibits peripheral conversion of T4 to T3

      ii. 0.1 mg/kg q12–24h

  4. Management of hypertension

    a. B-blockade may normalize blood pressure so try first

    b. Enalapril or benazapril 0.25–0.5 mg/kg q12–24hr

    c. Amlodipine: 0.625–1.25 mg PO or rectally q12–24h

    d. Nitroprusside: 0.5–5 μg/kg/min as a constant rate infusion

      i. Monitor blood pressure closely to avoid hypotension.

  5. Supportive care

    a. IV Fluid therapy +/– potassium chloride as necessitated by hydration status (see chap. 8)

    b. Potassium gluconate if hypokalemic at 0.5 mEq/kg PO per day

    c. B complex vitamins at 2–4 mL/L of IV fluids

    d. Aspirin 5 mg/cat q72h

    e. Unfractionated heparin 200–400 U/kg SQ q8h until aPTT 1.5–2 × > baseline

      i. Ensure patient is adequately hydrated and perfused prior to SQ injections.

II. Hypoadrenocorticism

  A. Hypoadrenocorticism is a rare disease in cats.

  B. Etiology

    1. Primary disease—most common

      a. Idiopathic

      b. Neoplastic infiltration, lymphoma

    2. Iatrogenic secondary disease—acute withdrawal of methylprednisolone acetate or other glucocorticoids at high doses

  C. Clinical presentation

    1. Signalment: young to middle-aged cats (range 1.5–14 yrs)

    2. History:

      a. Waxing and waning clinical signs

      b. Weight loss

      c. Anorexia

      d. Lethargy

      e. Intermittent vomiting

      f. High doses of glucocorticoids administered in repository form or acute withdrawal from short-acting glucocorticoids

    3. Clinical signs

      a. Depression

      b. Weakness

      c. Dehydration

      d. Hypothermia

      e. Collapse/weakness

      f. Bradycardia

    4. Clinicopathologic abnormalities

      a. CBC—nonregenerative anemia

      b. Chemistry

        i. Hyponatremia

            ii.   Hyperkalemia
            iii. Sodium-potassium ratio <27:1
            iv.   Hypochloridemia
            v.   Hypercalcemia
            vi.   Azotemia
            vii. Hyperphosphatemia
            viii. Metabolic acidosis
        c. Urinalysis: +/− isosthenuria
        d. Imaging studies
            i.   Microcardia
            ii.   Pulmonary hypoperfusion
            iii. Small or nonvisualized adrenal glands; may be enlarged with abnormal echogenicity if
                  infiltrative disease
    D. Diagnosis
        1. Major differential diagnoses
            a. Pleural, peritoneal, or bicavitary effusion (these are associated with low serum sodium and
                high serum potassium concentrations)
            b. Renal failure
            c. Gastrointestinal disease
            d. Diabetes mellitus
            e. Hyperthyroidism
        2. ACTH-stimulation test—tests adrenal reserve of cortisol secretion
            a. Synthetic ACTH (cortrosyn)
                i.   125 µg IM, serum cortisol samples 0, 30, 60 min.
                ii.   125 µg IV, serum cortisol samples 0, 60, 90 min. Use caution as vomiting and collapse have
                      been associated with IV administration in cats.
            b. ACTH gel: 2.2 U/kg IM, serum cortisol samples 0, 60, and 120 min
            c. To support a diagnosis of hypoadrenocorticism, baseline and post-ACTH serum cortisols
                should be below the cortisol reference range.
    E. Treatment
        1. Goals
            a. Correct hypovolemia
            b. Correct acid/base abnormalities
            c. Correct electrolyte deficiencies
            d. Correct adrenal cortical hormone deficiencies
        2. IV fluid therapy to correct hypovolemia
            a. 0.9% saline, replaces sodium and does not add potassium
            b. If serum sodium is very low, <125 mg/dL, raise sodium more slowly; consider using
                lactated Ringer's solution, which has a lower sodium than saline and lower potassium than
                many of the replacement fluids (see chap. 8—Fluid Therapy and chap. 34—Electrolyte
                Disorders).
            c. If severe hypovolemia, may need to bolus fluids to shock dose of 60 mL/kg/hr
        3. Initial glucocorticoid replacement
            a. Dexamethasone
                i.   Best choice until ACTH-stimulation test can be performed since it will not interfere with
                      cortisol assay
                ii.   Use quick-acting formulation, such as Dexamethasone SP.
                iii. 0.1 mg/kg IV to correct deficiencies and account for stress in the acutely ill animal
        4. Long-term glucocorticoid replacement
            a. Prednisolone

           i.   0.2–0.4 mg/kg PO q24h

           ii. Increase to 0.5 mg/kg PO q12–24h for stressful events

      b. Methylprednisolone acetate if oral medication prohibited

           i.   5–10 mg SQ per month

           ii. Increases possibility of diabetes mellitus

    5. Long-term mineralocorticoid replacement

      a. Desoxycorticosterone pivalate (DOCP; Percorten-V, Novartis Animal Health): 2.2 U/kg IM q 25–28 days

      b. Fludrocortisone acetate (Florinef, Bristol-Myers-Squibb): 0.1 mg q24h

  F. Monitoring

    1. Serum Na/K levels to determine mineralocorticoid therapy; adjust if necessary.

    2. Glucocorticoid therapy monitoring relies on the owner's reports of attitude, appetite, and energy levels at home. Weight gain can also be monitored. There is no need to repeat an ACTH-stimulation test.

  G. Prognosis—excellent long-term prognosis for hypoadrenocorticism if condition is recognized and treated appropriately

III. Hyperaldosteronism (Conn's Syndrome)

  A. Rare disease in cats

  B. Etiology

    1. Oversecretion of aldosterone

    2. Unilateral or bilateral adrenocortical tumors

    3. May be benign or malignant

  C. Clinical presentation

    1. Signalment

      a. Middle-aged to older cats (range 6–20 years)

      b. No breed/sex predilection

    2. History

      a. Episodic lameness or muscle weakness

      b. Polyuria/polydipsia

      c. Vision loss

      d. Polyphagia

      e. Weight loss

    3. Clinical signs

      a. Hypokalemic polymyopathy

           i.   Ventroflexion of neck

           ii. Hind limb weakness

           iii. Paresis

      b. Retinal abnormalities

           i.   Detachment

           ii. Tortuous vessels

           iii. Hemorrhages

           iv. Bullae

           v. Edema

      c. Hypertension

    4. Clinicopathologic changes

      a. Hypokalemia (common)

      b. Hypernatremia (uncommon)

      c. Azotemia

      d. Elevated CK

      e. Elevated plasma aldosterone

   5. Abdominal ultrasound
      a. Unilateral or bilateral adrenal mass(es)
      b. +/– mass extension into the vena cava
 D. Diagnosis
   1. Appropriate history and clinical signs
   2. Appropriate biochemical data, hypokalemia most important
   3. Elevated plasma aldosterone levels
   4. Presence of uni- or bilateral adrenal masses
 E. Treatment
   1. Correction of hypokalemia
      a. Oral potassium gluconate: 0.5 mEq/kg PO
      b. Potassium chloride IV not to exceed 0.5 mEq/kg/hr
   2. Blockage of aldosterone: spironolactone: 2–3 mg/kg PO q12h
   3. Treatment of hypertension
      a. Enalapril or benazepril: 0.5 to 2 mg/kg PO q12h
      b. Amlodipine: 0.625–1.25 mg PO or rectally q12–24h
      c. Nitroprusside: 0.5–5 μg/kg/min as a constant rate infusion
   4. Definitive treatment
      a. Surgical removal of tumor
      b. Ultrasound or MRI should be performed to determine whether tumor has invaded vessels.
 F. Prognosis
   1. Medical treatment improves clinical signs but will not normalize blood values.
   2. Medical treatment can preserve quality of life for 1–3 years; euthanasia is usually due to chronic renal failure.
   3. Surgical removal of nonmalignant tumor yields good response of up to 6 years.
IV. Hyperadrenocorticism
 A. Uncommon disorder in cats; being recognized more frequently
 B. Etiology
   1. Pituitary adenoma (85%)
   2. Adrenal adenoma
   3. Adrenal carcinoma
 C. Clinical presentation
   1. Middle-aged to older cats (5–16 years), no breed or sex predilection
   2. Concurrent insulin-resistant diabetes mellitus (80%)
   3. Thin, fragile skin
   4. Large, nonhealing cutaneous wounds
   5. Polyuria/polydipsia
   6. Polyphagia
   7. Recurrent cutaneous, upper respiratory, and urinary tract infections
   8. Lethargy
   9. Muscle atrophy
  10. Weakness
  11. Abdominal enlargement
  12. Alopecia/failure to regrow hair
 D. Clinicopathologic findings
   1. Elevated ALP and ALT
   2. Hypercholesterolemia
   3. Hyperglycemia
   4. Mature neutrophilia, lymphopenia, eosinopenia (stress leukogram)
   5. Glucosuria

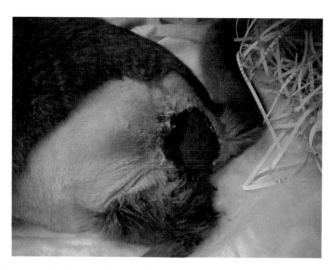

Fig. 32.1. Nonhealing wound of a cat with thin skin due to hyperadrenocorticism.

6. Lack of urine concentrating ability
7. Proteinuria
8. Bacteriuria, pyuria
E. Diagnosis
  1. Screening tests
    a. Low-dose dexamethasone suppression test
      i. 0.1 mg/kg dexamethasone IV (10× canine dose)
      ii. Serum cortisol measured 0, 4, 8 hr
      iii. Cortisol not suppressed at 4 and/or 8 hours—supports diagnosis of feline hyperadrenocorticism
      iv. Cannot be used as a differentiating test as in dogs
    b. ACTH-stimulation test
      i. 40–50% of cats with hyperadrenocorticism will show a normal response to ACTH
      ii. Synthetic ACTH (cortrosyn)
        1. 125 µg IM, serum cortisol samples 0, 60, 90 min.
        2. 125 µg IV (preferred), serum cortisol samples 0, 60, 90 min.
      iii. ACTH gel: 2.2 U/kg IM, serum cortisol samples 0, 60, and 120 min
      iv. An exaggerated response to ACTH of >19 µg/dL is consistent with a diagnosis of hyperadrenocorticism.
  2. Differentiating tests
    a. Plasma endogenous ACTH concentration
      i. Single plasma sample submitted
      ii. Special handling of sample (call lab for specifics)
      iii. Pituitary-dependent disease: ACTH concentrations normal to high
      iv. Adrenal-dependent disease: ACTH concentrations low or nondetectable
    b. Abdominal ultrasonography
      i. Unilaterally enlarged or calcified adrenal gland supports adrenal-dependent hyperadrenocorticism.
      ii. Bilaterally enlarged adrenal glands support pituitary-dependent hyperadrenocorticism.
    c. Magnetic resonance imaging—can detect presence of a pituitary tumor

F. Treatment
  1. Medical
    a. Mitotane (Lysodren)—do not use
      i.   Not effective in cats
      ii. Causes acute liver failure
    b. Trilostane
      i.   Begin with 5 mg/kg PO q24h and adjust as necessary.
      ii. Monitor with ACTH-stimulation test with the goal of having pre- and post-ACTH cortisol concentrations between 1 and 4 μg/dL.
      iii. Monitor serum Na/K levels
      iv. In cats with diabetes mellitus, reduce insulin by at least 25% before starting trilostane as insulin requirements will decrease.
  2. Surgical
    a. Unilateral adrenalectomy
    b. Bilateral adrenalectomy in cats that cannot be medicated orally
    c. Control clinical signs of hyperadrenocorticism with trilostane for at least 2 weeks before surgery to heal skin lesions and control diabetes mellitus if present; insulin dose should be decreased by at least 25% before initiating trilostane.
    d. If bilateral adrenalectomy, glucocorticoid and mineralocorticoid therapies will be necessary for life.
      i.   Desoxycorticosterone pivalate (DOCP; Percorten-V, Novartis Animal Health): 2.2 U/kg IM q 30 days
      ii. Prednisolone 0.4 mg/kg PO SID
      iii. Methylprednisolone acetate, Depomedrol, 10 mg IM q 30 days
    e. Unilateral adrenalectomy—glucocorticoid and mineralocorticoid therapies may be necessary for several weeks while the healthy adrenal gland regenerates.
G. Prognosis
  1. Successful treatment of hyperadrenocorticism will decrease or eliminate insulin requirement.
  2. Prognosis is good with successful control.

Recommended Reading

Bell R, Mellor DJ, Ramsey I, Knottenbelt C. Decreased sodium-potassium ratios in cats: 49 cases. Vet Clin Pathol, 2005; 34:110–114.

Chiaramonte D, Greco DS. Feline adrenal disorders. Clin Tech Sm Anim Prac, 2007; 1:26–31.

Dillmann WH. Thyroid storm. Curr Ther Endocrinol Metab, 1997; 6:81–85.

Flood SM, Randolph JF, Gelzer AR. Primary hyperaldosteronism in two cats. JAAHA, 1999; 35:411–416.

Lien YH, Huang HP, Chang PH. Iatrogenic hyperadrenocorticism in 12 cats. JAAHA, 2006; 42:423.

Neiger R, Witt AL, Noble A, Cerman AJ. Trilostane therapy for treatment of pituitary-dependent hyperadrenocorticism in 5 cats. JVIM, 2004; 18:160–164.

Peterson ME, Greco DS, Orth DR. Hypoadrenocorticism in ten cats. JVIM, 1989; 3:55–58.

Ward CR. Feline thyroid storm. Vet Clin Sm Anim, 2007; 37:745–754.

33
DIAGNOSTIC TESTING OF ENDOCRINE DISEASE IN THE CAT

Jennifer E. Prittie

Unique Features
- In cats, differential diagnoses are for weight loss and polyphagia together include hyperthyroidism, diabetes mellitus, and hyperadrenocorticism.
- Cats with hyperaldosteronism (Conn's syndrome) commonly present with the following constellation of signs: hypernatremia, hypokalemia and associated polymyopathy, metabolic alkalosis, and systemic hypertension.
- Atypical hypoadrenocorticism is not reported in cats; all cats with disease have demonstrated a low sodium:potassium ratio.

---

1. Introduction
    a. Feline endocrine and metabolic emergencies present a challenge to the attending clinician. Many of the endocrinopathies and ensuing electrolyte and cardiovascular abnormalities result in vague and episodic clinical signs, and routine laboratory tests rarely provide the veterinarian with a definitive diagnosis. Advanced imaging and less frequently utilized or provocative laboratory tests are often needed to elucidate the cause of the cat's clinical signs.
2. Clinical presentation
    a. Most cats with underlying endocrine disorders present with historical weight loss, changes in food consumption (inappetence or polyphagia), and general lethargy or malaise.
        i. Differential endocrine diagnoses for weight loss and polyphagia together include hyperthyroidism, diabetes mellitus, and hyperadrenocorticism.
    b. Polyuria and polydipsia may be associated with hyperthyroidism, diabetes mellitus, hyperadrenocorticism, hypoadrenocorticism, hyperaldosteronism, pheochromocytoma, and hyperparathyroidism.
    c. Cardiovascular abnormalities, including systemic hypertension, cardiac arrhythmias, cardiomyopathy with or without congestive heart failure, and hypertensive retinopathy, are most commonly associated with hyperthyroidism, hyperadrenocorticism, hyperaldosteronism, and pheochromocytoma.
    d. Neurologic or neuromuscular abnormalities accompany several endocrinopathies.
        i. Hypokalemia-induced polymyopathy, characterized by weakness, ataxia, dysphagia, respiratory depression, and ventroflexion of the neck, may occur secondary to diabetes ketoacidosis, hyperaldosteronism, or hyperthyroidism.
        ii. Both ionized hypocalcemia and hypercalcemia associated with hypoparathyroidism and hyperparathyroidism, respectively, may result in muscle tremors and fasciculations.

429

      iii. Seizure activity is most commonly reported with primary hypoparathyroidism and resultant hypocalcemia (tetany) and insulin-secreting tumors (neuroglycopenia).

          1. Hypocalcemic seizures are typically not associated with incontinence or a loss of consciousness.

          2. Hypocalcemic cats may also demonstrate mydriasis, lenticular cataracts, dysphagia, pruritus, ptyalism, panting, or protrusion of the nictitating membranes.

      iv. Irritability, nervousness, aggression, and an inability to sit still have been reported in hyperthyroid cats. Seizures have been infrequently reported.

    e. Patchy spontaneous alopecia or failure to regrow hair where it has been clipped and inelastic, fragile, thin skin that bruises easily are typical of hyperadrenocorticism.

    f. Cats with hyperthyroidism (>90%) or hyperparathyroidism may have a palpable cervical mass.

3. Routine laboratory findings

    a. Complete blood count in affected cats is typically unremarkable but may reveal:

      i.   Erythrocytosis and macrocytosis and the presence of Heinz bodies in hyperthyroid cats

      ii. Normocytic, normochromic anemia associated with hypoadrenocorticism

      iii. Lymphocytosis and eosinophilia in cats with hypoadrenocorticism

          1. The presence of an absolute lymphocytosis and/or eosinophilia in a sick cat should raise the clinician's suspicion that the patient is unable to mount an appropriate stress response, consistent with a diagnosis of hypoadrenocorticism.

    b. Abnormalities in serum biochemistry profile are typically more helpful diagnostically.

      i.   Hypokalemia

          1. Diabetes ketoacidosis

          2. Hyperaldosteronism

          3. Hyperthyroidism

      ii. Hyperkalemia

          1. Hypoadrenocorticism

          2. The hyperkalemia associated with hypoadrenocorticism in feline patients is milder than that documented in affected dogs.

      iii. Ionized hypocalcemia and concurrent hyperphosphatemia

          1. Primary hypoparathyroidism

          2. The main differential for hypocalcemia with hyperphosphatemia is renal insufficiency, which can easily be excluded with routine blood work.

          3. Other causes of hypocalcemia and hyperphosphatemia together, including acute pancreatitis, magnesium depletion, administration of phosphate-containing enemas, ethylene glycol toxicity, and intestinal malabsorption, should be excluded on a case-by-case basis.

      iv. Ionized hypercalcemia

          1. Primary hyperparathyroidism

            a. Concurrent hypophosphatemia is expected.

          2. Hypoadrenocorticism

          3. Other differentials for hypercalcemia in cats, including neoplasia, renal failure, idiopathic disease, granulomatous disease (deep fungal infection), and vitamin D toxicosis should be explored as deemed necessary on a case-by-case basis.

      v.   Hypoglycemia

          1. Insulin-producing islet cell tumor

          2. Less commonly associated with hypoadrenocorticism

      vi. Hyperglycemia

          1. Diabetes mellitus

          2. Hyperadrenocorticism

            a. 80% of cats with hyperadrenocorticism have concurrent diabetes mellitus.

vii. All cats with hypoadrenocorticism have demonstrated an abnormally low sodium-potassium ratio (<24:1).
1. Other differentials for this combination of electrolyte abnormalities include renal and urinary tract disease, liver failure, gastrointestinal infection with whipworms or salmonellosis, pleural effusion with repeat drainage, diabetes ketoacidosis, pancreatitis, and congestive heart failure.
viii. Metabolic alkalosis resulting from increased tubular bicarbonate transport is typical of cats with hyperaldosteronism.
ix. Less specific biochemical alterations include elevated liver enzymes, hyperbilirubinemia, and azotemia, which are associated to various degrees with hyperthyroidism, hyperadrenocorticism, hypoadrenocorticism, and hyperaldosteronism.
x. Siamese cats appear to be at increased risk for development of insulinoma and primary hyperparathyroidism, and at decreased risk for developing hyperthyroidism.
c. Urinalysis should be collected as part of a minimum database but is not often helpful in achieving a diagnosis.
i. Glucosuria is common in cats with diabetes mellitus and hyperadrenocorticism.
ii. Urine specific gravity varies drastically.
4. Ancillary diagnostics
a. Serial blood pressure evaluation is indicated for cats suspected to have hyperthyroidism, hyperadrenocorticism, pheochromocytoma, or hyperaldosteronism.
b. Electrocardiography may document arrhythmias in patients with derangements in calcium or potassium balance, hyperthyroidism, or catecholamine excess (pheochromocytoma).
c. Echocardiography may reveal concurrent cardiomyopathy, which has been reported in cats afflicted with hyperthyroidism, hyperaldosteronism, or pheochromocytoma.
d. Abdominal radiographs may reveal a cranial abdominal mass effect consistent with an adrenal tumor (adrenal-tumor–dependent hyperadrenocorticism, aldosterone-secreting tumor, or pheochromocytoma) or pancreatic neoplasia (insulinoma).
e. Thoracic radiographs are indicated in any feline patient suspected to have an endocrine disease of malignant origin.
f. Abdominal CT or MRI may confirm the presence of an abdominal mass and can be useful in ascertaining the extent of the tumor prior to surgical resection.
g. Brain CR or MRI may aid in visualization of a pituitary mass.
i. 50% of cats with pituitary-dependent hyperadrenocorticism have tumors that are large enough to visualize.
h. Cervical ultrasound may detect a thyroid or parathyroid mass but has not been shown to be useful or reliable for diagnosis of hyperthyroidism.
5. Definitive diagnosis of hyperthyroidism is achieved in most cases by measurement of serum thyroid hormones.
a. Basal total thyroid hormone concentrations
i. Thyroid hormone concentrations fluctuate, but basal total T4 concentration is above the reference range in greater than 90% of hyperthyroid cats.
ii. Infrequently, cats with hyperthyroidism have a normal total T4. This is most likely with:
1. Early or mild hyperthyroidism
2. Significant concurrent nonthyroid disease (euthyroid sick)
iii. Basal total T_3 is less sensitive than total T_4, diagnostic for hyperthyroidism in approximately 70% of affected cats.
iv. Most veterinary laboratories utilize human T_4 radioimmunoassay (RIA) kits for measurement of T_4.
1. Many are validated for use in cats.
2. Reference ranges should be established for feline patients.

b. Free thyroxine concentration (fT_4)
   i. 99% of thyroid hormone is protein bound and inactive; fT_4 is the hormone fraction (1%) that diffuses into the cell and is converted to T_3 to exert metabolic effects.
   ii. fT_4 is less affected by nonthyroid illness than is total T_4, and is therefore more sensitive for diagnosis of hyperthyroidism.
      1. fT_4 is elevated in greater than 98% of affected cats.
   iii. There is an increased likelihood of false positive fT_4 results, making this test less specific for diagnosis of hyperthyroidism than total T_4.
      1. 6–12% of cats with nonthyroidal disease demonstrate elevated fT_4 concentrations.
   iv. Free T_4 is typically assayed via equilibrium dialysis.
   v. If a clinician suspects hyperthyroidism and the total T_4 and/or T_3 are within the reference range, the current recommendation is as follows:
      1. Repeat the test days to weeks after initial testing.
      2. Rule out any concurrent nonthyroid illness.
      3. Measure the free T_4 concentration.
      4. Consider dynamic thyroid function tests.
c. Feline thyroid-stimulating hormone (TSH)
   i. There is currently no commercially available feline-specific assay.
   ii. Measurement of circulating TSH is not recommended as a screening test for feline hyperthyroidism.
d. Dynamic thyroid function tests should be considered in feline patients suspected of clinical hyperthyroidism when the serum T_4 concentration remains nondiagnostic.
   i. Triiodothyronine (T_3) suppression test
      1. Administration of T_3 to healthy cats should suppress pituitary TSH secretion and lower serum T_4 concentration.
      2. Cats with hyperthyroidism have chronic suppression of TSH secretion due to autonomous secretion of thyroid hormone from one or both thyroid glands. Administration of T_3 to these cats has little to no effect on serum T_4 concentration.
      3. Protocol: Baseline measurement of serum T_4 and T_3, administration of seven oral doses of liothyronine over a 2.5-day period, and subsequent measurement of serum T_4 and T_3 concentrations
      4. Interpretation: An increase in T_3 concentration confirms successful medication. Suppression of total T_4 concentration <50% of baseline, or <1.5 µg/dL (<20 nmol/L) does not occur in hyperthyroidism.
      5. The T_3 suppression test can be used to rule out hyperthyroidism, distinguishing between euthyroid and mildly hyperthyroid cats.
      6. A 3-day testing interval and reliance on owners to administer an oral medication seven times at home diminishes the practicality of this test.
   ii. Thyroid-stimulating hormone (TSH) response test
      1. This test is not recommended for diagnosis of hyperthyroidism in cats.
   iii. Thyrotropin-releasing hormone (TRH) stimulation test
      1. This test involves measurement of serum T_4 concentration before and 4 hours after administration of TRH (0.1 mg/kg IV).
      2. Hyperthyroid cats demonstrate a blunted response to TRH stimulation (<50% increase in T_4 over the baseline value) because of chronic suppression of TSH by thyroid hormone.
      3. This test compares favorably with the T_3 suppression test, requiring less time and with more convenience.
      4. Disadvantages include common adverse side effects associated with TRH administration, including vomiting, salivation, tachypnea, and defecation.
e. Radionuclide imaging

    i. Radionuclides available for thyroid scanning include radioactive technetium-99m (pertechnetate), iodine-131, and iodine-123.

    ii. Pertechnetate is the most readily available and inexpensive, exhibits the highest safety margin, and has the shortest half-life.

    iii. Tissue identified during subsequent scintigraphy includes all functioning thyroid tissue.

       1. Ectopic thyroid tissue in the anterior mediastinum, metastasis of functioning thyroid malignancies, and unilateral versus bilateral thyroidal disease can be identified via thyroid scan.

       2. Methimazole and related compounds may affect scintigraphy results.

    iv. This procedure requires specialized equipment, a licensed facility, and heavy sedation or general anesthesia, limiting its usefulness in most cases.

  f. Trial of antithyroid therapy

    i. A 30-day trial of antithyroid therapy while monitoring for improvement or resolution of clinical signs in a cat suspected as hyperthyroid may be considered when thyroid hormone testing is equivocal.

6. When hyperadrenocorticism, or feline Cushing's syndrome (FCS) is suspected, screening testing includes the following:

  a. Urine cortisol-to-creatinine ratio (UC:CR)

    i. A urine sample is collected, centrifuged, and the supernatant analyzed.

    ii. This test is highly sensitive and there is a high predictive value associated with a normal result.

       1. A UC:CR value $\geq 3.6 \times 10^{-5}$ in a cat with compatible clinical signs is supportive with a diagnosis of FCS.

       2. A UC:CR value between 1.3 and 3.6×10^{-5} in a cat with appropriate clinical signs is equivocal.

    iii. The low specificity of this test limits its usefulness in achieving a diagnosis.

       1. Elevated UC:CR values are seen with nonadrenal diseases, such as diabetes mellitus and hyperthyroidism.

       2. Collection of the urine at home may increase test reliability due to decreased patient stress.

  b. Low-dose dexamethasone suppression test

    i. Protocol: Serum cortisol is measured before (baseline cortisol) and then 4 and 8 hours after intravenous administration of 0.1 mg/kg dexamethasone.

    ii. Interpretation: Appropriate suppression of pituitary ACTH leads to a >50% decrease in serum cortisol from the baseline value.

       1. 80–90% of cats with FCS fail to suppress at 8 hours.

       2. Suppression at 4 hours but not 8 hours is consistent with a diagnosis of pituitary-dependent hyperadrenocorticism (PDH).

    iii. This is a highly sensitive screening test, outperforming the UC:CR and ACTH stimulation tests, but it does not consistently differentiate between adrenal-tumor-dependent hyperadrenocorticism (ATH) and PDH.

  c. ACTH stimulation test

    i. This test is not currently recommended as a screening test for feline FCS as it lacks the necessary sensitivity (60% of affected cats have cortisol responses within the reference range).

7. Discriminating tests for FCS include:

  a. High-dose dexamethasone suppression test (HDDST)

    i. Protocol: Serum cortisol is measured before (baseline cortisol) and then 4 and 8 hours after intravenous administration of 1.0 mg/kg dexamethasone.

    ii. Interpretation: Appropriate suppression of pituitary ACTH leads to a >50% decrease in serum cortisol from the baseline value.

       1. Cats with PDH may or may not suppress; cats with ATH will not suppress.

    iii. An alternative at-home HDDST protocol is now available that facilitates test implementation and interpretation and patient comfort.

        1. Protocol: The owner collects urine from the cat in the morning on days 1 and 2; administers three doses of dexamethasone (0.1 mg/kg PO) at 8-hour intervals at 8:00 a.m., 4:00 p.m., and 12:00 p.m. after collection of the second urine sample; then collects a urine sample on the morning of day 3. UC:CR values are obtained from the three urine samples.

        2. Interpretation: The mean of the first two UC:CR values acts as a screening test for FCS and serves as the baseline UC:CR value. If the UC:CR value on day 3 is <50% the baseline value, the cat has suppressed. Cats with PDH may or may not suppress, while cats with ATH will not suppress.

    b. Measurement of endogenous corticotropin (ACTH) concentration

      i. Protocol: Blood is collected in an EDTA tube (with aprotinin), the plasma immediately separated and placed in plastic, and shipped on ice or frozen for storage.

      ii. Interpretation: Cats with ATH typically have low to undetectable ACTH concentrations (<10 pg/mL), whereas cats with PDH have normal to high ACTH concentrations (often >45 pg/mL). ACTH concentrations of 10–45 pg/mL are equivocal.

    c. Abdominal ultrasound may correctly differentiate between ATH and PDH in up to 80% of afflicted cats.

8. Definitive diagnosis for hypoadrenocorticism (Addison's disease) in cats is achieved with the ACTH stimulation test.

    a. The ACTH stimulation test is the "gold standard" for diagnosis of hypoadrenocorticism in humans, dogs, and cats.

      i. Protocol A: With synthetic ACTH (cortrosyn), blood samples are obtained before and 30 and 60 minutes following administration of 0.125 mg IV or IM.

        1. This method is preferred because of more profound and consistent stimulation of the adrenal cortex.

      ii. Protocol B: Using ACTH gel, blood samples are collected before and 60 and 120 minutes following administration of 2.2 U/kg IM.

      iii. Interpretation: Cats with hypoadrenocorticism demonstrate both pre- and post-ACTH stimulated cortisol concentrations less than 2 µg/dL.

    b. Plasma endogenous ACTH concentration may aid in differentiation between primary and secondary adrenocortical destruction.

      i. Cats with naturally occurring primary hypoadrenocorticism will have elevated endogenous ACTH.

      ii. Rapid withdrawal of exogenous steroids results in iatrogenic secondary hypoadrenocorticism (from drug-induced inhibition of pituitary secretion of ACTH). These cats will exhibit low cortisol levels and low endogenous ACTH.

      iii. Naturally occurring secondary hypoadrenocorticism has not been reported in the cat.

      iv. Proper sample collection is important to avoid erroneous results, as ACTH is cleared from fresh whole blood rapidly.

        1. Blood is collected in an EDTA tube (with aprotinin), centrifuged, and the plasma stored in a plastic container (the ACTH molecule adheres to glass).

        2. The blood sample should be shipped at 4°C (or frozen if not collected in aprotinin).

      v. Normal endogenous ACTH concentration is 20–80 pg/mL (4.4–8.8 pmol/L).

9. Definitive diagnosis of primary hyperaldosteronism (Conn's syndrome) includes measurement of plasma aldosterone concentration.

    a. Plasma aldosterone concentration will be elevated in affected cats.

      i. A recent case series reports a mean aldosterone concentration of 5,820 pmol/l (reference range, 150–430).

    b. Primary hyperaldosteronism should result in suppressed plasma renin activity, or renin-aldosterone dissociation.

    i. When measured in affected cats, plasma renin activity has been variable, with 50% of cats having normal values. A normal renin level does not, therefore, rule out primary hyperaldosteronism.
    ii. A high plasma renin concentration is suggestive of secondary hyperaldosteronism.
        1. Diseases such as congestive heart failure and renal failure will lead to appropriate activation of the renin-angiotensin-aldosterone system.
    iii. The ratio of plasma aldosterone concentration to plasma renin activity may be more beneficial in confirming a diagnosis of Conn's syndrome.
  c. Histopathology will confirm a diagnosis of adrenocortical neoplasia.
  d. Increased urinary fractional excretion of potassium (FE_k) results from hyperaldosteronism and may facilitate with a diagnosis.
    i. FE_k in affected cats typically >50%, with normal FE_k <6% in hypokalemic animals
10. Definitive diagnosis of pheochromocytoma antemortem can be particularly challenging.
  a. Cytologic evaluation of the adrenal mass is consistent with neoplasia of endocrine or neuroendocrine origin.
    i. Histopathology following surgical resection or postmortem is necessary for definitive diagnosis.
  b. 24-hour urine collection and measurement of urinary catecholamines and their metabolites (vanillyl mandelic acid and metanephrines) may aid in diagnosis.
    i. Stress has been shown to increase catecholamine excretion in the urine in dogs and may affect test results if collection takes place in hospitalized patients.
    ii. ARUP, a national diagnostic laboratory in Utah, will measure urinary catecholamine levels:
        1. www.aruplab.com
    iii. Metanephrine-creatinine ratios from spot urine samples have been useful for diagnosis of pheochromocytoma in human patients. This test has not been evaluated in cats.
  c. The phentolamine test relies on the principal that administration of this alpha-adrenergic antagonist will lead to a predictable decrease in systemic blood pressure in affected patients.
    i. The potential for severe systemic hypotension and the availability of safer diagnostic modalities limits this test's clinical utility.
  d. The clonidine suppression test involves administration of an alpha-2 adrenergic agonist and subsequent documentation of failure of norepinephrine levels to suppress.
    i. Episodic release of catecholamines makes test results difficult to interpret, limiting its utility in the clinical setting.
  e. Provocative tests using glucagon, tyramine, or histamine are not recommended due to the potential of life-threatening complications and high cost.
11. Definitive diagnosis of insulinoma involves the following:
  a. Documentation of an inappropriately high serum insulin concentration despite the presence of hypoglycemia is confirmatory.
    i. Inappropriate hyperinsulinism is easiest to recognize when the blood glucose is <50–60 mg/dL.
        1. A 6–12-hour fast may be necessary prior to blood sample collection if the blood glucose is >60 mg/dL.
        2. Additionally, brief reduction or cessation of intravenous dextrose supplementation may be necessary to induce mild hypoglycemia for testing purposes.
    ii. Serum insulin and blood glucose concentrations should be evaluated simultaneously from the same blood sample.
    iii. An insulin concentration above the reference range or at the high-normal end of the reference range at the time of hypoglycemia supports the diagnosis of an insulin-secreting tumor.
    iv. There are radioimmunoassays utilized to measure serum insulin concentration that have been validated in cats (labs at Cornell University and Michigan State University).

b. The amended insulin-glucose ratio (AIGR) has previously been recommended as a diagnostic aid:

i. $\dfrac{\text{Serum insulin }(\mu U/mL)}{\text{Blood glucose }(mg/dL) - 30} \times 100$

1. An AIGR >30 is consistent with an insulin-secreting tumor.
2. This test is not specific for diagnosis of insulinoma. Elevated AIGR values have been documented in dogs with liver disease and sepsis, and in healthy dogs.
3. Dogs with confirmed insulinoma have had AIGR values <30, calling into question the sensitivity of this assay as well.

c. Histopathology will ultimately confirm the diagnosis of insulinoma.
d. Somatostatin receptor scintigraphy (utilizing radiolabeled octreotide) has been successful in identifying beta-cell neoplasia in dogs.
   1. Associated expense and need for specialized facilities and equipment limit the clinical utility of this diagnostic modality.

12. Definitive diagnosis of primary hyperparathyroidism requires documentation of:
   a. A serum parathyroid hormone (PTH) concentration that is either within or above the reference range in the face of hypercalcemia.
      i. Serum or EDTA plasma can be used to measure PTH concentration.
      ii. Utilization of an assay that detects intact PTH is important, as inactive PTH fragments may accumulate in the bloodstream in patients with concurrent renal dysfunction and confound results. This assay must be validated in cats.
      iii. Ionized calcium is the biologically active form that regulates PTH activity, and this is the recommended form to measure.
         1. Ionized calcium can be measured in serum or heparinized plasma.
      iv. Parathyroid hormone–related peptide (PTHrP) and vitamin D metabolites are also low in affected cats.
   b. Histopathology confirms parathyroid malignancy.

13. Definitive diagnosis of primary hypoparathyroidism involves documentation of:
   a. Lack of PTH during a period of profound, clinical hypocalcemia
      i. A PTH concentration that is in the low-normal range is also abnormal during periods of hypocalcemia.
      ii. Serum or EDTA plasma can be used to measure PTH.
      iii. Utilization of an assay that detects intact PTH is important, as inactive fragments may accumulate in the bloodstream in patients with concurrent renal dysfunction and confound results.
      iv. Ionized calcium is the biologically active form that regulates PTH activity, and this is the recommended form to measure.
         1. Ionized calcium can be measured in serum or heparinized plasma.
   b. Histological evaluation of a parathyroid gland biopsy provides additional supportive evidence but is no longer necessary to achieve a diagnosis.

Recommended Reading

Ash R, Harvey A, Tasker S. Primary hyperaldosteronism in the cat: a series of 13 cases. J Feline Med Surg, 2005; 7:173–182.

Bonczynski, J. Primary hyperparathyroidism in dogs and cats. Clin Tech Small Anim Pract, 2007; 22:70–74.

Feldman ES, Nelson RW. Beta-cell neoplasia: insulinoma. In Canine and Feline Endocrinology and Reproduction, 3rd ed, pp 616–644. Elsevier Science (USA), 2004.

Feldman ES, Nelson RW. Feline hyperthyroidism (thyrotoxicosis). In Canine and Feline Endocrinology and Reproduction, 3rd ed, pp 152–218. Elsevier Science (USA), 2004.

Feldman ES, Nelson RW. Hyperadrenocorticism in cats (Cushing's syndrome). In Canine and Feline Endocrinology and Reproduction, 3rd ed, pp 358–393. Elsevier Science (USA), 2004.

Feldman ES, Nelson RW. Hypercalcemia and primary hyperparathyroidism. In Canine and Feline Endocrinology and Reproduction, 3rd ed, pp 660–715. Elsevier Science (USA), 2004.

Feldman ES, Nelson RW. Hypoadrenocorticism (Addison's disease). In Canine and Feline Endocrinology and Reproduction, 3rd ed, pp 394–439. Elsevier Science (USA), 2004.

Feldman ES, Nelson RW. Hypocalcemia and primary hypoparathyroidism. In Canine and Feline Endocrinology and Reproduction, 3rd ed, pp 716–742. Elsevier Science (USA), 2004.

Feldman ES, Nelson RW. Pheochromocytoma and multiple endocrine neoplasia. In Canine and Feline Endocrinology and Reproduction, 3rd ed, pp 440–463. Elsevier Science (USA), 2004.

Greco DS. Hypoadrenocorticism in small animals. Clin Tech Small Anim Pract, 2007; 22:32–35.

Green SN, Bright RM. Insulinoma in a cat. JSAP, 2008; 49:38–40.

Gunn-Moore D. Feline endocrinopathies. Vet Clin Small Anim, 2005; 34:171–210.

Hendersen AK, Mahonay O. Hypoparathyroidism: pathophysiology and diagnosis. Compendium, 2005; 27(4):270–279.

Kallet A, Richter KP, Feldman EC, et al. Primary hyperparathyroidism in cats: seven cases (1984–1989). JAVMA, 1991; 199(12):1767–1771.

Lange MS, Galac S, Trip MRJ, et al. High urinary corticoid/creatinine ratios in cats with hyperthyroidism. J Vet Intern Med, 2004; 1:152–155.

McElravy BL, Brunker JD. Diagnosing and treating primary hypoparathyroidism in dogs and cats. Vet Med, January 2007; 40–50.

Peterson ME, Greco DS, Orth D. Primary hypoadrenocorticism in ten cats. J Vet Intern Med, 1989; 3:55–58.

Peterson ME, James KM, Wallace M, et al. Idiopathic hypoparathyroidism in five cats. J Vet Intern Med, 1991; 5:46–51.

Peterson ME, Ward CR. Etiopathologic findings of hyperthyroidism in cats. Vet Clin Small Anim, 2007; 37:633–645.

Redden B. Feline hypoadrenocorticism. Compendium, 2005; 27(9):697–706.

Shiel RE, Mooner CT. Testing for hyperthyroidism in cats. Vet Clin Small Anim, 2007; 37:671–691.

Syme HM. Cardiovascular and renal manifestations of hyperthyroidism. Vet Clin Small Anim, 2007; 37:723–743.

Ward CR. Feline thyroid storm. Vet Clin Small Anim, 2007; 37:745–754.

34
ELECTROLYTE DISORDERS

Linda G. Martin and Amanda E. Veatch

Unique Features

Electrolyte disorders are common in feline emergency and critically ill patients. Electrolyte disorders should be suspected in all patients predisposed to their development (disease processes or therapeutic modalities that can lead to alterations in electrolyte status) and exhibiting clinical signs consistent with electrolyte abnormalities.

A. Sodium
    a. General points
        i. Distribution
            1. Sodium is the primary cation in the extracellular fluid.
        ii. Functions of sodium
            1. Sodium is vital to the maintenance of extracellular fluid volume.
            2. Sodium is the major contributor to osmolality.
                a. Osmolality is calculated from the following formula:

$$Osmolality = 2(sodium) + BUN/2.8 + glucose/18$$

        iii. Homeostasis/regulation
            1. Osmoreceptors in the hypothalamus
                a. Regulate thirst and the release of antidiuretic hormone (ADH) and therefore indirectly regulate sodium concentration through regulation of body water content
            2. Kidney
                a. Responsible for balancing the excretion of salt and water under the control of ADH and aldosterone
                b. Sodium is filtered by the glomeruli and reabsorbed by the renal tubules.
    b. Hyponatremia
        i. Causes of hyponatremia (table 34.1)
            1. Hyponatremia can be real or artifactual (pseudohyponatremia).
                a. To determine if the hyponatremia is real, osmolality should ideally be measured. If the osmolality is low (<308 mOsm/L), then true hyponatremia is present.
            2. True hyponatremia
                a. Physical and historical assessment of vascular volume status can help determine the underlying cause (see table 34.1).

Table 34.1. Causes of hyponatremia.

Normal plasma osmolality
  Hyperlipidemia
  Hyperproteinemia
Elevated plasma osmolality
  Hyperglycemia
  Mannitol administration
Decreased plasma osmolality
  Concurrent hypovolemia
    Renal loss
      Hypoadrenocorticism
      Diuretic administration
    Extrarenal loss
      Gastrointestinal loss
        Vomiting
        Diarrhea
      Third-space loss
        Pleural effusion
          Chylothorax
          Lung lobe torsion
          Neoplasia
        Peritoneal effusion
          Pancreatitis
          Peritonitis
          Uroabdomen
          Neoplasia
      Cutaneous loss
        Severe burns
  Concurrent normovolemia
    Psychogenic polydipsia
    Syndrome of inappropriate ADH secretion
    Hypotonic fluid administration
    Antidiuretic drugs
      NSAIDs
      Narcotics
      Barbiturates
      Cholinergic drugs
      β-adrenergic drugs
      Vincristine
  Concurrent hypervolemia
    Severe liver disease
    Congestive heart failure
    Nephrotic syndrome
    Advanced renal failure

3. Pseudohyponatremia
   a. Normal plasma osmolality (308–355 mOsm/L)
   b. Occurs as a result of lipids, proteins, or high serum viscosity that causes sample dilution, resulting in spuriously low serum sodium concentrations.
4. Low serum sodium concentrations may occur in the presence of increased plasma osmolality (>355 mOsm/L) as a result of hyperglycemia or mannitol administration. Glucose and mannitol can cause fluid to shift from the intracellular to the extracellular fluid space with an accompanying decrease in serum sodium concentration as a result of dilution.

      a. Each 100-mg/dL increase in serum glucose concentration decreases serum sodium concentration by 2.4 mEq/L.
5. If a lipid layer is not noted in the supernatant of a centrifuged hematocrit tube or hyperglycemia is not present, the measurement of osmolality is not essential to make the diagnosis of true hyponatremia. It can be inferred by ruling out the conditions mentioned above.

ii. Clinical signs of hyponatremia
1. Clinical signs depend on the rapidity with which the sodium deficit develops. Most problems occur when sodium decreases acutely (<48 hours) and the body does not have sufficient time to compensate.
2. Clinical signs are generally attributable to CNS and neuromuscular dysfunction as rapid decreases in serum sodium result in rapid influx of water into the brain, causing cerebral edema.
   Signs include lethargy, weakness, weight gain, vomiting, incoordination, seizures, and coma.
3. If hyponatremia develops slowly (>48 hours), the brain has time to adjust by losing potassium, sodium, and organic osmolytes. Clinical signs are typically negligible under these circumstances.
4. Clinical signs are generally seen when serum sodium concentrations are <125 mEq/L.

iii. Diagnosis of hyponatremia
1. Normal feline serum sodium concentrations range from 149–162 mEq/L. Hyponatremia is defined as a serum sodium concentration <149 mEq/L.
2. If the serum sodium concentration is <120 mEq/L, it is unlikely that pseudohyponatremia or a hyponatremia secondary to hyperglycemia or mannitol administration is present.

iv. Therapy for hyponatremia (box 34.1)
1. Correct underlying problem.
2. Replace volume and electrolyte deficits by administering 0.9% NaCl or a balanced electrolyte solution such as Normosol-R or lactated Ringer's solution intravenously. Rapid correction with hypertonic saline (3–7.5%) is contraindicated.
3. The speed of correction depends on the speed with which the hyponatremia developed and the patient's clinical signs. Hyponatremia that is corrected too quickly can result in demyelinization of the central pons and other areas of the CNS. Cerebral dehydration and hemorrhage may also occur as the brain shrinks and tears subarachnoid blood vessels. To minimize these complications, hyponatremia should be corrected at a rate of no faster than 0.5–0.7 mEq/L/hr.

Box 34.1.   Highlights of therapy for hyponatremia.
1. Correct underlying disease process.
2. Replace volume and electrolyte deficits.
   a. 0.9% NaCl
   b. Normosol-R
   c. Lactated Ringer's solution
3. Slowly correct hyponatremia
   a. Increase sodium no faster than 0.5–0.7 mEq/L/hr
4. Monitor sodium concentrations q1–2h initially.
5. Restrict water intake in normovolemic hyponatremic cats.
6. Discontinue drugs that may stimulate release of ADH.
   a. NSAIDs
   b. Narcotics
   c. Barbiturates

4. Sodium concentrations should be checked every 1–2 hours until a consistent trend of change has been established, then sodium monitoring can be adjusted accordingly.
5. In normovolemic cats, restrict water so that water intake is less than urine output.
6. Discontinue any drugs that might stimulate the release, or enhance the effects, of ADH (i.e., NSAIDs, narcotics, or barbiturates).
7. If pseudohyponatremia is diagnosed, no specific therapy for hyponatremia is necessary. If hyponatremia with high plasma osmolality is diagnosed, treat the underlying cause (e.g., treat diabetes mellitus with insulin therapy).

c. Hypernatremia
   i. Causes of hypernatremia (table 34.2)
      1. Hypernatremia can result from sodium-free fluid (pure water) loss, hypotonic fluid (low sodium containing fluid) loss, or from sodium gain.
      2. In feline patients, hypernatremia is most commonly caused by sodium-free and hypotonic fluid loss.

Table 34.2. Causes of hypernatremia.

Sodium-free fluid loss
Renal loss
Diabetes insipidus
Respiratory loss via panting
Fever
High environmental temperatures
Major body cavity loss during surgery
Lack of free water intake
Lack of access to water
Neurological disease with altered thirst mechanism
Primary hypodipsia
Hypotonic fluid loss
Gastrointestinal loss
Vomiting
Diarrhea
Renal loss
Osmotic diuresis
Diabetes mellitus
Mannitol administration
Intravenous glucose supplementation
Third-space loss
Pleural effusion/inflammation
Peritoneal effusion/inflammation
Sodium gain
Administration of high-sodium–containing fluids or drugs
0.9% NaCl
Hypertonic saline
Sodium bicarbonate
Sodium phosphate enema
Ingestion of high-sodium–containing food or water
Sea water
Rock salt
Sodium retention (rare in the cat)
Decreased renal excretion
Hyperaldosteronism
Hyperadrenocorticism

  ii. Clinical signs of hypernatremia
     1. Signs are manifested primarily as disorders of the CNS. Hypernatremia causes a shift of water from the cells of the brain to the intravascular space. Decreases in cell volume can cause vascular rupture, cerebral and subarachnoid hemorrhage, and irreversible neurological damage.
     2. Clinical signs are generally seen when serum sodium concentrations are >170 mEq/L. The severity of the signs is determined by the rate of change in the serum sodium concentration.
        a. A slow increase in serum sodium concentration is associated with a higher sodium level before neurological signs develop.
        b. A rapid rise in serum sodium concentration is associated with a lower sodium level when neurological signs develop.
     3. Early signs can appear as weakness, lethargy, depression, vomiting, and abnormal behavior.
     4. Later signs can develop into twitching, tremors, seizures, coma, and death.
 iii. Diagnosis of hypernatremia
     1. Hypernatremia is defined as a serum sodium concentration >162 mEq/L in cats.
     2. The underlying pathophysiologic cause of hypernatremia can be inferred from the patient's volume status.
        a. If the patient is hypovolemic, the most likely cause of hypernatremia is hypotonic fluid loss.
        b. If the patient is normovolemic, the most likely cause of hypernatremia is a result of sodium-free fluid (pure water) loss or decreased free water intake.
        c. If the patient is hypervolemic, the most likely cause of hypernatremia is due to sodium gain.
 iv. Therapy for hypernatremia (box 34.2)
     1. Correct underlying problem.
     2. Correct hypovolemia and replace water deficits.
        a. Correction of hypovolemia can be accomplished by the intravenous administration of isotonic saline (0.9% NaCl). Giving sodium-containing fluids may seem illogical. However, with prolonged hypernatremia, the brain lessens cellular fluid loss by generating idiogenic osmoles. The presence of these osmoles causes cerebral edema if plasma sodium levels are corrected too rapidly. This can be avoided by administering fluids at a rate that does not decrease serum sodium concentrations by more than 0.5–0.7 mEq/L/hr. In hypernatremia, 0.9% NaCl (containing 154 mEq/L of sodium) often has a lower sodium concentration than that of the patient, resulting in gradual dilution of sodium as the intravascular volume is replaced (table 34.3).

Box 34.2. Highlights of therapy for hypernatremia.
1. Correct underlying disease process.
2. Correct hypovolemia and replace water deficits.
   a. 0.9% NaCl
3. Correct remaining free water deficits only after correction of hypovolemia.
   a. 0.45% NaCl
   b. 5% dextrose in water
4. Slowly correct hypernatremia.
   a. Decrease sodium no faster than 0.5–0.7 mEq/L/hr.
5. Monitor sodium concentrations q1–2h initially.
6. Administer furosemide only to hypervolemic hypernatremic cats.

Table 34.3. Sodium concentration of intravenous fluids.

Fluid Solution	mEq/L
7% NaCl	1,197
3% NaCl	513
0.9% NaCl	154
Normosol-R	140
Lactated Ringer's	130
0.45% NaCl	77
5% dextrose in water	0

  b. Only after the hypovolemia is corrected should the remaining free water deficit be addressed. Residual free water deficits should be replaced slowly, correcting the serum sodium concentration gradually over 48–96 hours. The free water deficit can be replaced by giving hypotonic crystalloids such as 0.45% NaCl or 5% dextrose in water intravenously.
  c. To estimate the effect of 1 L of a crystalloid solution on the patient's serum sodium concentration, see the following equation:

$$\text{Change in Serum Sodium} = \frac{\text{Crystalloid [Sodium]} - \text{Patient's Serum [Sodium]}}{[\text{Body Weight (kg)} \times 0.6] + 1}$$

  d. Regardless of the crystalloid fluid solution given or the rate of intravenous fluid administration, hypernatremic patients need frequent monitoring and reassessment. Fluid therapy should be adjusted and individualized to best meet the patient's needs. It is difficult to predict how fast or even in what direction the sodium concentration will change. Therefore, sodium concentrations should be checked every 1–2 hours until a consistent trend is established, then sodium monitoring can be adjusted accordingly.
  3. Increase sodium excretion.
  a. Hypernatremia secondary to sodium gain is often associated with normovolemia or hypervolemia. In these cases, the administration of furosemide at 1–2 mg/kg q8–24h PO, SC, IM, or IV will help increase sodium elimination and decrease volume.
B. Potassium
  a. General points
   i. Distribution
    1. Most abundant intracellular cation in the body; 95–98% located intracellularly
    2. Concentrated most in muscle tissue
   ii. Functions of potassium
    1. Generation of the resting cell membrane potential (sodium-potassium ATPase pump)
    2. Various enzyme systems for cell growth
   iii. Homeostasis
    1. Intake
     a. Primarily from dietary ingestion
    2. Excretion
     a. Primarily renal excretion
    3. Translocation
     a. Potassium movement into intracellular space is stimulated by several factors, including insulin, catecholamines, metabolic alkalosis, and increased extracellular potassium.
     b. Extracellular translocation of potassium is stimulated by a metabolic acidosis, which then results in increased potassium excretion.

Table 34.4. Causes of hypokalemia.

Decreased intake
  Anorexia
  Vomiting
  Potassium-deplete diet
  Administration of potassium-deplete IV fluids
Increased excretion
  Vomiting
  Diarrhea
  Chronic renal failure
  Renal tubular acidosis
  Postobstructive diuresis
  Dialysis
  Hyperadrenocorticism
  Primary hyperaldosteronism
  Drugs
    Diuretics
      Furosemide
      Thiazides
    Mineralocorticoids
    Amphotericin B
    Penicillins
    Aminoglycosides
Intracellular translocation
  Insulin and glucose
  Alkalosis
  Albuterol overdose
  Catecholamines
  Hyperthyroidism
  Hypokalemic periodic paralysis (Burmese kittens)

b. Hypokalemia
  i. Causes of hypokalemia (table 34.4)
    1. General causes of hypokalemia include decreased intake, increased excretion, and intracellular translocation.
      a. Chronic renal failure is one of the most common causes of hypokalemia in cats.
      b. Hyperaldosteronism
  ii. Clinical signs of hypokalemia
    1. Clinical signs may be absent or nonspecific, such as anorexia, lethargy, ileus, or weakness.
    2. Musculoskeletal weakness manifested by ventroflexion of the neck, forelimb hypermetria, or a wide-based hind limb stance, may progress to respiratory muscle paralysis with severe hypokalemia.
    3. Hypokalemic nephropathy, with impaired urinary concentrating ability, polyuria, and polydypsia, may occur.
    4. Potassium depletion has been associated with the development of metabolic acidosis in cats.
    5. Abnormal cardiac conduction can occur.
      a. The ECG changes of ST segment depression, reduced T-wave amplitude, and prolonged QT intervals are not consistently seen in feline hypokalemic patients but may occur.
      b. Ventricular or supraventricular arrhythmias may occur and may be refractory to Class I antiarrhythmics (lidocaine and procainamide) until hypokalemia is corrected.

Table 34.5. Potassium supplementation guidelines.

Serum Potassium Concentration (mEq/L)	mEq KCl to Add to 1 L Fluids	Maximum Fluid Rate (mL/kg/hr) Not Exceeding 0.5 mEq/kg/hr KCl
3.6–5.0	20	25
3.1–3.5	30	18
2.6–3.0	40	12
2.1–2.5	50	10
<2.0	60	6

      6. With chronic hypokalemia, inhibited cell growth is manifested by weight loss, poor hair coat, and decreased muscle mass. Potassium-deficient cats may develop taurine deficiency and associated cardiovascular disease.

  iii. Diagnosis of hypokalemia

      1. Normal feline serum potassium concentrations range from 3.5–5.5 mEq/L. Hypokalemia occurs when serum potassium concentrations fall below 3.5 mEq/L.

  iv. Therapy for hypokalemia

      1. Correct underlying problem.

      2. Intravenous potassium supplementation

         a. Potassium chloride (2 mEq/mL) and potassium phosphate (4.36 mEq/mL) solutions are available for parenteral use. These solutions must be diluted in a parenteral fluid solution and mixed well to avoid oversupplementation. Rate of administration should not exceed 0.5 mEq/kg/hr. See table 34.5 for appropriate supplementation amounts and rates of administration.

         b. Higher rates of potassium supplementation may be essential during fluid therapy for diabetic ketoacidotic patients, as the body is usually potassium depleted and administration of insulin causes serum potassium concentrations to decrease even further due to intracellular translocation (See Chap. 31—Management of Specific Endocrine and Metabolic Diseases: Diabetes).

         c. Hypokalemia that fails to respond to supplementation may indicate the presence of concurrent hypomagnesemia.

      3. Oral potassium supplementation

         a. Potassium gluconate is most commonly recommended for oral supplementation. It can be administered at 5–8 mEq/cat/day PO divided BID or TID initially, then reduced to 2–4 mEq/cat/day for maintenance therapy.

      4. Serial potassium measurements are recommended when supplementing.

  c. Hyperkalemia

    i. Causes of hyperkalemia (table 34.6)

      1. Extreme leukocytosis or thrombocytosis can falsely elevate serum potassium concentrations and are considered to be causes of pseudohyperkalemia.

      2. Sustained hyperkalemia is almost always associated with impaired urinary excretion of potassium (urethral obstructions, bladder rupture, anuric or oliguric renal failure).

      3. Cats in a diabetic ketoacidotic state may be hyperkalemic because of insulin deficiency or hyperosmolarity. However, an overall hypokalemia may be present that can become apparent when insulin therapy is started due to movement of potassium into the cells.

      4. Drugs associated with hyperkalemia usually are not clinically significant unless other factors that potentiate hyperkalemia are present, such as decreased urinary excretion.

Table 34.6.   Causes of hyperkalemia.

Iatrogenic—potassium-rich IV fluid administration
Extracellular translocation
   Diabetic ketoacidosis
   Tumor lysis syndrome
   Massive tissue trauma
   Mineral acidosis
   Reperfusion injury—after aortic thromboembolism
   Lysine or arginine (TPN)
   Drugs
      Beta-blockers (propranolol)
      Cardiac glycosides
Decreased urinary excretion
   Urethral obstruction
   Bilateral ureteral obstruction
   Urinary bladder rupture
   Anuric/oliguric renal failure
Hypoadrenocorticism
Gastrointestinal disease
   Severe whipworms
   Salmonellosis
   Duodenal perforation
Effusions
   Chylothorax—repeated drainage
   Peritoneal effusion
   Pericardial effusion
Pseudohyperkalemia
   Thrombocytosis
   Acute lymphoblastic leukemia
Drugs promoting hyperkalemia
   Potassium-containing drugs
   ACE inhibitors
   Potassium-sparing diuretics
   NSAIDs
   Heparin
   Succinylcholine

  ii.   Clinical signs of hyperkalemia
     1.   The most significant and life-threatening effects of hyperkalemia are changes in cardiac conduction, associated with characteristic ECG changes.
        a.   The first abnormality seen is a T wave increased in amplitude with a "tented" appearance. A decrease in R wave amplitude, a prolonged P-R interval, and a decreased QT interval may be seen.
        b.   The P waves decrease in amplitude, widen, and eventually become absent (atrial standstill) with increasing hyperkalemia. Widening of the QRS complex and bradycardia are also seen with higher levels.
        c.   Ventricular fibrillation, asystole, and cardiac arrest can also occur.
     2.   Hyperkalemia may be associated with generalized skeletal muscle weakness.
  iii.   Diagnosis of hyperkalemia
     1.   Hyperkalemia should be suspected in cats with appropriate underlying diseases or showing associated clinical signs. Potassium concentrations should be measured in every sick cat presenting with a urethral obstruction.
     2.   Hyperkalemia occurs when feline serum potassium concentrations rise above 5.5 mEq/L.

Box 34.3. Highlights of therapy for hyperkalemia.
1. Correct underlying disease process.
2. In cases of hyperkalemic crisis administer one or more of the following:
   a. Sodium bicarbonate
   b. Dextrose and regular insulin
   c. Calcium gluconate
3. Discontinue all sources of potassium (IV fluids, medications).
4. Start IV fluid therapy with a low-potassium–containing crystalloid.
   a. 0.9% NaCl
   b. Lactated Ringer's solution
5. Consider furosemide to enhance renal potassium excretion.
   a. Do not give to hypovolemic or dehydrated cats.
6. Consider peritoneal dialysis or hemodialysis in cases of anuric or oliguric renal failure.

---

    iv. Therapy for hyperkalemia (box 34.3)
1. The presence of cardiac conduction abnormalities may require treatment before the cause of hyperkalemia is identified. Treatment of hyperkalemia involves intracellular translocation of potassium and protection of the myocardium.
   a. Calcium gluconate (50–100 mg/kg IV slowly over 5–10 minutes) is cardioprotective by making the threshold potential less negative. This should be administered to any cat with life-threatening ECG changes due to hyperkalemia. Doses should be administered slowly and the patient's ECG should be monitored during administration as changes in heart rate or cardiac arrhythmias may occur with administration that is too fast. Effects will last 30 minutes to 1 hour.
   b. Sodium bicarbonate (1–2 mg/kg IV slowly over 15–20 minutes) causes intracellular movement of potassium. This treatment method is often recommended in cats with urethral obstruction after administration of calcium, as hypocalcemia may also be present and seizures may be induced by further lowering the ionized calcium concentration with sodium bicarbonate administration.
   c. Glucose also causes intracellular movement of potassium. Dextrose-containing solutions or a combination of regular insulin with dextrose solutions can be used. Twenty-five percent dextrose can be administered as an IV bolus. Additionally, 0.25–1.0 U/kg of regular insulin can be diluted in IV fluids containing dextrose (2 g/U insulin), or 0.25–1.0 U/kg of regular insulin can be administered as an IV bolus followed by a 25% dextrose IV bolus (1–2 g/U insulin).
2. Correct the underlying cause of hyperkalemia (i.e., establishing urine outflow).
3. Discontinue all sources of potassium intake (intravenous fluids, medications).
4. Intravenous fluid therapy with low-potassium crystalloids (lactated Ringer's solution, 0.9% NaCl) provides a dilutional effect on extracellular potassium.
5. Loop or thiazide diuretics may be considered as adjunctive therapy to enhance renal potassium excretion.
6. Peritoneal dialysis or hemodialysis should be considered if other treatments are ineffective in lowering potassium concentrations, and they may be necessary in cases of anuric or oliguric renal failure.

C. Calcium
    a. General points
       i. Distribution

1. Ninety-nine percent of the body's calcium is found in the skeletal system as a component of hydroxyapatite, and 1% is present in extracellular fluid (<1% is intracellular).
2. For extracellular calcium, 52% is in an ionized form, 40% is bound to albumin or globulins, and 8% is chelated with phosphate, citrate, or bicarbonate. The ionized form is thought to be the physiologically active component.
3. In the presence of acidosis, a shift toward ionized over protein-bound calcium occurs, and the opposite occurs with alkalosis.

ii. Functions of calcium
1. Calcium is a major component of bone, important for stability and formation.
2. Calcium is necessary for muscle contraction, including skeletal, smooth, and cardiac muscle, and is required for cardiac pacemaker cell excitation.
3. At a molecular level, calcium is involved in enzyme activation and second messenger systems that promote neurotransmitter and hormone release, coagulation, and cellular motility, secretion, differentiation, and permeability.

iii. Homeostasis
1. Parathyroid hormone (PTH) is the primary regulator of calcium, and its release causes increased serum calcium concentrations. (Increased serum calcium serves as a negative feedback for PTH release.)
   a. GI tract—PTH causes increased absorption of calcium.
   b. Bone—PTH causes bone resorption and mobilization of calcium and phosphate.
   c. Kidney—PTH causes decreased excretion of calcium, inhibits reabsorption of phosphate, and stimulates synthesis of calcitriol.
2. Calcitriol is an active metabolite of vitamin D produced by the kidney. Its major action is on the gastrointestinal tract to increase calcium and phosphate absorption.

b. Hypocalcemia
i. Causes of hypocalcemia (table 34.7)
1. Hypoalbuminemia will cause total serum calcium to decrease; however, ionized calcium (iCa) concentrations should be normal.

ii. Clinical signs of hypocalcemia
1. Musculoskeletal manifestations of hypocalcemia include muscle fasiculations or tremors, stiffness, or tetany. Severe hypocalcemia can result in seizures. True seizures can be differentiated from severe muscle tremors in that seizures are typically accompanied by hypersalivation, tonic-clonic limb motion, loss of consciousness, and other signs of central nervous system dysfunction.
2. Cardiovascular signs include hypotension, tachyarrhythmias, or prolonged Q-T interval.
3. Other signs may include prolapsed nictitating membrane, facial rubbing, behavioral changes (restlessness, excitation, aggression, hypersensitivity to stimuli, disorientation), laryngeal or bronchospasm, panting, or apnea in severe cases.

iii. Diagnosis of hypocalcemia
1. Obtaining iCa concentrations is the preferred method of measuring calcium, and reference ranges are 4.5–5.5 mg/dL or 1.1–1.4 mmol/L. (In order to convert mg/dL to mmol/L, multiply mg/dL by 0.25; to convert mmol/L to mg/dL, multiply mmol/l by 4.)
   a. Clinical signs usually do not manifest if iCa is >0.8 mmol/L or 3.2 mg/dL.
   b. Results can be altered by processing samples aerobically, overheparinizing samples, or using silicone separator tubes.
2. Normal feline serum total calcium concentrations range from 8.0–10.5 mg/dL or 2.0–2.6 mmol/L.
   a. Consider albumin level and protein-bound calcium. The albumin correction formula (calcium − albumin + 3.5) is typically not accurate in cats.

Table 34.7. Causes of hypocalcemia.

Hypoproteinemia/hypoalbuminemia (normal iCa)
Renal failure
   Acute or chronic
   Ethylene glycol toxicity
Hypoparathyroidism
   Iatrogenic (parathyroidectomy, thyroidectomy)
   Primary (rare, may be congenital)
   Cervical trauma
   Severe hypomagnesemia
Nutritional or renal secondary hyperparathyroidism
Vitamin D deficiency
   Hepatic insufficiency
   Intestinal malabsorption or malnutrition
   Renal disease
Redistribution
   Alkalosis
   Eclampsia (1–3 weeks postpartum)—rare in cats
   Hyperphosphatemia causing Ca-P precipitation
      Phosphate-containing enemas
      Renal or postrenal causes
Massive blood transfusions (citrate anticoagulant)
   Massive soft-tissue trauma/rhabdomyolysis
   Tumor lysis syndrome
   Sodium bicarbonate therapy
   Urethral obstruction
   Acute pancreatitis
   Extensive IV fluid or furosemide diuresis
Hyperthyroidism
Hypoadrenocorticism (rare in cats)
Sepsis/SIRS

3. Additional tests to establish the cause of hypocalcemia may be necessary, such as PTH concentrations, T4 concentrations, chemistry profile, urinalysis, or bone marrow aspirates or biopsy.

iv. Therapy for hypocalcemia

1. Correct underlying problem.

2. Calcium can be administered intravenously for severe hypocalcemia, or orally in mild or chronic cases of hypocalcemia. Parenteral supplementation is recommended only if degree of hypocalcemia is severe or clinical signs are present.

3. Calcium gluconate or calcium chloride can be administered intravenously. Ten percent calcium gluconate (50–150 mg/kg IV slowly) contains 9.2 mg/mL elemental calcium and is safer than 10% calcium chloride, which contains 27.2 mg/mL elemental calcium. Additionally, calcium chloride is very irritating if given perivascularly.

   a. Administration should be over at least 10–30 minutes. Monitor patient's ECG during administration, as rapid administration can cause bradyarrhythmias, asystole, and death.

   b. Repeat as needed until neuromuscular signs resolve.

   c. Subcutaneous administration is not recommended, as tissue irritation and necrosis can occur (most commonly associated with calcium chloride).

4. Isotonic intravenous fluids can be administered to correct hypovolemia or hyperthermia.

5. Oral vitamin D can be used adjunctively if hypocalcemia is secondary to hypoparathyroidism or renal disease. Serum calcium concentrations should be monitored while using vitamin D preparations.

Table 34.8.   Causes of hypercalcemia.

Hypercalcemia of malignancy
  Lymphoma
  Anal sac apocrine gland adenocarcinoma
  Carcinomas
  Multiple myeloma
  Leukemia
  Metastatic or primary bone neoplasms
Renal failure—acute or chronic
Hypervitaminosis D
  Toxic plants
    Cestrus diurnum—day-blooming jessamine
    Solanum malacoxylon—nightshade
    Triestum flavescens—yellow oatgrass
  Cholecalciferol rodenticides
  Calcipotriene—psoriasis medication
  Excessive dietary supplementation
Excessive calcium ingestion
  Calcium-containing intestinal phosphate binders
  Excessive calcium supplementation
Hyperparathyroidism
  Primary—neoplasic (adenoma), hyperplasia
  Secondary—renal, nutritional
Skeletal lesions
  Neoplastic
  Osteomyelitis—esp. fungal
  Hypertrophic osteodystrophy
  Disuse osteoporosis
Nonpathologic or transient causes
  Hyperproteinemia/hemoconcentration
  Lipemia
  Hemolysis
  Postprandial
  Physiologic growth of young animals
  Laboratory error
Hypoadrenocorticism
Acromegaly
Postrenal transplantation
Idiopathic hypercalcemia of cats

6. For oral supplementation, several formulations are available, the most common being calcium carbonate (dose: 25–50 mg/kg/day divided BID–QID on the basis of elemental calcium content). Other formulations include calcium chloride, gluconate, or lactate.
7. Correct hyperphosphatemia prior to calcium administration to prevent precipitation and soft tissue mineralization.
8. If eclampsia is the cause of hypocalcemia, wean kittens.
9. Serial monitoring of serum calcium concentrations is recommended while supplementing.

c. Hypercalcemia
  i. Causes of hypercalcemia (table 34.8)
    1. Hypercalcemia of malignancy is less common in cats than in dogs but can occur with several neoplasms, the most common being lymphoma.
    2. In the condition of idiopathic hypercalcemia of cats, no etiology is identified. Young to middle-aged cats are affected. The hypercalcemia is usually not progressive and is associated with

   minimal clinical signs but may be associated with azotemia, nephrocalcinosis, and calcium
   oxalate urolithiasis.
 ii. Clinical signs of hypercalcemia
    1. Clinical signs are due to alterations of cellular membrane permeability and calcium pump
       activity causing cellular dysfunction or death. The most affected organs include the central
       nervous system (CNS), gastrointestinal system, heart, and kidney.
    2. CNS signs range from depression or lethargy to seizures or coma.
    3. Peripheral neuromuscular signs include muscle weakness or wasting, tremors, shivering, stiff
       gait, decreased reflexes, or soft tissue calcification.
       a. Soft tissue calcification occurs when concurrent hypercalcemia and hyperphosphatemia
          result in a calcium phosphorus product that is greater than $70 \, mg^2/dL^2$.
    4. Cardiovascular effects may be a direct consequence of hypercalcemia or secondary to tissue
       calcification. ECG changes (prolonged PR interval, shortened QT interval) or ventricular
       arrhythmias can be seen, and hypertension and vasoconstriction can occur peripherally.
       a. Hypercalcemia can cause an increased sensitivity to digitalis.
    5. Renal effects from hypercalcemia include polyuria/polydipsia, isosthenuria, azotemia,
       decreased renal blood flow, nephrocalcinosis, urolithiasis, or interstitial nephritis. Hypercalcemia
       can cause renal damage or it can develop as a consequence of existing renal damage.
    6. Gastrointestinal signs associated with hypercalcemia include anorexia, weight loss, vomiting,
       diarrhea, constipation, ulceration, and pancreatitis.
iii. Diagnosis of hypercalcemia
    1. Hypercalcemia occurs when feline serum total calcium concentrations rise above 10.5 mg/dL
       and when iCa concentrations rise above 1.4 mmol/L or 5.6 mg/dL.
    2. Additional tests to establish the cause of hypercalcemia may be necessary, such as electrolytes,
       BUN, and creatinine to identify nonneoplastic causes; PTH or PTH-related peptide assays;
       imaging of the cervical region, chest, or abdomen; lymph node or bone marrow aspirates; or
       measurement of vitamin D metabolites.
 iv. Therapy for hypercalcemia (box 34.4)
    1. Definitive treatment for hypercalcemia involves treating the underlying cause. Goals of treat-
       ment include increasing urinary excretion of calcium, inhibiting bone resorption, and prevent-
       ing intestinal absorption.
    2. Volume expansion and calciuresis with 0.9% NaCl given intravenously at 100–125 mL/kg/
       day is often sufficient to cause a significant decrease in calcium concentrations. For mild eleva-
       tions, fluids can be administered subcutaneously at 75–100 mL/kg/day.

Box 34.4. Highlights of therapy for hypercalcemia.
 1. Correct underlying disease process.
 2. Diurese using 0.9% NaCl.
 3. Consider furosemide to enhance diuresis and calciuresis.
    a. Do not give to hypovolemic or dehydrated cats.
 4. Consider glucocorticoids if appropriate.
    a. Do not give if concern of neoplasia or infection.
 5. Consider calcitonin if appropriate.
 6. Consider sodium bicarbonate if appropriate.
 7. Consider bisphosphonates if appropriate.
 8. Consider antineoplastic agents if appropriate.
 9. Consider peritoneal dialysis or hemodialysis in cases of anuric or oliguric renal failure.
10. Consider calcium channel antagonists to protect against cardiac arrhythmias.

3. Furosemide (2–4 mg/kg PO, SC, IM, or IV q8–12 hr) can be given after adequate volume re-expansion. Avoid thiazide diuretics because they may result in hypocalciuria and aggravate hypercalcemia.

4. Glucocorticoids cause inhibition of bone resorption and intestinal absorption and increase renal excretion. Their use is most effective in hypercalcemia of malignancy, hypervitaminosis D, and hypoadrenocorticism. Glucocorticoids should not be used in cases of suspect neoplasia or infection, as administration can make a diagnosis of lymphoma difficult or worsen infectious diseases.
   a. Prednisone, 1.0–2.2 mg/kg q12–24h PO, SC, IM, or IV
   b. Dexamethasone, 0.1–0.22 mg/kg q12–24h PO, SC, IM, or IV

5. Calcitonin (4–6 IU/kg SC q8–12h) causes inhibition of bone resorption and increases renal excretion; it is indicated for cholecalciferol toxicity. Its analgesic properties may provide relief in malignancy.
   a. Calcitonin has a rapid onset and causes moderate decreases in calcium concentrations.
   b. If resistance develops, coadminister glucocorticoids or discontinue use for 24–48 hours.
   c. Vomiting can occur secondary to calcitonin administration.
   d. Since calcitonin is a foreign protein, allergic reactions can occur. Pretreat with Benadryl. Some clinicians recommend an intradermal test first to check for wheal formation.

6. Sodium bicarbonate is used for reversal of acidosis. It causes some calcium binding to proteins and can also directly bind calcium. It can be used in an acute crisis.
   a. Bicarbonate dose (mEq) = 0.4 × BW(kg) × (12 − patient's bicarbonate). Give ½ of the calculated dose over 3–4 hours in IV fluids.

7. Bisphosphonates (etidronate, pamidronate) inhibit bone resorption. They have a slow onset of action and are indicated for long-term treatment.
   a. Etidronate, 5–20 mg/kg/day PO divided BID.
   b. Pamidronate, 1.3–2.0 mg/kg IV in 0.9% NaCl given over 2 hours; repeat in 1–3 weeks PRN.

8. Antineoplastic agents (plicamycin, gallium nitrate) are used to inhibit bone resorption. Significant side effects can be associated with their use, and clinical experience for some drugs is limited in cats.

9. Hemodialysis or peritoneal dialysis can be used in patients with renal insufficiency. A low-Ca dialysate should be used.

10. Calcium channel antagonists (diltiazem, verapamil) protect against cardiac arrhythmias that hypercalcemia may induce, and they may help to stabilize calcium concentrations.
    a. Diltiazem, 0.5–1.5 mg/kg PO q8h.
    b. Verapamil, 0.025 mg/kg IV q 10–30 min; max. cumulative dose 0.15 mg/kg.

11. Prostaglandin synthesis inhibitors/NSAIDs have been historically used for hypercalcemia of malignancy but are largely ineffective for the majority of patients. These therapies should be avoided if the hypercalcemia has resulted in renal damage and worsening of renal function.

12. Diet changes (calcium-restricted, high fiber, alkalinizing) can be implemented for long-term control.

D. Phosphorus
   a. General points
      i. Distribution
         1. Phosphorus is the most plentiful intracellular anion and is a major component of the phospholipid bilayer of cellular membranes.
         2. Approximately 85–90% of the body's phosphorus is present as a structural component of teeth and bone, as a component of hydroxyapatite.
         3. Approximately 1% of the body's phosphorus is present in extracellular fluid.
      ii. Functions of phosphorus
         1. Phosphorus is a major component of cellular and extracellular structure, present in cellular membranes, bone, and teeth.

    2. Two of the most important phosphorus-containing compounds are ATP and 2,3-DPG, necessary for cellular energy, membrane integrity, and oxygen delivery.

    3. Phosphorus is also necessary for several metabolic processes and secondary messenger systems.

iii. Homeostasis

    1. Phosphorus is absorbed by the gastrointestinal tract by passive diffusion, and by active absorption mediated by calcitriol.

    2. The kidney is the primary regulator of phosphate levels.

      a. Low phosphorus concentrations stimulate calcitriol production and enhanced reabsorption by the kidney.

      b. Reabsorption by the kidney is inhibited by PTH, hypercalcemia, calcitonin, cortisol, and expanded ECF volume.

    3. Several factors influence the intracellular or extracellular transport of phosphorus.

      a. Entry into cells is stimulated by insulin, glucose, carbohydrates, alkalosis, amino acids, corticosteroids, sodium bicarbonate, or diuretics.

      b. Efflux from cells is promoted by glucagon, acidosis, or proteins.

b. Hypophosphatemia

  i. Causes of hypophosphatemia (table 34.9)

    1. General mechanisms for hypophosphatemia include intracellular translocation, decreased intake, or increased renal loss.

Table 34.9. Causes of hypophosphatemia.

Intracellular translocation
Insulin administration
Hyperventilation with respiratory alkalosis
CNS disorders
Sepsis
Pain
Eclampsia and postprandial
Refeeding syndrome/nutritional recovery syndrome
Hyperalimentation
Severe hypothermia
Salicylate toxicity
Decreased intake/absorption
Vomiting
Starvation
Enteropathies
Intestinal binding agents
Malabsorption syndromes
Hypovitaminosis D
Increased renal loss
Renal tubular loss
Dialysis
Drugs promoting urinary excretion
Corticosteroids
Diureics
Sodium bicarbonate
Hyperparathyroidism
Diabetes mellitus
Hyperadrenocorticism
Hyperaldosteronism
Laboratory error
Mannitol therapy

    ii. Clinical signs of hypophosphatemia
       1. Severe hypophosphatemia can affect all blood cell lines, causing hematologic dysfunction.
          a. Erythrocyte fragility and hemolysis results from decreased membrane integrity and is most likely when phosphorus concentrations are <1.0 mg/dL.
          b. Leukocyte dysfunction results in leukocyte chemotaxis and phagocytosis.
          c. Platelet dysfunction and thrombocytopenia can occur with hypophosphatemia.
       2. Skeletal muscle weakness, fasciculations, or pain can occur with hypophosphatemia, and if severe enough can result in respiratory failure and death. Rhabdomyolysis and myoglobinuria can occur.
       3. Cardiac muscle dysfunction can occur and results in decreased cardiac contractility and stroke volume.
       4. CNS signs include ataxia, paresthesia, altered mental status, seizures, or coma.
       5. Gastrointestinal signs include intestinal ileus, nausea, or vomiting.
       6. With chronic hypophosphatemia, bone demineralization can occur.
   iii. Diagnosis of hypophosphatemia
       1. A feline serum phosphorus concentration <2.5 mg/dL indicates hypophosphatemia.
       2. Cats are more susceptible to clinical signs with mild decreases in phosphorus.
       3. Diabetic ketoacidotic patients may have normal or elevated serum phosphorus concentrations despite total body depletion.
          a. Monitor serum phosphorus concentrations 12–24 hours after beginning insulin therapy, as insulin can cause intracellular translocation of phosphorus.
   iv. Therapy for hypophosphatemia
       1. Intravenous phosphate replacement, in the form of potassium phosphate solution, is indicated for feline patients with a serum phosphorus <1.5 mg/dL. (Dose: 0.01–0.03 mmol/kg IV over 6 hours.) It should be administered in calcium-free fluids (0.9% NaCl) and is contraindicated in oliguric or hypocalcemic patients.
          a. Recheck at 6 and 12 hours, and continue constant rate infusion if necessary.
          b. Discontinue when serum phosphorus >2.5 mg/dL.
          c. Complications of supplementation include hyperphosphatemia, hypocalcemia, tetanic seizures, soft tissue mineralization, or hypotension.
       2. Oral phosphorus (0.5–2.0 mmol/kg/day) is indicated for mild hypophosphatemia or long-term supplementation.
       3. Gradual refeeding of patients with chronic anorexia is recommended to avoid a rebound hypophosphatemia.
          a. Feed 1/3 daily caloric requirement on first day, 2/3 on second day, then the full amount on third day (see chap. 9—Nutritional Support for the Critically Ill Feline Patient).
          b. Avoid high-carbohydrate diets during refeeding.
E. Magnesium
  a. General points
    i. Distribution
       1. Magnesium is the second most abundant intracellular cation.
       2. The vast majority of magnesium is present in bone (60%) and muscle (20%).
       3. Less than 1% of total body magnesium is present in the serum.
       4. In the serum, magnesium exists in three distinct forms: a protein-bound fraction (30%), an anion-complexed fraction (4%), and an ionized fraction (66%).
          a. The ionized fraction is believed to be the physiologically active component.
    ii. Functions of magnesium
       1. Magnesium is required for many cellular metabolic processes, such as those involved in the production and use of ATP. This electrolyte is a coenzyme for the membrane-bound sodium-potassium ATPase pump and functions to maintain the sodium-potassium gradient

across all membranes. Calcium ATPase and proton pumps also require magnesium as a coenzyme.

2. Magnesium participates in the synthesis and degradation of DNA, the binding of ribosomes to RNA, and the production on intracellular second messengers such as cyclic adenosine monophosphate (cAMP).

3. Magnesium is involved in the regulation of vascular smooth muscle tone and signal transduction.

4. Magnesium also exerts an influence on lymphocyte activation and cytokine production.

iii. Homeostasis

1. Magnesium homeostasis is achieved through intestinal absorption and renal excretion.
   a. Magnesium absorption occurs primarily in the small intestine (jejunum and ileum).
   b. The kidney is the main regulator of serum magnesium concentration and total body magnesium content. This is achieved by glomerular filtration and tubular reabsorption.

2. Lactation also plays a role in gut and renal handling of magnesium. Increased concentrations of PTH, in addition to calcium concentration, likely play a role in magnesium conservation during lactation to supply the mammary glands with sufficient magnesium.

3. No primary regulatory hormone has been identified for magnesium homeostasis, although parathyroid, thyroid, and adrenal glands are likely involved.

b. Hypomagnesemia

i. Causes of hypomagnesemia (table 34.10)

1. The causes of magnesium deficiency can be divided into three categories: decreased intake, increased losses, and redistribution by intracellular translocation, chelation, or sequestration.

ii. Clinical signs of hypomagnesemia

1. Often relate to magnesium's effect on the cell membrane, which results in changes in the resting membrane potential, signal transduction, and smooth muscle tone. This is most commonly manifested as cardiovascular and neuromuscular abnormalities.

2. Cardiovascular signs include arrhythmias comprising atrial fibrillation, supraventricular tachycardia, premature ventricular contractions, ventricular tachycardia, and ventricular fibrillation. Magnesium deficiency can also cause hypertension, coronary artery vasospasm, and platelet aggregation.

3. Magnesium decreases acetylcholine release from nerve terminals and depresses the excitability of nerve and muscle membranes. This electrolyte also plays a role in muscle contraction and relaxation by regulating calcium channels. Neuromuscular signs of magnesium deficiency include muscle weakness (which can be manifested by dysphagia or dyspnea if esophageal or respiratory muscles are affected respectively), muscle fasciculations, seizures, ataxia, and coma.

4. Since magnesium is necessary for the movement of sodium, potassium, and calcium into and out of cells, other manifestations of hypomagnesemia include metabolic abnormalities such as concurrent hypokalemia (often refractory to potassium supplementation), hyponatremia, and hypocalcemia.

iii. Diagnosis of hypomagnesemia

1. Determination of serum magnesium concentrations is usually the most readily available technique for estimation of magnesium status. However, the precise clinical diagnosis of hypomagnesemia can be difficult. Since greater than 99% of total body magnesium is located in the intracellular compartment, serum magnesium concentrations do not always reflect total body magnesium stores. Therefore, a normal serum magnesium concentration can occur in the presence of a total body magnesium deficiency. The reported reference range for serum magnesium in cats is 1.9–2.6 mg/dL. Hypomagnesemia occurs when serum magnesium concentrations fall below 1.9 mg/dL.

Table 34.10.   Causes of hypomagnesemia.

Decreased intake
   Inadequate nutritional intake
   Administration of magnesium-deplete IV fluids
   Administration of magnesium-deplete TPN or PPN
Increased losses
   Gastrointestinal
      Malabsorption syndromes
      Extensive small bowel resection
      Chronic diarrhea
      Inflammatory bowel disease
      Cholestatic liver disease
   Renal
      Intrinsic tubular disorders
         Glomerulonephritis
         Acute tubular necrosis
         Postobstructive diuresis
         Drug-induced tubular injury
            Aminoglycosides
            Amphotericin B
            Carbenicillin
            Cisplatin
            Cyclosporine
      Extrarenal factors influencing renal magnesium handling
         Diuretic-induced states
            Furosemide
            Thiazides
            Mannitol
         Digitalis administration
         Diabetic ketoacidosis
         Hyperthyroidism
         Primary hyperparathyroidism
Alterations in distribution
   Extracellular to intracellular shifts
      Glucose, insulin, or amino acid administration
   Chelation
      Elevation in circulating catecholamines
         Sepsis/shock
         Trauma
         Hypothermia
      Massive blood transfusion
   Sequestration
      Pancreatitis

2. Measurement of ionized magnesium may provide a more accurate reflection of intracellular ionized magnesium status. Ionized magnesium appears to equilibrate rapidly across the cell membrane; thus, extracellular ionized magnesium may be reflective of intracellular stores. The feline reference range for ionized magnesium is 0.43–0.70 mmol/L. Ionized hypomagnesemia occurs when ionized magnesium concentrations fall below 0.43 mmol/L.

  iv. Therapy for hypomagnesemia

    1. The amount and route of magnesium replacement depends on both the degree of hypomagnesemia and the patient's clinical condition. Mild hypomagnesemia may resolve with treatment of the underlying disorder and modification of intravenous fluid therapy. Animals

receiving long-term diuretic and/or digoxin therapy may benefit from oral magnesium supplementation. Supplementation should be considered if serum magnesium concentrations are below 1.5 mg/dL and at higher concentrations if clinical signs (cardiac arrhythmias, muscle tremors, refractory hypokalemia) are present.

2. Renal function and cardiac conduction should be assessed prior to magnesium administration. Since magnesium is primarily excreted by the kidneys, the dose of magnesium should be reduced by 50% in azotemic patients and serum concentrations should be monitored to prevent the development of hypermagnesemia. Magnesium also prolongs the conduction through the AV node. Patients with cardiac conduction disturbances should have judicious supplementation of magnesium and continuous ECG monitoring.

3. Both magnesium sulfate and magnesium chloride are available for parenteral supplementation. Parenteral administration of magnesium sulfate may result in hypocalcemia due to chelation of calcium with the sulfate. Therefore, magnesium chloride should be given when hypocalcemia is already present.

4. The intravenous route is preferred for rapid repletion of magnesium concentrations. (The intramuscular route is generally painful.)

5. For rapid repletion of magnesium concentrations, an initial dose of 0.75–1.0 mEq/kg/day can be administered for the first 24–48 hours by continuous rate infusion in 0.9% NaCl or 5% dextrose in water. A lower dose of 0.3–0.5 mEq/kg/day can be used for an additional 3–5 days.

6. For the treatment of life-threatening ventricular arrhythmias, a dose of 0.15–0.3 mEq/kg of magnesium diluted in normal saline or 5% dextrose in water can be slowly administered IV over 5–15 minutes.

7. Side effects of magnesium therapy include hypotension and atrioventricular and bundle-branch blocks. Adverse effects are usually associated with intravenous boluses rather than continuous rate infusions.

c. Hypermagnesemia
 i. Causes of hypermagnesemia
  1. Renal failure
   a. Magnesium excretion decreases as GFR declines. Acute renal failure is more likely to be associated with hypermagnesemia than chronic renal failure, but it may occur in the latter.
   b. Hypermagnesemia has also been reported in cats with urethral obstruction.
  2. Endocrinopathies
   a. Hyperparathyroidism
   b. Hypoadrenocorticism
   c. Hypothyroidism
   d. These diseases are rare in cats and cause hypermagnesemia less frequently and to a milder degree than other causes of hypermagnesemia. The mechanisms that lead to hypermagnesemia are not well understood in these endocrine disorders.
  3. Iatrogenic overdose of magnesium
   a. Improper dosing of magnesium replacement therapy or lack of consideration of the underlying renal function generally plays a role in the development of iatrogenic hypermagnesemia.
   b. Many cathartics, laxatives, and antacids contain magnesium, and care should be exercised if multiple doses are given to a patient with underlying renal disease.
 ii. Clinical signs of hypermagnesemia
  1. Nonspecific clinical signs may include:
   a. Lethargy, depression, and weakness
  2. Neuromuscular signs include:
   a. Hyporeflexia and flaccid paralysis

      b. Profound magnesium toxicity has been associated with respiratory depression secondary to respiratory muscle paralysis. Severe respiratory depression can result in hypoventilation and subsequent hypoxemia.

      c. Dull mentation, absent menace and palpebral reflex

   3. Cardiovascular effects include:

      a. Hypotension secondary to relaxation of vascular resistance vessels

      b. Bradycardia, complete heart block, and asystole

      c. Hypothermia

 iii. Diagnosis of hypermagnesemia

   1. Hypermagnesemia occurs when feline serum magnesium concentrations rise above 2.6 mg/dL. Ionized hypermagnesemia occurs when ionized magnesium concentrations rise above 0.70 mmol/L.

   2. Unlike magnesium deficiency, serum concentrations cannot hide increased magnesium stores.

 iv. Therapy for hypermagnesemia (box 34.5)

   1. Correct underlying problem.

   2. Stop all exogenous magnesium administration.

   3. Diurese using 0.9% NaCl at 2–4 mL/kg/hr IV.

      a. Consider peritoneal dialysis or hemodialysis in patients with severely impaired renal function.

   4. Furosemide, 1–4 mg/kg q8–12h, PO, SC, IM, or IV to increase renal magnesium excretion.

      a. Do not use in a dehydrated or hypotensive patient.

Box 34.5.   Highlights of therapy for hypermagnesemia.
1. Correct underlying disease process.
2. Stop all exogenous magnesium therapy.
3. Diurese using 0.9% NaCl.
4. Consider furosemide to enhance renal magnesium excretion.
   a. Do not give to hypovolemic or dehydrated cats.
5. Consider calcium gluconate to reverse the cardiotoxic effects of hypermagnesemia.
6. Consider physostigmine to reverse the neurotoxic effects of hypermagnesemia.
7. Intubate and provide positive pressure ventilation and/or vasopressor therapy in severe cases.

Electrolyte disorders: Algorithmic overview

Suspicion of an electrolyte abnormality.

↓

Confirm electrolyte abnormality by appropriate diagnostic method.

↓

Institute emergency therapy.

↓

Determine etiology of electrolyte abnormality.

↓

Correct underlying disease process.

Fig. 34.1.   Electrolyte disorders: algorithmic overview.

Table 34.11. Drug table.

Drugs	Classes	MOAs	Side Effects	Contraindications or Precautions	Routes of Administration and Doses	General Uses
Calcitonin	Hormone	Inhibits osteoclastic resorption	Vomiting, diarrhea, anorexia, allergic reaction/anaphylaxis	Caution in young animals	4–6IU/kg SC q8–12h	Adjunctive therapy for hypercalcemia
Calcitriol	Vitamin D analog (hormone)	Promote GI absorption, renal reabsorption, and bone resorption of calcium	Hypercalcemia, nephrocalcinosis, hyperphosphatemia	Hypercalcemia, vitamin D toxicity, malabsorption syndrome; caution with hyperphosphatemia	2.5–3.5 ng/kg PO q24h	Hypocalcemia from hypoparathyroidism or renal disease
Calcium carbonate	Calcium salt	Increase extracellular calcium	Hypercalcemia, if in combination with vitamin D or increased PTH	Hypercalcemia, ventricular fibrillation; caution with digitalis	25–50mg/kg/day divided BID-QID on the basis of elemental calcium content	Hypocalcemia
Calcium chloride	Calcium salt	Increase extracellular calcium	Hypercalcemia, vascular irritation; hypotension, arrhythmias, arrest if rapid administration	Hypercalcemia, ventricular fibrillation; caution with digitalis, cardiac or renal disease, respiratory acidosis or failure	50–300 mg/cat IV slowly over 10–30min	Hypocalcemia
Calcium gluconate	Calcium salt	Increase extracellular calcium, normalize cardiac membrane excitability	Hypercalcemia, vascular irritation; hypotension, arrhythmias, arrest if rapid administration	Hypercalcemia, ventricular fibrillation; caution with concurrent digitalis use, cardiac or renal disease	50–150mg/kg IV slowly over 5–30 minutes; 60–90 mg/kg/day IV CRI for refractory hypocalcemia	Hyperkalemic crisis, correction of hypocalcemia, decrease cardiotoxic effects of hypermagnesemia
Dexamethasone	Glucocorticoid	Multiple mechanisms	Symptoms of hyperadrenocorticism, GI ulceration, growth retardation of young animals	Systemic fungal infections; will complicate diagnosis of lymphoma	0.1–0.22 mg/kg PO, SC, IM, IV q12–24h	Hypercalcemia

Drug	Class	Mechanism	Adverse effects	Cautions/contraindications	Dosing	Indications
Dihydrotachysterol	Vitamin D analog (hormone)	Promote GI absorption, renal reabsorption, and bone resorption of calcium	Hypercalcemia, nephrocalcinosis, hyperphosphatemia	Hypercalcemia, vitamin D toxicity, malabsorption syndrome; caution with hyperphosphatemia	0.03 mg/kg/day PO divided BID for 2–5 days, then 0.01 mg/kg/day divided BID	Hypocalcemia from hypoparathyroidism or renal disease
Dilitazem	Calcium-channel blocker	Inhibit influx of extracellular calcium	Bradycardia, GI distress, hypotension, heart block, CNS effects	Hypotension, sick sinus syndrome, AV block; caution in heart failure, hepatic and renal impairment	0.5–1.5mg/kg PO q8h; for acute management 0.125–0.35mg/kg IV	Hypercalcemia— cardioprotective
Ergocalciferol	Vitamin D analog (hormone)	Promote GI absorption, renal reabsorption, and bone resorption of calcium	Hypercalcemia, nephrocalcinosis, hyperphosphatemia	Hypercalcemia, vitamin D toxicity, malabsorption syndrome; caution with hyperphosphatemia	4,000–6,000U/kg/day PO, then 1,000–2,000 U/kg/day once daily to once weekly PO	Hypocalcemia from hypoparathyroidism or renal disease
Etidronate	Bisphosphonate	Inhibit osteoclastic resorption	Diarrhea, nausea, bone pain	Impaired renal function; caution with bone fractures, enterocolitis, cardiac failure	5–20 mg/kg/day PO divided BID	Adjunctive therapy for hypercalcemia
Furosemide	Loop diuretic	Increase renal excretion of magnesium and calcium	Electrolyte abnormalities due to renal loss, dehydration, ototoxicity, GI disturbances, weakness	Dehydration, hypotension, preexisting electrolyte imbalances, hepatic dysfunction, diabetes mellitus	After volume reexpansion, 1–4mg/kg PO, SC, IM, or IV q8–24h	Hypercalcemia, hypermagnesemia
Magnesium chloride	Magnesium salt	Increase extracellular magnesium	Usually the result of overdose. Hypermagnesemia, hypotension, bradycardia, vomiting, weakness, respiratory depression, CNS depression, hyporeflexia	Caution with heart block and impaired renal function	Rapid repletion: 0.75–1 mEq/kg/day for 1st 24–48 hrs; slow repletion: 0.3–0.5mEq/kg/day for 3–5 days; life-threatening ventricular arrhythmias: 0.15–0.3mEq/kg over 5–15 minutes. Dilute in 0.9% NaCl or 5% dextrose in water.	Hypomagnesemia

461

Table 34.11. Continued.

Drugs	Classes	MOAs	Side Effects	Contraindications or Precautions	Routes of Administration and Doses	General Uses
Magnesium sulfate	Magnesium salt	Increase extracellular magnesium	See magnesium chloride. Hypocalcemia	See magnesium chloride. Hypocalcemia	See magnesium chloride.	Hypomagnesemia
Pamidronate	Bisphosphonate	Inhibit osteoclastic resorption	Nephrotoxicity	Hypomagnesemia, arrhythmias, impaired renal function, anemia, thrombocytopenia	1.3–2.0 mg/kg IV in 0.9% NaCl given over 2 hrs; repeat in 1–3 wks PRN	Adjunctive therapy for hypercalcemia
Physostigmine	Anticholinesterase	Reverses anticholinergic effects or agents	Vomiting, nausea, miosis, salivation, sweating, lacrimation, bronchospasm, dyspnea, pulmonary edema, respiratory paralysis, irregular pulse, bradycardia or tachycardia, hypotension or hypertension, restlessness, weakness, muscle twitching, seizures, collapse, paralysis	Epilepsy/seizures, bradycardia, tachycardia, asthma, diabetes mellitus, cardiovascular disease, gastrointestinal or urinary obstruction	0.02 mg/kg IV q12h	Decrease neurotoxic effects of hypermagnesemia
Plicamycin (Mithramycin)	Antineoplastic	Inhibit osteoclastic resorption	GI, thrombocytopenia, hepatotoxicity, nephrotoxicity	Impaired renal function	25 μg/kg IV in 5% dextrose in water over 2–4 hrs	Hypercalcemia
Potassium chloride (2 mEq/mL)	Potassium salt	Increase extracellular potassium	Hyperkalemia, vascular irritation	Hyperkalemia, renal impairment, hemolytic reactions, acute dehydration, digitalized patients	If IV, do not exceed 0.5 mEq/kg/hr. If SC, do not exceed 30 mEq/L.	Hypokalemia treatment or prevention
Potassium gluconate	Potassium salt	Increase extracellular potassium	Hyperkalemia, GI irritation	Hyperkalemia, renal impairment, hemolytic reactions, acute dehydration, digitalized patients	5–8 mEq/cat/day PO divided BID or TID initially, then 2–4 mEq/cat/day maintenance	Hypokalemia treatment or prevention

Drug	Class	Mechanism	Adverse effects	Contraindications/Cautions	Dose	Indication
Potassium Phosphate (4.36 mEq/ml)	Potassium salt	Increase extracellular potassium	Hyperkalemia, vascular irritation, hyperphosphatemia, hypocalcemia, hypotension, renal failure, soft tissue mineralization, seizures	Hyperkalemia, renal impairment, hemolytic reactions, acute dehydration, digitalized patients, hyperphosphatemia, hypocalcemia, oliguric or anuric renal failure, tissue necrosis	For potassium supplementation: If IV, do not exceed 0.5 mEq/kg/hr. If SC, do not exceed 30 mEq/L. For phosphorus supplementation: 0.01–0.03 mmol/kg IV over 6 hours in calcium-free fluids	Hypokalemia treatment or prevention, hypophosphatemia treatment
Prednisone/prednisolone	Glucocorticoid	Multiple mechanisms	Symptoms of hyperadrenocorticism, GI ulceration, growth retardation of young animals	Systemic fungal infections, Will complicate diagnosis of lymphoma	1.0–2.2 mg/kg PO, SC, IM, IV q12–24h	Hypercalcemia
Regular insulin	Endocrine pancreatic hormone	Facilitates intracellular nutrient uptake	Hypoglycemia	Hypoglycemia	0.25–1.0 U/kg diluted in IV fluids containing dextrose (2 g/U insulin)	Hyperkalemic crisis
Sodium bicarbonate	Alkalinizing agent	Extracellular buffer, calcium binding	Metabolic alkalosis, hypokalemia, hypocalcemia, hypernatremia, volume overload, decreased oxygenation	Alkalosis, hypochloremia, hypocalcemia; caution in CHF, volume overload, nephrotic syndrome, oliguria, hypertension	For hyperkalemic crisis: 1–2 mg/kg IV slowly. For metabolic acidosis or hypercalcemia: Bicarbonate dose (mEq) = $0.4 \times BW$ (kg) $\times$ (12 – patient's bicarbonate). Give ½ of the calculated dose over 3–4 hours in IV fluids.	Hyperkalemic crisis, metabolic acidosis, hypercalcemia
Verapamil	Calcium-channel blocker	Inhibit influx of extracellular calcium	Hypotension, brady/tachycardia, AV block, worsening of CHF, nausea, constipation	Hypotension, sick sinus syndrome, AV block; caution in heart failure, hepatic and renal impairment	0.025 mg/kg IV q 10–30 min; max cumulative dose 0.15 mg/kg	Hypercalcemia—cardioprotective

5. Calcium gluconate, 50–100 mg/kg IV over 10 minutes
   a. Direct antagonist of magnesium at the neuromuscular junction
   b. May be beneficial in reversing the cardiotoxic side effects of hypermagnesemia
6. Physostigmine, 0.02 mg/kg q12h IV
   a. May offset the neurotoxic side effects of hypermagnesemia.
7. Severe cases may require intubation, positive pressure ventilation, and vasopressor therapy to maintain blood pressure.

Recommended Reading

Adams LG, Hardy RM, Weiss DJ, Bartges JW. Hypophosphatemia and hemolytic anemia associated with diabetes mellitus and hepatic lipidosis in cats. J Vet Int Med, 1993; 7(5):266–271.

Bateman S. Disorders of magnesium: magnesium deficit and excess. In DiBartola SP, ed, Fluid, Electrolyte, and Acid-Base Disorders in Small Animal Practice, pp 210–226. St. Louis: Saunders Elsevier, 2006.

Bruskiewicz KA, Nelson RW, Feldman EC, Griffey SM. Diabetic ketosis and ketoacidosis in cats: 42 cases (1980–1995). J Am Vet Med Assoc, 1997; 211(2):188–192.

Dhupa N. Magnesium therapy. In Bonagura JD, Kirk RW, eds, Kirk's Current Veterinary Therapy XII, pp 132–133. Philadelphia: W.B. Saunders, 1995.

Dhupa N, Proulx J. Hypocalcemia and hypomagnesemia. Vet Clin North Am Sm Anim Pract, 1998; 28(3):587–598.

DiBartola SP. Disorders of sodium and water: hypernatremia and hyponatremia. In DiBartola SP, ed, Fluid, Electrolyte, and Acid-Base Disorders in Small Animal Practice, pp 47–79. St. Louis: Saunders Elsevier, 2006.

DiBartola SP, Morais HA de. Disorders of potassium: hypokalemia and hyperkalemia. In DiBartola SP, ed, Fluid, Electrolyte, and Acid-Base Disorders in Small Animal Practice, pp 91–121. St. Louis: Saunders Elsevier, 2006.

DiBartola SP, Willard MD. Disorders of phosphorus: hypophosphatemia and hyperphosphatemia. In DiBartola SP, ed, Fluid, Electrolyte, and Acid-Base Disorders in Small Animal Practice, pp 195–209. St. Louis: Saunders Elsevier, 2006.

Drobatz KJ, Hughes D. Concentration of ionized calcium in plasma from cats with urethral obstruction. J Am Vet Med Assoc, 1997; 211(11):1392–1395.

Hackett T. Endocrine and metabolic emergencies. In King L, Hammond R, eds, Manual of Canine and Feline Emergency and Critical Care, pp 177–189. Shurdington, Cheltenham, United Kingdom: British Small Animal Veterinary Association, 1999.

Jackson CB, Drobatz KJ. Iatrogenic magnesium overdose: 2 case reports. J Vet Emerg Crit Care, 2004; 14(2):115–123.

Justin RB, Hohenhaus AE. Hypophosphatemia associated with enteral alimentation in cats. J Vet Int Med, 1995; 9(4):228–233.

Kimmel SE, Washabau RJ, Drobatz KJ. Incidence and prognostic value of low plasma ionized calcium concentration in cats with acute pancreatitis: 46 cases (1996–1998). J Am Vet Med Assoc, 2001; 219(8):1105–1109.

Macintire DK, Drobatz KJ, Haskins SC, Saxon WD. Endocrine and metabolic emergencies. In Manual of Small Animal Emergency and Critical Care Medicine, pp 296–333. Philadelphia: Lippincott Williams and Wilkins, 2005.

Manning AM. Electrolyte disorders. Vet Clin North Am Sm Anim Pract, 2001; 31(6):1289–1321.

Martin LG. Hypercalcemia and hypermagnesemia. Vet Clin North Am Sm Anim Pract, 1998; 28(3):565–585.

Martin LG, Matteson VL, Wingfield WE, Van Pelt DR, Hackett TB. Abnormalities of serum magnesium in critically ill dogs: incidence and implications. J Vet Emerg Crit Care, 1994; 4(1):15–20.

Martin LG, Van Pelt DR, Wingfield WE. Magnesium and the critically ill patient. In Bonagura JD, Kirk RW, eds, Kirk's Current Veterinary Therapy XII, pp 128–131. Philadelphia: W.B. Saunders, 1995.

Martin LG, Wingfield WE, Van Pelt DR, Hackett TB. Magnesium in the 1990's: implications for veterinary critical care. J Vet Emerg Crit Care, 1993; 3(2):105–114.

Norris CR, Nelson RW, Christopher MM. Serum total and ionized magnesium concentrations and urinary fractional excretion of magnesium in cats with diabetes mellitus and diabetic ketoacidosis. J Am Vet Med Assoc, 1999; 215(10):1455–1459.

Phillips SL, Polzin DJ. Clinical disorders of potassium homeostasis. Vet Clin North Am Sm Anim Pract, 1998; 28(3):545–563.

Schenck PA, Chew DJ. Understanding recent developments in hypocalcemia and hypomagnesemia. Proceedings of the 23rd American College of Veterinary Internal Medicine Forum, 2005; 23:666–668.

Schenck PA, Chew DJ, Nogode LA, Rosol TJ. Disorders of calcium: hypercalcemia and hypocalcemia. In DiBartola SP, ed, Fluid, Electrolyte, and Acid-Base Disorders in Small Animal Practice, pp 122–194. St. Louis: Saunders Elsevier, 2006.

Toll J, Erb H, Birnbaum N, Schermerhorm T. Prevalence and incidence of serum magnesium abnormalities in hospitalized cats. J Vet Int Med, 2002; 16(3):217–221.

Wooldridge JD, Gregory CR. Ionized and total serum magnesium concentrations in feline renal transplant recipients. Vet Surg, 1999; 28(1):31–37.

35
REPRODUCTIVE EMERGENCIES

Page E. Yaxley and L. Ari Jutkowitz

Unique Features
- Cats are seasonally polyestrous, induced ovulators.
- A working knowledge of normal parturition is essential to recognition of dystocia.
- Uterine prolapse generally results from severe straining during or post parturiation.
- Uterine torsion is rare in cats but should be suspected in cases of dystocia with persistent severe straining.
- Endometritis, mastitis, and eclampsia are the most frequently reported postparturient complications.
- Pyometra may be successfully managed medically or surgically, but ovariohysterectomy is the treatment of choice.

A. Normal feline reproduction
- a. Seasonally polyestrous
  - i. Normal breeding season is February through October in the Northern Hemisphere.
    - 1. Heat cycles are typically repeated unless interrupted by pregnancy, pseudopregnancy, or illness.
    - 2. Queens can produce two litters per season.
- b. Estrous cycle
  - i. Proestrus
    - 1. 1–2 days in length
    - 2. Ovarian follicles increase in size.
    - 3. Estrogen is dominant hormone produced.
    - 4. Queens attract males but are unreceptive to copulation.
  - ii. Estrus (box 35.1)
    - 1. 3–16 days (average 7 days) in length
    - 2. Estrogen levels increase due to follicular growth and maturation.
    - 3. Females become receptive to males and sexual behaviors are noted (see box 35.1).
    - 4. Cats are induced ovulators.
      - a. Only ovulate in response to mating
  - iii. Interestrus
    - 1. 1–2 weeks (8 days average)
    - 2. Follicles from previous estrogen wave regress.

Box 35.1. Signs of estrus.
Vocalization
Affectionate, rolling behavior
Lordosis (elevation of hindquarters while in sternal recumbency)

       3. No copulation occurs during this time.
       4. Low estrogen, low progesterone levels
       5. Ends when a new follicular wave starts
    iv. Diestrus
       1. Uterus is prepared for implantation of fertilized ovum.
       2. Progesterone is released from corpus luteum.
       3. Pseudopregnancy
         a. Queen ovulated but failed to become pregnant.
         b. Triggers 35–45-day period of luteal activity
         c. May be clinically inapparent
       4. Pregnancy
         a. Gestation is approximately 63–67 days.
         b. Queens can have two litters per season.
    v. Seasonal anestrus
       1. Reproductive quiescence with onset in late fall through winter
       2. Females do not exhibit sexual behavior or attraction of males.
B. Pregnancy diagnosis
  a. History of breeding
  b. Abdominal palpation
    i. Fetuses are first palpable at approximately 21–28 days.
  c. Abdominal radiographs
    i. Mineralization of the feline fetus at 45 days allows for skeletal detection on radiographs.
    ii. Most useful for assessment of fetal numbers and position
  d. Ultrasonography
    i. Gestational sacs visible by 11 days, fetal poles by 15 days
    ii. Fetal heart rate detectable at 23–26 days
    iii. Useful for assessment of fetal viability
    iv. Assessment of fetal numbers may be inaccurate due to miscounting.
C. Normal parturition
  a. Stage 1 labor (box 35.2)
    i. May be preceded by a drop in rectal temperature 12 hours prior to parturition, though this finding is unreliable in queens
    ii. Lasts approximately 2–12 hours

Box 35.2. Signs of stage 1 labor.
Vocalization
Restlessness
Tachypnea
Nesting
Purring
Milk secretion from developed mammary glands

      iii. Subclinical uterine contractions and progressive dilation of cervix
- b. Stage 2 labor
  - i. Average 2–6 hours but can be up to 24–42 hours
  - ii. Rapid abdominal contractions
  - iii. First fetal delivery usually occurs 1–2 hours after onset of stage 2 labor.
  - iv. Generally there is less than 30 minutes between births of kittens.
  - v. Queens will nurse while continuing parturition.
  - vi. Presentation
    1. Anterior
       a. Head, neck, and forelimbs extended through canal
    2. Posterior
       a. Rear limbs extended through canal
       b. Up to 40% of kittens born in this position
  - vii. Queens can stop parturition for 12–24 hours
    1. Queens will shut down labor if they feel threatened.
  - viii. Lochia (presence of greenish vaginal discharge) can be present shortly before the onset of stage 2 labor and is suggestive of placental separation.
- c. Stage 3 labor
  - i. Period of placental expulsion
    1. This follows fetal delivery closely in the queen.
  - ii. The placenta is frequently attached to fetus by umbilical cord
  - iii. Placental expulsion within 15 minutes of each kitten
    1. Alternate delivery between uterine horns allows for two placental deliveries after two kittens are delivered.
  - iv. Queens remove amniotic membranes and placenta from the kittens by licking and chewing.
    1. Ingestion of too many placentas can lead to vomiting or black, watery diarrhea.
  - v. Queens lick and clean the kitten, stimulating normal respiration.
- d. Bloody vaginal discharge can be seen normally for 7–10 days postpartum.
  - i. Discharge can become darker brown and slowly decrease over 4–6 weeks as uterine involution takes place.

D. Dystocia
- a. Inability to expel fetuses through the birth canal during parturition
- b. Maternal factors leading to dystocia:
  - i. Uterine inertia is the most common cause of dystocia (box 35.3).
    1. Complete uterine inertia
       a. Gestation that has exceeded 67 days post suspected breeding date with no progression to active labor
    2. Partial uterine inertia
       a. Parturition is initiated with subsequent failure to deliver all fetuses.
    3. Secondary uterine inertia
       a. Prolonged attempts to expel an obstructed fetus result in myometrial failure that persists following relief of obstruction.
  - ii. Morphologic (obstructive) factors
    1. Primary morphologic factors
       a. The birth canal is too small to pass a fetus of normal size for the breed.
          i. Brachycephalic breeds
    2. Secondary morphologic factors
       a. Abnormal influence within or upon birth canal
          i. Previous pelvic fractures
          ii. Pelvic canal neoplasia

Box 35.3. Factors associated with uterine inertia.
Myometrial fatigue
Hypoglycemia
Calcium/magnesium imbalance
Old age of queen
Obesity of queen
Hereditary factors
Stress or environmental disturbances
Inadequate oxytocin secretion
Prematurity
Uterine overdistension
  Large litter size
  Large fetus size
Uterine underdistension
  Small litter size
  Inadequate fetal fluids
Estrogen/progesterone imbalance

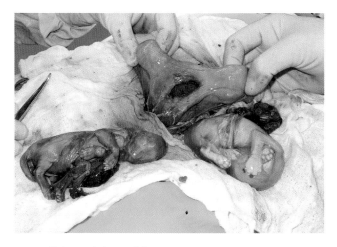

Fig. 35.1. Uterine rupture with intra-abdominal fetuses in a queen.

        iii. Uterine torsion
        iv. Uterine rupture (see fig. 35.1)
        v.   Uterine prolapse
        vi. Fibrosis of uterus, cervix, or vagina
        vii. Vaginal septum
   c. Fetal factors leading to dystocia
        i.   Malpresentation (Box 35.4)
             1. Second most common cause for dystocia
        ii. Oversize
             1. Uncommon in cats
             2. Single, large fetus

Box 35.4.   Common malpresentations.

Transverse
Lateral or ventral flexion of neck
Anterior presentation with flexion of one or both forelimbs
Posterior presentation with retention of both hind limbs
Simultaneous presentation of two fetuses

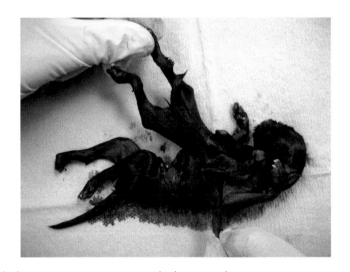

Fig. 35.2.   Fetal duplication in a cat presenting with obstructive dystocia.

    iii. Fetal malformation
        1. Anasarca (generalized subcutaneous edema)
        2. Hydrocephalus
        3. Cerebral or cerebrospinal hernias
        4. Abdominal hernias
        5. Duplication (fig. 35.2)
        6. Rib cage malformations (Pectus Excavatum)
    iv. Fetal death
        1. Increases the likelihood of malpresentation because of failure to posture normally
  d. Diagnosis of dystocia
    i.   Obtain an accurate breeding history (box 35.5).
    ii. Perform a thorough physical exam.
        1. Rule out systemic illness.
        2. Abdominal palpation
            a. Assess the size and tone of uterus.
            b. Estimate the number of remaining fetuses.
            c. Evaluate for presence of fetus in birth canal.
        3. Vaginal exam
            a. Use a sterile glove, well lubricated with sterile lubricant.
            b. Determine:
                i.   Vaginal or cervical abnormalities

Box 35.5. Taking a good reproductive history.

Previous queening history
Earliest and latest breeding dates
Male animal used
Time of temperature drop
Time of onset of parturition
Frequency and intensity of expulsive efforts
Number and viability of kittens already delivered
Interventions utilized

Box 35.6. Radiographic findings associated with fetal death.

Intrafetal gas patterns
Hyperextension of extremities (rigor mortis)
Collapse of spinal column due to loss of muscular support
Overlapping bones of fetal skull
Accumulation of intrauterine gas

---

            1. Finger should pass easily on digital exam.
            2. Due to patient size, digital exam may not be possible.
         ii. Fetal presentation
         iii. Fetal viability
      c. Gentle stroking (feathering) of dorsal vaginal wall stimulates contractions (Ferguson reflex).
         i. Allows assessment of contraction strength
   iii. Rule out underlying systemic causes.
      1. Measure blood glucose and calcium levels.
   iv. Obtain radiographs for:
      1. Rapid, accurate assessment of number, size, location, and position of fetuses
      2. Detection of maternal pelvic abnormalities
      3. Assessment of fetal viability (box 35.6)
   v. Abdominal ultrasound
      1. More useful than radiographs for assessing fetal viability, fetal malformations, fetal distress
      2. Average normal fetal heart rate is 228 +/- 35 bpm in the cat.
      3. Deceleration of heartbeat to less than 180 bpm or the presence of fetal bowel movements on ultrasound indicate fetal distress and necessitate rapid intervention.
  e. Medical management of dystocia
   i. If a fetus is lodged in the birth canal, digital manipulation is recommended.
      1. Use copious amounts of sterile lubricant.
      2. Apply digitally or infuse around fetus with a red rubber catheter and syringe.
      3. Grasp fetus around the head and neck, or pelvis, or *proximal* portions of hind limbs.
         a. Be careful not to exert too much traction.
         b. Fetal limbs are easily torn or damaged.
      4. Apply gentle traction posterior-ventral with queen standing.
      5. Rock fetus back and fourth and twist diagonally to free shoulders and hips locked in the pelvic canal.
   ii. For nonobstructive dystocia

1. Oxytocin
   a. Increases the frequency and strength of uterine contraction by promoting the influx of calcium into myometrial cells
   b. Dose: 0.5–1 units IM in the cat
   c. May be repeated every 30 minutes as needed for expulsion of fetuses
      i. If two doses have not resulted in production of fetus, surgical intervention is warranted.
   d. Contraindicated in obstructive dystocia and uterine inertia secondary to overstretching
   e. Although higher oxytocin doses have been previously recommended, these can cause ineffective or tetanic uterine contraction and lead to decreased fetal blood flow.
2. Calcium gluconate
   a. Enhances uterine tone through influx of calcium
   b. Used when contractions are weak or infrequent, if initial oxytocin dose was nonproductive, or if laboratory results reveal hypocalcemia
   c. Dose: calcium gluconate 10% solution
      i. 0.5–1.5 mL/kg IV slowly
   d. Monitor ECG for arrhythmias.
3. Dextrose
   a. Should be considered when laboratory results reveal hypoglycemia
   b. Dose: dextrose 50% solution, 0.5–1 mL/kg IV or 2 mL/kg PO
4. Failure of the queen to clean kittens should prompt human intervention.
   a. Remove amnion by cleaning carefully with a soft dry towel.
   b. Remove fluid from nasal passage with a bulb syringe.
   c. Clamp, transect, and ligate umbilicus approximately 1–2 cm from the newborn's body.
   d. Disinfect the umbilical stump with iodine to prevent infection.
iii. Prognosis
   1. 29–40% successful for vaginal delivery following dystocia in cats
   2. Stillbirth rates rise when dystocia continues for 4.5–6 hours from the onset of stage 2 labor.
   3. Caesarian section should therefore not be delayed.
f. Surgical management (box 35.7)
   i. Preanesthetic considerations
   1. Provide intravenous fluid therapy as needed to prevent or correct hypovolemia.
   2. Perform CBC and serum biochemistry to assess maternal status.
   3. Minimize fetal drug exposure by avoiding premedications.

Box 35.7.   Indications for C-section.

Complete primary uterine inertia
Partial primary or secondary uterine inertia with poor response to medical therapy
Fetal oversize
Gross maternal pelvic abnormalities
Fetal malformations
Malpresentation not amenable to manipulation
Past history of dystocia or caesarian section
Fetal putrefaction
Maternal systemic illness
Suspicion of uterine torsion, rupture, prolapse, or herniation
Evidence of fetal distress

Box 35.8. Drugs associated with higher mortality.
Thiopental
Ketamine
Xylazine
Medetomidine
Methoxyflurane

---

    4. Clip hair and perform surgical prep with the queen awake to minimize anesthesia time.
    5. Preoxygenate via mask for 3–5 minutes
  ii. Anesthetic considerations (box 35.8)
    1. Equipment and personnel (surgical team) should be ready prior to induction.
    2. Induction agents should be given *to effect*.
      a. Choose drugs with a short duration of action or drugs that can be reversed.
        i. Propofol 4–6 mg/kg IV to effect, or
        ii. Mask induction with isoflurane or sevoflurane
      b. Use the lowest possible concentration of inhalant.
        i. Inhalant anesthetics can cause vasodilation and reduction of uterine blood flow, leading to neonatal depression.
    3. Protect the maternal airway.
      a. Delayed gastric emptying results in an increased risk of aspiration pneumonia in gravid animals.
      b. The use of cuffed endotracheal tubes is recommended.
      c. Do not tilt the table head downward as this may cause undue pressure on the diaphragm and impair ventilation.
    4. Regional anesthetic techniques
      a. Useful for limiting fetal exposure by decreasing maternal anesthetic requirements
      b. Line block
        i. Lidocaine 2%, 1–2 mg/kg infused along the midline
        ii. Cats may be more sensitive to lidocaine.
        iii. Minimal effect on fetus
      c. Alternatively epidural anesthesia
        i. Lidocaine: 2–3 mg/kg
          1. Preferable to bupivicaine because of a more rapid time of onset and shorter duration of action
 iii. Surgical techniques
    1. General considerations
      a. The linea alba will be much thinner due to abdominal stretching, and care should be taken to avoid incising the underlying uterus or bladder.
      b. Avoid incision of mammary tissue.
      c. Caesarian section or en-bloc hysterectomy (see 3) may be utilized.
      d. En-bloc hysterectomy has comparable neonatal survival rates to C-section and will not interfere with lactation.
    2. Hysterotomy (Caesarian section)
      a. Make a ventral midline incision.
      b. Exteriorize the uterus.
      c. Pack off the abdominal cavity with moistened laparotomy sponges to minimize contamination from fetal fluids.

Box 35.9.   Consider en-bloc ovariohysterectomy if:
Uterine disease is present
Speed is necessary due to instability of queen
Morphological abnormalities prevent vaginal delivery of further litters
Owner does not plan to breed animal again

---

       d. Create a single, longitudinal incision in an avascular area of uterine body with a scalpel. This incision can be opened further with scissors if needed to prevent incision of fetus.
       e. Milk fetuses down each uterine horn and remove one at a time.
       f. Handle the umbilicus carefully to prevent body wall tearing.
       g. Once all fetuses are removed, the uterus is closed with a double layer continuous inverting suture pattern using absorbable monofilament suture material.
       h. Copious lavage of abdominal cavity with warmed sterile saline should be performed to remove any fetal fluids.
       i. Close abdominal wall and skin routinely.
       j. Nonabsorbable monofilament suture should be used in the skin to prevent wicking and breakdown from nursing neonates.
   3. En-bloc ovariohysterectomy (box 35.9)
       a. Make a ventral midline incision.
       b. Exteriorize the uterus.
       c. Gently manipulate intracervical or vaginal fetuses back into uterus.
       d. Break down the suspensory ligaments on both sides prior to placing clamps to minimize the duration of fetal hypoxia.
       e. Place double clamps on the body of the uterus just cranial to cervix and across each ovarian pedicle.
       f. Remove the entire uterus by incising between the clamps.
          i. The uterus is rapidly handed off to a team of assistants prepared for neonatal resuscitation.
         ii. Resuscitation of fetuses should be performed within 60 seconds of clamping pedicles to prevent fetal hypoxia and maximize survival.
       g. Double ligate the ovarian and uterine pedicles and perform routine abdominal closure.
E. Neonatal resuscitation
   a. Preparedness
     i. Have ready a warmed incubator (90°F), hemostats, suture material, suction bulb syringes, emergency drugs, and an adequate supply of soft dry towels.
   b. Clamp the umbilical cord 1–2 cm away from body wall and ligate.
   c. Address hypothermia.
     i. Fetal fluids should be removed by rubbing briskly with a soft, dry, clean towel.
     ii. Radiant heat and warmed air maintain body temperature better than circulating water blankets.
       1. Use a warmed and humidified incubator or warm air blanket.
       2. Use prewarmed towels.
   d. Stimulate ventilation.
     i. Suction oral cavity and nares with a bulb syringe.
     ii. Avoid "swinging" kittens as this increases the risk for cerebral hemorrhage.
     iii. If vigorous rubbing fails to stimulate respirations, positive pressure ventilation using a snug-fitting oxygen mask should be instituted.

        1. Because isoflurane is not metabolized, ventilation is necessary to eliminate the anesthetic gas from the body.

        2. Keep head and neck extended to facilitate lung inflation.

        3. Patients should be carefully monitored for gastric distention as this technique may result in gastric insufflation.

    iv. Intubation may also be performed using a red rubber catheter or small uncuffed endotracheal tube.

    v. Jen Chung Acupuncture (GV 26) has been reported to stimulate respiration.

        1. For adjunctive use only—should *not* replace traditional therapy

        2. Insert 25-gauge needle in nasal philtrum at base of nares.

        3. When bone is contacted, rotate needle to stimulate respiratory center.

e. Cardiac massage

    i. Institute cardiac massage if no heartbeat is detected, once rubbing, warming, and ventilatory measures have been started.

        1. Goal is approximately 200 bpm, compressing the chest by approximately 33%

f. Routes of fluid and drug administration

    i. Intravenous

        1. Difficult to access—jugular or umbilical veins preferred

    ii. Intraosseous

        1. A 22–25-gauge needle can be inserted into proximal femur for administration of drugs and fluids.

    iii. Endotracheal

        1. For administration of:

          a. Atropine, epinephrine, lidocaine, naloxone

        2. Drugs should be diluted to increase the area of mucosal contact and improve uptake.

g. Resuscitation drugs

    i. Atropine

        1. Atropine may cause increased myocardial oxygen demand and is therefore not routinely recommended in the hypoxic neonate.

    ii. Epinephrine

        1. Drug of choice for neonatal resuscitation

        2. 0.02–0.2 mg/kg administered IV, IO, IT if warming, ventilating, and chest compressions are not effective

    iii. Naloxone

        1. Consider if queen received opioid anesthesia

          a. Dose: 0.1 mg/kg IV, IM, or sublingual

    iv. Doxapram

        1. Once thought to aid in respiratory stimulation

        2. No longer recommended due to lack of evidence to support its use

        3. May significantly decrease cerebral blood flow in vulnerable hypoxemic newborns

    v. 50% dextrose

        1. If clinical signs of hypoglycemia are noted or suspected

          a. Seizures

          b. Flaccidity

          c. Weakness

          d. Coma

        2. Doses: 0.25–1 mL/kg IV (dilute if given peripherally), 2 mL/kg PO

h. Fluid therapy

    i. Preferred method IO or IV

    ii. Warm fluids to 37°C (96.8°F).

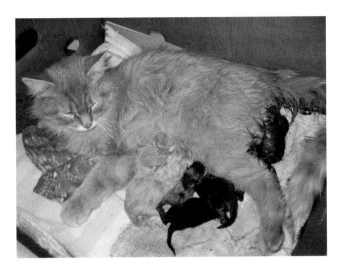

Fig. 35.3.   Uterine prolapse in a postpartum queen.

           iii. Rate dependent on severity of fluid deficits
               1. Bolus doses of 10 mL/kg may be administered as needed to address hypovolemia
               2. Neonatal maintenance crystalloid fluid requirements 60–180 mL/kg/day
                  a. Neonatal requirements higher due to higher total body water percentage and inability to concentrate their urine
F. Uterine prolapse
   a. Rare postpartum complication in cats
   b. Clinical signs
      i. Seen during or immediately following parturition as cervical dilation is necessary for prolapse to occur (fig. 35.3)
   c. Risk factors for prolapse
      i. Severe straining during or after parturition
      ii. Incomplete placental separation
      iii. Relaxation or atony of the uterus
      iv. Excessive relaxation of the pelvic and perineal region
   d. Physical exam
      i. Nonspecific signs of abdominal pain and straining may indicate prolapse into cranial vagina (incomplete prolapse).
      ii. A large mass may be seen protruding from vaginal orifice (fig. 35.3).
      iii. Variable degrees of tissue edema, ulceration, or necrosis may be present.
      iv. Undelivered fetuses may remain within the retained horn.
      v. Hemorrhagic shock may result from ovarian or uterine vessel rupture.
   e. Treatment
      i. Lubricate and protect exposed tissues.
      ii. Stabilization
         1. Intravenous fluids to correct shock
         2. Blood transfusion
            a. Required if signs consistent with severe hemorrhage are noted
               i. Packed cells 10 mL/kg
               ii. Whole blood 20 mL/kg
         3. Systemic antibiotic therapy

    iii. General anesthesia should be performed after stabilization is achieved.

    iv. Clean tissue gently and determine viability.

    v. If tissue appears healthy, lubricate copiously with sterile lubricant.

    vi. Manual reduction may be attempted as follows:

        1. Apply external pressure to manually replace uterus within the body.

        2. A test tube can be used to help invert and replace the uterus.

        3. Hydropulsion with a red rubber catheter and warmed sterile saline may aid in proper positioning of the uterine horns.

        4. Dorsal episiotomy may be performed to aid in reduction when severe edema is present.

        5. Oxytocin (0.5 U IM) administered after replacement will promote uterine involution.

    vii. Surgical reduction is indicated if manual reduction attempts have failed, severe hemorrhage is present, tissues are deemed nonviable, or animal is not intended for future breeding.

        1. Make a caudoventral midline incision.

        2. Apply intraabdominal traction to the uterus while an assistant applies external pressure to replace the uterus within the abdomen.

        3. Routine ovariohysterectomy may then be performed.

        4. If tissue is viable and future breeding is desired, uterus may alternately be pexied to the ventrolateral body wall to prevent reoccurrence.

        5. If reduction is impossible due to severe tissue swelling or necrosis, amputation of traumatized external tissue may be necessary.

           a. Urethral catheterization is recommended to prevent accidental trauma.

           b. Identify and ligate bleeding uterine vessels.

           c. After excision of necrotic tissue, the remainder is reduced via laparotomy and a complete ovariohysterectomy is performed.

G. Uterine torsion

  a. Rare in cats

    i. Can involve one or both uterine horns

    ii. Most commonly involves a single horn that twists at its base

    iii. 180-degree torsion can be present for weeks without clinical signs.

  b. Risk factors

    i. Multiparous animals

        1. Caused by previous stretching of broad ligament

    ii. Mid to late pregnancy or at parturition

    iii. Pyometra

  c. Etiology

    i. Unknown

    ii. Suspected to be related to fetal movement, rough handling during pregnancy, uterine contraction, lack of uterine tone, lack of fetal fluid, flaccid mesometrium, or previous stretching of the broad ligament of the uterus

  d. Clinical signs

    i. Depression, anorexia, lethargy

    ii. Abdominal pain

    iii. Abdominal distension

    iv. Shock

    v. Hypothermia

    vi. Hemorrhagic vaginal discharge

    vii. Dystocia with severe persistent straining

    viii. Vomiting

    ix. Restlessness

  e. Radiographic or ultrasonographic findings
   i. Fluid-filled uterus
   ii. Fetal death
   iii. Intrauterine gas
   iv. Peritoneal effusion
  f. Treatment
   i. Intravenous fluid therapy to address shock
   ii. Perioperative antimicrobial use
   iii. Exploratory surgery is required for definitive diagnosis and treatment.
    1. Ovariohysterectomy is the technique of choice.
    2. The uterus should be removed without untwisting to prevent release of endotoxin and inflammatory mediators.
  g. Prognosis
   i. Good for the queen, provided shock is corrected and surgery is performed in a timely fashion
   ii. Fetal survival is unlikely.
H. Mastitis
  a. Uncommon postpartum complication in cats resulting from bacterial infection of the mammary gland
  b. Etiology
   i. Bacterial entrance through nipple secondary to nursing, trauma, or poor hygiene
   ii. May be spread hematogenously
   iii. May develop in immunosuppressed animals
    1. Feline leukemia
    2. Feline immunodeficiency virus
    3. Feline infectious peritonitis
  c. Clinical signs
   i. Discomfort
   ii. Swelling and inflammation of mammary gland
   iii. Systemic illness in severe cases
    1. Fever
    2. Anorexia
    3. Lethargy
   iv. Reluctance to lie down
   v. Refusal to nurse offspring
    1. This results in vocalization and failure to thrive of neonates.
    2. Vocalization of neonates often prompts owner's phone call to veterinarian.
   vi. Abscessation and necrosis of mammary gland
  d. Diagnosis
   i. Generally based on history and clinical signs
   ii. Complete blood count
   iii. Chemistry
   iv. Milk evaluation
    1. Gross examination may yield milk that appears fibrinous, purulent, hemorrhagic, or gray colored.
    2. Cytology
     a. Large number of white blood cells
     b. Degenerative neutrophils with intracellular bacteria
    3. Culture
     a. *Escherichia coli*, *Staphylococcus*, and *Streptococcus* most commonly isolated
  e. Treatment

      i. Broad-spectrum antibiotics
         1. Amoxicillin-clavulanic acid
            a. Safe for nursing neonates
            b. Dose: 62.5 mg/cat PO BID
         2. Cephalexin
            a. Safe for nursing neonates
            b. Dose: 22 mg/kg PO BID
         3. Clindamycin
            a. Achieves good levels in milk
            b. Gastroenteritis may develop in nursing neonates.
            c. Dose: 5–11 mg/kg PO BID
      ii. Warm compresses
      iii. Frequent milk stripping
         1. Kittens should be allowed to continue nursing as this will promote drainage of affected glands.
      iv. Lancing of abscess pocket if palpable
      v. Mastectomy of necrotic glands
         1. Controversial
         2. May aid in rapid resolution
         3. Acceptable cosmesis by most owners
I. Endometritis (box 35.10)
   a. Bacterial infection of the uterus generally seen within 3 days of parturition
   b. Etiology
      i. Retention of fetus or placenta
      ii. Abortion
      iii. Uterine trauma secondary to dystocia or obstetrical instrumentation
      iv. Ascending infection from vaginal vault
   c. Diagnostics
      i. Complete blood count
         1. Leukocytosis with left shift
         2. Leukopenia
         3. Thrombocytopenia
      ii. Serum chemistry profile
         1. Elevated liver values
         2. Hypoalbuminemia
      iii. Coagulation panel
         1. Rule out disseminated intravascular coagulation (DIC).

Box 35.10. Clinical signs of metritis.

Fever
Lethargy
Anorexia
Vomiting
Diarrhea
Poor lactation
Neglect of offspring
Fetid, malodorous vaginal discharge
Purulent vaginal discharge

      iv. Imaging (radiographs or abdominal ultrasound)
         1. Evaluate for fetal death, retained placentas, or evidence of uterine enlargement
      v. Cytology of vaginal discharge
         1. Degenerate neutrophils and macrophages with intracellular bacteria
   d. Treatment
      i. For sepsis
         1. Intravenous fluid therapy
         2. Broad-spectrum antibiotic combinations
            a. Ampicillin/enrofloxacin
            b. Ampicillin/aminoglycoside
            c. Cefazolin/aminoglycoside/metronidazole
               i. Aminoglycosides should only be used after the patient is rehydrated to avoid nephrotoxicity.
         3. Supportive measures
      ii. Surgical intervention
         1. After stabilization, ovariohysterectomy should be performed.
      iii. Medical therapy
         1. May be considered in nonseptic, breeding animals
         2. Evacuation of uterine contents achieved through prostaglandin $F_{2\alpha}$ ($PGF_{2\alpha}$; lutalyse)
            a. See discussion of $PGF_{2\alpha}$ in pyometra section below

J. Eclampsia
   a. Life-threatening hypocalcemia in the periparturient period
   b. Uncommon in cats
   c. Can be seen as early as 3–17 days prior to parturition
   d. More commonly develops 2–3 weeks postparturition
   e. Pathophysiology
      i. Loss of calcium through lactation and fetal skeletal mineralization in excess of that entering the extracellular fluid through gastrointestinal absorption and bone resorption
   f. Risk factors
      i. Increased ratio of litter size to maternal body weight has been associated with the development of hypocalcemia.
   g. Clinical signs (may be subtle)
      i. Hypothermia
      ii. Hyperexcitability
      iii. Hypersensitivity
      iv. Flaccid paralysis
      v. Clonic-tonic muscle spasms
      vi. Ptyalsim
      vii. Ataxia
      viii. Mydriasis
   h. Diagnosis
      i. Based on history and physical exam
      ii. Low ionized or total calcium levels
   i. Treatment
      i. Place an intravenous catheter.
      ii. Initiate intravenous fluid therapy.
      iii. Administer calcium gluconate (10%) 0.5–1.5 mL/kg IV slowly to effect, until cessation of tremors is noted.
      iv. Monitor an ECG during calcium administration.
         1. Slow or discontinue calcium infusion if bradycardia or ventricular arrhythmias are noted.

     v.   Monitor ionized calcium levels after administration to ensure adequate replacement.

     vi. Monitor temperature, as hyperthermia is common with eclampsia.

  j. Prevention of recurrence

     i.   Remove the kittens from the queen and bottle feed or wean.

     ii. Feed the queen a high-quality kitten food.

     iii. Oral calcium supplementation is necessary if continued nursing is permitted.

        1. Calcium carbonate: 50–100 mg/kg divided into three doses daily until weaning.

           a. Regular strength Tums contains 200 mg calcium per tablet.

        2. Supplementation prior to parturition is not recommended as this may promote calcium wasting during pregnancy leading to increased risk of eclampsia postpartum.

  k. Prognosis

     i.   Good

K. Ectopic pregnancy

  a. Rare, but reported in cats

  b. Primary ectopic pregnancy

     i.   Results from fertilized ova entering peritoneal cavity and attaching to mesentery or abdominal viscera

  c. Secondary ectopic pregnancy

     i.   Results from rupture of uterus following trauma

  d. Clinical signs

     i.   Mechanical interference with abdominal organs

     ii. Necrosis of intra-abdominal ectopic tissue

     iii. Incidental finding

  e. Treatment

     i.   Surgical removal +/- ovariohysterectomy

L. Abortion (fig. 35.4)

  a. May result from maternal, fetal, or placental abnormalities

     i.   Systemic illness of queen

        1. Viral disease is the most common cause of abortion in cats

           a. Feline leukemia virus

           b. Feline immunodeficiency virus

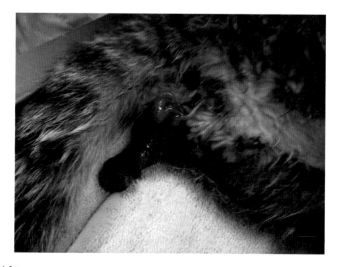

Fig. 35.4. Aborted fetus.

        c. Feline infectious peritonitis

        d. Feline herpesvirus

    2. *Toxoplasma gondii*

  ii. Early embryonic death

    1. Generally occurs before 45 days of pregnancy

    2. Cause is often undetermined

    3. Chromosomal abnormalities have been identified in aborted kittens.

  iii. Placental problems

    1. Placental necrosis of unknown cause has been reported in cats.

  iv. Drugs

    1. Chloramphenicol

    2. Glucocorticoids

    3. Prostaglandins

  b. Partial abortion may occasionally be seen.

   i. The rest of the litter may be carried to term.

  c. Treatment

   i. Treat underlying cause of abortion.

    1. Supportive and symptomatic care of queen

    2. Baseline lab analysis

      a. CBC

      b. Serum chemistry profile

      c. Urinalysis

      d. Serological testing of queen for infectious agents

   ii. Establish status of uterine contents.

    1. Radiography or ultrasonography

      a. Determine viability of remaining fetuses

   iii. Evacuate nonviable uterine contents.

    1. PGF$_{2\alpha}$ 0.1–0.25 mg/kg SC

    2. Oxytocin 0.5–3 units IM

   iv. Queens may attempt to consume aborted fetus.

   v. Abortus and placenta should be submitted for gross, microbiological, and histopathological analysis.

  d. Prognosis

   i. Dependent on underlying cause of abortion

   ii. May put other colony members at risk

M. Pyometra

  a. Accumulation of purulent exudate within the uterine lumen

  b. Hormonally mediated disease seen in diestrus

  c. Risk factors

   i. Rare in cats

    1. Require intercourse for luteal activity

   ii. Cystic endometrial hyperplasia may play a role.

    1. Abnormal uterine response to progesterone results in hypertrophy of mucus-producing glands in the endometrium, endometrial thickening, and decreased myometrial activity.

    2. The combination of increased mucus production and decreased myometrial activity leads to fluid accumulation within the uterus.

      a. Hydrometra: low-viscosity uterine fluid

      b. Mucometra: high-viscosity uterine fluid

    3. Establishes favorable environment for bacterial growth

      a. Opportunistic invasion by bacteria from vaginal vault

     iii. Most commonly affects middle-aged cats, though cats of any age may be affected

     iv. More common in cats treated with megestrol acetate (ovaban) and cats with retained corpora lutea or cystic ovaries

d. Clinical signs

     i. Anorexia

     ii. Sanguineous to mucopurulent vulvar discharge

        1. May be subtle due to grooming behaviors

     iii. Depression

     iv. Polyuria/polydipsia

     v. Vomiting

     vi. Diarrhea

     vii. History of estrus 28–60 days ago

        1. 80% may be within 28 days of last estrus

        2. Higher frequency during breeding season

     viii. Abdominal distension

     ix. Uveitis

     x. Perineal soiling

     xi. Dehydration

     xii. Sepsis/septic shock

e. Physical exam

     i. Palpably enlarged uterus

        1. Caution should be taken to not rupture uterus with aggressive palpation, as the uterus may be friable.

     ii. Rectal temperature can be low, normal, or high depending on degree of morbidity.

     iii. Evidence of shock may be noted.

f. Diagnostics

     i. Complete blood count

        1. Anemia

        2. Leukocytosis

           a. Degenerative left shift

        3. Leukopenia

     ii. Serum chemistry profile

        1. Hyper- or hypoproteinemia

        2. Hyperglobulinemia

        3. Hyper- or hypoglycemia

        4. Azotemia

           a. May result from prerenal or renal causes

        5. Elevations in alanine aminotransferase and alkaline phosphatase

     iii. Urinalysis

        1. Concurrent urinary tract infections are common.

        2. Cystocentesis should be avoided to prevent risk of uterine rupture.

        3. Midstream voided urine sample should be obtained if possible, or cystocentesis can be obtained at surgery for evaluation.

        4. Proteinuria

           a. Can be indicative of urinary tract infections or immune complex deposition in the glomeruli resulting in glomerulonephropathy

           b. Typically resolves with treatment of pyometra

        5. Isosthenuria

           a. *E. coli* endotoxin causes decreased ability of renal tubules to concentrate urine in response to ADH.

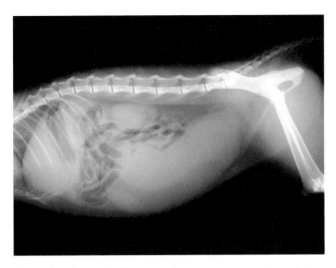

Fig. 35.5. Lateral abdominal radiograph of a cat with pyometra. Note the mid-abdominal, large, fluid-filled tubular structure.

        b. Specific gravity is therefore not helpful in differentiating prerenal from renal causes of azotemia.

        c. Differentiation of prerenal from renal causes of azotemia may be accomplished by assessing response to fluid therapy.

    iv. Vaginal cytology

        1. Large number of degenerative neutrophils with intracellular bacteria

        2. Obtain sample from anterior vagina via use of a shielded swab.

          a. Aids in antibiotic sensitivity for medical management

        3. Vaginal and uterine cultures

          a. *Escherichia coli* most common isolate

          b. Reported to be negative in 10–30% cases

    v. Radiographs

        1. A tubular soft tissue opacity may be seen in the caudal abdomen (fig. 35.5).

        2. Loss of abdominal detail may suggest uterine rupture.

        3. Inability to identify the uterus does not rule out pyometra, as open pyometra may prevent significant distension.

        4. Differential diagnosis of pregnancy should also be considered.

          a. Uterus normally visible on radiographs by day 28 of pregnancy

          b. Difficult to differentiate from pyometra as fetal skeletal development does not occur until day 45

    vi. Ultrasonography

        1. May reveal increased wall thickness and presence of uterine fluid (fig. 35.6)

        2. Useful for identification of gravid uterus

  g. Patient stabilization and perioperative considerations

    i. Administer fluid therapy with goals of correction of shock, normalization of electrolyte and acid base abnormalities, and correction of hypoglycemia.

        1. Colloids may also be administered to address hypotension and peripheral edema resulting from hypoproteinemia.

          a. Indicated when total protein <4.0 g/dL

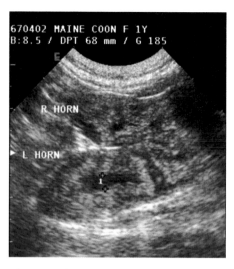

Fig. 35.6. Abdominal ultrasound image of the horns of a cat with pyometra. Note increased thickness of the uterine wall.

    ii. Broad-spectrum antibiotic therapy
        1. Administer preoperatively.
        2. Continue 7–10 days postoperatively.
    iii. Treatment of coagulopathy
        1. Fresh frozen plasma (10 mL/kg) is indicated when clotting times are prolonged.
  h. Surgical management
    i. Ovariohysterectomy is the treatment of choice.
        1. Surgical considerations:
           a. Large, friable uterus may be easily ruptured.
           b. Caution should be taken to avoid uterine laceration on entry, or accidental rupture or spillage during manipulation.
           c. The uterus should be exteriorized and packed off with laparotomy sponges to avoid contamination of the abdomen.
           d. The uterine stump should not be oversewn as this may increase the chance of uterine stump abscessation.
    ii. Surgical complications
        1. Anesthetic complications
           a. Correct electrolyte abnormalities prior to surgery.
        2. Uterine rupture
        3. Hemorrhage
        4. Peritonitis
        5. Dehiscence
        6. Uterine stump pyometra
           a. Incomplete removal of the uterine body or horns
           b. Progesterone source from ovarian remnant or exogenous administration necessary for development.
    iii. Prognosis
        1. 92% survival with surgical management
        2. Development of peritonitis results in more guarded prognosis and may necessitate closed suction drain placements or management as an open abdomen

i. Medical management of pyometra
   i. Generally discouraged due to potential for complications
      1. High rate of recurrence
      2. Increased risk of uterine rupture
      3. Less effective in closed pyometra
         a. Potential for retrograde expulsion of exudate through oviducts into abdomen
   ii. May be of value in animals whose sole purpose is for breeding
   iii. Prostaglandin $F_{2\alpha}$ ($PGF_{2\alpha}$; lutalyse) is medical therapy of choice
      1. Mechanism of action
         a. Causes contraction of the myometrium and relaxation of the cervix leading to evacuation of the uterine contents
         b. Decreases progesterone levels through luteolysis
      2. May require greater than 48 hours for clinical improvement to be seen
         a. Should not be attempted in systemically ill animals
      3. Dose: 0.1–0.25 mg/kg subcutaneously, diluted in equal volume of saline, once daily for 5 days
         a. Start at lower dose and titrate upward based on animal's response.
            i. Increase frequency of administration to twice daily if increased volume of discharge is not noted following administration.
         b. Only naturally occurring $PGF_{2\alpha}$ should be used.
         c. Synthetic analogues more potent and can be fatal
      4. Not approved for use in queens
         a. Owners should be informed of extralabel usages.
      5. Associated with numerous side effects (box 35.11), typically lasting 30–60 minutes following injection
   iv. Concurrent use of broad-spectrum antibiotics recommended for 14 days (based on anterior vaginal culture)
      1. Amoxicillin-clavulanate: 13.75–27 mg/kg every 12 hours
      2. Fluoroquinolone: enrofloxacin 5 mg/kg every 24 hours, combined with another drug such as ampicillin 22 mg/kg every 12 hours
   v. Hospitalize animal during medical management to allow for continued monitoring.
      1. Resolution of clinical signs, cessation of vaginal discharge, and resolution of neutrophilia indicate good response to medical management.

Box 35.11.   Side effects seen following $PGF_{2\alpha}$ administration.

Restlessness
Panting
Pacing
Ptyalism
Tachycardia
Abdominal pain
Fever
Vomiting
Mydriasis
Vocalization
Excessive grooming
Lordosis
Tenesmus

      2. Acute onset of signs of systemic illness should prompt immediate surgical intervention.
        a. Suggestive of uterine rupture or peritonitis
  vi. Reevaluation 2 weeks after completion of treatment
      1. If persistent clinical signs, repeat second course of treatment
  vii. Prognosis
      1. Reported 95% cats with open pyometra good outcome after single course of therapy
      2. Breeding is recommended next estrus cycle to maximize reproductive potential of queen.
      3. Ovariohysterectomy is recommended once animal is no longer used for breeding.

References

Adeyanju JB. Eclampsia in a cat. Vet Rec, 1984; 114:1296–1297.

Berepubo NA, Long SE. A study of the relationship between chromosome anomalies and reproductive wastage in domestic animals. Theriogenology, 1983; 20:177–190.

Biller DS, Haibel GK. Torsion of the uterus in a cat. J Am Vet Med Assoc, 1987; 19:1128–1129.

Bjerkas E. Eclampsia in the cat. J Anim Pract, 1974; 15:411–414.

Darvelid AW, Linde-Forsberg C. Dystocia in the bitch: a retrospective study of 182 cases. J Small Anim Pract, 1994; 35:402–407.

Davidson AP, Feldman EC, Nelson RW. Treatment of pyometra in cats using prostaglandin F2α: 21 cases (1982–1990). J Am Vet Med Assoc, 1992; 200:825–828.

Davidson AP, Nyland TG, Tsutsui T. Pregnancy diagnosis with ultrasound in the domestic cat. Vet Radiol, 1986; 27:109–114.

Drobatz KJ, Casey KK. Eclampsia in dogs: 31 cases (1995–1998). J Am Vet Med Assoc, 2000; 217:216–219.

Ekstrand C, Linde-Forsberg C. Dystocia in the cat: a retrospective study of 155 cases. J Small Anim Pract, 1994; 35:459–464.

Farrow CS. Maternal-fetal evaluation in suspected canine dystocia: a radiographic perspective. Can Vet J, 1978; 19:24–26.

Fascetti AJ, Hickman MA. Preparturient hypocalcemia in four cats. J Am Vet Med Assoc, 1999; 215:1127–1129.

Funkquist PME, Nyman GC, Lofgren AMJ, et al. Use of propofol-isoflurane as an anesthetic regimen for cesarian section in dogs. J Am Vet Med Assoc, 1997; 211:313–317.

Gunn-Moore DA, Thrusfield MV. Feline dystocia: prevalence and association with cranial conformation and breed. Vet Rec, 1995; 136:350–353.

Huxtable CR, Duff BC, Bennett AM, et al. Placental lesions in habitually aborting cats. Vet Pathol, 1979; 16:283–291.

Johnston SD. Management of pregnancy disorders in the bitch and queen. In Kirk, RW, ed, Current Veterinary Therapy VIII, pp 952–955. Philadelphia: W.B. Saunders, 1983.

Kenney KJ, Matthiesen DT, Brown NO, Bradley RL. Pyometra in cats: 183 cases (1979–1984). J Am Vet Med Assoc, 1987; 191:1130–1132.

Linde-Forsberg C, Eneroth A. Parturition. In Simpson GM, ed, Manual of Small Animal Reproduction and Neonatology, pp 127–142. Cheltenham: British Small Animal Veterinary Association, 1998.

Marretta SM, Matthiesen DT, Nichols R. Pyometra and its complications. Prob Vet Med, 1989; 1:50–61.

Maxon FB, Krausnick KE. Dystocia with uterine prolapse in a Siamese cat. Vet Med Small Anim Clin, 1969; 64:1065–1066.

Moon PF, Erb HN, Ludders JW, et al. Perioperative management and mortality rates of dogs undergoing cesarian section in the United States and Canada. J Am Vet Med Assoc, 1998; 213:365–369.

Moon PF, Massat BJ, Pascoe PJ. Neonatal critical care. Vet Clin N Am Small Anim Pract, 2001; 31:343–367.

Moon-Massat PF, Erb HN. Perioperative factors associated with puppy vigor after delivery by cesarian section. J Am Anim Hosp Assoc, 2002; 38:90–96.

Nelson RW, Feldman EC. Pyometra. Vet Clin N Am Small Anim Pract, 1986; 16:561–575.

Pascoe PJ, Moon PF. Periparturient and neonatal anesthesia. Vet Clin N Am Small Anim Pract, 2001; 31:315–341.

Potter K, Hancock DH, Gallina AM. Clinical and pathologic features of endometrial hyperplasia, pyometra, and endometritis in cats: 79 cases (1980–1985). J Am Vet Med Assoc, 1991; 198:1427–1431.

Ridyard AE, Welsh EA, Gunn-Moore DA. Successful treatment of uterine torsion in a cat with severe metabolic and haemostatic complications. J Feline Med Surg, 2000; 2:115–119.

Robbins MA, Mullen HS. En bloc ovariohysterectomy as a treatment for dystocia in dogs and cats. Vet Surg, 1994; 23:48–52.

Roll C, Horsch S. Effects of doxapram on cerebral blood flow velocity in preterm infants. Neuropediatrics, 2004; 35:126–129.

Root MV, Johnston SD, Olson PN. Estrous length, pregnancy rate, gestation and parturition lengths, litter size and juvenile mortality in the domestic cat. J Am Anim Hosp Assoc, 1995; 31:429–433.

Skarda RT. Anesthesia case of the month. J Am Vet Med Assoc, 1999; 214:37–39.

Verstegen JP, Silva LDM, Onclin K, et al. Echocardiographic study of heart rate in dog and cat fetuses in utero. J Reprod Fertil Suppl, 1993; 47:175–180.

Wallace LJ, Henry JD, Clifford JH. Manual reduction of uterine prolapse in a domestic cat. Vet Med Small Anim Clin, 1970; 65:595–596.

Wallace M. Management of parturition and problems of the periparturient period of dogs and cats. Sem Vet Med Surg, 1994; 9:28–37.

Zone MA, Wanke MM. Diagnosis of canine fetal health by ultrasonography. J Reprod Fertil Suppl, 2001; 57:215–219.

36
PEDIATRIC EMERGENCIES

Maureen McMichael

> **Unique Features**
> - Hct decreases from 47.5% at birth to 27% at 4–6 weeks of age and then slowly begins to normalize.
> - Albumin is also lower in pediatric felines; expect a lower total solids in this age group.
> - Urine is isosthenuric in neonates, and there is a decreased capacity to concentrate or dilute urine.
> - Meticulous monitoring for both under- and overhydration is essential via accurate pediatric gram scales, frequent checks of weight, Hct/TS, urine SG, and respiratory rate.

A. Overview
   a. There are significant differences in biochemical, hematological, radiographic, pharmacologic, and monitoring parameters in feline neonates compared to their adult counterparts. This chapter will discuss these differences and stress the importance of knowing the variations from normal. In addition, hemodynamic parameters, drug dosages, laboratory data, and diagnostic imaging differ considerably in feline neonatal and pediatric patients. Interpretation of certain parameters can be quite challenging, and familiarity with normal values will assist in accurate assessment.
   b. For the purposes of this chapter, the term *neonate* encompasses birth to 2 weeks of age, and the term *pediatric* encompasses 2 weeks to 6 months of age.
B. Initial examination
   a. Environment
      i. Keep stress low and the environment warm.
      ii. Warmed towels on cold steel table
      iii. Essential equipment—pediatric and neonatal stethoscopes and appropriate-sized blood pressure cuffs, accurate gram scale, digital thermometer
C. History
   a. Should have a strong suckle reflex at birth
   b. Should nurse and sleep constantly first 2–3 weeks
   c. Constant crying may signal insufficient milk ingestion.
D. Physical examination and normal parameters
   a. Normal body temperature in kittens is 98°F at birth
   b. Increases to 100°F by the end of the first week
   c. Pain sensation present at birth, analgesia essential for all procedures that are anticipated to be painful
   d. Kittens have less muscle tone than puppies, so weakness should be assessed in comparison to other normal kittens.

    e. Heart rate (200–220 bpm) and respiratory rate (15–35 bpm) are higher in neonates than adults.

    f. Eyes open by day 12–14, vision normalizes by the end of the first month.

    g. Menace reflex not present until 2–3 months of age.

    h. Physical examination should include
- i. Oral examination to check for a cleft palate
- ii. Abdominal palpation to check for an umbilical hernia
- iii. Skull palpation to check for an open fontanel
- iv. Verification of the presence of patent urogenital openings
- v. Umbilical cord area should be free of redness, swelling, and discharge.

E. Nutrition

    a. Weight gain should be progressive; kittens should gain ~10 g per day and should double their birth weight in the first 10 days of life.

    b. If amount of ingestion is questionable, the kittens should be weighed on a gram scale before and after feeding.

    c. Options for supplemental feedings include surrogate dam, bottle feeding, and tube feeding.

    d. Tube feeding is done using a 5-Fr red rubber catheter for neonates under 300 g and should only be done by experienced personnel. The gag reflex may not develop until after the first week of life, so it is essential that experienced personnel perform tube feeding to avoid aspiration.

    e. Address nutritional issues early.

F. Laboratory values

    a. This section will discuss the variations in the laboratory values that may be encountered in the feline neonatal or pediatric patient. It is essential to be familiar with these parameters to avoid misdiagnoses.

    b. Hematology and coagulation changes
- i. Hct decreases from 47.5% at birth to 27% at 4–6 weeks of age and then begins to increase to adult values.
- ii. During this time period, a rise in the Hct may indicate significant dehydration.
- iii. Clotting factors and antithrombin are decreased at birth and increase to normal values by the end of the first week.
    1. Prothrombin time is increased and normalizes by 7 days. Partial thromboplastin time is also increased but may not normalize by day 7.

    c. Biochemical changes
- i. Elevation in alkaline phosphatase (ALP 123 IU/L, normal adult range 9–42) is three times adult values at birth and decreases to adult ranges in the first weeks of life.
- ii. Bile acids are normal in kittens at 2 weeks of age.
- iii. Serum blood urea nitrogen (BUN), creatinine, albumin, cholesterol, and total protein are lower in neonates than adults.
- iv. Lower creatinine due to decreased muscle mass
- v. Lower BUN and cholesterol due to immature liver function
- vi. Knowledge of these values is critical to prevent a misdiagnosis of liver disease in the neonate (elevated liver enzymes and low levels of BUN, cholesterol, and albumin can mimic liver dysfunction).
- vii. Elevations in calcium and phosphorous due to bone growth

    d. Renal changes
- i. Urine is isosthenuric in neonates, as the capacity to concentrate and dilute urine is limited in this age group.
- ii. Key point in fluid resuscitation—overhydration is just as much a concern as underhydration.

G. Radiographic imaging

    a. In this section the differences in neonatal radiographic imaging are highlighted. In order to maximize radiographic diagnosis, consider decreasing the KVP below the adult range.

    b. The thymus is in cranial thorax on the left side and can mimic a mediastinal mass or lung consolidation.

    c. The heart takes up more space in the thorax than in adults, and it can falsely appear enlarged.

    d. The lung parenchyma has increased water content and is therefore more opaque in neonates.

    e. Absence of costochondral mineralization makes liver appear falsely enlarged.

    f. Loss of abdominal detail due to lack of fat and a small amount of abdominal effusion can mimic peritonitis.

H. Pharmacology

    a. Some of the significant differences in the pharmacology of various drugs are highlighted here. It is imperative that the practitioner with a feline pediatric patient base become familiar with these differences in order to avoid toxicity.

    b. General differences in feline neonatal and pediatric patients

        i. Cats have a longer intestinal transit time, a shorter intestinal tract, and increased intestinal permeability to drugs compared with dogs.

        ii. Dog dosages cannot be extrapolated directly to cats for most drugs.

        iii. Differences in body fat, total protein and albumin, immature renal and hepatic mechanisms contribute to differences in drug metabolism compared with adult cats.

        iv. Decreased body fat may cause increased potency of certain drugs (e.g., thiopental).

        v. Decreased total protein and albumin may cause increased potency in drugs that are highly protein bound.

        vi. Renal excretion of many drugs (e.g., diazepam, digoxin) is diminished, increasing the half-life in circulation.

        vii. Drugs requiring activation via hepatic metabolism have lower plasma concentrations, while drugs requiring metabolism for excretion have higher plasma concentrations.

        viii. Cardiovascular drugs (e.g., epinephrine, dopamine, dobutamine, etc.) are difficult to dose in neonates due to individual variations in maturity of the autonomic nervous system.

        ix. Response to treatment, continuous monitoring of hemodynamic variables essential

        x. The blood brain barrier is more permeable in neonates, allows drugs that do not normally cross over to enter the central nervous system.

    c. Routes of delivery

        i. Oral drug absorption is higher in first 72 hours (increased permeability of GI).

        ii. Intestinal flora is very sensitive to disruption by oral antimicrobials.

        iii. Intravenous routes most predictable, preferred over intramuscular or subcutaneous routes.

    d. Specific recommendations

        i. Aminoglycosides cause histologic damage to kidneys in neonates—avoid.

        ii. Chloramphenicol causes changes in hematopoietic parameters and collapse in neonates—avoid.

        iii. Potassium bromide can cause bronchitis in cats—avoid.

        iv. Tetracyclines cause skeletal growth abnormalities, staining of teeth—avoid.

        v. Lidocaine—cats are very susceptible to toxicity and neonates have a decreased response—avoid.

        vi. Oral diazepam can cause hepatic failure in cats—avoid.

        vii. Fluoroquinolones can cause blindness in cats and destructive lesions of cartilage in long bones—caution.

        viii. Sulfonamides can suppress bone marrow—caution.

        ix. Metronidazole preferred for giardiasis and anaerobes, decrease dose or increase interval in neonates.

        x. B-lactam antibiotics is made safe in neonates by decreasing dose or increasing interval (from q8h to q12h).

        xi. Avoid drugs that depress respiration and heart rate (neonates are very dependent on high heart rate to increase cardiac output).

xii. For drugs with decreased clearance or increased response, reduce dose.

xiii. Thiopental can cause an increased response in neonates due to the lower percentage of body fat and decreased hepatic clearance. Titrate to effect.

xiv. For inotropes and vasopressors titrate drug dosages to individual kitten.

xv. Opioids good for analgesia due to reversibility, but kittens more susceptible to excitement and dysphoria—use lower dosage and monitor heart rate and respiratory rate very closely.

I. Catheter placement

a. Intravenous (IV) route is preferred.

b. Neonates often require very small–gauge catheters (i.e., 24 ga), which can burr easily when being driven through skin.

    i. Small skin puncture with 20-ga needle can be made while the skin is kept elevated and then the catheter can be fed through skin hole.

c. If attempts at IV catheter placement fail, an intraosseous catheter (IO) should be placed.

    i. An IO catheter can be inserted in the proximal femur or humerus using an 18–22-gauge spinal needle or an 18–25-gauge hypodermic needle.

    ii. Can be used for fluid and blood administration

    iii. Area must be prepared in a sterile manner, needle inserted into bone parallel to the long axis of the bone.

    iv. Gently aspirate to assure patency and secure with sterile bandage.

    v. Ideal for neonates because they have a large portion of "red" marrow compared with adults who have more "yellow" marrow consisting of fat

    vi. Intravenous access must be established as soon as possible, ideally within 2 hours, and the IO catheter should be removed to minimize intraosseous infection.

    vii. Intraosseous catheter complications correlate with duration of use.

J. Fluid requirements

a. Neonates have higher fluid requirements than adults due to a higher percentage of total body water, a greater surface area to body weight ratio, a higher metabolic rate, decreased renal concentrating ability, and decreased body fat. This section discusses the fluid requirements and monitoring of fluid therapy in feline pediatric patients.

b. Assessing requirements

    i. Dehydration and overhydration are concerns; kidneys cannot concentrate or dilute urine adequately.

    ii. Monitor for under- or overhydration via accurate pediatric gram scale, weigh patient 3–4 times per day.

    iii. Baseline weight, Hct/TS (Hct decreases in first 4–6 weeks of life and TS are lower than adult levels in normal neonate), urine specific gravity, and thoracic are radiographs helpful.

    iv. Fluid overload diagnosis difficult (heart takes up more of thoracic cavity and normal neonate lungs have more interstitial fluid) without baseline thoracic radiographs.

c. Specific recommendations

    i. A fluid bolus of 10–15 mL/kg in moderately dehydrated neonates is recommended.

    ii. Rapid reassessment of perfusion via mentation, urine output, pulse quality, and possibly lactate levels should be done after each bolus. Lactate levels are higher in neonatal dogs, but normal values have not been reported in kittens.

    iii. Repeat bolus if perfusion remains compromised.

    iv. Follow with constant rate infusion of 50–70 mL/kg/day of warm crystalloids.

    v. A fluid warmer placed in line is a good option to keep fluids warmed.

    vi. Lactated Ringer's solution is ideal (lactate is the preferred metabolic fuel in neonate during times of hypoglycemia).

K. Hypothermia

a. Hypothermia, defined as a temperature below 95°F, is common in the neonatal patient. Depending on the degree of temperature decrease, hypothermia can cause hypoventilation, bradycardia, gastrointestinal ileus, and mentation changes.

b. The shivering reflex is not present at birth and may take up to a full week to develop, so frequent temperature checks are essential.

c. Rewarming should proceed slowly and should always be completed prior to drug administration (many drugs will not be active until rewarming) and feeding (to prevent hypothermia-induced ileus).

d. The kitten should be placed in a neonatal incubator set at 85–90°F and approximately 60% humidity, and all IV fluids should be warmed with an in-line warmer. Heat lamps and heating pads are best avoided as they can lead to burns and overheating easily in the neonate with limited ability to move away from the heat source.

L. Hypoglycemia

   a. Hypoglycemia is very common in the pediatric patient, and the etiology and treatment are discussed in this section.

   b. Clinical signs of hypoglycemia are challenging to recognize due to inefficient counterregulatory hormone release during hypoglycemia in neonates.

   c. In adults, counterregulatory hormones are released in response to low blood glucose and facilitate euglycemia by increasing gluconeogenesis and antagonizing insulin. These hormones are responsible for the majority of clinical signs of hypoglycemia.

   d. Neonates have immature glucose feedback mechanisms, inefficient hepatic gluconeogenesis, decreased liver glycogen stores, and loss of glucose in urine.

   e. Urinary glucose reabsorption does not normalize until ~3 weeks.

   f. Brain requires glucose for energy in neonate, brain damage can occur with prolonged hypoglycemia.

   g. Neonatal myocardium uses carbohydrate (glucose) for energy rather than long chain fatty acids used by adult.

   h. In summary, the healthy neonate has increased demand for, increased loss of, and decreased ability to synthesize glucose compared with adults.

   i. Vomiting, diarrhea, infection, and decreased intake contribute to hypoglycemia.

   j. Clinical signs of hypoglycemia, if present, may include lethargy and anorexia.

   k. Treatment for hypoglycemia

      i. Infusions of 1 mL/kg of 12.5% dextrose (i.e., dilute 50% dextrose 1:4) followed by a CRI of isotonic fluids supplemented with 1.25% to 5.0% dextrose for hypoglycemia

      ii. Always follow dextrose bolus with a CRI that is supplemented with dextrose or there is a risk of rebound hypoglycemia.

      iii. Refractory hypoglycemia may only respond to hourly boluses of dextrose in addition to a CRI of crystalloid with supplemental dextrose.

      iv. Consider carnitine supplementation in these cases (in some studies, carnitine supplementation improved hypoglycemia). Carnitine can be supplemented at 200 mg/kg PO q24h.

M. Hypovolemia and dehydration

   a. Depletion of body fluids via dehydration alone or dehydration accompanied by hypovolemia is very common in the sick kitten. The following section discusses the most common causes and appropriate treatment of these conditions.

   b. Causes of hypovolemia/dehydration

      i. Diarrhea, vomiting, and decreased intake are the most common causes.

      ii. Diarrhea is most commonly due to parasites, viruses, and dietary issues.

      iii. Parasites

         1. Common parasites in kittens include roundworms, hookworms, and a protozoal parasite, *Tritrichomonas fetus* (often seen in co-infections with *Giardia* species).

2. GI parasites can be a complicating factor and secondary to a primary disease or immunodeficiency.

3. Roundworms can be transmitted via milk and can cause diarrhea, poor hair coat, abdominal effusion, and failure to thrive.

   a. Diagnosis made with fecal float

   b. Treatment with Pyrantel (20 mg/kg orally once and then repeated in 3 weeks) or Fenbendazole (50 mg/kg q24h orally for 3 days) is safe and effective in kittens that are at least 2 weeks of age.

4. Hookworms can cross via placenta and in milk and cause fatal anemia at 2–3 weeks of age—before patent infection; do not rely on fecal. Clinical signs include lethargy, anemia, and melena. Hookworms are treated with the same drugs as roundworms.

5. *Tritrichomonas fetus* causes large intestinal diarrhea which may be accompanied by hematochezia. Diagnosis is difficult but may be improved if multiple direct smears of fresh feces are made.

   a. There is no treatment for Trichomoniasis in cats, but the diarrhea is usually self-limiting and clears within 9 months.

   b. Diagnostic yield improved with fresh fecal specimen and a zinc sulfate float with centrifugation.

6. For *Giardia* spp. and *Cryptosporidium* spp., immunoassays may be needed.

iv. Viral causes

1. Viral causes of diarrhea in kittens usually from feline panleukopenia

2. Feline panleukopenia can cause vomiting, fever, and diarrhea.

3. Similar to canine parvovirus, and the agent of canine parvovirus has been shown to cause diarrhea in kittens.

4. Treatment is supportive and includes warm IV fluids if dehydration is present, nutritional support, antibiotics if infection is suspected, and antiemetics if indicated.

v. Dietary

1. One of the most common dietary causes of diarrhea in kittens is owner overfeeding with kitten milk replacer.

2. Owners should be instructed on how to properly feed kittens. A 3–5 French red rubber feeding tube should be used and the placement checked via injection of a small amount of saline (coughing suggests tube is in trachea). Due to the absence of a gag reflex for up to 10 days after birth, improper placement of the feeding tube in the trachea is a frequent complication.

c. Recognition and monitoring of hypovolemia/dehydration

i. Hypovolemia results in decreased perfusion and subsequent decreases in oxygen delivery to tissues.

ii. In adults, hypovolemia is compensated for by increasing HR, concentrating urine, and decreasing urine output.

iii. In neonates, compensatory mechanisms may not be existent.

iv. Autonomic nervous system

1. Fetal and neonate myocardium has less contractile elements (30% vs. 60% in adult)—difficult to increase cardiac contractility in response to hypovolemia.

2. Immature sympathetic nerve fibers in myocardium prevents maximal increases in heart rate in response to hypovolemia.

3. Complete maturation of the autonomic nervous system occurs at ~8 weeks.

v. Blood pressure and central venous pressure

1. Mean arterial pressure lower in normal neonates, normalizing by 9 months of age.

2. Muscular component of arterial wall immature at birth, thought to be the cause of the low MAP.

      3. Central venous pressure higher in neonates

      4. In adult kidneys BP is autoregulated over wide range of systemic arterial pressures. No autoregulation in neonate kidneys so GFR decreases as systemic blood pressure decreases.

   vi. Renal regulation

      1. Immature kidneys not capable of concentrating urine in response to hypovolemia.

      2. Adequate concentration and dilution of urine not seen until ~10 weeks of age.

      3. Causes include inefficient countercurrent mechanisms, decreased sodium resorption in the thick ascending loop of Henle, short loops of Henle, and decreased urea concentration.

d. Clinical and laboratory parameters of hypovolemia/dehydration

   i. Skin turgor cannot be used to assess dehydration due to increased fat and decreased water content compared with adults.

   ii. Mucous membranes cannot be used to assess dehydration as they remain moist in the face of severe dehydration in neonates and may be hyperemic during the first week of life. However, pale or cyanotic mucous membranes are indicative of an abnormality.

   iii. A heart murmur may be indicative of sepsis, anemia, fever, a congenital cardiac defect, or may be an innocent murmur. Innocent murmurs may be present during the first 3 months of life.

   iv. BUN and creatinine lower in neonates—monitoring of azotemia very challenging.

e. Specific recommendations

   i. Dehydration can progress rapidly due to higher neonatal fluid requirements and increased losses (decreased renal concentrating ability, higher respiratory rate, higher metabolic rate).

   ii. Weigh at least every 12 hours, preferably every 8 hours.

   iii. Monitor urine specific gravity. Dehydration is likely when urine specific gravity reaches 1.020; monitor as an indicator of rehydration.

   iv. It should be assumed (due to difficulties in assessment in neonates) that all neonates with severe diarrhea, inadequate intake, or severe vomiting are dehydrated and potentially hypovolemic.

   v. Treatment should be initiated immediately with fluid therapy, monitoring of electrolyte and glucose status, temperature regulation, and nutritional support.

   vi. Start with a bolus of 25 mL/kg of warm isotonic fluids in severely dehydrated or hypovolemic kittens.

   vii. Follow with a CRI of maintenance fluids (50–70 mL/kg/day) together with losses.

   viii. Estimate losses (i.e., 2 tablespoons of diarrhea is equal to 30 mL of fluid).

   ix. If hypoglycemic or not able to eat, add dextrose to IV fluids at lowest amount that will maintain normoglycemia (i.e., start with 1.25% dextrose).

   x. Monitor perfusion parameters (mentation, urine output/specific gravity). Lactate and Hct should not be increasing.

N. Viral infections

a. Upper respiratory infections

   i. Feline herpesvirus type I and calicivirus are most common causes of viral URI in kittens.

   ii. These are most common at 3–4 weeks of age but can occur earlier.

   iii. Clinical signs range from mild (nasal discharge, ocular discharge) to severe (dyspnea, anorexia, dehydration).

   iv. Treatment is symptomatic and may include oxygen therapy (no higher than FiO$_2$ of 40%), restoration of fluid volume, gentle cleaning of nasal secretions, vaporizer or nebulizer treatments, antibiotics for secondary bacterial infections, nutritional support, and antiviral therapy.

b. Other viral infections

   i. Feline leukemia virus—can be transmitted by dam or in contact cats. Can cause thymic atrophy and slow wasting of kittens. Treatment is supportive and includes IV fluid therapy for dehydration, antibiotics for secondary bacterial infections, and nutritional support if indicated.

      ii. Coronavirus can cause diarrhea and FIP. Treatment is supportive and includes broad spectrum anthelminth treatment (e.g., praziquantel/pyrantel pamoate) since secondary parasitic infections are commonly a source of increased morbidity in these cases.

O. Neonatal alloimmune hemolytic anemia

    a. Three feline blood types: A, B, and AB

    b. Type A most common in U.S. (~99% of cats in U.S.)

    c. Type B not common (higher percentage in Abyssinian, Birman, Persian, Somali, Scottish fold, Exotic and British Shorthair, Cornish, and Devon Rex)

    d. Type AB very rare

    e. Cats have naturally occurring antibodies against other blood types at birth.

        i. Type B cats have very strong antibodies against type A antigen.

        ii. Transfusion of type A blood into type B cat causes rapid, often fatal, severe hemolytic reaction.

        iii. All cats must be typed before transfusing.

    f. Essentially no transfer of antibodies from queen to fetus via placenta.

    g. Passive transfer of antibodies occurs in first 12–24 hours of life through ingestion of colostrum.

    h. If type B queen mates with a type A tom, the kittens can be born with type A blood.

    i. When type A kitten ingests colostrum from type B queen, it ingests anti-A antibodies—destruction of red blood cells of kitten.

    j. Clinical signs include pale mucous membranes, weak pulses, lethargy, red or brown urine, icterus, and death. Occasionally sloughing of ear tips, tail tip, and toenails can occur.

    k. Diagnosis via blood type of queen and kittens.

    l. If queen is type B, all type A kittens should be removed immediately and fed with milk replacer.

    m. If clinical signs warrant, a blood transfusion of type A blood can be given via the intravenous or intraosseous route.

    n. Serum from a healthy, well-vaccinated, type A adult cat can be given to kittens that are prevented from ingesting colostrum.

        i. The serum can be given orally (within the first 24 hours of life) or subcutaneously. Dosages of 5 mL/kitten given in three increments (at birth, 12 hours, and 24 hours) have been shown to augment IgG levels in kittens.

P. Sepsis

    a. Neonatal sepsis is most often secondary to wounds, such as umbilical cord ligation and respiratory, urinary, and GI infections. Commonly isolated bacterial organisms include *Escherichia coli*, *Klebsiella* spp., *Enterococcus* spp., *Enterobacter* spp., *Campylobacter* spp., *Streptococcus* spp., *Staphylococcus* spp., *Bartonella henselae*, and Mycoplasmas. This section will highlight the difficulty of diagnosing, monitoring, and treating sepsis in kittens.

    b. Clinical and laboratory values often subtle, and sepsis can be difficult to detect due to immature autonomic nervous system (inconsistent cardiac response to hypovolemia), lower MAP, higher CVP in normal neonate, and lack of urinary concentration.

    c. Clinical signs may include crying, reluctance to nurse, decreased urine output, and cold extremities.

    d. Treatment of sepsis

        i. Aggressive fluid resuscitation associated with decreased mortality in children with sepsis and in several animal models of sepsis.

        ii. Large volumes of fluid often needed in septic patients due to increased capillary permeability (increased losses) and vasodilation.

        iii. Start with a bolus of 25 mL/kg of warm isotonic fluids.

        iv. Consider a CRI of fresh or fresh frozen plasma (5–10 mL/kg at 1–3 mL/kg/hour) from a well-vaccinated adult cat to attempt to augment immunity and augment colloid oncotic pressure.

     v.   Or consider giving serum from a vaccinated adult subcutaneously at 5 mL q12h for three dosages.

     vi.   Submit culture and susceptibility of area of concern before beginning antibiotics.

     vii. Broad-spectrum antibiotics may be required if the source of infection cannot be identified.

     viii. First-generation cephalosporins are a good choice in the neonate and provide coverage for gram-positive and some gram-negative organisms.

     ix.   Oxygen therapy should be kept at or below an FiO_2 of 0.4 to avoid oxygen toxicity.

         1. Excess oxygen supplementation in neonates can cause retrolental fibroplasias and blindness.

     x.   Avoid hypothermia, provide safe heat source (i.e., warm water blanket, Bair Hugger, etc.).

     xi.   Consider nutritional supplementation early if not eating.

     xii. Consider vasopressor and/or inotropic support if hypoperfusion is refractory to IV fluid loading (i.e., cold extremities, high lactate levels, low urine output).

     xiii. Due to variations in the maturity of the autonomic nervous system, all inotropic drugs need to be individually tailored to each kitten.

  e. Monitoring the septic kitten

     i.   Monitor serial checks of perfusion via mucous membrane color (should be less pale), pulse quality (should get stronger), extremity temperature (should go up), lactate levels (should go down), and mentation.

     ii.   Frequent electrolyte and blood glucose checks every 4–6 hours are essential with supplementation as needed.

     iii. Acceptable endpoints of perfusion include increases in extremity temperature, decreases in lactate levels, increased urine production, and improved mentation.

     iv.   An index of suspicion for sepsis should be maintained for all neonates with risk factors, and aggressive treatment should be instituted rapidly. In people, the incidence of pediatric sepsis is highest in premature newborns. Respiratory infections (37%) and primary bacteremia (25%) were the most common infections.

Q. Respiratory distress of the newborn kitten

  a. Respiratory distress encountered at birth may be due to pulmonary hypertension, decreased surfactant levels (prematurity), aspiration of meconium, or excess fluid in the airways.

  b. Congenital defects may cause persistent pulmonary hypertension and respiratory distress that is refractory to treatment.

  c. In people, ventilation of the lungs is the single most effective step in cardiopulmonary resuscitation of the compromised infant.

  d. Emergency treatment of a newborn in respiratory distress includes reversal of any drugs that were used during anesthesia if a Cesarean section was performed. Bulb suctioning of the airways to clear out accumulated fluid.

  e. Avoid aggressive suctioning of airways (i.e., with a suctioning device)—can cause a vagal response or laryngospasm.

  f. Gentle rubbing of the neonate all over can also help stimulate respirations.

  g. Do not shake or hit newborn—can cause loss of surfactant among other complications.

  h. Doxapram hydrochloride (1–5 mg/kg IV or 1–2 drops under the tongue) can be given under tongue to stimulate respirations in a newborn with no respiratory drive, although some clinicians don't advocate this anymore.

  i. At birth, physical expansion of the lungs causes release of prostacyclin, which increases pulmonary blood flow through pulmonary vasodilation.

  j. Nitric oxide contributes to pulmonary vasodilation and is thought to be released in response to oxygenation at birth.

  k. Surfactant reduces the tension of the air-fluid interface of the alveoli and prevents collapse. It is essential to improve compliance (i.e., reduce stiffness) and therefore the work of breathing.

    i. Surfactant is released at birth in response to lung inflation.

    ii. Dramatic decreases in pulmonary vascular resistance and adequate surfactant synthesis and release are essential to neonatal survival at birth.

l. The two most important interventions for respiratory distress at birth are oxygenation and lung expansion. These will maximize the release of prostacyclin and nitric oxide and surfactant release.

m. Oxygen should be supplied via face mask or endotracheal tube, as adequate lung expansion is crucial for pulmonary blood flow.

n. A tight-fitting face mask is often easier than intubation of a newborn and can be lifesaving.

o. Overexpansion can cause damage so it is essential to use the minimal amount of pressure not to exceed 15–20 mmHg for ventilation.

    i. We use an ambubag designed for pediatric use and intubate and ventilate if there are no spontaneous respirations at birth. Intubation is attempted with an 18–20-ga short IV catheter (remove stylet first), and if unsuccessful after 1–2 minutes a tight-fitting face mask if attached.

    ii. The neonate should be ventilated at 20–30 bpm to a maximum pressure of 20 mmHg, and this should be done for ~30 seconds before cardiac compressions are started if required.

    iii. If the chest is not expanding, check the seal on the face mask or the ET tube placement, resuction the airway.

R. Cardiopulmonary cerebral resuscitation

a. Compressions

    i. Cardiac compressions are done with the thumb and forefinger on either side of the thorax with approximately 100–120 compressions per minute.

    ii. In neonates, thoracic compressions actually cause cardiac compression (vs. generalized thoracic compression seen in larger animals).

b. Venous access

    i. Intravenous access is ideal for delivery of drugs for resuscitation, but intraosseous routes work well also.

    ii. When an IO catheter is placed it is essential to remove it as soon as possible.

    iii. The goal is to use the IO catheter as a bridge to increase volume and make placement of an IV catheter possible.

c. Drugs

    i. Epinephrine has both alpha and beta adrenergic activity and is the first-line drug during cardiopulmonary arrest.

    ii. It is started after 30 seconds of chest compressions while the animal is effectively ventilated.

    iii. The dose is 0.01 mg/kg for the first dose and then 0.1 mg/kg for subsequent doses.

    iv. Recently, vasopressin has been advocated for cardiopulmonary arrest in humans with asystole.

        1. In a pediatric porcine model, vasopressin combined with epinephrine was better for resuscitation than either drug alone.

        2. Vasopressin is an accepted treatment for children with vasodilatory shock after cardiac surgery and for neonatal congestive heart failure.

        3. Vasopressin can be administered intravenously, via the endotracheal tube, or through an intraosseous catheter.

        4. The suggested dosage of vasopressin for CPCR is 0.8 units/kg body weight intravenously. There are no published dosages for kittens.

    v. Acidosis due to decreased perfusion (i.e., lactic acidosis) and decreased ventilation (i.e., respiratory acidosis) is common during cardiopulmonary arrest.

        1. Ideally should be addressed by treating the primary problems (i.e., increasing perfusion and ventilation).

        2. Severe acidosis can decrease myocardial contractility; this could be critical in neonates, who have a lower percentage of myocardial contractile fibers than adults.

3. It can also blunt responses to catecholamines, which again is critical in neonates, who have a lower percentage of sympathetic fibers in their myocardium compared to adults.

4. The use of buffers (e.g., sodium bicarbonate) is controversial because they increase sodium levels, cause hyperosmolality, can cause paradoxical CNS and intracellular acidosis, and increase carbon dioxide.

5. The guidelines from the American Heart Association *Manual of Neonatal Advanced Life Support* in humans do not recommend bicarbonate as frontline therapy due to lack of evidence for its efficacy.

vi. Glucose is the main energy substrate of the neonatal brain and myocardium and should be monitored frequently during an arrest and supplemented as needed, but avoid oversupplementation and hyperglycemia, as this can lead to further brain cellular damage post cardiac resuscitation.

vii. Ionized calcium has been shown to be low in human neonates.

1. Neonates also have an increased requirement for calcium for contractility than adults.

2. Calcium is not recommended for cardiopulmonary arrest in human neonates, however.

S. Head trauma

a. Children have a higher percentage of diffuse brain injury during trauma compared with adults, and this is thought to be due to their greater head-to-torso ratio.

b. The neonatal brain also has a higher water content, lacks complete axonal myelinization, and may be more susceptible to hypoxia and hypotension than adults.

c. There may also be a greater susceptibility to apoptosis and delayed cell death during head trauma in children compared with adults.

d. With all head trauma cases, the goals are to improve oxygen delivery, decrease intracranial pressure (ICP), and maximize cerebral perfusion pressure (CPP).

e. Children have a lower ICP as well as a lower MAP compared with adults.

i. The author is unaware of ICP values in normal kittens.

f. Since CPP is equal to the MAP minus the ICP, it can be seen that MAP must be kept high and ICP kept low in order to maximize CPP.

g. Appropriate fluid therapy to keep the systolic blood pressure above 90 mmHg is suggested in adult head trauma and has been associated with improved survival.

h. Since CPP depends on adequate cardiac output and adequate ventilation, these should be optimized in head trauma patients.

i. Both hyper- and hypoventilation should be avoided in favor of normocarbia.

j. Hyperventilation to reduce $PaCO_2$ to less than 35 mmHg may be helpful as a temporary bridge (usually to surgery to remove a subdural hemorrhage) in an emergency patient with impending signs of brain herniation.

k. The resulting vasoconstriction caused by the hyperventilation can decrease the CPP in the healthy brain (due to intact autoregulation), leading to decreased oxygen delivery and hypoxia.

l. Once volume has been addressed (i.e., fluid therapy), vasopressors may be administered if MAP is still low—dosage must be tailored to each neonate. Starting at the lowest dosage for the drug chosen (dopamine, dobutamine, epinephrine, etc.), the dosage is increased in 5–10-minute increments depending on response (i.e., increased heart rate, increased blood pressure, improved urine output, improved mentation, etc.).

m. Seizures after head trauma appear to be more common in children than in adults and can occur with minimal brain damage.

n. Elevation of the head to 30 degrees has been suggested, but this must be done without compressing the jugular veins (i.e., using a tilt table or a foam wedge).

i. The habit of placing a rolled up towel under the neck to elevate the head is potentially dangerous, as compression of the jugular veins may increase ICP.

o. Jugular catheters or neck bandages should not be placed in head trauma patients. Any blood needed should be drawn from a peripheral vein or a long saphenous catheter.

p. In people, measurement of ICP can be made directly, but this is impractical in most veterinary situations.

q. The Cushing's reflex can be helpful to gauge increasing ICP. In adults when ICP increases, the systemic blood pressure rises, and as a response the heart rate decreases.

   i. Unfortunately, this reflex has not been evaluated in neonatal and pediatric patients. Since the autonomic nervous system does not mature until 9–10 weeks of age, there is reason to believe that the Cushing's reflex may be unreliable in this age group.

r. In summary, the magnitude of head trauma can be difficult to assess in kittens.

s. Treatment involves optimizing systemic blood pressure using IV fluids and vasopressors as needed, raising the head 30 degrees without compression of the jugular veins, and optimizing oxygenation and ventilation.

T. Conclusion

a. The unique anatomic and physiologic characteristics of kittens make diagnosis, monitoring, and treatment a challenge. Adult parameters cannot be relied upon in these patients, and an awareness of these unique characteristics is essential for any practitioner with a feline neonatal and pediatric patient base. In addition, many laboratory and pharmacological data differ dramatically in neonates compared with adults of the same species. Familiarity with these variations is essential in the monitoring and treatment of the neonatal and pediatric illness such as hypovolemia, shock, and sepsis.

37
OCULAR EMERGENCIES

Deborah C. Mandell

Unique Features

1. Cats will prolapse their third eyelid in response to pain, and topical anesthetic may be needed to evaluate the eye.
2. Clinically normal cats can have low Schirmer tear test results.
3. Feline herpesvirus can cause dendritic corneal ulcers.
4. Anaphylaxis and severe chemosis can occur secondary to topical neomycin administration.
5. Debride nonhealing corneal ulcers; do not perform keratotomy.
6. Corneal sequestra are unique to cats and are more common in brachycephalic breeds. An area of black pigment will be seen on the cornea.
7. Anterior uveitis usually has a serious underlying cause.
8. Secondary glaucoma is more common and may be due to anterior uveitis or intraocular neoplasia. The eye is usually blind and not painful.
9. It takes significant blunt force to propose a cat's eye; therefore, there is usually significant concurrent head trauma.
10. Be very careful not to pull on the eye that is being enucleated; the contralateral eye can become blind because the optic chiasm is very short.
11. Systemic hypertension is a common cause of retinal detachments and blindness.
12. Enrofloxacin can cause nonreversible retinal degeneration.
13. Secondary lens luxation is more common and due to chronic uveitis, chronic glaucoma, or trauma.
14. Conjunctivitis most commonly has an infectious cause. FHV-1 and *Chlamydophila felis* are common pathogens.
15. Keratoconjunctivitis sicca is not common and may be secondary to FHV-1.
16. Ocular trauma, intraocular surgery, trauma to the lens, and chronic uveitis may all lead to post-traumatic sarcoma, an extremely malignant intraocular neoplasia.

Most, if not all, feline ocular emergencies can be diagnosed by clinical signs and very few diagnostic tests. If an eye is not responding to treatment or there are multiple disease processes in the same eye, an ophthalmologist should always be consulted.

I. Clinical signs
   A. Red eye
   B. Grey or cloudy eye
   C. Acute blindness—unilateral or bilateral
   D. Big or enlarged eye
   E. Ocular discharge
   F. Blepharospasm/squinting

II. Ophthalmic examination
   A. Look for asymmetry of face, orbits, and globes.
   B. Evaluate periorbital structures, conjunctiva, sclera, cornea, anterior chamber, lens, vitreous, and fundus.
   C. Neurological exam—menace (may be difficult to evaluate in cats), pupillary light reflex (direct and consensual), and palpebral or corneal reflex.
   D. Cats will protrude the third eyelid, which makes visualization of the globe difficult. Gentle restraint and a dim light may help. Topical anesthetic (proparacaine 0.5%) can be used to push the third eyelid out of the way if needed.

III. Diagnostic and monitoring procedures
   A. Schirmer tear test
      1. Should be first diagnostic test performed on all cases.
      2. Normal is about 17 mm/minute (see KCS below).
   B. Fluorescein stain test
      1. Extremely important for all feline ocular emergencies
      2. Diagnoses and outlines extent of corneal ulcers, lacerations, chemical injuries, and trauma
      3. Multiple techniques for performing fluorescein stain
         a. Put drop of eye wash onto strip and let stain drip into eye.
         b. Put fluorescein stain strip into 3-cc syringe with eye wash and put drop of stain into eye.
         c. Place strip directly onto sclera/conjunctiva.
      4. A descemetocele or perforation in the cornea will not take up stain.
      5. If there is leakage of aqueous humor, can see rivulets of stain where the perforation occurs (Seidel test).
      6. Also tests patency of tear duct (will see stain coming out of nostril).
      7. Rose Bengal stain is reported to be superior to fluorescein stain for herpetic dendritic corneal ulcers.
   C. Tonometry—useful to diagnose glaucoma and anterior uveitis; normal intraocular pressure (IOP) is 15–25 mmHg.
      1. Indentation tonometry—measures intraocular pressure by determining the distance the plunger can indent the cornea.
         a. Schiotz tonometer (Miltex, Germany)—more difficult in cats than dogs (fig. 37.1)
            i. 1–2 drops of topical anesthetic (proparacaine 0.5%) is placed in eye(s).
            ii. Lightest weight is placed on Schiotz.
            iii. The cornea must be parallel with ground, so cat must be in dorsal recumbancy with head up or sitting with head tilted toward ceiling.
            iv. Place Schiotz on cornea, read scale, compare scale reading on chart to IOP number.
            v. Can use the chart established for humans (fig. 37.2).
      2. Applanation tonometry—measures IOP by determining the amount of force needed to flatten the cornea.
         a. Tonopen (Mentor, Norwell, MA)—much easier to use, flattens a small region of cornea. Cornea does not need to be parallel to ground.
         b. 1–2 drops of topical anesthetic (proparacaine 0.5 %) is instilled in eye(s). Wait 5 minutes for full effect.
         c. Place tonopen probe tip cover on tip of tonopen.
         d. Holding the tonopen like a pencil, gently touch the cornea with the tip.
         e. A beep will sound with each of three readings and then an average will appear after a longer beep.
         f. Tonopen should be calibrated once a day.

IV. Management of specific conditions
   A. Corneal ulcer (box 37.1)

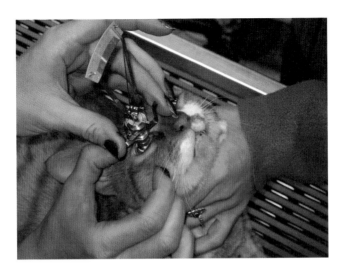

Fig. 37.1. Using the Schiotz tonometer on a cat.

1. Causes include trauma, infectious (viral, bacterial), decreased tear production, underlying ocular conditions (entropion), foreign body, and topical irritants/chemical injury.
2. Clinical signs include blepharospasm, corneal edema, corneal neovascularization, conjunctival hyperemia/congestion and possibly a miotic pupil.
3. Diagnosed based on fluorescein stain results
    a. Classification of corneal ulcer depends on amount or depth of cornea affected, whether secondary infection is present, or if there is nonadhered epithelium (nonhealing).
4. Feline herpes virus (FHV-1) causes classic "dendritic" corneal ulcers (look like branches on a tree; fig. 37.3).
5. Can have a reflex uveitis and miotic pupil.
6. If the cornea has perforated, then additional clinical signs can include a misshapen cornea, iris protruding to and potentially through the cornea, a shallow anterior chamber, aqueous flare or fibrin strands in the anterior chamber, and a fibrin clot (red and white/tan piece of tissue) on the area of cornea that ruptured (see below). Rivulets of fluorescein stain where the perforation is on the cornea can also be seen, if not sealed as well.
7. Treatment depends on depth and cause of ulcer.
8. For deep to penetrating corneal ulcers, an ophthalmologist should be consulted to discuss surgical options.
9. Anaphylaxis has been reported in a cat secondary to the neomycin in triple antibiotic ophthalmic preparations. More commonly, chemosis and conjunctivitis can occur. Thus, other topical antibiotics are preferred (i.e., erythromycin 0.3% ointment) for uncomplicated corneal ulcers.
    a. Superficial ulcer—involves the epithelium of the cornea (fig. 37.4)
        i.   Topical antibiotics (erythromycin 0.3%) every 6–8 hours for 1 week
        ii. Topical atropine ointment (1%) every 12 hours if miotic pupil present. Atropine ointment is much less irritating than suspension for cats.
        iii. Elizabethan collar
        iv. Topical antiviral therapy may be indicated if recurrent, dendritic, or feline herpes virus is suspected. Trifluridine 1% or idoxuridine 0.1% can be compounded at a pharmacy, use every 6–8 hours for 1–2 weeks.

	Weight, grams			
	5.5 g	7.5 g	10 g	15 g
Schiotz Measurement	Intraocular Pressure, mmHg			
0.0	41.5	59.1	81.7	127.5
0.5	37.8	54.2	75.1	117.9
1.0	34.5	49.8	69.3	109.3
1.5	31.6	45.8	64.0	101.4
2.0	29.0	42.1	59.1	94.3
2.5	26.6	38.8	54.7	88.0
3.0	24.4	35.8	50.6	81.8
3.5	22.4	33.0	46.9	76.2
4.0	20.6	30.4	43.4	71.0
4.5	18.9	28.0	40.2	66.2
5.0	17.3	25.8	37.2	61.8
5.5	15.9	23.8	34.4	57.6
6.0	14.6	21.9	31.8	53.6
6.5	13.4	20.1	29.4	49.9
7.0	12.2	18.5	27.2	46.5
7.5	11.2	17.0	25.1	43.2
8.0	10.2	15.6	23.1	40.2
8.5	9.4	14.3	21.3	38.1
9.0	8.5	13.1	19.6	34.6
9.5	7.8	12.0	18.0	32.0
10.0	7.1	10.9	16.5	29.6
10.5	6.5	10.0	15.1	27.4
11.0	5.9	9.0	13.8	25.3
11.5	5.3	8.3	12.6	23.3
12.0	4.9	7.5	11.5	21.4
12.5	4.4	6.8	10.5	19.7
13.0	4.0	6.2	9.5	18.1
13.5		5.6	8.6	16.5
14.0		5.0	7.8	15.1
14.5		4.5	7.1	13.7
15.0		4.0	6.4	12.6
15.5			5.8	11.4
16.0			5.2	10.4
16.5			4.7	9.4
17.0			4.2	8.5
17.5				7.7
18.0				6.9
18.5				6.2
19.0				5.6
19.5				4.9
20.0				4.5

Fig. 37.2. The conversion table for the Schiotz tonometer, redrawn from the human conversion/calibration table that accompanies the Schiotz tonometer.
The 5.5-g weight is the plunger, not an added weight.

> **Box 37.1.** Corneal ulcers.
> 1. Look for underlying cause (Schirmer tear test for KCS).
> 2. Fluorescein stain to diagnose and evaluate extent of ulcer.
> 3. All corneal ulcers are treated with topical antibiotics.
>   a. Erythromycin is a common first-line topical antibiotics.
>   b. Topical ciprofloxacin should be used if very deep or if a descemetocele or melting or perforated corneal ulcer is present.
> 4. Topical atropine should always be used if there is a reflex uveitis (miotic pupil), descemetocele, or melting or perforated cornea.
> 5. Systemic antibiotics and topical autologous serum should be used if the ulcer is infected/melting.
> 6. Systemic antibiotics and nonsteroidal anti-inflammatory medications should be added if there is a perforated cornea.
> 7. May need topical antiviral medications if secondary to FHV-1.
> 8. Only debride—do not perform a grid/punctate keratotomy on nonhealing corneal ulcers.

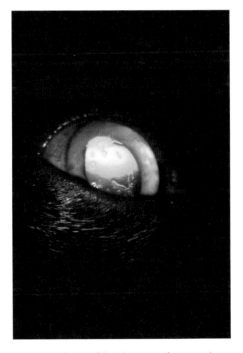

Fig. 37.3. Dendritic corneal lesions secondary to feline herpes infection (photograph courtesy of Dr. Steve Gross).

      v. The eye should be fluorescein stained in 1 week to evaluate response to treatment. An uncomplicated superficial ulcer should heal in 5–7 days.
    b. Deep ulcer—involves the corneal stroma (fig. 37.5)
      i. Topical antibiotics (ciprofloxacin 0.3%) every 2–4 hours
      ii. Topical atropine ointment (1%) every 12 hours
      iii. Elizabethan collar

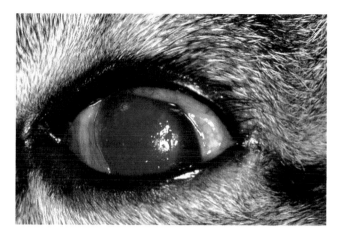

Fig. 37.4. A superficial ulcer in a cat. Reproduced from the *Manual of Canine and Feline Emergency and Critical Care*, 2nd ed., edited by L. King and A. Boag. With permission of BSAVA.

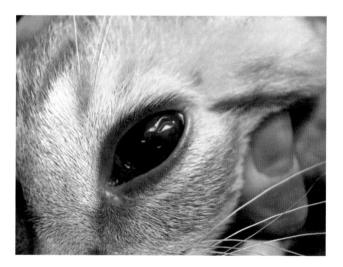

Fig. 37.5. A deep corneal ulcer secondary to a cat fight.

     iv. Deep ulcers can take up to 4 weeks to heal. The eye should be fluorescein stained in weekly intervals to monitor response to treatment.

     v. Surgery (e.g., conjunctival flap) is recommended if 50% or more of the corneal stroma is involved. A slit lamp can help determine the percentage of corneal stroma involved.

  c. Descemetocele—ulcer is down to Descemet's membrane; will see a clear or black area in the center of the ulcer.

     i. Topical antibiotics (ciprofloxacin 0.3%) every 2 hours

     ii. Topical atropine solution every 6 hours. Do not use ointment if the cornea is perforated. The oily base can cause severe intraocular inflammation.

    iii. Systemic antibiotics (amoxicillin-clavulonic acid 15 mg/kg orally every 12 hours)

    iv. Elizabethan collar

    v. Surgery (i.e., conjunctival flap) is the ideal treatment and should be performed as soon as possible.

  d. Melting ulcer—involves an infected ulcer, most commonly with Gram-negative bacteria (*Pseudomonas aeruginosa, Proteus* spp. *E. coli*) that produce collagenases

    i. Should obtain a swab for cytology and aerobic culture and sensitivity

    ii. Topical antibiotics (ciprofloxacin 0.3%) every 2 hours

    iii. Topical atropine solution (1%) every 4–6 hours

    iv. Topical autologous serum—one drop every 2 hours; needs refrigeration; contains anti-collagenases/alpha macroglobulins

    v. Systemic antibiotics (amoxicillin-clavulonic acid 15 mg/kg orally every 12 hours or doxycycline 10 mg/kg orally every 24 hours)

    vi. Elizabethan collar

    vii. Surgery may be required if not responding or if underlying ulcer is deep or perforated.

  e. Perforated corneal ulcer (fig. 37.6)—can be managed medically until surgery (e.g., conjunctival flap) can be performed.

    i. Topical antibiotics (ciprofloxacin 0.3%) every 2 hours

    ii. Topical atropine solution (do not use ointment if cornea is perforated; the oily base can cause severe intraocular inflammation) every 6 hours

    iii. Systemic antibiotics (amoxicillin-clavulonic acid 15 mg/kg orally every 12 hours)

    iv. Elizabethan collar

    v. Systemic nonsteroidal anti-inflammatory medication (meloxicam 0.01 mg/kg orally once a day for 3–5 days)

    vi. If the anterior capsule of the lens was disturbed when the corneal perforation occurred (may see tract of fibrin in the anterior chamber or fibrin or opacity on the anterior lens capsule), then systemic corticosteroids (prednisone 0.5 mg/kg every 12 hours) are

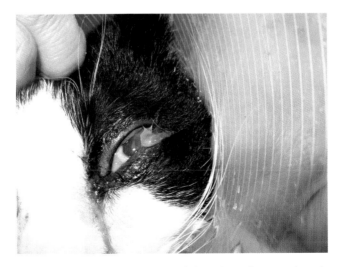

Fig. 37.6. A perforated corneal ulcer. This cat was in a fight with another cat. The only injury he sustained was to his eye.

indicated due to the extreme and intense lens-induced anterior uveitis that can follow. The owner should be warned that if the anterior uveitis cannot be controlled with medical management or is leading to secondary glaucoma, the lens may need to be removed in the future. The eye should be reevaluated in 1–2 days.

      vii. Surgery is the ideal treatment and should be performed if the rupture is not sealing or the corneal reruptures after attempting medical management.

   f. Nonhealing, indolent, or recurrent corneal ulcer

      i. Brachycephalic breeds may be more predisposed.

      ii. May be secondary to feline herpes virus.

      iii. Less common in cats than dogs.

      iv. Fluorescein stain extends beyond the edges of the ulcer due to non adhered epithelium.

      v. After instillation of a topical anesthetic (proparacaine 0.5 %), use a cotton swab to gently debride nonadhered epithelium (fig. 37.7).

      vi. Do not perform a grid or punctate keratotomy as would be performed next in dogs. Studies have shown longer healing times and increased risk of developing a sequestrum when this is done.

   g. Corneal sequestrum (fig. 37.8)

      i. Unique to cats

      ii. Clinical signs include blepharospasm and pain, corneal edema, protrusion of third eyelid, and an area of thick black pigment, which is the sequestrum.

      iii. The cause is unknown, but it is more common in brachycephalic breeds.

      iv. Treatment involves removing the sequestrum with a lamellar keratectomy by an ophthalmologist.

10. All corneal ulcers should be restained and rechecked in 5–7 days to ensure healing. A superficial ulcer should be healed at this time. A deep ulcer may take 2–4 weeks to heal and should be checked weekly to ensure that it is not becoming a complicated or nonhealing ulcer.

11. An ophthalmologist should always be consulted if the ulcer is not responding to treatment or if there is more than one disease process in the same eye making treatment more challenging.

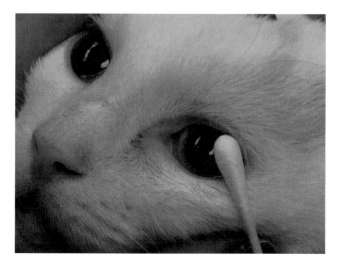

Fig. 37.7. Placement of a cotton swab to debride a nonhealing corneal ulcer.

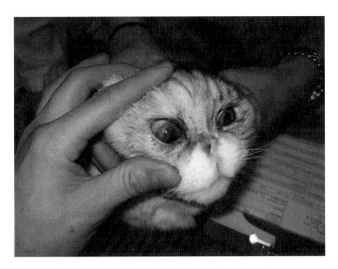

Fig. 37.8.   A corneal sequestrum. Note the corneal edema, corneal neovascularization, and black pigment located ventral and medial.

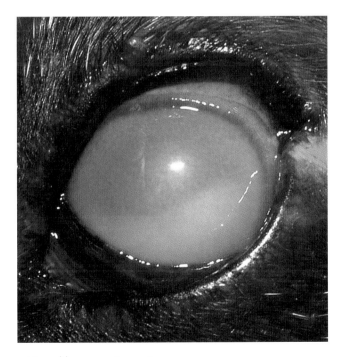

Fig. 37.9.   Anterior uveitis and hypopyon in a cat.

  B.   Anterior uveitis—inflammation of the iris and ciliary body (fig. 37.9; box 37.2)
    1.   As opposed to that in dogs, anterior uveitis in cats usually has a serious underlying cause.
    2.   A complete ocular examination including fundus examination should be performed to look for chorioretinitis lesions or panophthalmitis (hyporeflexive or brown fuzzy areas in tapetal area; fig. 37.10).

Box 37.2. Anterior uveitis.
1. Clinical signs include a swollen, "fluffy" iris, aqueous flare, blepharospasm, and a miotic pupil.
2. Always look for retinal lesions.
3. Most common causes are infectious and neoplastic.
4. All cats should have a thorough medical workup.
5. Treatment includes topical corticosteroids, topical atropine, and treating the underlying cause.
6. Prognosis is guarded.
7. Can develop secondary glaucoma.

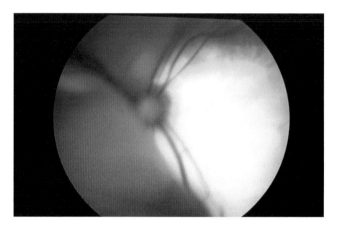

Fig. 37.10. Chorioretinitis in a 6-year-old cat diagnosed with lymphosarcoma.

3. Causes include infectious (FIP, FeLV, FIV, *Toxoplasmosis gondii*, *Bartonella* spp., fungal), sepsis, idiopathic, neoplastic (lymphosarcoma, iris melanoma), lens-induced, immune-mediated, and trauma.
4. Can have a spectrum of inflammation from mild inflammation of the iris to severe hypopyon (fig. 37.9).
5. Clinical signs include blepharospasm; photophobia; conjunctival hyperemia; a red, inflamed, "fluffy" iris; prolapsed nictatans; aqueous flare; hyphema; hypopyon; and a miotic pupil due to ciliary spasm.
6. Can measure IOP, which will be low (<10 mmHg) due to decreased aqueous production in acute anterior uveitis. In chronic or severe uveitis, the IOP can be elevated and secondary glaucoma can be present due to decreased drainage (see "C. Glaucoma," below).
7. The diagnostic plan for any cat presenting with anterior uveitis includes viral serology (FIV, FeLV, FIP), toxoplasmosis titers (IgM and IgG), *Bartonella* spp. titer, complete blood count, serum chemistry panel, chest radiographs for metastatic disease, fungal titers, possible abdominal ultrasound for underlying neoplasia, and possible aspirates of the aqueous for cytology.
8. Treatment includes topical corticosteroids (prednisone acetate 1%) every 6–8 hours once a concurrent corneal ulcer is ruled out, topical atropine ointment (1%, every 12 hours) if the IOP is low, and treating the underlying cause. If the IOP is normal or elevated, then atropine is contraindicated (see C. Glaucoma below).
9. If secondary to lens injury, the lens may need to be removed if the anterior uveitis cannot be controlled with medical management or is leading to secondary glaucoma for the best chance to preserve vision.

> **Box 37.3.** Glaucoma.
> 1. Primary glaucoma is uncommon in cats.
> 2. Secondary glaucoma is more common and due to anterior uveitis, neoplasia, or trauma.
> 3. An IOP of >25 mmHg is indicative of glaucoma.
> 4. Cats usually present with chronic secondary glaucoma.
> 5. The most common sign is buphthalmia.
> 6. The eye is usually irreversibly blind and nonpainful.
> 7. Treatment for secondary glaucoma includes treating the underlying cause and topical carbonic anhydrase inhibitors.
> 8. Latanoprost may not be effective in cats.

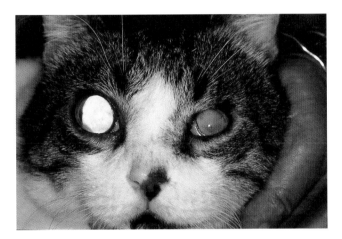

Fig. 37.11. Secondary glaucoma. Note the buphthalmia and fixed, dilated pupil in the right eye. The left eye has anterior uveitis. Reproduced from the *Manual of Canine and Feline Emergency and Critical Care*, 2nd ed., edited by L. King and A. Boag. With permission of BSAVA.

    10. The eye should be reevaluated in 5–7 days to determine the response to treatment and to determine if further therapy or surgery is indicated.

    11. The prognosis for resolution and vision is more guarded due to the prognosis of the underlying diseases. Recurrence and secondary glaucoma are common.

  C. Glaucoma—increased intraocular pressure (box 37.3)
    1. Normal intraocular pressure in cats is 15–25 mmHg.
    2. Primary or congenital glaucoma is rare in cats but has been reported in Siamese, Burmese, and Persian cats.
    3. Secondary glaucoma (fig. 37.11) is much more common in cats.
      a. Causes include anterior uveitis, intraocular neoplasia (lymphosarcoma, iris melanoma), anterior lens luxation, hyphema, trauma with lens injury, and corneal ulcer.
      b. Cats usually present with chronic secondary glaucoma.
      c. The eye is usually irreversibly blind by the time the animal presents to a veterinarian.
    4. The most common clinical sign of secondary glaucoma is buphthalmos. There will also be a fixed and dilated pupil with a negative menace. Other less common clinical signs include blepharospasm, corneal edema, and scleral injection. There can also be a secondary lens luxation. The eye is usually not painful if chronic.
    5. The underlying cause of the secondary glaucoma may also be seen.

6. Diagnosis is based on IOP measurement. An IOP measurement of >25 mmHg is indicative of glaucoma.
7. Treatment involves treating the underlying cause, increasing drainage, and decreasing production of aqueous humor.
8. If acute glaucoma is secondary to anterior lens luxation, then removal of the lens is indicated. If the owner cannot afford lens extraction surgery, treatment with topical carbonic anhydrase inhibitors and beta-blockers three times a day can be tried.
9. Since acute glaucoma is less common, aggressive emergency treatment to rapidly decreased IOP may not be indicated as in dogs. However, if the eye is painful and there are no underlying causes seen, then treatment for acute glaucoma is indicated.
10. If a cat is presenting with acute glaucoma, emergency treatment is similar to that for dogs. Drugs used to increase drainage include mannitol and latanoprost.
    a. Intravenous mannitol at 1–2 g/kg over 20–30 minutes. This is an osmotic diuretic that increases drainage of the aqueous humor.
        i. Use cautiously in dehydrated animals or animals with renal or cardiac disease. Serum sodium, packed cell volume, total solids, and renal values should be checked before giving mannitol in dehydrated patients or patients with a history of renal disease. If moderately to severely dehydrated, if azotemic or if the patient has a history of congestive heart failure or signs of congestive heart failure, mannitol should not be used.
        ii. It can significantly decrease IOP within an hour.
    b. Latanoprost is a prostaglandin analog that has been shown to significantly decrease IOP in humans, dogs, and horses.
        i. It works by increasing drainage through the alternate uveoscleral route. This route is only responsible for 3% of aqueous drainage in cats.
        ii. It also causes an intense miosis, and some feel that this is the major factor in increasing drainage (constricting the pupil opens the drainage angle).
        iii. Studies have mixed results in whether latanoprost significantly decreases IOP in cats.
        iv. It is contraindicated if there is an anterior lens luxation and should not be used if there is an anterior uveitis.
        v. However, many ophthalmologists will use it in cases of primary glaucoma.
11. Drugs that decrease aqueous production are more commonly used in feline glaucoma.
    a. Dorzolamide 2% topically every 8–12 hours. This is a topical carbonic anhydrous inhibitor that has fewer side effects than the systemic carbonic anhydrous inhibitors.
    b. Timolol 0.5% topically every 8–12 hours (for timolol). This is a beta blocker that decreases aqueous production. It should be used cautiously in cats with asthma due to the potential of an increase in airway smooth muscle tone and bronchoconstriction.
    c. Pilocarpine 1% topically every 15–30 minutes initially. This constricts the pupil, thus opening the drainage angle but is used uncommonly because it is very irritating.
    d. Methazolamide 2 mg/kg orally every 12 hours. This is a systemic carbonic anhydrous inhibitor and thus side effects such as anorexia and vomiting are more common.
12. Medical management should be attempted and may maintain a normal IOP and comfortable eye. Due to the chronic nature of glaucoma in cats, if medical management has failed and if the eye is irreversibly blind and painful, surgery may be the best option.
    a. Enucleation or exenteration (removing the entire contents of the bony orbit) is indicated on any eye where intraocular neoplasia may be the underlying cause of the glaucoma.
    b. If primary glaucoma is suspected and the eye is not responding to medical management, then an ophthalmologist can perform a procedure that creates selective damage to the ciliary body (which produces aqueous humor). Laser cycloablation uses a Nd:YAG or diode laser, whereas cyclocryotherapy freezes the area of the ciliary body with either liquid nitrogen or nitrous oxide.

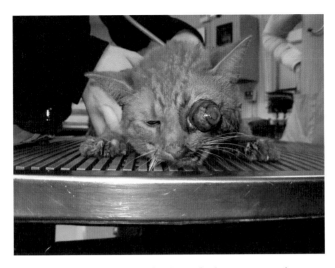

Fig. 37.12. Severe proptosis. This cat presented after being hit by a car. He also sustained a symphyseal mandibular fracture. This eye was eventually enucleated after the cat was stabilized.

13. Prognosis is dependent on underlying cause and response to treatment.
14. Aqueous humor misdirection glaucoma is another less common cause of glaucoma. The aqueous is being directed into the vitreous or posterior chamber instead of the anterior chamber. This occludes the iridocorneal angle. Clinical signs include a uniformly shallow anterior chamber and an anteriorly displaced lens. The exact cause is unknown, but one theory is that there is an abnormal anterior hyaloid. Referral to an ophthalmologist is recommended for medical management and possible lens extraction and anterior vitrectomy.

D. Proptosis—forward displacement of the globe with the eyelid margins caudal to the globe (fig. 37.12).
1. It occurs secondary to head trauma, most commonly secondary to hit by car, bite wounds, high-rise syndrome, or blunt-force injuries.
   a. The amount of force required to proptose a cat's eye is much greater than the more common brachycephalic dog. This means there is usually significant head trauma with other injuries along with the proptosed eye.
2. Must treat and manage head trauma before attempting surgery for the eye.
3. Apply sterile lubricant every 1–2 hours (artificial tears) while waiting for surgery to prevent the globe from drying out.
4. The two options for any proptosed eye include enucleation or replacement with tarsorrhapy.
   a. The decision is based on integrity of the globe and extraocular muscles and owner compliance.
   b. The prognosis for return of vision is guarded to poor in a proptosed eye; it is replaced for cosmetic reasons only.
   c. If there is a penetrating wound in the globe, the majority (more than two) of the extraocular muscles are avulsed, there is infected tissue, or the owners would be unable to medicate, then enucleation is the best option.
   d. If the globe is intact, the majority of the extraocular muscles are intact (still attached to the sclera) and healthy and the owners are able to medicate yet understand that enucleation may still be needed, then replacement with tarsorrhaphy can be performed.

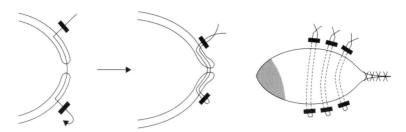

Fig. 37.13. Suture and stent placement for replacement and tarsorrhapy. The suture should go through a stent, enter 6–8 mm away from the upper eyelid margin, exit through the Meibomian glands, enter the lower lid Meibomian glands, and exit 6–8 mm away from the lower eyelid margin, go through a stent. The needle then goes back in the reverse direction forming a horizontal mattress suture. Rubber bands, IV tubing, or French red rubber catheters can be used for stents.

5. Replacement of the globe with temporary tarsorrhapy
   a. Avoid anesthetics that can increase intraocular pressure (i.e., ketamine).
   b. The cat should be placed under general anesthesia once it is deemed systemically stable.
   c. The periorbital area is clipped and gently scrubbed with betadine solution.
   d. A lateral canthotomy is performed.
   e. Using 2-0 nylon, about 0.5–1 cm away from the lid margins, a stay suture is placed in the upper and lower lid.
   f. A generous amount of sterile lubricant is placed on the globe.
   g. While lifting out and up on the stay sutures, the globe is gently pushed back into the orbit using a scalpel handle.
   h. The stay sutures are crossed and held to prevent reproptosis.
   i. Using 3-0 to 4-0 nylon or silk suture and tension-relieving stents, horizontal mattress sutures are placed as shown in figure 37.13.
   j. Pieces of intravenous tubing, extension sets, sterile rubber bands, or red rubber catheters can be used for the stents.
   k. The medial canthus is left open to allow placement of medications.
   l. The lateral canthotomy is closed using 4-0 braided absorbable suture or silk in a simple interrupted pattern.
   m. Aftercare is crucial to prevent infection and inflammation.
      i. Topical antibiotics—tobramycin or gentamycin 0.3 % solution every 6 hours
      ii. Topical atropine solution 1% every 12 hours
      iii. Systemic antibiotics—amoxicillin-clavulonic acid twice a day for 2 days and once a day for 3–4 days or enrofloxacin (5 mg/kg once a day)
      iv. Short, weaning course of anti-inflammatory doses of corticosteroids (0.5 mg/kg orally twice a day for 1–2 days then once a day for 2 days then every other day for two treatments)
   n. Remove sutures in 14 days.
   o. Postreplacement complications/sequelae
      i. Infection/abscess
      ii. Reproptosis
      iii. Exposure keratitis—the cornea loses innervation and thus is susceptible to irritation.
      iv. Dorsolateral strabismus—may correct itself over time
      v. May require a permanent partial tarsorrhaphy if persistent corneal disease
      vi. May ultimately need enucleation if complications occur

6. Enucleation—consult a surgery text for descriptions and methods of enucleation. The most important aspect to remember about enucleation in cats is that their optic chiasm is very short compared to dogs. When transecting the extraocular muscles off of the sclera and lifting the eye out of the orbit, if the eye is pulled out too vigorously or far, the optic chiasm can be stretched to a point where the contralateral eye becomes blind.

E. Ocular foreign body

   1. The most common ocular foreign bodies are little pieces of wood, grass awns, or sticks that get imbedded in the conjunctiva or cornea.

   2. Clinical signs include blepharospasm, conjunctival hyperemia, and corneal edema around the foreign body if it is in the cornea.

   3. May need to place a topical anesthetic agent (proparacaine 0.5%) in the eye to allow visualization of the entire globe.

   4. Will most likely see the foreign body in the conjunctiva or cornea.

   5. Techniques to dislodge the foreign body depend on the depth of the penetration.

     a. First, try flushing copious amounts of sterile eye wash to dislodge the foreign body. May need to place 1–2 drops of a topical anesthetic (proparacaine 0.5%) for the cat to allow this.

     b. If this is unsuccessful, the next technique will most likely require sedation.

     c. If in the conjunctiva, try to remove it with small forceps. If it will not dislodge, the area of conjunctiva that is affected may be removed, if small enough, with the foreign body.

     d. Treat the conjunctival wound with topical antibiotics (erythromycin 0.3%) every 6 hours for 1 week. If there is significant inflammation or infection, then systemic antibiotics should be started as well (amoxicillin-clavulonic acid 15 mg/kg orally twice a day for 1 week). The eye should be rechecked in 1 week.

     e. If in the cornea, can try to lift the foreign body out of the cornea using a cotton swab or 25-ga needle, being careful not to push it deeper into the cornea.

     f. Fluorescein stain the cornea once the foreign body is removed.

     g. Treat the remaining corneal ulcer with topical antibiotics (erythromycin 0.3% every 8 hours) and topical atropine (1%) ointment or solution every 12 hours if there is a reflex uveitis for 7–14 days. The eye should be rechecked in 3–5 days and then weekly until resolved.

     h. If the foreign body spans most of the cornea or penetrates the cornea into the anterior chamber, then the cornea will have to be sutured and a conjunctival flap may be needed once the foreign body is removed. Consultation with an ophthalmologist is recommended.

F. Acute blindness (box 37.4)

Box 37.4.   Acute blindness.

1. Clinical signs include dilated pupils with negative menace.
2. Can be due to primary ocular disease (e.g., glaucoma), primary neurologic disease (e.g., brain tumor), or systemic disease (e.g., infectious).
3. A common cause of acute blindness is retinal detachment secondary to systemic hypertension.
   a. The retina can reattach and vision may return if the underlying cause can be treated successfully.
4. Can visualize detached retina with focal penlight source directed through the pupil.
5. Always perform an indirect systemic blood pressure measurement.
6. If not hypertensive, then a more aggressive medical workup searching for infectious and neoplastic causes is warranted.
7. Enrofloxacin can cause an irreversible retinal degeneration.

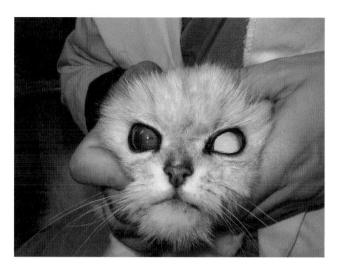

Fig. 37.14. A 16-year-old cat that presented with a 2-day history of acute blindness. Note the bilateral fixed and dilated pupils.

1. Determine if it is truly acute or if it appears acute to owner but actually is a chronic process (i.e., progressive retinal atrophy).
2. Causes include retinal detachment, panuveitis, anterior uveitis, enrofloxacin, taurine deficiency, encephalitis (i.e., FIP), cerebral vascular accident, brain tumor, retinal hemorrhage, and glaucoma.
3. Clinical signs include fixed and dilated pupils (fig. 37.14) and a negative menace response. Other clinical signs are dependent on the underlying cause (i.e., negative menace but possible positive PLR and neurologic signs [e.g., cortical blindness] vs. signs of anterior uveitis, glaucoma, etc). Kittens will have a negative menace response until 10–12 weeks of age.
4. A thorough fundic examination should be performed in any animal that presents with blindness. Look for evidence of retinal detachment, chorioretinitis, optic neuritis, or papilledema.
5. Retinal detachment is a very common cause of acute blindness in cats and is discussed below.
6. Enrofloxacin causes a nonreversible retinal degeneration. Fundic exam will reveal tapetal hyper-reflectivity and vascular attenuation. This is thought to be a rare and idiosyncratic reaction to the outer retinal tissues. Doses should not exceed 5 mg/kg once a day.
7. Diagnostic tests include intraocular pressure measurement, complete blood count, serum chemistry panel, thyroid hormone level, urinalysis, and indirect blood pressure measurement. Once systemic hypertension and glaucoma are ruled out, more extensive diagnostic tests, including viral serology (FIV, FeLV, FIP), toxoplasmosis titers (IgM and IgG), chest radiographs to rule out metastatic disease, and abdominal ultrasound to rule out neoplasia, may be indicated. Likewise, if primary neurologic disease is suspected, a cerebrospinal fluid tap and MRI may be indicated.
8. Prognosis is dependent on underlying cause (e.g., grave for FIP encephalitis) and whether the retinal lesions can resolve.
G. Retinal detachment—retinal pigment epithelium separates from photoreceptors.
   1. Clinical signs include fixed and dilated pupils and negative menace response. May be unilateral or bilateral.
   2. An indirect or direct lens is usually not required to diagnose a detached retina. It can usually be seen with a focal pen light source directed through the pupil. An indirect lens can then be used to fully evaluate the fundus.

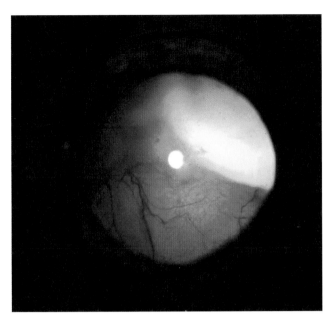

Fig. 37.15. The fundus in the cat in Fig. 37.8. Note the ballooning out of the retina in multiple planes. His systemic blood pressure was 280 mmHg. (Photograph courtesy of Dr. Mary Lassaline.)

3. The retina will be "ballooning" out and in multiple planes (fig. 37.15). The vessels will not be on a smooth surface. May also see retinal hemorrhages.
4. The most common cause of retinal detachment is systemic hypertension. Other causes include infectious (FeLV/FIV/FIP/fungal), neoplastic (lymphosarcoma), and trauma.
5. If systemic hypertension is present (Doppler blood pressure usually >200 mmHg), amlodipine (Norvasc 0.625 mg once a day) should be started.
6. If due to systemic hypertension, the prognosis for vision is fair to guarded. The retina can reattach and vision can return once systemic blood pressure is under control.
7. Other causes of retinal detachment have a more guarded prognosis.

H. Chemical injury
1. The most common causes are topical products (shampoos, flea treatments, etc.) that accidentally get into the eye.
2. Smoke secondary to being in a house fire can also lead to severe chemical injury to the corneas.
3. It leads to diffuse corneal irritation and abrasions to ulcers. Other clinical signs include chemosis and conjunctivitis.
4. Treatment includes flushing the eyes out with copious amounts of sterile eye wash and topical antibiotics (erythromycin 0.3% every 6–8 hours). Topical atropine ointment (1% every 12 hours) should be started if there is a reflex uveitis and miosis present.
5. The eye should be rechecked every 5–7 days to determine response to treatment, and medications should be continued until the injury is healed.

I. Anterior lens luxation
1. Due to stretching of the zonules that suspend the lens
2. Clinical signs include abnormal depth to anterior chamber, corneal edema if the lens touches the cornea, and visualizing the lens in the anterior chamber. If the lens is subluxated, may see an aphakic crescent (the lens is shifted down or to one side so there is an area of pupil where

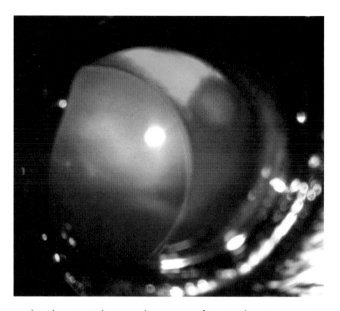

Fig. 37.16. An anterior lens luxation (photograph courtesy of Dr. Andras Komaromy).

there is no lens (fig. 37.16). There may also be signs consistent with anterior uveitis and/or glaucoma.

3. Primary lens luxation is less common in cats but can occur due to senile zonular degeneration.

4. Secondary lens luxation is more common and is due to chronic uveitis, chronic glaucoma, or trauma.

5. Glaucoma secondary to anterior lens luxation is less common in cats as opposed to dogs due to a deeper anterior chamber.

6. Surgery to remove the lens is not usually recommended in a secondary lens luxation since the lens is not the primary problem. If there is a primary lens luxation and the eye is visual, then surgery to remove the lens is recommended. There is still the potential for postintraocular surgery glaucoma and intraocular sarcoma (see below).

J. Prolapsed nictatans

1. True prolapsed nictatans or third eyelid gland or "cherry eye" is uncommon in cats but requires surgery to replace the third eyelid gland as in dogs. There is one report that suggested a Burmese breed predilection (fig. 37.17); however, it is now reported in other breeds. As in dogs, it is not a true emergency.

2. Clinical signs include a red eye and an enlarged, prolapsed third eyelid gland. The edge of the third eyelid will not be visible.

3. Cats can have prolapsed nictatans very commonly secondary to a variety of diseases including dehydration, loss of orbital fat (especially in geriatric cats), and anything that produces pain.

4. "Haws," or a prolapsed nictatans secondary to a disparity of sympathetic innervation, can be caused by GI disease, especially parasites, *Chlamydophilia felis*, or herpes infection. Horner's syndrome can also be seen. A drop of phenylephrine can be used to diagnose neurologic causes if the nictatans returns to normal position. This usually spontaneously resolves in 4–6 weeks.

5. This should be differentiated from a true prolapsed third eyelid gland where the cartilage is prolapsed.

K. Corneal laceration

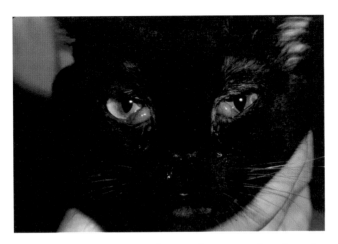

Fig. 37.17   Bilateral cherry eye in a Burmese cat (photograph courtesy of Dr. Steve Gross).

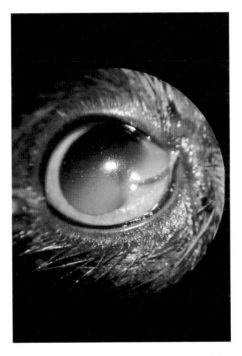

Fig. 37.18.   A corneal laceration. Note the corneal edema. A twig caused this cat's laceration. Reproduced from the *Manual of Canine and Feline Emergency and Critical Care*, 2nd ed., edited by L. King and A. Boag. With permission of BSAVA.

1. Due to trauma
2. Clinical signs depend on the depth of the laceration and include corneal edema, blepharospasm, conjunctival hyperemia, anterior uveitis (either secondary or primary if the laceration is full thickness), and visualization of the laceration (fig. 37.18).
3. Treatment is also dependent on the depth of the laceration.

4. If a superficial laceration, treat with topical antibiotics (erythromycin 0.3%, gentamycin 0.3%) every 6 hours and topical atropine ointment (1%) every 12 hours.

5. The eye should be rechecked in 1 week. If uncomplicated, the laceration should heal in 1–2 weeks.

6. If a deep or full-thickness laceration is present, then surgery to debride the edges and then suture the cornea with 6-0 to 9-0 absorbable (polyglactin or braided) may be needed. This may need to be followed with a conjunctival flap/pedicle graft.

7. If the owners are financially unable to have surgery performed or surgery cannot be performed in the near future, then treat aggressively similar to a perforated corneal ulcer—topical antibiotics (ciprofloxacin 0.3% suspension) every 2 hours, topical atropine solution (1%) every 6–8 hours, systemic antibiotics (amoxicillin-clavulonic acid 15 mg/kg every 12 hours), and systemic nonsteroidal anti-inflammatory medications (meloxicam 0.01 mg/kg once a day). The eye should be rechecked every 1–2 days to monitor response to treatment initially to ensure that the cornea has sealed and then weekly until resolved.

8. If the anterior lens capsule was disrupted when the laceration occurred (may see tract of fibrin in anterior chamber or fibrin on lens), then a tapering dose of systemic anti-inflammatory doses of corticosteroids, instead of NSAIDs, is warranted due to the stronger anti-inflammatory properties. An extreme and intense anterior uveitis can occur and the owner should be warned that the lens may need to be removed in the future if the eye does not respond to medical management or if secondary glaucoma occurs. The eye should be rechecked every 1–2 days to monitor response to treatment.

9. An Elizabethan collar should also be used.

L. Eyelid laceration
  1. Due to trauma, for example, bite wounds
  2. Clinical signs depend on depth and cause of laceration and include blood at the site of the injury, blepharospasm, and pawing at the eye.
  3. Treatment depends on the depth of the laceration.
  4. If very superficial and the eyelid margins are apposed normally, then can treat as a superficial wound with topical (erythromycin 0.3% every 6–8 hours) and systemic antibiotics (amoxicillin-clavulonic acid 15 mg/kg every 12 hours). The eye should be rechecked in 5–7 days.
  5. If deep or full thickness, then surgery to reappose the eyelid margins is needed (fig. 37.19).
  6. A simple interrupted pattern is used with 4-0 to 7-0 absorbable suture (braided or polyglactin) in the subconjunctiva and then skin.
  7. Extreme care must be taken to align the Meibomian glands on both sides of the wound. Once in place, the sutures must not touch or rub against the cornea.
  8. Topical and systemic antibiotics as described above are then instituted.
  9. An Elizabethan collar should always be used.
  10. The eye should be rechecked in 3–5 days and the cornea fluorescein stained to ensure that the sutures are not irritating the cornea.
  11. If the eyelid laceration involves the medial canthus and nasolacrimal system, an ophthalmologist should perform the repair.

M. Hyphema—blood in the anterior chamber (fig. 37.20).
  1. Can see flecks of blood to a pool of blood in the ventral aspect of the anterior chamber, to the entire chamber filled with blood.
  2. Causes include trauma, coagulapathy (thrombocytopenia or clotting factor deficiency), or neoplasia (e.g., LSA).
  3. May also be secondary to anterior uveitis or systemic hypertension.
  4. Need to look for other signs of trauma or coagulapathy/bleeding.
  5. If no other signs of trauma, then diagnostic tests include complete blood count, serum chemistry panel, full coagulation panel, systemic blood pressure measurement, and possibly diagnostic tests for anterior uveitis (see above).

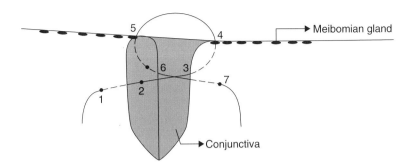

1) Enter eyelid about 3-4 mm away from margin
2) Exit through the middle of the eyelid width
3) Enter other eyelid (other part of laceration) about 2-3 mm from the margin
4) Exit through Meibomian glands
5) Enter first eyelid through Meibomian glands
6) Exit through middle of eyelid width
7) Enter and exit other eyelid about 3-4 mm away from margin

Fig. 37.19. Eyelid laceration repair. Enter the eyelid about 3–4 mm away from the margin. Exit through the middle of the eyelid width. Enter the other eyelid about 2–3 mm from the margin. Exit through the Meibomian glands. Enter first eyelid through the Meibomian glands. Exit through middle of eyelid width. Enter and exit other eyelid about 3–4 mm away from the margin.

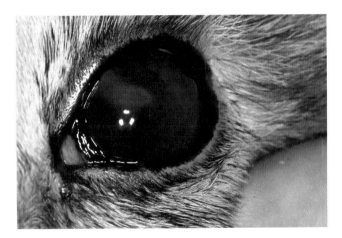

Fig. 37.20. Hyphema. Trauma, coagulapathy, and neoplasia are the most common causes of hyphema. This cat also has thrombocytopenia and mesenteric lymphadenopathy secondary to lymphosarcoma. Reproduced from the *Manual of Canine and Feline Emergency and Critical Care*, 2nd ed., edited by L. King and A. Boag. With permission of BSAVA.

6. Ultrasound of the eye may also diagnose an intraocular mass.
7. An IOP measurement should be taken due to the potential of secondary glaucoma.
8. Treatment involves treating the underlying cause. If anterior uveitis is suspected, then treat as described above. If secondary to intraocular neoplasia, then enucleation or exenteration is warranted.
9. Topical corticosteroids (predisolone acetate 1%) can be used three times a day once a corneal ulcer is ruled out. Atropine ointment twice a day should be used if the IOP is low or low-normal (i.e., due to anterior uveitis). Atropine is contraindicated if the IOP is normal or elevated.

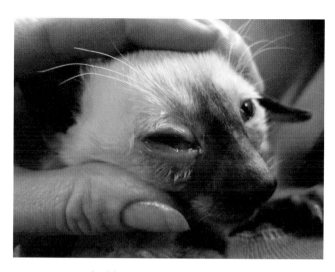

Fig. 37.21. Conjunctivitis in a 4-month-old Siamese cat. He also had nasal discharge and sneezing.

   10. Prognosis is dependent on the underlying cause.
   11. The eye must be monitored to ensure that secondary glaucoma is not occurring. If the initial IOP is high or high normal, then topical dorzolamide and topical timolol (see "Glaucoma" above) should be started at three times a day. The eye should be rechecked in 1–2 days. If the IOP is low or low normal, the eye should be rechecked in 5–7 days.
   12. The blood in the anterior chamber will slowly resorb over days to weeks if the cause of the bleeding can be controlled. Injection of "clot busters" into the anterior chamber can have multiple complications and should be discussed with an ophthalmologist.
   N. Conjunctivitis—inflammation of the conjunctiva (fig. 37.21).
   1. Clinical signs include purulent ocular discharge, blepharospasm, swollen and red conjunctiva, conjunctival hyperemia, and chemosis. There may be signs consistent with an upper respiratory infection (e.g., nasal discharge and sneezing). Systemic signs such as fever, lethargy, and anorexia may also be noted.
   2. In cats, as opposed to dogs, it is almost always secondary to an infectious cause.
   3. Common infectious agents that lead to conjunctivitis include feline herpes virus (FHV-1), *Chlamydophilia felis*, and *Mycoplasma* spp.
   4. Treatment includes topical antibiotics (erythromycin 0.3%) every 6–8 hours for 7–14 days and supportive care.
   5. Topical antiviral medications (idoxuridine 0.1%, trifluridine 1% compounded at a pharmacy) every 6–8 hours can be used for 1–2 weeks if FHV-1 is suspected.
   6. Famcyclovir, a systemic antiviral medication, can be used in adult cats with suspected FHV-1. The dose is ¼ of a 250-mg tablet once a day for 20 days. It is metabolized by the liver and excreted through the kidneys; thus, patients must have normal liver and kidney function.
   O. Exophthalmos—abnormal protrusion of globe (i.e., globe is pushed forward)
   1. Causes include a retrobulbar abscess or retrobulbar mass
      a. Retrobulbar abscess
         i. Clinical signs include pain on opening the mouth, pain on retropulsion of the eye, facial asymmetry, exposure keratitis and secondary corneal ulcer, and prolapsed nictatans. A red or swollen area behind the last upper molar may be seen.

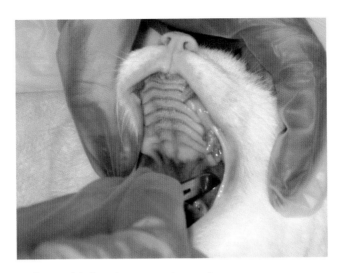

Fig. 37.22.   Placement of a #11 blade to lance a tooth root abscess.

ii.   Systemic signs such as anorexia, lethargy, and fever may also be seen.

iii.   One of the most common causes of a retrobulbar abscess is a tooth root abscess. A swelling ventral to the eye with or without a draining tract may be seen.

iv.   Treatment involves establishing drainage under general anesthesia. A #11 blade is used to make an incision in the mucosa behind the last upper molar tooth (fig. 37.22). The tips of mosquito hemostats are then pushed into the incision and opened to create drainage of the abscess. An aerobic and anaerobic culture and sensitivity should ideally be submitted. Sterile saline can then be used to gently flush the wound and abscess.

v.   Systemic antibiotics (amoxicillin-clavulonic acid 15 mg/kg every 12 hours) are prescribed for 14 days.

vi.   If the retrobulbar abscess is secondary to a tooth root abscess, then extraction of the tooth may be needed.

  b.   Retrobulbar mass

i.   Clinical signs include decreased ability to retropulse the eye, prolapsed nictatans, blindness, exposure keratitis with secondary corneal ulcer, and possible retinal changes. There is usually NO pain when opening the mouth.

ii.   Ultrasound of the eye and/or CT scan can help diagnose and delineate the mass.

iii.   Chest radiographs should be performed if neoplasia is suspected.

iv.   A needle aspirate may be feasible to diagnose the cause of the mass.

v.   Exploratory orbitotomy may be needed for surgical removal of the mass.

vi.   Prognosis is dependent on the type of neoplasia. Types of neoplasia reported include squamous cell carcinoma, fibrosarcoma, lymphosarcoma, meningioma, and osteosarcoma/osteoma.

P.   Keratoconjunctivis sicca (KCS)—decreased tear production with secondary inflammation of the conjunctiva and cornea

1.   KCS is not as common in cats as in dogs.

2.   Clinical signs include blepharospasm, mucoid to mucopurulent discharge, a visibly dry cornea, conjunctival hyperemia, mild corneal opacification, conjunctivitis, and possibly a secondary corneal ulcer.

3. It is diagnosed based on Schirmer tear test results (<5 mm/min). Normal Schirmer tear test is 17 mm/minute. However, cats with normal tear production can have low Schirmer tear test results (less than 5 mm/min), thus diagnosis is based mostly on clinical signs.

4. Fluorescein stain should then be used to diagnose and delineate a corneal ulcer.

5. The most common cause of KCS is chronic conjunctivitis secondary to feline herpes virus (FHV-1) infection.

6. It can also be secondary to other causes of chronic conjunctivitis, sulfa drugs, anesthesia, trauma, surgical removal of the gland, or idiopathic.

7. Treatment involves protecting the cornea, treating the underlying cause, and treating a secondary corneal ulcer if present.

    a. The most important treatment is an artificial tear preparation every 4–6 hours.

    b. There are longer-acting artificial tear solutions that can be used at night.

    c. Topical cyclosporine (0.2%) every 12 hours to decrease immune-mediated destruction of lacrimal glands. This can be started on a trial basis for 1 month to see if there is resolution of clinical signs.

    d. Topical antibiotics (erythromycin 0.3%) every 6–8 hours if secondary corneal ulcer present and to prevent secondary bacterial infections.

    e. Topical antiviral medications (e.g., idoxuridine solution 0.1% compounded at a pharmacy every 6–8 hours) should be started if feline herpes infection is thought to be the underlying cause.

    f. Some ophthalmologists will use a topical antibiotic-steroid combination if there is no corneal ulcer yet chronic disease present.

Q. Posttraumatic sarcoma

1. Extremely malignant intraocular neoplasia

2. Thought to be secondary to ocular trauma, intraocular surgery, trauma to lens, and chronic uveitis

3. Clinical signs include anterior uveitis, glaucoma, hyphema, and intraocular mass(es).

4. Can use ultrasound to help diagnose an intraocular mass.

5. The neoplasia will invade the optic nerve and retina and will metastasize to regional lymph nodes and distant sites.

6. Chest radiographs to rule out pulmonary metastasis are recommended.

7. Exenteration, where the entire contents of the bony orbit are removed, is recommended.

8. Prognosis is guarded to poor for long-term survival.

Recommended Reading

Attali-Soussay K, Jeqou JP, Clerc B. Retrobulbar tumors in dogs and cats: 25 cases. Vet Ophthalmology, 2001; 4(1):19–27.

Blocker T, van der Woerdt A. The feline glaucomas: 82 cases (1995–1999). Vet Ophthalmology, 2001; 4(2):81–85.

Brooks DE. Glaucoma in the dog and cat. Vet Clin North Am Sm Anim Pract, 1990; 20(3):775–797.

Chahory S, Crasta M, Trio S, Clere, B. Three cases of prolapse of the nictatans gland in cats. Vet Ophthalmology, 2004; 7(6):417–419.

Colitz CM. Feline uveitis: diagnosis and treatment. Clin Tech Small Anim Pract, 2005; 20:117–120.

Crispin SM, Mould JR. Systemic hypertensive disease and the feline fundus. Vet Ophthalmology, 2001; 4(2):131–140.

Czederpiltz JMC, La Croix NC, van der Woerdt A, et al. Putative aqueous humor misdirection syndrome as a cause of glaucoma in cats: 32 cases (1997–2003). J Am Vet Med Assoc, 2005; 227(9): 1434–1441.

Dietrich U. Feline glaucomas. Clin Tech Small Anim Pract, 2005; 20:108–116.

Featherstone HJ, Sansom J. Feline corneal sequestra: a review of 64 cases (80 eyes) from 1993–2000. Vet Ophthalmology, 2004; 7(4):213–227.

Gelatt KN, van der Woerdt A, Ketring KL, et al. Enrofloxacin-associated retinal degeneration in cats. Vet Ophthalmology, 2001; 4(2);99–106.

Gionfriddo JR. Identifying and treating conjunctivitis in dogs and cats. Vet Med, 1995; 90:242–253.

Giuliano EA. Feline ocular emergencies. Clin Tech Small Anim Pract, 2005; 20:135–141.

Glaze MB, Gelatt KN. Feline ophthalmology. In Gelatt KN, ed, Veterinary Ophthalmology, 3rd ed, pp. 997–1052. Baltimore: Lippincott Williams & Wilkins, 1999.

Komaromy AM, Andrew SE, Denis HM, et al. Hypertensive retinopathy and choroidopathy in a cat. Vet Ophthalmology, 2004; 7(1):3–9.

La Croix NC. Ocular manifestations of systemic disease in cats. Clin Tech Small Anim Pract, 2005; 20:121–128.

La Croix NC, van der Woerdt A, Olivero DK. Nonhealing corneal ulcers in cats: 29 cases (1991–1999). J Am Vet Med Assoc, 2001; 218(5):733–735.

Maggs DJ. Update on pathogenesis, diagnosis, and treatment of feline herpesvirus type 1. Clin Tech Small Anim Pract, 2005; 20:94–101.

Mandell DC. Ophthalmological emergencies. In King L, Hammond R, eds, Manual of Canine and Feline Emergency and Critical Care, pp. 117–126. Cheltenham, England: British Small Animal Veterinary Association, 1999.

Mandell DC, Holt E. Ophthalmic emergencies. Vet Clin North Am Small Anim Pract, 2005; 35:455–480.

Moore PA. Feline corneal disease. Clin Tech Small Anim Pract, 2005; 20:83–93.

Plunkett SJ. Anaphylaxis to ophthalmic medication in a cat. J Vet Emerg Crit Care, 2000; 10(3):169–171.

Rainbow ME, Dziezyc J. Effects of twice daily application of 2% dorzolamide in intraocular pressure in normal cats. Vet Ophthalmology, 2003; 6(2):147–150.

Sapienza JS. Feline lens disorders. Clin Tech Small Anim Pract, 2005; 20:102–107.

Strubbe DT, Gelatt KN. Ophthalmic examination and diagnostic procedures. In Gelatt KN, ed, Veterinary Ophthalmology, 3rd ed, pp. 427–466. Baltimore: Lippincott Williams & Wilkins, 1999.

Sykes JE. Feline chlamydiosis. Clin Tech Small Anim Pract, 2005; 20:129–134.

Whitley RD, Hamilton HL, Weigand CM. Glaucoma and disorders of the uvea, lens and retina in cats. Vet Med, 1993; 88:1164–1173.

Whitley RD, Whitley EM, McLaughlin SA. Diagnosing and treating disorders of the feline conjunctiva and cornea. Vet Med, 1993; 8:1138–1149.

Willis AM, Diehl KA, Robbin TE. Advances in topical glaucoma therapy. Vet Ophthalmology, 2002; 5(1):9–17.

38
DERMATOLOGIC EMERGENCIES

Jill L. Abraham

> **Unique Features**
> Many skin diseases present with similar clinical signs. A thorough dermatologic history, dermatologic exam, and initial dermatologic tests, such as flea combing, skin or ear cytology, skin scrapings, and fungal culture, may help rule in or rule out common disorders and guide the need for further workup, treatment, or referral. The most common skin diseases encountered in cats are bite wound abscesses or other traumas, ectoparasite infections, ringworm, and allergies such as flea bite allergy, food allergy, and atopy.

A. Overview, common presenting complaints and clinical signs
  a. Overview
    i. Many skin diseases present with similar clinical signs, so the diagnosis may not be apparent based solely on the history and dermatologic exam findings. Basic dermatologic tests allow for immediate identification of secondary infections or ectoparasites and guide initial treatment until further workup can be provided.
    ii. A basic dermatologic diagnostic workup includes:
      1. Skin scrapings for ectoparasites
      2. Cytology for bacterial infections
      3. Ear cytology and ear mite preps in cases of otitis
      4. Fungal culture for dermatophytes
      5. Historical, clinical, and laboratory findings will guide the need for additional tests such as bacterial cultures and skin biopsies.
    iii. Severe compromise to the barrier function of the skin, as occurs with generalized ulcerative dermatoses, burns, or trauma (bite wounds, degloving injuries), may predispose to sepsis.
    iv. Wear gloves when handling any cat with skin lesions, as some diseases have zoonotic potential.
    v. Most skin disorders are not life-threatening but may significantly impact patient comfort and quality of life, and disrupt the human-animal bond.
  b. Presenting complaints and clinical signs
    i. Pruritus
      1. An unpleasant sensation that provokes the desire to scratch.
        a. Manifests as licking, scratching, biting, or excessive grooming.
        b. Some cats hide to lick and scratch, so owners may not think that their cats are itchy.

2. Dermatologic exam may reveal:
   a. Broken hairs, alopecia
   b. Erythema, excoriations
   c. Crusts, erosions, ulcers
3. Seasonal pruritus can be due to atopy to outdoor allergens (e.g., pollens).
4. Nonseasonal pruritus can be due to food allergy or atopy to indoor allergens (e.g., house dust mites).
5. Ectoparasites (fleas, *Cheyletiella*, *Notoedres*, *Demodex gatoi*), flea allergy dermatitis, and secondary bacterial infections can cause seasonal or nonseasonal pruritus.
   a. Caudal-dorsal distribution of pruritus is seen most commonly with flea allergy dermatitis.
6. Less common causes of pruritus include:
   a. Dermatophytosis
   b. Pemphigus foliaceus
   c. Overgrooming secondary to hyperthyroidism
7. Most causes of pruritus are dermatologic rather than behavioral in origin.
   a. Self-trauma can perpetuate the itch-scratch cycle.

ii. Alopecia
1. The most common cause of alopecia is self-trauma due to pruritus (allergies and ectoparasites most commonly).
   a. Dermatologic exam may reveal:
      i. Broken hairs or other lesions associated with pruritus
      ii. Or there may be minimal clinical inflammation.
2. Dermatophytosis can cause focal, multifocal, or generalized alopecia, often with scaling or crusting. Pruritus is variable.
3. Uncommon to rare causes of alopecia in cats include:
   a. Behavioral overgrooming
   b. Cutaneous lymphoma
   c. *Demodex cati*
   d. Endocrinopathies (iatrogenic or spontaneous hyperadrenocorticism)
   e. Paraneoplastic alopecia
      i. Typically affects the abdomen and limbs. Affected skin has a glistening appearance.
      ii. Most often secondary to pancreatic carcinoma

iii. Eosinophilic granuloma complex lesions
1. These are cutaneous reaction patterns to various underlying causes, not final diagnoses, and are very common presenting complaints. They include:
   a. Eosinophilic plaques (fig. 38.1)
      i. Raised flat alopecic erythematous moist to dry or crusted lesions. May be called "hot spots" by owners.
   b. Eosinophilic granulomas
      i. Linear cutaneous granulomas or oral granulomas
      ii. Chin edema ("fat chin" syndrome)
   c. Indolent (rodent) lip ulcers (fig. 38.2).
2. Common underlying causes include allergies:
   a. Flea bite allergy
   b. Food allergy
   c. Atopy
   d. Other insect hypersensitivities
3. Embedded insect or mite parts (foreign bodies) or a genetic predilection may be part of the etiology.

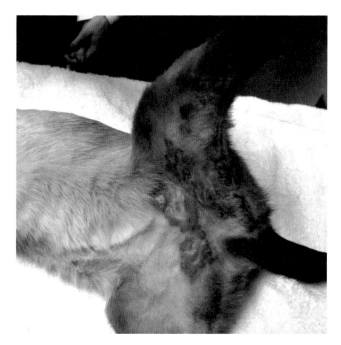

Fig. 38.1. Alopecia and multiple eosinophilic plaques in the inguinal region. Possible underlying causes include flea allergy, food allergy, and atopy. Secondary bacterial infection may occur.

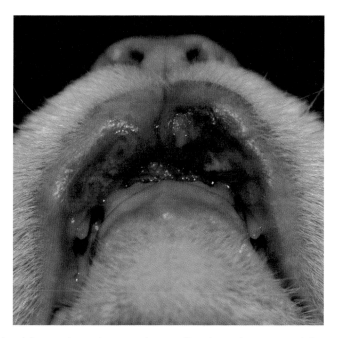

Fig. 38.2. Bilateral indolent (rodent) ulcers on the maxillary lips. This is part of the eosinophilic granuloma complex. Possible underlying causes include food allergy and atopy. Secondary bacterial infection may occur.

    4. Secondary bacterial or concurrent dermatophyte infections may complicate lesions and intensify pruritus.

    5. A peripheral blood eosinophilia may be present.

iv. Papules and intact pustules are rare in cats but may be seen with:

    a. Feline acne

    b. Pemphigus foliaceus

    c. Ectoparasites

    d. Dermatophytosis

    e. Cutaneous adverse drug reactions

v. Crusting dermatitis, miliary dermatitis

    1. Crusts are formed when dried exudate, serum, blood, pus, or cells adhere to the skin surface.

    2. Miliary dermatitis consists of small punctate crusts and commonly occurs along the dorsum.

    3. Causes include:

       a. Allergies (flea allergy, food allergy, and atopy) and associated pruritus and self-trauma

       b. Ectoparasites

         i. Fleas, *Cheyletiella*, *Notoedres*, *Otodectes*, *Demodex*

       c. Infections

         i. Bacteria, fungal (yeasts or dermatophytes), or viral

           1. Herpes viral infections on the face are typically erosive or ulcerative but may have overlying crusts.

       d. Autoimmune diseases (pemphigus)

       e. Cutaneous adverse drug reaction

vi. Erosions and ulcers

    1. An erosion is a disruption of the epidermis with an intact basement membrane.

    2. An ulcer is a disruption of the epidermis through the basement membrane into the dermis.

    3. Possible causes include:

       a. Severe pruritus and subsequent self-trauma from allergies or ectoparasites

       b. Eosinophilic granuloma complex

       c. Autoimmune diseases

       d. Cutaneous adverse drug reactions

       e. Mycobacterial, fungal, or viral infections

       f. Neoplasia (e.g., squamous cell carcinoma, mast cell tumor, cutaneous lymphoma, lymphangiosarcoma/angiosarcoma)

       g. Ischemic injury or vasculitis

       h. Burns, frostbite, other trauma

    4. Skin biopsies may aid in diagnosing the underlying cause.

vii. Nodules, abscesses, and draining tracts can be classified as:

    1. Infectious inflammatory

       a. Bite wound abscesses

       b. Actinomyces/nocardia infections

       c. Mycobacterial infections

       d. Fungal granulomas

         i. Sporotrichosis

         ii. Cryptococcosis

         iii. Dermatophyte pseudomycetoma

         iv. Blastomycosis

    2. Sterile inflammatory

       a. Foreign body reactions

       b. Eosinophilic granulomas

       c. Injection site reactions

   3. Neoplastic
   4. Excisional biopsy of a nodule and macerated tissue cultures for bacteria (aerobic and anaerobic), mycobacteria, and fungi are often indicated.
B. Diagnostic procedures
   a. Basic dermatologic diagnostics help guide initial antimicrobial or antiparasitic therapy and may support the need for further workup including cultures, biopsies, or referral to a veterinary dermatologist.
   b. Flea combing is indicated in every cat with skin disease.
      i. If no fleas seen, rub collected debris onto a wet paper towel.
         1. Flea "dirt" (feces = digested blood) will turn orange-red.
      ii. Place collected debris onto a glass slide with mineral oil under a cover slip and examine microscopically for ectoparasites.
   c. Skin cytology is indicated in all cases to rule out infections. Otic cytology is indicated in all cases of otitis.
      i. Methods of cytology collection include:
         1. Direct glass slide impression smear
         2. Acetate (clear) tape impression
            a. Press the sticky side of the tape to the skin 3–5 times.
            b. Useful for dry lesions, lesions difficult to sample with glass slides or swabs, and identification of *Malassezia*.
         3. Fine needle aspiration
            a. Used to sample fluctuant swellings, nodules, or tumors
            b. Two techniques are used most often.
               i. Repeatedly insert into the lesion a 22–25-gauge needle without a syringe attached. Redirect the needle with each insertion. Remove the needle and attach it to a 6-cc syringe filled with air, aim the needle bevel down at a slide, and press the plunger to "blow" the material onto the slide. Gently smear the sample using another slide, allow to air dry, and stain with cytology stain.
               ii. Insert a 22–25-gauge needle attached to a 6-cc syringe into the center of the lesion. Pull back on the plunger to apply pressure, release, then redirect and repeat 1–3 times. Release the plunger before removing the needle from the lesion so that negative pressure doesn't pull cells from the hub of the needle into the syringe. If blood is seen in the hub, remove the needle and start again, as blood will dilute the cellular sample. Then, remove the needle from the syringe, fill the syringe with air, reattach the needle, and "blow" the material onto a slide. Gently smear and stain the slide.
         4. Otic swabs
      ii. Cytological evaluation
         1. Heat-fix glass slides with waxy or thick exudates and stain with modified Wright's stain (Diff-Quick).
         2. Press sticky side of tape onto a drop of blue cytology stain (e.g., blue stain of Diff-Quick) on a slide.
         3. Evaluate for (fig. 38.3):
            a. Inflammatory cells
            b. Bacteria
            c. Fungal organisms (yeasts)
            d. Neoplastic cells
            e. Acantholytic cells
   d. Skin scrapings are indicated in all cases to rule out ectoparasites. Negative skin scrapings do not rule out the presence of mites.
      i. Procedure

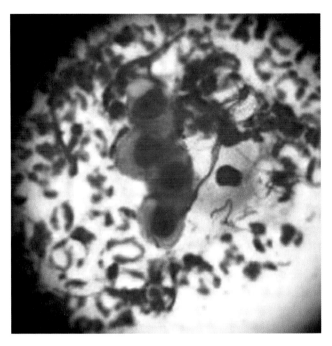

Fig. 38.3. Acantholytic keratinocytes surrounded by neutrophils. Impression smear cytology from a cat with pemphigus foliaceus.

1. Gently clip hair.
2. Use a No. 10 scalpel blade held at a 45-degree angle. Dull the scalpel blade by rubbing it against the edge of a metal table 10–15 times.
3. Coat scalpel blade and skin with mineral oil. Place a drop of oil onto a glass slide.
4. Superficial scrapings (fig. 38.4)
   a. To identify mites that live in the hair coat or superficial layers of the skin
      i. *Notoedres cati, Sarcoptes scabiei, Cheyletiella* spp., *Otodectes cynotis, Demodex gatoi.*
   b. Scrape the surface of the skin in broad strokes in the direction of hair growth.
   c. Scrape multiple sites. New lesions are preferred.
5. Deep scrapings
   a. To identify mites that live in hair follicles (*Demodex cati*). Performed less often in cats since *D. cati* is rarely encountered.
   b. Gently pinch the skin prior to scraping to extrude mites from follicles.
   c. Scrape small area in the direction of hair growth until capillary oozing is seen.
6. Transfer material to glass slide and place a coverslip. Examine the entire area under coverslip with the 10x objective for mites, ova, and mite feces.
7. Lower the microscope condenser and light intensity to enhance visualization.
   e. Otic mite preps are used to evaluate for *Otodectes cynotis* or otic demodicosis, and are indicated in all cases of otitis.
      i. Swab ear canals as for otic cytology and roll swabs in a drop of mineral oil placed on a glass slide. Examine as for skin scrapings.
   f. Trichogram (microscopic examination of plucked hairs) can be used to evaluate for evidence of pruritus and dermatophyte spores and/or hyphae.
      i. Gently grasp a small number of hairs with fingertips or rubber-covered hemostats and epilate hairs in direction of growth.

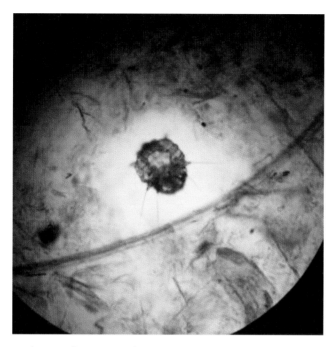

Fig. 38.4. *Sarcoptes scabei* mite from a superficial skin scraping. *Notoedres cati,* the cause of "head mange," are similar in appearance.

   ii. Place hairs in mineral oil under a coverslip and evaluate with the 10x objective.
      1. Broken hair tips indicate pruritus and self-induced or traumatic alopecia.
      2. Distorted, swollen, or fuzzy hair shafts with ectothrix spores or hyphae may be seen with dermatophytosis (fig. 38.5)
      3. *Demodex cati* mites may be found at the roots of hairs in infected cats (fig. 38.6).
   g. Wood's lamp evaluation may be used for any cat with skin lesions to screen for dermatophytosis.
      i. Emits ultraviolet light causing fluorescence of tryptophan metabolites of approximately 50% of *Microsporum canis* strains.
      ii. Warm up the lamp for 5 minutes prior to use because the stability of the light's wavelength and intensity depends upon its temperature.
      iii. Positive fluorescence is apple-green color fluorescence along the hair shafts.
         1. Use fluorescent hairs for microscopic evaluation (trichogram) and fungal culture.
      iv. Lack of fluorescence does not rule out dermatophytosis, as 50% of *M. canis* strains and other important ringworm species will not show fluorescence.
      v. False positive fluorescence is typically white or blue and can be seen with scales or crusts, topical medications, and some bacteria.
   h. Fungal culture is indicated in any cat with skin lesions to confirm or rule out dermatophytosis, particularly because of zoonotic concerns.
      i. Procedure
         1. Lightly disinfect the area to be sampled with 70% alcohol. Allow to air dry.
         2. Pluck hairs and scale from the periphery of lesions with sterile hemostats and place onto (don't bury into) dermatophyte test medium (DTM).
            a. DTM = Sabouraud's dextrose agar with a color indicator and ingredients to inhibit bacterial and saprophytic fungal overgrowth.

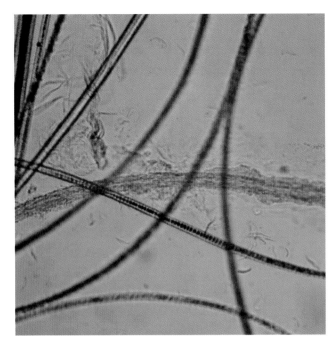

Fig. 38.5. Trichogram (hair pluck) from a cat with patchy alopecia and mild scaling. There is a distorted, swollen hair shaft in the center with ectothrix fungal spores.

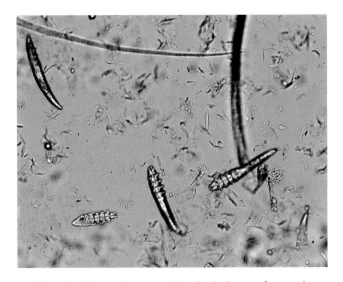

Fig. 38.6. *Demodex cati* (long-bodied) and *D. gatoi* (short-bodied) mites from a skin scraping.

3. For cats without lesions (resolving infections or asymptomatic carriers), brush the entire hair-coat with a sterile or new toothbrush. Place collected hairs/scale onto the media.
4. Incubate samples with moisture
   a. In the dark at room temperature or in a closed shoebox with a cup of water to provide humidity
   b. Check samples daily for 21 days.

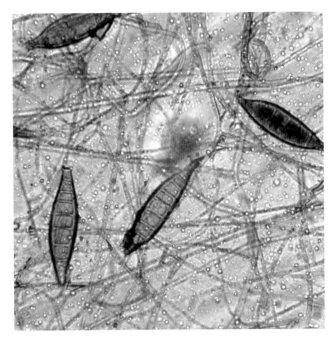

Fig. 38.7. *Microsporum canis* macroconidia. This is a tape stripping from a fungal colony grown on a DTM culture plate that was placed onto a glass slide with a drop of blue stain.

5. Positive result
   a. Pathogenic dermatophytes produce alkaline metabolites that turn the DTM pH indicator red as soon as a white- or beige-colored fluffy colony develops.
   b. Some contaminants cause a red color change after several days, so always confirm the diagnosis with microscopic evaluation.
      i. Touch a piece of acetate tape sticky side down onto the colony, then place the tape sticky side down onto a drop of blue cytology stain on a glass slide and examine with the 10× objective for macroconidia (fig. 38.7).
   i. Bacterial culture and sensitivity
      i. Indications include:
         1. Deep cellulitis-like lesions
         2. Nodules and draining tracts
         3. Bacterial infection unresponsive to empirical therapy
      ii. Methods to obtain sample
         1. Sample an intact pustule.
         2. Sample under crust.
         3. Express fresh exudate from lesion.
         4. Swab ears as for otic cytology.
         5. Submit a skin biopsy for macerated tissue culture.
      iii. Perform cytology to correlate with culture results.
   j. Skin biopsies
      i. Indications include:
         1. Suspected neoplasia
         2. Vesicles or persistent ulcers

       3. Unusual or severe lesions

       4. Conditions failing to respond to empirical therapy

       5. Dermatoses most readily diagnosed by biopsy (suspected autoimmune disease)

       6. A disease that requires therapy which may be expensive, of extended duration, or carries significant side effect risks (e.g., autoimmune diseases, some neoplasms, or paraneoplastic syndromes) is suspected.

  ii. Perform biopsies during the initial exam with any of the above conditions, or within 3 weeks of therapy in unresponsive cases.

       1. If possible, resolve secondary pyoderma and discontinue glucocorticoids for 2–3 weeks prior to biopsy.

  iii. Procedure

       1. Site selection is important.

          a. Newly formed and primary lesions (vesicles, papules, pustules, etc.) are preferred over older or secondary lesions (crusts).

          b. Biopsy the center of lesions unless lesions are necrotic or ulcerated; then biopsy the edge of the lesion.

          c. Always biopsy at least three representative sites.

       2. Punch biopsy using a disposable Bakers punch (0.4–0.8 mm) and local anesthesia, with or without sedation, is acceptable for most lesions.

       3. Use heavy sedation or general anesthesia to biopsy the nose, foot pads, or pinnae.

       4. Excisional or wedge biopsy is recommended for nodules or deep lesions.

       5. Clip fur gently or cut fur with scissors, but do not prep the skin in any other way to avoid distorting histology. NEVER scrub a skin biopsy site. If area is alopecic, draw a line in the direction of hair growth with a permanent marker (to orient the pathology lab when the skin biopsy sample is processed).

       6. Apply moderate pressure and twist the biopsy punch in one direction only. When the punch penetrates the full thickness of the skin, remove the punch, grasp the SQ tissue with forceps (NEVER grasp the dermis or epidermis) and cut the SQ attachments.

       7. Blot gently to remove blood. Place sample immediately into 10% formalin.

       8. Suture biopsy sites with simple interrupted or cruciate pattern.

       9. Submit skin biopsies to an experienced dermatopathologist and bacterial or fungal cultures for suspected infections.

C. Management of specific conditions

  a. Bite wound abscesses

    i. Overview

       1. More common in intact males due to roaming behavior and aggression

       2. Microorganisms from the oral cavity are introduced under the skin.

          a. Infection develops within 2–7 days.

          b. Resident feline oral cavity organisms such as *Streptococci*, *Bacteroides*, and *Pasturella* are the most common bacteria involved.

       3. Small wounds often seal over and may not be visible upon initial examination.

    ii. Clinical signs and diagnosis

       1. The history may include exposure to the outdoors or other animals or a witnessed fight.

       2. Physical examination may reveal:

          a. Fever, bite wound(s), pain, firm or fluctuant SQ swelling, or purulent discharge

          b. Nonspecific signs (lethargy, anorexia, lameness) and regional lymphadenopathy

       3. Common locations include the face and neck, tail base, shoulder, or distal limb.

       4. Clip hair to help detect small wounds and determine the extent of involved tissue.

          a. Two adjacent punctures suggest a bite injury.

          b. A single wound more likely indicates another cause of penetrating injury.

5. Cellulitis develops prior to abscess formation, so the absence of pus does not rule out a bite wound. Cellulitis can often appear as just mild diffuse swelling or just pain on palpation of the affected area.
   a. Early bite wound–related cellulitis is one of the more common causes of lameness in cats.
6. Differential diagnoses include fungal or atypical bacterial infections, so always wear gloves.

iii. Treatment
   1. Use light sedation or general anesthesia, depending upon the extent and severity of the wound.
   2. Liberally clip fur and surgically prepare the area.
   3. Lance the abscess at the ventralmost aspect with a No. 11 or 15 blade.
   4. Flush with copious volumes of sterile saline.
   5. Probe the SQ space to fully assess the amount of dead space.
      a. Dead space is often much larger than the area evident on initial exam.
   6. Debride any necrotic tissue.
   7. Place penrose drains in large wounds or wounds with excessive dead space.
      a. Multiple drains may be needed (e.g., wounds that extends across dorsal midline of neck or lumbar area).
      b. Establishing adequate ventral drainage is of utmost importance.
         i. Incomplete treatment of the initial wound is the most common cause of recurrence.
   8. Bite wounds should never be completely sutured closed.
   9. Large wounds can be partially closed with nonabsorbable monofilament sutures, leaving an opening for the Penrose drain.
      a. Drains should not exit through the incision but through a separate site.
   10. Place an Elizabethan collar to prevent self-trauma and self-removal of drains.
   11. Administer SQ or IV fluids to cats that are febrile, anorectic, or that undergo prolonged anesthesia for wound treatment.
   12. Administer broad spectrum antibiotics effective against feline oral microflora for 7–10 days:
      a. Amoxicillin 22 mg/kg PO q12h
      b. Amoxicillin/clavulanate 13.75–22 mg/kg PO q12h
      c. Clindamycin 5–11 mg/kg PO q12h
   13. Remove drain(s) in 3–5 days; remove sutures in 7–10 days.

iv. Prognosis
   1. Castrate intact males to minimize the incidence of recurrence by reducing aggression and roaming.
   2. Refractory or recurrent abscesses most commonly result from:
      a. Inadequate debridement or drainage
      b. Foreign body
      c. Resistant or atypical infection
      d. Underlying retroviral or other immunosuppressive disease
      e. Osteomyelitis
   3. Consider further diagnostics such as culture/susceptibility testing, biopsy, radiographs, or surgical exploration if there is a poor response to initial therapy, if drainage persists greater than 10 days, or if the abscess recurs within 1–3 weeks of apparent resolution.

b. Burns
   i. Overview
      1. Causes of thermal injury include hot water, grease, tar, fire, heating pads, electrical cords, heated metal (automobile mufflers), and chemical burns.
      2. Burns are classified as
         a. Partial thickness

      i. Superficial
        1. Affects epidermis only
        2. Wounds with an intact basal epidermal layer may heal completely or with minimal scarring or permanent hair loss.
      ii. Deep
        1. Extend to dermis
    b. Full thickness
      i. Affects entire dermis with destruction of adnexae, nerves, and vessels
      ii. May destroy subcutaneous tissue including muscle and bone
      iii. Deep partial-thickness and full-thickness wounds require extensive wound management followed by surgical closure or grafting.
      iv. Significant scarring and permanent hair loss may occur.
  3. Mortality is often due to systemic complications such as sepsis and multiple organ failure.
ii. Clinical signs and diagnosis
  1. Superficial and deep partial thickness burns
    a. Erythema, edema, +/– vesicles, +/– singed hairs or hair loss, varying degrees of inflammation, erosion, and ulceration
  2. Full-thickness burns
    a. May appear dry or leathery; abscessed area may be covered by an eschar.
    b. Often do not bleed and are not painful due to destruction of blood vessels and sensory nerves.
  3. Chemical burns are often ulcerative and necrotic.
  4. Singed facial hairs and whiskers and corneal lesions suggest possible smoke inhalation.
    a. Careful monitoring of respiratory status is indicated.
  5. Various systemic signs, hematologic, biochemical, or blood gas abnormalities may be present depending upon the severity and extent of the burn.
  6. The full extent of injury may not be evident for 2–3 days or longer, so liberal clipping and careful monitoring during initial management is indicated.
  7. Biopsy may help distinguish a burn from other diseases such as severe erythema multiforme, autoimmune disease, vasculitis, or cutaneous lymphangiosarcoma/angiosarcoma. Preferred biopsy sites are areas of erythema without ulceration.
iii. Treatment
  1. Apply cool water to wounds immediately if exposure is recent to possibly minimize extent of injury.
  2. Superficial partial thickness wounds
    a. Clip hair and lavage with sterile saline to remove surface heat, debris, and chemicals.
    b. Apply silver sulfadiazine 1% cream/Silvadene 1% cream (King Pharmaceuticals, Inc., Bristol, TN) or Thermazene 1% cream (Tyco Healthcare/Kendall, Mansfield, MA) to keep the wound moist and prevent secondary bacterial colonization.
      i. Apply a thin layer 1–2 times daily until a healthy bed of granulation tissue develops.
      ii. Do not use in cats with known hypersensitivities to sulfa drugs.
    c. Cover with sterile occlusive dressing.
  3. Deep partial-thickness or full-thickness wounds
    a. Resuscitate patient as indicated (supplemental oxygen, IV fluids, etc.) and provide appropriate supportive care.
    b. Sedation or anesthesia is required for adequate wound management.
    c. Aggressive pain management is necessary throughout the healing process.
      i. Use injectable or transdermal narcotics and/or nonsteroidal anti-inflammatory medications (NSAIDs; see chap. 7—Pain Management in Critically Ill Feline Patients).
        1. NSAIDs should only be administered after the patient is fluid resuscitated and normotensive to prevent renal damage.

d. Perform aggressive lavage and debridement to remove debris and necrotic, nonviable tissue.
e. Apply silver sulfadiazine cream and cover the wound with sterile occlusive dressing.
f. Daily debridement is indicated until a healthy bed of granulation tissue develops.
   i. Sugar, honey, silver sulfadiazine cream mixed with insulin (anecdotal reports suggest mixing 100 U NPH into 1 oz. of silver sulfadiazine 1% cream), or synthetic matrix materials may help promote granulation tissue formation.
      1. Apply a thin layer of silver sulfadiazine cream, soak gauze with honey, or apply enough sugar to coat wound. Change dressings once to twice daily and rinse thoroughly with sterile saline before reapplication. Apply until a healthy bed of granulation tissue develops.
g. Sterile technique is critical to prevent infection.
h. Use splints when necessary to prevent excessive movement during healing.
i. Surgical closure or skin grafts may ultimately be needed.
j. Systemic antibiotics are not indicated in most cases and may predispose to infection with resistant organisms.
   i. Choose antibiotics for wound infections based on full-thickness biopsy culture and sensitivity.
   ii. Administer broad-spectrum antibiotics if sepsis occurs.
k. Once healed, protect scarred or hairless skin from sun exposure by applying zinc oxide cream.

iv. Prognosis
   1. Humans with burns involving more than 40–50% of body surface area have a high mortality rate, and survival is rare when greater than 80% of body surface area is involved.
   2. Warn owners that large areas of skin loss will require multiple rechecks and bandage changes with or without sedation. This can be relatively expensive over the period of care.

c. Degloving injuries
i. Overview
   1. Traumatic shear wounds that cause avulsion of skin and exposure of deep soft tissue structures and bone most often occur on distal extremities when limbs are compressed between an automobile tire and the pavement.

ii. Clinical signs, diagnosis
   1. Loss of skin and soft tissues to varying degrees. Usually occurs on medial aspects of distal limbs. Bleeding is often minimal due to traumatic injury to blood vessels.
   2. Severe injury commonly results in extensive damage to ligament and bone leading to exposed and unstable joints.
   3. Wounds are often contaminated with dirt, hair, and other debris.
   4. Signs of other traumatic injuries such as shock, long bone/pelvis fractures, and respiratory distress are often present and should be treated first (see chap. 1—Approach to the Critically Ill Cat).

iii. Treatment
   1. Stabilize life-threatening traumatic injuries first (see chap. 1—Approach to the Critically Ill Cat).
   2. Clip and lavage the wound and place a protective stabilizing bandage +/– splint until the patient is stabilized.
   3. Sedation or anesthesia is required for adequate wound management.
   4. Aggressive pain management is necessary throughout the healing process (see "Burns"; see chap. 7—Pain Management in Critically Ill Feline Patients).
   5. Treat severe injuries as open wounds with copious lavage and aggressive debridement.
   6. Tendons, ligaments, or bone with soft tissue attachments are left in place.
   7. Remove bone fragments that are not connected to tissue or blood vessels.
   8. Evaluate muscle for viability.

      a. Consistency (firm, not friable)

      b. Color (pink/red, not gray/brown)

      c. Contractility (should contract when pricked—not always a reliable test for viability)

      d. Circulation (should bleed when cut)

         i. If viability is questioned, leave tissue and reassess at next bandage change.

    9. Preserve as much skin as possible to facilitate wound closure.

  10. Initially, wound edges should be partially opposed using nonabsorbable suture to permit drainage, minimize exposure of deep tissues, and provide some stability.

  11. Lavage, debride, apply sterile wet-to-dry bandages, +/- matrix materials such as sugar, honey, or insulin mixed with silver sulfadiazine 1% cream (see above).

      a. Change bandages daily until granulation tissue forms (moist, soft, dark pink to light red, glistening, highly vascularized tissue with a granular appearance), then use nonadherent dressings and change bandages less frequently.

  12. Surgical closure or grafts may ultimately be needed.

  13. Temporarily stabilize orthopedic injuries with splints or external pin splints.

      a. Pins should be placed in healthy bone above and below the fracture and should be placed as far from the wound as possible if secondary fixation is anticipated.

  14. Use broad-spectrum antibiotics with efficacy against skin flora:

      a. Cefazolin/Cephalexin 22 mg/kg IV or PO q12h; Cefadroxil 20 mg/kg PO q2h

      b. Amoxicillin-clavulanate (Clavamox) 13.75–22 mg/kg PO q12h

  15. Perform culture/sensitivity in refractory tissue infections.

    iv. The prognosis is dependent upon extent of injuries and may not be evident at initial presentation. Limb amputation may be required.

d. Parasitic diseases

  i. Overview

    1. All of the following parasites except *Demodex* spp. have zoonotic potential.

    2. People may develop a transient pruritic papular rash.

      a. Always ask if any in-contact person has an itchy rash as part of a dermatologic history.

      b. If so, direct people to their physicians for evaluation.

    3. Any suspected zoonotic parasitic disease should be empirically treated, even if diagnostic test results are inconclusive. A therapeutic trial is often needed to confirm or negate a diagnosis.

    4. Always treat in-contact animals.

    5. Hypersensitivity reactions to fleas and mites may contribute to inflammation and pruritus.

  ii. Fleas

    1. Overview, clinical signs, and diagnosis

      a. *Ctenocephalides felis felis* (cat flea) is the most common species.

      b. Diagnosis is based on presence of fleas or flea dirt.

      c. Cats are excellent groomers, so lack of fleas does not rule out a flea infestation or a flea allergy.

      d. Severe infestation can lead to life-threatening anemia in very young kittens.

      e. Secondary tapeworm infections may occur and should be treated.

    2. Treatment

      a. Nitenpyram (Capstar) orally (kittens ≥4 weeks old and ≥2 lbs). Give one dose or repeat up to every other day as needed until resolution.

      b. Imidocloprid (Advantage), fipronil (Frontline), or selamectin (Revolution) topically (kittens ≥8 weeks).

      c. Young kittens may require manual flea removal with flea comb.

      d. Indoor and/or outdoor environmental treatment may be necessary in severe infestations.

  iii. Flea allergy dermatitis is the most common allergic skin disease and may be seen in combination with food allergy or atopy.

1. Cats may present with alopecia, miliary dermatitis, eosinophilic granuloma complex lesions, or open wounds secondary to severe pruritus.
2. The caudal dorsum is commonly affected, but lesions may be seen on the ventrum, hind limbs, flanks, or neck.
3. Diagnosis and treatment
   a. Presence of fleas or flea dirt and/or resolution of clinical signs with strict flea control trial
      i. Nitenpyram (see above)
      ii. Imidocloprid, fipronil, or selamectin q 2–3 weeks for at least 8 weeks
         1. Continue q 3–4 weeks year-round for treatment.
         2. Only imidocloprid is labeled for up to weekly use.
   b. Treat in-contact animals.
   c. Anti-inflammatory doses of glucocorticoids may be needed acutely or periodically to control pruritus and other clinical signs. Example doses:
      i. Prednisolone 1–2 mg/kg PO q24h × 5–7 days, then taper
      ii. Depo-medrol 5 mg/kg SQ or IM once
   d. Antibiotics are indicated if secondary bacterial infections are present.
      i. Treat superficial bacterial infections for at least 21 days.
      ii. Cephalexin 22–30 mg/kg PO q12h or Cefadroxil 20 mg/kg PO q12h
      iii. Cefpodoxime proxetil (Simplicef) 5–10 mg/kg PO q24h (off-label use in cats)
      iv. Amoxicillin-clavulanate 15–22 mg/kg PO q12h
      v. Clindamycin 5–11 mg/kg PO q12h
      vi. Enrofloxacin 5 mg/kg or Marbofloxacin 2.2–5.5 mg/kg q24h
iv. *Otodectes cynotis* (ear mites)
   1. Overview
      a. The most common cause of otitis externa in cats.
   2. Clinical signs may be variable and include:
      a. Erythema, aural pruritus, black waxy to dry aural exudates, and excoriations of pinnae, head, or neck
      b. Lesions may occur rarely on the body, as mites can be found outside of the ear canals.
   3. Diagnosis
      a. Otic mite preparations or superficial skin scrapings (see fig. 38.8)
      b. Otic cytology to rule out secondary bacterial and/or *Malassezia* infections.
   4. Treatment
      a. Daily to every other day ear cleanings to remove exudate and dead mites for 1–3 weeks.
         i. Examples of routine ear cleansers include Epi-otic (Virbac) and Oti-Clens (Pfizer Animal Health).
      b. Systemic treatment should be given as mites can reside on the body, and this may be the only treatment needed in addition to ear cleanings.
         i. Selamectin 6–12 mg/kg topically q 2 wks for 2–3 treatments (kittens >8 wks age; off-label use at this frequency)
         ii. Ivermectin 200–300 µg/kg SQ or PO q 2–3 wks for 3–4 treatments (off-label use)
      c. Topical otic mitacides are alternatives to systemic treatment.
         i. Tresaderm (thiabendazole)
            1. 2–4 drops into each ear twice daily for 7 days, stop for 7 days, then treat for 7 days, then stop.
            2. Or, treat daily to every other day for 21 days.
         ii. Acarexx (ivermectin 0.01%) or MilbeMite OTIC (milbemycin oxime 0.1%)
            1. One dose applied in each ear (0.5 mL of Acarexx or 0.25 mL of MilbeMite).
            2. Repeat treatment in 3–4 weeks if necessary. Reported safe in kittens >4 wks.

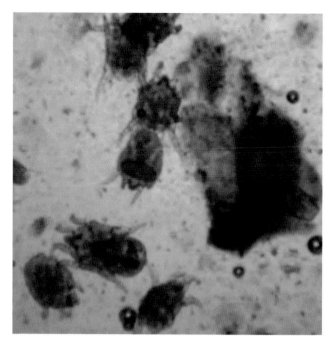

Fig. 38.8. *Otodectes cynotis* (ear mites) from an otic swab rolled in mineral oil on a glass slide.

d. Treat secondary otic infections (see "Otitis externa"). If infections are mild, ear cleanings alone are usually sufficient.
v. *Cheyletiella*
    1. Overview
        a. *Cheyletiella blakei* is the most common species found on cats.
        b. Adult mites live on the stratum corneum and move through the epidermal debris. Eggs are attached to the host's hairs.
    2. Clinical signs
        a. Excessive and often large scales, erythematous papules, miliary dermatitis, or alopecia
        b. Dorsal midline is commonly affected.
        c. Pruritus is highly variable.
    3. Diagnosis
        a. Presence of mites and/or response to treatment. Use flea combing, superficial skin scrapings, or tape impressions to collect hair and scales (see fig. 38.9).
        b. Fecal floatation may reveal mites or eggs due to grooming and ingestion of mites.
    4. Treatment
        a. Selamectin 6–12 mg/kg topically q 2 weeks for a minimum of three treatments (off-label use)
        b. Ivermectin 300 μg/kg PO or SQ q 2 weeks for a minimum of three treatments (off-label use)
        c. Lime sulfur dips q 5–7 days for a minimum of 4–6 weeks. Place an E collar until dry to prevent licking the dip, which may cause salivation or vomiting.
        d. Environmental treatment (bedding, carpets, insecticidal sprays, etc.) is recommended.
            i. Wash bedding or other linens in hot water with regular laundry detergent and dry in a hot dryer.

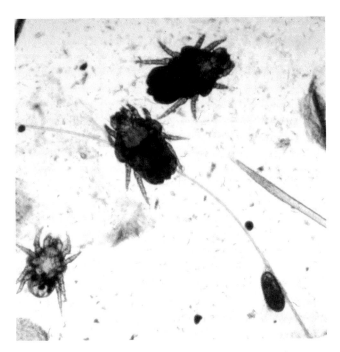

Fig. 38.9. *Cheyletiella* mites and an egg attached to a hair shaft from a cat with pruritus and dorsally distributed large white scales.

    vi. Feline mange (head mange)
        1. Overview
           a. *Notoedres cati* is the cause of head mange in cats.
           b. *Sarcoptes scabiei* (dog scabies) infections occur less commonly in cats.
           c. Mites burrow into the superficial layers of the skin (stratum corneum).
        2. Clinical signs
           a. Intense pruritus, alopecia, papules, excoriations, erosions, and crusts
           b. Pinnae often affected first, then upper ears, face, eyelids, and neck
        3. Diagnosis
           a. Superficial skin scrapings are likely to demonstrate mites or mite eggs.
           b. Fecal floatation may reveal mites or eggs due to grooming and ingestion of mites.
           c. Perform skin cytology to rule out secondary bacterial infections.
        4. Treatment
           a. Same as for *Cheyletiella* (see above)
           b. Treat secondary bacterial infections (see "Flea allergy dermatitis").
           c. Anti-inflammatory doses of glucocorticoids may be necessary to alleviate the intense pruritus (see "Flea allergy dermatitis").
    vii. Demodicosis occurs uncommonly in cats.
        1. Overview and clinical signs
           a. *Demodex cati* live in hair follicles and have long and slender bodies.
              i. Infection is often associated with underlying immunosuppressive or metabolic disease.
                 1. FIV, FeLV, or diabetes mellitus
              ii. Clinical signs include:
                 1. Patchy alopecia, erythema, scaling, crusting, or comedones with variable pruritus

   2. Common locations include the periocular skin, head, neck, ear canals (ceruminous otitis), or trunk.
   b. *Demodex gatoi* inhabit the epidermal surface and have short stubby bodies.
      i. May be contagious to other cats, so suspect *D. gatoi* if multiple cats in a household are affected.
      ii. Clinical signs include:
         1. Symmetric alopecia, scaling, excoriations, or crusts
         2. Pruritus is variable but can be severe.
         3. Common locations include the trunk, abdomen, head, neck, or elbows.
2. Diagnosis
   a. Skin scrapings or trichograms
   b. *D. gatoi* may not be readily found on skin scrapings; negative findings do not rule out infection.
   c. A workup for underlying disease is indicated with *D. cati* infection.
3. Treatment
   a. Lime sulfur dips q 5–7 days for a minimum of 4–6 weeks is the treatment of choice for both types of demodicosis.
   b. Treat in-contact cats for *D. gatoi*.
e. Dermatophytosis
   i. Overview
      1. *Microsporum canis* is the most commonly encountered dermatophyte in cats.
      2. Persians, cattery cats, and cats that travel to shows are predisposed.
      3. Transmission occurs by direct contact and via contaminated environment and fomites.
   ii. Clinical signs
      1. Focal, multifocal, or generalized alopecia
      2. Scaling, crusting, erythema, papules, or miliary dermatitis may be seen.
      3. Pruritus is variable.
   iii. Diagnosis
      1. Wood's lamp and trichography may be helpful for screening.
      2. Fungal culture is needed for definitive diagnosis.
   iv. Treatment
      1. Inform owners of zoonotic potential.
      2. Isolate infected cat(s) to one room.
         a. Spores shed into the environment may remain infective for nearly 2 years.
      3. Clip long-haired cats or cats with generalized infection.
         a. May help shorten the course of disease and reduce environmental contagion.
         b. Personnel involved must wear protective gear, dispose of hairs in biohazard waste, and disinfect or dispose of clippers.
         c. Lesions may worsen 7–10 days postclipping.
      4. All cats should receive systemic treatment.
         a. Itraconazole 5–10 mg/kg PO q24h (off-label use)
            i. Give daily until cure, or give daily for 28 days, then as alternate week pulse therapy (1 week on treatment, 1 week off, etc.) until cure.
            ii. Usually tolerated well by cats, but monthly to every other monthly monitoring of liver enzymes is recommended.
            iii. Use capsules or Sporanox suspension. A suspension compounded from bulk powder may have markedly reduced bioavailability in cats.
         b. Griseofulvin
            i. Microsized (Fulvicin or GriFulvin V) 50–120 mg/kg PO divided twice daily and given with a fatty meal

        ii. Ultramicrosized (Gris-PEG) 5–15 mg/kg PO divided twice daily
           1. Teratogenic
           2. Test for FIV prior to starting treatment due to potential for bone marrow suppression.
      c. Terbinafine 30–40 mg/kg PO q24h
        i. May be an effective alternative therapy (off-label use)
      d. Lufenuron is often ineffective for treatment or prevention and is not recommended.
    5. Adjuvant topical therapy is recommended once to twice weekly.
      a. May shorten the course of disease and reduce environmental contagion.
        i.   Lime sulfur dips
        ii. Miconazole shampoo
        iii. Enilconazole 0.2% solution is an effective topical treatment but is not licensed for small animal use in USA.
    6. Environmental decontamination
      a. 1:10 diluted bleach solution
      b. Enilconazole (Clinafarm EC disinfectant) used as a sprayer or fogger is very effective but is not licensed for small animal use in the USA.
      c. Destroy bedding, brushes, etc.
      d. Frequent vacuuming
    7. Repeat fungal cultures every 2–4 weeks.
      a. Owners can use the toothbrush technique at home and bring in the toothbrushes for culture.
    8. Cats may appear clinically normal prior to mycologic cure. Treat until three negative successive cultures taken 2–4 weeks apart are obtained.
  f. Otitis externa
    i.   Overview: The causes of otitis can be divided into the following categories. Any causes from each category must be addressed for complete resolution of otitis. On an emergency basis, attempts should be made to rule out ear mites, secondary infections, foreign bodies, polyps/masses, and topical drug reactions.
      1. Predisposing and primary underlying causes
        a. Ear mites (most common cause of otitis in cats)
        b. Nasopharyngeal polyps (second most common cause of otitis in cats)
        c. Allergies
        d. Foreign bodies (e.g., foxtail)
        e. Neoplasia
      2. Secondary causes
        a. Bacterial or yeast infections
        b. Topical medication reactions
      3. Perpetuating factors
        a. Progressive pathologic changes in ear canals (hyperplasia, stenosis)
        b. Otitis media (often underdiagnosed)
    ii. Clinical signs are variable.
      1. Head shaking, scratching, pinnal erythema, aural exudates, malodor, or self-trauma to the pinnae, head, or neck.
      2. Topical drug reactions often present with severe erythema and scaling +/– ulcers of inner surface of pinna and opening of external ear canal. Discontinue use of medication and do not use related products in the future.
      3. Otitis media may present with pain upon opening the mouth, Horner's syndrome or peripheral vestibular disease, or just a history of chronic or recurrent external ear infections.
      4. Cats with allergic disease may have concurrent dermatitis, so perform a thorough dermatologic exam.

     5. Aural hematomas occur uncommonly in cats.
  iii. Diagnosis
     1. Otic cytology and mite preps
     2. Perform otoscopy to assess the patency of the ear canal, the tympanic membrane, and to rule out polyps, other masses, or foreign bodies, especially in cases of unilateral otitis.
       a. Sedation or general anesthesia may be needed.
     3. Bacterial culture and sensitivity is indicated when rods are present on cytology (suspect *Pseudomonas* spp.) or when initial therapy fails.
     4. Bulla radiography or CT imaging is indicated in cases of suspected otitis media, polyps, or neoplasia.
     5. A workup for underlying allergic disease is necessary if other causes of otitis are ruled out.
  iv. Treatment
     1. Otitis externa
       a. Ear cleansing/flushing with large volumes to fill ear canal is the key to proper ear cleaning. As cats appear to be more vulnerable to ototoxicity than dogs, be less aggressive with ear cleanings in cats.
         i. Frequency is based on the severity of otitis. Severe cases may require daily cleanings initially.
         ii. Many acidifying ear cleansers such as Epi-otic (Virbac) have mild antibacterial or antifungal properties and may be used as the sole treatment for mild infections.
         iii. Avoid chlorhexidene-based flushes, as they have the potential to cause ototoxicity.
       b. Acute otitis externa
         i. Apply at least 3–4 drops of medication per dose, typically BID. Medicate topically for minimum of 7–14 days.
       c. Chronic or recurrent otitis externa
         i. Medicate topically for minimum of 21–30 days.
         ii. Use systemic anti-inflammatory glucocorticoids if edema, stenosis, or other progressive changes are present.
         iii. Use systemic antibiotics if extensive swelling, ulceration, periaural dermatitis, or otitis media is present.
       d. Bacterial and yeast infections
         i. Neomycin (Tresaderm)
         ii. Gentamicin (Gentocin otic or ophthalmic, Otomax, Mometamax)
         iii. For resistant *Pseudomonas* infections:
            1. Silver sulfadiazine: compound powder into 1% solution or mix cream 50/50 with water.
            2. Enrofloxacin injectable mixed with tris-EDTA ear flush. Achieve a 10 mg/mL concentration of enrofloxacin and flush ears BID.
            3. Tobramycin or polymyxin B ophthalmic drops.
       e. Yeast infection (without bacteria)
         i. Miconazole (Conofite drops)
       f. Use topical corticosteroids if moderate to severe inflammation or stenosis is present.
         i. Combination products containing corticosteroids (Tresaderm, Otomax)
         ii. Mix injectable dexamethasone with silver sulfadiazine or Conofite (8–12 mL dex per 30 mL antimicrobial).
     2. Treatment of otitis media usually requires either a middle ear lavage (deep ear flush) under general anesthesia or ventral bulla osteotomy followed by antimicrobial therapy.
       a. Topical and systemic antimicrobial therapy based on middle ear bacterial culture, and sensitivity is indicated for a minimum of 4–6 weeks.

3. Recurrence of otitis is likely if underlying cause(s) are not addressed.

g. Autoimmune skin diseases (pemphigus foliaceus)

  i. Overview

    1. Pemphigus foliaceus is the most common autoimmune skin disease seen in cats.

      a. Pemphigus vulgaris, discoid or systemic lupus erythematosus, and other autoimmune skin diseases occur rarely.

    2. The pathogenesis is not well characterized in cats, but in dogs and humans it involves the breakdown of keratinocyte adhesion molecules following autoantibody targeting. This leads to acantholysis (keratinocytes break apart from one another).

    3. Drug-induced pemphigus may occur rarely.

    4. Perform skin biopsies at initial visit prior to glucocorticoid therapy if autoimmune disease is suspected.

  ii. Clinical signs

    1. Intact pustules are fragile and transient, so the most common lesions seen are:

      a. Crusts, erosions, scale, and alopecia

      b. Pruritus is variable.

    2. Common locations include:

      a. Face/head (especially pinnae), paws/clawbeds/footpads, periareolar, or other body regions

      b. Lesions may be bilaterally symmetric.

    3. Lethargy, anorexia, fever, or other nonspecific clinical signs may occur.

  iii. Diagnosis

    1. Skin cytology is needed to rule out secondary infections and may reveal acantholytic cells:

      a. Round nucleated epithelial cells alone or in clumps surrounded by neutrophils (larger than neutrophils; fig. 38.10).

    2. Confirm diagnosis with histopathology. Biopsy intact pustules or multiple representative lesions.

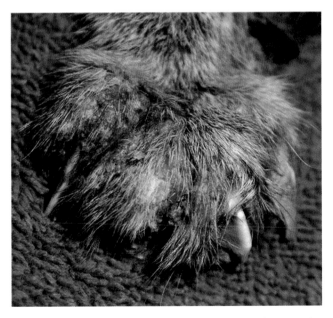

Fig. 38.10. Alopecia, erythema, crusting, and swelling of the claw folds of a cat with pemphigus foliaceus and secondary bacterial infection.

iv. Treatment options
1. Glucocorticoids
   a. Triamcinolone 0.2–0.4 mg/kg PO q12h
   b. Dexamethasone 0.1–0.2 mg/kg PO q12h
   c. Prednisolone 1–2 mg/kg PO q12h
2. Chlorambucil (Leukeran) 0.1–0.2 mg/kg PO q24h
   a. Can combine with glucocorticoids initially, and then taper to EOD once clinical remission is achieved.
   b. Potential side effects include myelosuppression and gastrointestinal toxicity.
3. Modified cyclosporine (Neoral or Atopica) 5 mg/kg q12–24h has been anecdotally reported to be effective in more than half of feline pemphigus cases.
   a. May be effective as monotherapy, but if disease is severe combine with corticosteroids initially.
   b. Perform FIV, FeLV, and toxoplasmosis titers (IgG and IgM) prior to cyclosporine therapy in cats.
      i. Anecdotal reports of cyclosporine use in either FIV- or FeLV-positive cats have not described an increase in side effects, but closer hematologic and biochemical monitoring is recommended.
      ii. Toxoplasma-positive cats have been treated concurrently with cyclosporine and clindamycin.
   c. Potential side effects include anorexia, vomiting, diarrhea, hirsutism, and at extremely high doses hepato- or nephrotoxicity. Hyperglycemia and diabetes mellitus have been reported anecdotally in some cats.
   d. Long-term use, especially when combined with other immunosuppressive medications, may predispose to opportunistic infections or neoplasia.
4. Treat secondary bacterial infections for at least 21 days.
   a. Cephalexin 22–30 mg/kg PO q12h or Cefadroxil 20 mg/kg PO q12h
   b. Cefpodoxime proxetil (Simplicef) 5–10 mg/kg PO q24h (off-label use in cats)
   c. Amoxicillin-clavulanate 15–22 mg/kg PO q12h
   d. Clindamycin 5–11 mg/kg PO q12h
   e. Enrofloxacin 5 mg/kg or Marbofloxacin 2.2–5.5 mg/kg q24h
5. Slowly taper medications to q48h then q72h when clinical remission is achieved.
v. Prognosis
1. Often a good prognosis, although cats may need lifelong therapy.
2. Routine monitoring of complete blood counts, serum biochemical analysis, and urine analysis is recommended throughout treatment.
h. Cutaneous adverse drug reactions
   i. Overview
   1. Nonimmunologic or predictable
      a. Dose-dependent reaction
      b. Due to pharmacologic properties of the drug
   2. Immunologic or unpredictable
      a. Idiosyncratic, non–dose-dependent
      b. Caused by a variety of host and drug factors
   3. May occur with topical, oral, or injectable medications
      a. Sulfonamides, cephalosporins, penicillins, and topical neomycin are mostly commonly involved.
   4. Usually occur within 1–3 weeks after initiating therapy
   ii. Clinical signs are highly variable and can mimic nearly any dermatosis.

1. Pruritus, macular-papular rashes, exfoliative erythroderma, urticaria/angioedema, or hypersensitivity vascultitis
2. Injection site reaction
3. Pinnal dermatitis/otitis secondary to topical otic medications
4. Erythema multiforme (EM)
   a. May present with erythematous maculae or patches in various shapes, often with central clearing (bull's-eye appearance). Commonly seen on the ventrum.
5. Toxic epidermal necrolysis (TEN)
   a. Occurs very rarely
   b. Extensive necrosis and sloughing of the epidermis, which also predisposes the patient to sepsis
   c. EM or TEN may be triggered by factors other than drugs, including infections, systemic disease, neoplasia, vaccines, or adverse reactions to food; or may occur as an idiopathic immune-mediated dermatosis.
   iii. Diagnosis
1. History of recent medication use
2. Abatement of symptoms following drug withdrawal
3. Skin biopsies are indicated and may confirm the diagnosis.
   iv. Treatment
1. Discontinue use of prior drug(s).
   a. Often symptoms begin to subside within 1–2 weeks.
2. Avoid chemically similar drugs.
3. Severe EM or TEN requires intensive supportive care including fluid/nutritional support.
   a. Attempt to diagnose and treat an underlying cause of EM or TEN if a drug reaction is not suspected.
4. The use of glucocorticoids is controversial and may predispose to sepsis.
5. Chlorambucil (Leukeran) 0.1–0.2 mg/kg PO q24h or modified cyclosporine (Neoral or Atopica) 5 mg/kg PO q24h
   a. Both medications have been used with variable success.
6. Systemic antibiotics are used for secondary bacterial infections or suspected sepsis.
   a. If an antibiotic is suspected as causing a reaction, select an antibiotic from a different class.
   v. The prognosis is variable. Some drug reactions persist for days to weeks after the offending drug is withdrawn.
   i. Tapazole (methimazole) reaction
   i. Overview
1. Cutaneous adverse reactions to methimazole occur uncommonly.
2. When they occur, it is usually within 3–8 weeks of starting treatment.
3. The exact pathogenesis is currently unknown.
   ii. Clinical signs include facial and/or neck pruritus and self-induced trauma, which may lead to erythema, alopecia, excoriations, erosions, or ulcers and crusts.
   iii. Diagnosis
1. History of methimazole use
2. Presence of facial and/or neck pruritus or dermatitis
3. Rule out differential diagnoses
   a. Ectoparasites; allergies; bacterial, fungal, and viral infections; immune-mediated diseases; neoplastic diseases; and behavioral disorders
   b. Perform skin scrapings, skin and otic cytology, otic mite preps, and fungal culture.
4. Skin biopsies may help rule out differential diagnoses.
   iv. Treatment

        1. Requires cessation of methimazole treatment

           a. May occur with transdermal formulations of methimazole as well

        2. May be partially responsive to glucocorticoids at anti-inflammatory doses

    v. Prognosis

        1. Good to excellent for resolution of dermatologic signs when methimazole treatment is stopped

        2. Alternative therapy for hyperthyroidism is required.

  j. Feline acne

    i. Overview

        1. Thought to be a localized keratinization disorder of the hair follicles

        2. Poor grooming habits, production of abnormal sebum, stress, or other factors (allergies) may play a role in the pathogenesis.

        3. Commonly complicated by secondary bacterial infection

        4. Outbreaks have been seen in multiple-cat households and catteries, but attempts to isolate viral or other infectious causes have been unsuccessful.

    ii. Clinical signs

        1. The most commonly affected site is the chin, but lesions may also be seen on the lips.

        2. Lesions may include:

           a. Comedones, crusts, alopecia, erythema, papules, pustules, nodules/fistulae, chin swelling, or regional lymphadenopathy

           b. Pruritus is variable.

           c. Cysts and scarring may occur in chronic cases.

    iii. Diagnosis

        1. Often based on clinical appearance, but cytology, deep skin scrapings, and fungal cultures are needed to rule out differential diagnoses and to identify secondary or concurrent infections.

        2. Bacterial culture/sensitivity and skin biopsies are indicated in persistent, refractory, or unresponsive cases.

        3. Differential diagnoses include bacterial or fungal (yeast or dermatophytes) infections, demodicosis, eosinophilic granuloma (allergy), contact dermatitis, or idiopathic keratinization disorders.

    iv. Treatment

        1. Don't make the treatment worse than the disease, as some cats are asymptomatic or mildly affected.

        2. Avoid plastic food and water bowls; wash bowls daily.

        3. Mild cases

           a. Benign neglect if asymptomatic

           b. Wash affected areas 1–3 times per week with benzoyl peroxide, chlorhexidine-based, or sulfur-based (antiseborrheic) shampoos or wipes.

              i. Benzoyl peroxide may lead to overdrying.

        4. Moderately affected cases

           a. Mupirocin 2% ointment topically q12h × 3–6 weeks

           b. More frequent topical cleansing (frequency depends upon severity)

        5. Severe cases

           a. Sedate, clip, and gently scrub with chlorhexidene or benzoyl peroxide cleanser. Warm compress with magnesium sulfate (Epsom salt) solution (2 tbsp/quart or 30 mL/L water) for 5–10 minutes.

           b. Manually express comedones and cystic lesions.

           c. Topical mupirocin ointment or metronidazole gel

           d. Systemic antibiotics are indicated with pustules, furuncles, or when intracellular bacteria are seen on cytology.

              i. See "Flea allergy dermatitis."

  e. Instruct owners not to express lesions at home. That may lead to internal rupture of comedones and more inflammation.

 6. Daily oral fatty acid supplementation may benefit recurrent or persistent cases.

  a. Administer a supplement containing EPA (eicospentaenoic acid) at 180 mg EPA/10 pounds body weight/day either in capsule, liquid, or powder form.

 v. Prognosis

  1. Many affected cats have recurrent or persistent disease and require maintenance topical therapy on a twice weekly or more frequent basis.

k. Eosinophilic granuloma complex

 i. Overview and clinical signs

  1. See "Clinical signs," and "Diagnosis" above.

 ii. Diagnosis

  1. Often based upon clinical appearance

  2. Skin cytology

   a. Often reveals a predominance of eosinophils, but neutrophils or bacteria may be present as well

  3. Rule out ectoparasitic infection

   a. Trial of selamectin topically q 2 weeks for a minimum of three treatments.

   b. Trial of lime sulfur dips q 5–7 days for 4–6 treatments (to rule out *D. gatoi*).

  4. Skin biopsies may provide the final diagnosis and aid in ruling out differential diagnoses such as squamous cell carcinoma or other neoplasia or herpes viral dermatoses.

 iii. Treatment

  1. Treat ectoparasite and/or secondary bacterial infections.

  2. Anti-inflammatory doses of oral or injectable glucocorticoids can be very helpful in acute situations, but steroid therapy is not a replacement for the diagnosis and management of the underlying cause (see "Flea allergy dermatitis").

  3. Modified cyclosporine (Neoral or Atopica) 5–7.5 mg/kg PO q24h

   a. Treat daily × 4–6 wks and then taper over 2–4 months to lowest effective frequency.

Dermatologic history

Dermatologic exam

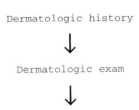

Initial dermatologic diagnostics: skin/ear cytology, flea combing, skin scrapings, trichograms, DTM (fungal) culture

If results are positive, treat with appropriate antimicrobials and/or antiparasitic medications; consider allergy workup/treatment.

If results are negative, consider antiparasitic treatment, allergy workup/treatment (rule out flea allergy first, then food allergy, then atopy), skin biopsies.

Fig. 38.11. General approach to the cat with skin disease: Algorithmic overview.

Table 38.1. Drug table.

Drugs	Classes	MOAs	Side Effects	Contraindications or Precautions	Routes of Administration and Doses	General Uses
Amoxicillin	Aminopenicillin antibiotic	Inhibits bacterial cell wall synthesis	GI side effects	Known hypersensitivity to beta-lactams	11–22 mg/kg PO or SQ q12h	Bite wound infections; not useful for staph pyoderma
Amoxicillin-clavulanate	Aminopenicillin antibiotic with beta-lactamase inhibitor	Inhibits bacterial cell wall synthesis	GI side effects	Known hypersensitivity to beta-lactams	13.75 mg/kg PO for bite wound infections, up to 22 mg/kg PO q12h for pyoderma	Bite wound infections; pyoderma
Cefadroxil	1st generation cephalosporin antibiotic	Inhibits bacterial cell wall synthesis	GI side effects	Known hypersensitivity to beta-lactams	20–22 mg/kg PO q12h × 3 wks minimum for pyoderma	Pyoderma, trauma to skin with secondary bacterial infection
Cefazolin	1st generation cephalosporin antibiotic	Inhibits bacterial cell wall synthesis	GI side effects	Known hypersensitivity to beta-lactams	22–30 mg/kg IV q12h × 3 wks minimum for pyoderma	Pyoderma, trauma to skin with secondary bacterial infection
Cefpodoxime	3rd generation cephalosporin antibiotic	Inhibits bacterial cell wall synthesis	GI side effects	Known hypersensitivity to beta-lactams, off-label use in cats	5–10 mg/kg PO q24h × 3 wks minimum for pyoderma	Pyoderma
Cephalexin	1st generation cephalosporin antibiotic	Inhibits bacterial cell wall synthesis	GI side effects	Known hypersensitivity to beta-lactams	22–30 mg/kg PO q12h × 3 wks minimum for pyoderma	Pyoderma, trauma to skin with secondary bacterial infection
Chlorambucil (Leukeran®)	Alkylating antineoplastic/immunosuppressive agent	Cross-links cellular DNA	GI side effects, myelosuppression	Known hypersensitivity; pre-existing bone marrow disease; infections; pregnancy	0.1–0.2 mg/kg PO q24–48h	Eosinophilic granuloma complex lesions, pemphigus foliaceus, erythema multiforme/cutaneous drug reactions

Drug	Class	Mechanism	Side effects	Contraindications/cautions	Dosage	Indications
Chlorpheniramine	Alkylamine antihistamine	H1-receptor antagonist	GI side effects, CNS depression, paradoxical excitement, anticholinergic effects	Known hypersensitivity; caution with hyperthyroidism or cardiovascular disease	2–4 mg/cat PO q12h	Atopy
Clindamycin	Lincosamide antibiotic	Inhibits bacterial peptide bond formation by binding to 50 S ribosomal subunit	GI side effects	Known hypersensitivity to clindamycin or lincomycin	5–11 mg/kg PO q12h or 11–22 mg/kg PO q24h × 3 wks minimum for pyoderma	Pyoderma, otitis media
Cyclosporine A (modified, Neoral® or Atopica®)	Immunosuppressant	Inhibits T cell activation by inhibiting calcineurin	GI side effects; hepatotoxicity or renal toxicity may occur at extremely high blood levels; hirsutism	Toxoplasmosis; several drug interactions; hepatic or renal disease; caution in cats with viral diseases	5–7.5 mg/kg PO q24h for allergies or eosinophilic granuloma complex lesions, 5 mg/kg PO q12–24h for immunosuppression (Atopica® is off-label in cats)	Allergies, eosinophilic granuloma complex lesions, erythema multiforme/cutaneous drug reactions, pemphigus foliaceus
Dexamethasone	Corticosteroid	Glucocorticoid activity	Polyuria, polydipsia, polyphagia, diarrhea, weight gain, iatrogenic hyperadrenocorticism, diabetes mellitus	Diabetes, severe cardiovascular disease, systemic fungal infection, viral infection, renal failure	0.2–0.4 mg/kg PO q24h initially, taper to alternate day or less frequent therapy; combine 2–3 mL injectable dexamethasone with 30 mL otic antimicrobial	Autoimmune disease, otitis externa
Enrofloxacin	Fluoroquinolone antibiotic	Inhibits bacterial DNA-gyrase	Potential cartilage abnormalities in young animals; ocular toxicity (blindness)	Known hypersensitivity to fluoroquinolones; caution in cats <1 year old; do not use >5 mg/kg; caution with known CNS disease; flavor tabs contain soy and pork	5 mg/kg PO q24h, or 10 mg/mL concentration in tris-EDTA as an otic antimicrobial	Pyoderma, resistant Pseudomonas otitis media

Table 38.1. Continued

Drugs	Classes	MOAs	Side Effects	Contraindications or Precautions	Routes of Administration and Doses	General Uses
Fipronil	Antiparasitic agent	Inhibits GABA-regulated chloride channels	Rarely irritation or alopecia at site of administration	Kittens <8 wks	Topically q 2–4 wks (off-label at >q 4 wk frequency)	Fleas, ticks
Griseofulvin	Fungistatic antibiotic	Arrests metaphase of cell division by disrupting structure of cell's mitotic spindle	GI side effects, bone marrow suppression, hepatotoxicity, photosensitivity	Known hypersensitivity; liver disease; FIV; pregnancy; kittens more sensitive to side effects	Fulvicin/GriFulvin (microsized) 50–120 mg/kg PO divided daily with fatty meal; Gris-PEG (ultramicrosized) 5–15 mg/kg PO divided twice daily	Dermatophytosis
Imidocloprid	Antiparasitic agent	Binds to nicotinic acetylcholine receptors	Rarely irritation or alopecia at site of administration	Kittens <8 wks	Topically q 1–4 wks	Fleas
Itraconazole	Triazole antifungal	Inhibits fungal cell membrane ergosterol synthesis	GI signs, rarely hepatotoxicity	Known hypersensitivity; hepatic disease; pregnancy	5–10 mg/kg PO q24h	Dermatophytosis
Ivermectin (injectable and Acarexx®)	Avermectin antiparasitic agent	Enhances release of GABA	Large safety margin in cats but neurotoxicity with massive overdoses have been reported	Age restrictions for cats not reported by manufacturers	200–400 µg/kg SQ or PO q 1–3 wks (off-label use as ectoparasiticide)	Otodectes, Notoedres, Cheyletiella, Demodicosis
Lime sulfur (LymDyp®)	Antimicrobial, antiparasitic	Unknown, thought to be combo of keratolytic effects and formation of miticidal chemicals	May stain light-colored coats, stains jewelry, unpleasant odor; salivation or vomiting if licked off hair coat	Apply E collar until dry to prevent licking	Dilute according to label; use as a dip every 5–7 days × 3–6 wks	Notoedres, Cheyletiella, Demodicosis, Dermatophytosis
Marbofloxacin	Fluoroquinolone antibiotic	Inhibits bacterial DNA-gyrase	Potential cartilage abnormalities in young animals; unknown ocular toxicity	Known hypersensitivity to fluoroquinolones; caution in cats <1 year old; caution with known CNS disease	2.2–5.5 mg/kg PO q24h	Pyoderma, otitis medis

Drug	Class	Mechanism	Side Effects	Contraindications	Dose	Indications
Methylprednisolone (Depo-medrol®)	Corticosteroid	Glucocorticoid activity	Polyuria, polydipsia, polyphagia, diarrhea, weight gain, iatrogenic hyperadrenocorticism, diabetes mellitus	Diabetes, severe cardiovascular disease, systemic fungal infection, viral infection, renal failure	5 mg/kg SQ or IM; do not repeat more frequently than q 2wks, check blood glucose prior to injection	Allergies, eosinophilic granuloma complex lesions, hypersensitivity reactions to mites, oral corticosteroids preferred for autoimmune diseases
Miconazole Conofite® or shampoo	Imidazole antifungal	Inhibits fungal cell membrane ergosterol synthesis	Topical contact reaction	Known hypersensitivity	3–4 drops into ear canal q12h × 14–30 days	Yeast (Malassezia) otitis externa
MilbeMite OTIC (milbemycin 0.1%)	Antiparasitic agent	Inhibits GABA	None reported; consider topical otic reaction	Kittens <4wks	1 tube topically in each ear canal, repeat in 3–4wks if needed	Ear mites
Mupirocin 2% ointment	Antibiotic ointment	Inhibits bacterial protein synthesis	Potential nephrotoxicity due to polyethylene glycol content of vehicle	Known sensitivity; avoid use on extensive deep lesions; limit ingestion by cats	Thin layer applied topically q12h × 3–6wks	Feline acne, localized bacterial skin infections
Nitenpyram (Capstar®)	Neonicotinoid anti-parasitic agent	Binds to nicotinic acetylcholine receptors	No serious side effects reported	Kittens <4wks and <2 lbs.	11.4 mg tablet PO once; repeat as needed	Immediate kill of adult fleas
Polymyxin B	Polypeptide antibiotic	Increases permeability of bacterial cell membrane	Potential ototoxicity	Known hypersensitivity	3–4 drops in ear canal q12h × at least 30 days	Resistant *Pseudomonas* otitis
Prednisolone	Corticosteroid	Glucocorticoid and mineralocorticoid activity	Polyuria, polydipsia, polyphagia, diarrhea, weight gain, iatrogenic hyperadrenocorticism, diabetes mellitus	Diabetes, severe cardiovascular disease, systemic fungal infection, viral infection, renal failure	1–4 mg/kg PO q12–24h, eventually taper (lower dose for anti-inflammatory effects, higher dose for immunosuppression)	Allergies, eosinophilic granuloma complex lesions, autoimmune disease (pemphigus)

Table 38.1. *Continued*

Drugs	Classes	MOAs	Side Effects	Contraindications or Precautions	Routes of Administration and Doses	General Uses
Otomax®/ Mometamax®	Otic product combining gentamicin, clotrimazole, and betamethasone or mometasone	Antibacterial, antifungal, and corticosteroid effects	Topical contact reaction	Known hypersensitivity	3–4 drops into ear canal q12h × 14–30 days	Bacterial +/− yeast otitis
Selamectin	Avermectin anti-parasitic agent	Enhances release of GABA	Rarely irritation or alopecia at site of administration	Kittens <8wks	Topically q 2–4wks (off-label at >q 4wk frequency)	Fleas, Otodectes, Notoedres, Sarcoptes, Cheyletiella
Silver sulfadiazine	Topical sulfonamide antibiotic	Prevent bacterial replication by interfering with folic acid synthesis	Topical irritation; rarely bone marrow, GI, liver, or renal toxicities if large amounts are absorbed	Known hypersensitivity to sulfonamides	Thin layer applied topically q12–24h; 1% solution or mixed 50:50 with water as an otic solution	Burns, ulcers, skin trauma, resistant otitis externa/media
Terbinafine	Allylamine antifungal	Inhibits fungal cell membrane ergosterol synthesis and inhibits fungal squalene metabolism	Limited reports in cats; consider GI side effects, neutropenia, hepatotoxicity, cutaneous drug reaction	Known hypersensitivity; hepatic or severe renal disease	30–40mg/kg PO q24h	Dermatophytosis

Tobramycin	Aminoglycoside antibiotic	Inhibits protein synthesis by binding 30s ribosomal subunit	Topical contact reaction, potential for ototoxicity	Known hypersensitivity	3–4 drops into ear canal q12h × at least 30 days (ophthalmic drops)	Resistant gram-negative bacterial otitis
Tresaderm®	Otic product combining neomycin, thiabendazole, and dexamethasone	Antibacterial, antifungal, and corticosteroid effects	Topical contact reaction, potential for ototoxicity	Known hypersensitivity	3–4 drops into ear canal q12h × 14–30 days	Bacterial +/− yeast otitis
Triamcinolone acetonide	Corticosteroid	Glucocorticoid activity	Polyuria, polydipsia, polyphagia, diarrhea, weight gain, iatrogenic hyperadrenocorticism, diabetes mellitus	Diabetes, severe cardiovascular disease, systemic fungal infection, viral infection, renal failure	0.4–0.8 mg/kg PO q24h, taper as soon as possible to alternate day then twice weekly therapy; 0.11–0.22 mg/kg PO may be used for atopy	Autoimmune disease (pemphigus), atopy
Tris-EDTA	Carrier vehicle or presoak ear wash	Tris = buffer, EDTA increases permeability and sensitization of gram-negative bacteria to antibiotics	Topical contact reaction	Known hypersensitivity	Fill ear canals with flush q12h prior to topical antibiotics or mix with injectable enrofloxacin (10mg/mL concentration)	Gram-negative bacterial otitis, especially resistant Pseudomonas

4. Chlorambucil (Leukeran) 0.1–0.2 mg/kg PO q24–48h may be useful in refractory cases.
5. Diagnose and manage the underlying allergic disease.
    a. Rule out a flea allergy with strict frequent flea control.
    b. Rule out a food allergy with a 10–12 week strict hydrolyzed (e.g., Hills Prescription Diet z/d Low Allergen Feline) or novel (e.g., Royal Canin Veterinary Diet [formerly IVD] Green Peas and Rabbit or Green Peas and Duck) protein diet trial.
    c. If signs persist or recur, pursue intradermal and/or serum allergy testing to formulate allergen-specific immunotherapy.
    d. Antihistamines (e.g., chlorpheniramine 2–4 mg PO q12h per cat) and oral fatty acid supplementation may help reduce the clinical signs of allergic dermatitis in some cats.

Recommended Reading

Campbell KL, guest ed. Updates in dermatology. Vet Clin North Am Sm Anim Pract, 2006; 36(1).

Greene. Infectious diseases of the dog and cat, 3rd ed. Philadelphia: Saunders, Elsevier, 2006.

Gross TL, Ihrke PJ, et al. Skin Diseases of the Dog and Cat: Clinical and Histopathologic Diagnosis, 2nd ed. Ames, Iowa: Blackwell, 2005.

Guaguère E, Prélaud P. A Practical Guide to Feline Dermatology. Oxford: Merial, 1999.

Matousek JL, guest ed. Ear disease. Vet Clin North Am Sm Anim Pract, 2004; 34(2).

Medleau L, Hnilica KA. Small Animal Dermatology: A Color Atlas and Therapeutic Guide, 2nd ed. St. Louis: Saunders, 2006.

Moriello K. Treatment of dermatophytosis in dogs and cats: review of published studies. Vet Derm, 2004; 15:99–107.

Preziosi DE. et al. Feline pemphigus foliaceus: a retrospective analysis of 57 cases. Vet Derm, 2003; 14:313–321.

Rhodes K. The 5-Minute Veterinary Consult Clinical Companion: Small Animal Dermatology. Philadelphia: Lippincott Williams & Wilkins, 2002.

Scott DW, Miller WH, Griffin CE. Muller & Kirk's Small Animal Dermatology, 6th ed. Philadelphia: W.B. Saunders, 2001.

Swaim SF, Henderson RA, Jr. Small Animal Wound Management, 2nd ed. Philadelphia: Williams & Wilkins, 1997.

White SD et al. Feline acne and results of treatment with mupirocin in an open clinical trial: 25 cases (1994–96). Vet Derm, 1997; 8:157–164.

39
TOXICOLOGICAL EMERGENCIES

Robert H. Poppenga

Unique Features
- Cats are potentially exposed to a wide variety of toxicants and are uniquely sensitive to several, including acetaminophen and pyrethrins.
- The incidence of intoxication in cats is low compared to dogs; this is likely due to their more discriminating palate.
- There are few specific antidotes for treating intoxicated cats.
- For the large majority of poisoning cases, timely decontamination and appropriate symptomatic and supportive care will greatly increase the chances of a favorable outcome.

1. Telephone triage
   a. The immediate aims of the initial telephone triage are to determine if the patient needs to be examined and what the owner can do for the pet.
   b. Animals with respiratory distress, neurologic abnormalities, protracted vomiting, slow or rapid heart rates, hemorrhage, weakness, or pale mucous membranes should be seen as soon as possible.
   c. If there is any question about poisoning, the animal should be evaluated.
   d. The owner should be instructed to bring any packages or material that the patient might have had access to, as well as any material the patient might have vomited. The material should be placed in a plastic bag or plastic or glass container for possible evaluation.
2. Home management
   a. In most instances, it is more efficient and safer to have the patient brought into the clinic rather than managed at home by the owner.
   b. Initial assessment of the poisoned cat involves applying the basic principles for assessment of emergency patients.
3. Diagnosis
   a. A working diagnosis is based on a history of witnessed exposure; characteristic, suggestive, or suspicious signs; and chemical analysis.
      i. Unfortunately, results from chemical analysis are generally not available quickly enough to influence initial case management.
   b. Intoxication with some chemicals causes a characteristic group of clinical signs called toxidromes that may narrow the list of differentials.

      i. Acetaminophen: depression, emesis, cyanosis, facial edema, tachycardia, tachypnea

      ii. Anticholinergics: agitation, dry mucous membranes, urinary retention, tachycardia, increased body temperature, mydriasis, decreased peristalsis

      iii. Cholinesterase inhibitors and cholinergics: DUMBELS—diarrhea, urination, miosis, bronchospasm, emesis, lacrimation, and salivation

      iv. Sympathomimetics: agitation, tremors, seizures, increased blood pressure, tachycardia, tachypnea, increased body temperature, mydriasis

  c. Although the majority of toxicants affect more than one organ system, identification of affected organ systems based upon clinical signs and early diagnostic testing can substantially narrow the differential list

  d. It is common for owners to think that their pets have been poisoned whenever they become sick. This can often be discounted based on detailed questioning of the owner.

4. Exposure assessment

  a. Proper exposure assessment is important to avoid unnecessary decontamination and/or treatment.

      i. Essential information includes identification of a chemical and its concentration (e.g., in a product), the amount of chemical/product ingested, the weight of the animal, and the toxicity of the chemical (e.g., an oral LD_{50}).

      ii. In many cases this information is not available.

      iii. Conservative estimates of exposure need to be made.

      iv. Toxicity information specific to cats is often unavailable, and information from other species needs to be extrapolated to cats.

        1. This can be problematic due to metabolic or other unique physiologic differences in cats.

  b. Sources of information

      i. National Animal Poison Control Center: 1 (900) 680-000 or 1 (800) 548-2423 (charge per case; credit cards only)

      ii. Regional human poison control centers

        1. Many human poison control centers accept calls related to animals.

        2. Useful for obtaining product and toxicity information

        3. Expertise to manage veterinary cases is variable

      iii. Web resources can be extremely valuable to obtain information regarding the identification of active ingredients and their toxicities.

5. General decontamination strategies

  a. Decrease further absorption

      i. Skin

        1. Bathe the cat with a mild pet shampoo or mild liquid dishwashing detergent. Patients with exposure to powder should have their hair coat combed or vacuemed if possible to remove significant amounts of the toxicant prior to bathing. Persons performing the vacuuming and/or bathing need to wear appropriate clothing and protective gear.

      ii. Eyes should be flushed with copious amounts of water if ocular exposure has occurred.

      iii. Gastrointestinal decontamination

        1. Induction of emesis

          a. Emesis should be considered if the toxin has been ingested within the last 1–2 hours.

            i. Beyond this time, it is likely that a significant amount of toxicant has either been absorbed or has moved farther down the GI tract. Some exceptions include large ingestions of tablets or capsules that may form concretions in the stomach or ingestion of toxicants that delay gastric emptying.

          b. Use of an emetic should be balanced with the resulting delay in ability to administer activated charcoal that their use causes.

          c. Toxicant ingestions often cause spontaneous vomiting. If this has occurred, induction of further vomiting is questionable.

Box 39.1.   Contraindications to the use of emetics.
- Prior, significant vomiting
- Respiratory distress
- Ingestion of corrosives (acids or alkalies)
- Ingestion of petroleum hydrocarbons
- Decreased or loss of gag reflex
- Seizures or the likelihood of the occurrence of seizures
- Extreme weakness
- CNS depression or coma
- Largyngeal paralysis
- Foreign body ingestion
- Ingestion of a known toxicant with a rapid onset of action that might compromise the airway or stimulate or depress the CNS

---

    d. The efficacy of emesis declines rapidly if ingestion has occurred less than 1 hour prior to induction.

    e. There are a number of contraindications to inducing emesis (see box 39.1)

    f. Emetics

       i. Syrup of ipecac (3.3 mL/kg diluted 1:1 with water to increase acceptability)

          1. Induces emesis by local irritation of gastric mucosa and activation of the chemo-receptor trigger zone

          2. Advantages—often available in the home, few side effects with single use

          3. Disadvantages—delayed onset of emesis (up to 30 minutes) or prolonged emesis (30–60 minutes)

          4. In-home use of syrup of ipecac has largely been abandoned in human medicine.

       ii. 3% hydrogen peroxide

          1. Induces emesis by local irritation of gastric mucosa at doses of 1–2 mL/kg

          2. Advantages—often available in the home, few side effects with 1–2 doses

          3. Disadvantages—inconsistent induction of emesis, often not readily acceptable by cat

       iii. Apomorphine

          1. Reputation for being contraindicated for use in cats due to adverse reactions; however, used successfully by many veterinarians

          2. Safe and effective emetic doses have not been firmly established for cats.

          3. CNS and respiratory depression can be reversed by naloxone but not the emetic effect.

       iv. Xylazine

          1. Injectable emetic of choice for cats

          2. Induces emesis through centrally mediated mechanisms

          3. Advantages: in cats (0.44 mg/kg IM), emesis is often rapid (3 to 5 minutes); can be reversed (yohimbine HCl at 0.5 mg/kg IV or atapamazole at 0.32 mg/kg IV).

          4. Disadvantages: sedation, decreased cardiac output and prolonged hypotension resulting in delay in administration of activated charcoal and/or oral antidotes and the absence of evidence that use of an emetic alters case outcome. Their use should be seriously questioned.

       v. Other possible emetics (e.g., table salt, liquid dishwashing detergent, etc.) should NEVER be used.

   2. Gastric lavage (GL)

   a. The main indication for GL is the presence of a contraindication to the use of an emetic.
   b. The efficacy of GL declines rapidly if ingestion has been >1 hour previously.
   c. Technique
      i.   Anesthesia sufficient to allow placement of an endotracheal tube. Close monitoring
           is essential.
      ii. End of endotracheal tube should be such that gastric contents cannot be accidentally
           aspirated.
      iii. Premeasure as large a bore stomach tube as possible from the tip of the nose to the
           end of the last rib.
      iv. Lubricate the tube with K-Y gel and gently pass down the esophagus into the
           stomach.
      v.   Ten to 20 mL of tepid normal saline or water should be administered through the
           stomach tube. The free end of the stomach tube is then lowered below the level of the
           stomach and placed into a container to allow gravity flow. Aspiration can be facilitated
           by use of an aspiration bulb or 60-mL syringe. Vigorous aspiration should be avoided.
      vi. Gentle manipulation of the stomach may assist with lavage fluid drainage.
      vii. Lavage should be repeated with the animal in different positions until the lavage fluid
           is visually clear of gastric contents.
      viii. Use of water has resulted in hyponatremia in human pediatric patients; for this reason
           use of normal saline is preferred.
      ix. In theory, mixing the lavage fluid with activated charcoal may enhance the effective-
           ness of GL, although this has not been verified.
      x.   The stomach tube should be kinked when removed to prevent any drainage of lavage
           fluid into the esophagus, oropharynx, or mouth.
      xi. The esophagus, oropharynx, and mouth should be suctioned to prevent aspiration
           of any remaining fluid.
3. Activated charcoal (AC)
   a. Effective adsorbent for many organic compounds
   b. Toxicants that are not well absorbed to AC include ethanol, methanol, ethylene glycol,
      isopropanol, and most metals.
   c. Standard dose is 1–4 g/kg body weight mixed in ~6 to 12 mL/kg water
   d. Some formulations contain sorbitol.
   e. May be given orally or via stomach tube following GL
   f. Multiple doses of activated charcoal are indicated when the ingested toxicant undergoes
      significant enterohepatic recirculation (if multiple doses of AC are administered, only one
      dose of a cathartic should be given).
      i.   AC should be given every 4 to 6 hours until there is a significant clinical improvement
           or AC is noted in the feces.
   g. The efficacy of activated charcoal declines with time after ingestion.
   h. Constipation or concretion formation are rarely reported side effects.
   i. AC can be very messy to administer.
   j. Owner should be advised that feces will be black for several days.
4. Cathartics
   a. Assist in hastening the elimination of ingested toxicants and AC-toxicant complexes from
      GI tract
   b. Administer orally or via stomach tube
      i.   Saccharide (sorbitol) and saline cathartics (sodium or magnesium sulfate) are most
           commonly used.
      ii. Sorbitol (70%)—1–3 mL/kg PO; often found in combination with AC
      iii. Sodium sulfate (Glauber's salt)—250–500 mg/kg mixed in 5–10 times as much water

> **Box 39.2.**   Contraindications to the use of cathartics.
> - Prior, significant diarrhea
> - Very young or very old patients
> - Patients with preexisting renal disease or known ingestion of nephrotoxicants
> - Patients with volume depletion
> - Hemodynamic instability
> - Existing GI pathology such as ileus, perforation, colitis, megacolon, hemorrhage, or obstruction
> - Recent GI surgery

    iv. Magnesium sulfate (Epsom's salt)—250–500 mg/kg mixed in 5–10 times as much water
  c. Contraindications to using cathartics are in box 39.2.
  d. There is no good evidence that the use of AC + cathartic is superior to the use of AC alone.
 5. Whole bowel irrigation
  a. Involves the use of large volumes of polyethylene glycol (PEG) isosmotic solution to flush the bowel and increase toxicant elimination.
  b. Concentration of PEG and electrolytes in solution causes no net absorption or secretion of ions so there are no significant changes in water or electrolyte balance.
  c. Potentially useful following ingestion of iron, lead, or zinc-containing materials
  d. Contraindicated in patients with bowel obstruction or perforations, ileus, hemodynamic instability, or compromised unprotected airways
  e. Technique has not been evaluated in veterinary patients. The need to administer large volumes of PEG solution complicates its use unless patient has an orogastric tube in place.
iv. Facilitating toxicant clearance (box 39.3)
 1. Diuresis
  a. The efficacy of forced diuresis by volume expansion with isotonic sodium-containing solutions such as 0.9% NaCl or lactated Ringer's solution has not been established and its routine use is not recommended.
  b. Complications of forced diuresis include hyponatremia, hypokalemia, fluid overload, pulmonary and/or cerebral edema, and alkalemia or acidemia depending on the agent used.
 2. Ion trapping
  a. Weak acids or weak bases can be ionized and therefore retained within renal tubules by increasing or decreasing urine pH, respectively.
  b. Urinary acidification should not be attempted due to possible complications and relative lack of efficacy.
  c. Urinary alkalinization (without forced diuresis) is only recommended to increase the clearance of salicylates.
   i. Alkalinization is achieved by the intravenous administration of sodium bicarbonate infused at 1–2 mEq/kg over 3–4 hours.
   ii. The goal is to achieve a urine pH of 7–8.
   iii. The more alkaline the urine (up to a pH of ~8), the greater the excretion.
 3. Other extracorporeal methods
  a. Although not widely available, hemodialysis and hemoperfusion are options at several veterinary hospitals.
   i. The relative efficacy of either technique is toxicant specific. Toxicant classes that are effectively removed either by hemodialysis or hemoperfusion include barbiturates,

---

Box 39.3. Decontamination procedures.
- Need to be matched to the individual patient's situation
- Few evidence-based studies in veterinary medicine to judge the efficacy of specific decontamination strategies
- With a few exceptions, the efficacy of emetic and AC +/– a cathartic declines with increasing time since ingestion.
- The efficacy of emetic + AC use compared to AC use alone has not been established.
- Facilitating clearance of absorbed toxicants can be useful for some toxicants.

Box 39.4. Acetaminophen.
- Decontamination strategy must balance potential efficacy with seriousness of presenting clinical signs.
- Respiratory signs are more life-threatening early compared to other species.
- Hepatotoxicity should not be overlooked.
- Early administration of NAC is critical to case outcome.

---

analgesics, nonbarbiturate hypnotics and tranquilizers, alcohols, paraquat, cardio-vascular drugs, antidepressants, methylxanthines, amanitin, PCBs, and some metals.
   b. Peritoneal dialysis can be used in lieu of hemodialysis.
4. Acetaminophen (box 39.4)
   a. Widely available analgesic and antipyretic
      i.   Formulations: capsules, tablets, chewable tablets, granules, liquids, powders, suspensions, suppositories
          1. Available in extended-release formulations
          2. Up to 650-mg strengths
          3. Often found in combination with other drugs
   b. Toxicity
      i.   Cats: typically 50–100 mg/kg is toxic, although doses as low as 10 mg/kg may be associated with signs.
   c. Relevant kinetics
      i.   Rapid absorption
      ii. Rapid metabolism in liver by glucuronidation and sulfation
          1. Cats have low UDP-glucuronosyltransferase activity and thus have diminished ability to conjugate acetaminophen
      iii. Liver metabolism results in the formation of N-acetyl benzoquinoneimine (NAPQI)
          1. NAPQI is detoxified via glutathione conjugation.
          2. Overdoses cause glutathione depletion, thus preventing NAPQI detoxification.
   d. Mechanism of action
      i.   Unconjugated NAPQI is electrophilic and combines with numerous proteins.
      ii. Damage to proteins, including structural and regulatory proteins and numerous enzymes, disrupts hepatocellular function.
      iii. Decreased glutathione increases susceptibility of cells to oxidative damage.
          1. Sensitivity of feline red blood cells to oxidative damage results in oxidation of hemoglobin to methemoglobin.
   e. Clinical signs
      i.   Acute signs in cats are less commonly associated with hepatic injury than for other species.

           1. Cyanotic or muddy mucous membranes, methemoglobinemia, respiratory distress, open-mouth breathing, anxiety, edema of face and paws, depression, hypothermia, vomiting

           2. Hepatotoxicity more common with higher doses and in male cats

           3. Methemoglobinemia imparts a brownish color to blood image

      ii. Clinical pathology: methemoglobinemia, anemia, hemoglobinemia, hemoglobinuria, ↑ ALT and AST, and bilirubinemia

           1. Later hepatic failure may result in coagulopathy with ↑ PT and APTT

   f. Diagnosis

      i. Often relies on history of exposure and occurrence of typical signs

      ii. Plasma, serum, and urine can be tested for presence of acetaminophen

           1. Test results are not rapidly available to assist in case management

   g. Treatment

      i. Stabilize vital signs

           1. Supplemental oxygen

      ii. Appropriate decontamination should be considered.

           1. Weigh risk of handling hypoxic animal with likely efficacy of decontamination procedures

      iii. N-acetylcysteine (NAC) is "antidotal"

           1. Provides cysteine, which is the rate-limiting amino acid for glutathione production.

           2. Available as 10% or 20% sterile solution (Mucomyst)

           3. Also available in a 200 mg/mL product (Acetadote) marketed specifically as an antidote to acetaminophen intoxication

           4. Administer undiluted or diluted in a 5% dextrose solution.

             a. Loading dose: 140 mg/kg IV or PO (IV administration preferred if the cat is vomiting)

             b. Maintenance dose: 70 mg/kg IV or PO q6h for 5–7 treatments

           5. Studies have shown that NAC is still efficacious when given PO at recommended doses following AC administration despite adsorption to AC

      iv. Efficacy of other sulfur donors (SAMe), antioxidants (ascorbic acid), or P-450 inhibitors (cimetidine) is unknown and should not substitute for NAC administration.

           1. SAMe administered at 180 mg PO g12h for 3 days followed by 90 mg PO q12h for 14 days has shown protective effects in cats.

      v. Early treatment is critical to survival.

7. Amphetamines

  a. There are a number of prescription, OTC, and illicit amphetamine compounds.

    i. Prescription amphetamines are used to treat obesity, narcolepsy, and attention deficit–hyperactivity disorder.

      1. Examples include methylphenidate, phendimetrazine, and sibutramine, among others

    ii. OTC drugs include phenylpropanolamine and pseudoephedrine.

    iii. Illicit amphetamines include methamphetamine and a variety of "designer" drugs (MDMA, MDEA).

  b. Toxicity

    i. An oral LD_{50} for amphetamine sulfate and methamphetamine chloride for dogs is 20–27 mg/kg and 9–11 mg/kg, respectively. Toxicity is unknown for cats.

  c. Relevant kinetics

    i. Well absorbed following oral exposure

    ii. Sustained release formulations have slower absorption rate

    iii. Undergo liver metabolism and are eliminated via the kidneys

   d. Mechanism of toxic action
      i.   Not known with certainty; sympathomimetic effect via release of catecholamines such as nor-
           epinephrine or direct stimulation of α- and β-adrenergic receptors
   e. Clinical signs
      i.   Hyperactivity, restlessness, mydriasis, hypersalivation, vocalization, tachypnea, tremors, hyper-
           thermia, ataxia, seizures, and tachycardia. Some animals may be depressed, weak, and
           bradycardic.
   f. Diagnosis
      i.   Possible confirmation via testing of blood or urine (testing not widely available from veterinary
           diagnostic laboratories; human drug testing laboratories are more likely to be of assistance)
   g. Treatment
      i.   Decontamination protocol if deemed appropriate
      ii. Control seizures with diazepam or midolazepam (0.5–1 mg/kg IV)
           1. Benzodiazepines may exacerbate neurologic effects.
              a. Chlorpromazine (10–18 mg/kg IV) may be effective.
      iii. Control hyperthermia.
      iv. Tachycardias respond to β-blockers such as propanolol.
8. Anticoagulant rodenticides (box 39.5)
   a. Most common type of rodenticide in use and widely available
   b. First-generation anticoagulant rodenticides include warfarin, diphacinone, and chlorophacinone.
      i.   Warfarin is not commonly used due to rodent resistance.
   c. Second-generation anticoagulant rodenticides (those effective against warfarin-resistant rats) include
      brodifacoum and bromodiolone.
   d. Available in a variety of formulations, including pellets, wax blocks, and tracking powders
   e. Secondary intoxication via ingestion of poisoned rodents is possible with the second-generation
      compounds, although there are no documented cases involving cats.
   f. Relevant kinetics
      i.   Readily absorbed with high-protein binding
      ii. Variable half-lives, with second-generation anticoagulants having prolonged half-lives
   g. Toxicity
      i.   Not well defined in cats; based on limited toxicity information, cats are less sensitive than dogs.
      ii. Acute oral LD_{50}s for warfarin, bromodiolone, diphacinone, and brodifacoum are 5–30 mg/kg,
           >25 mg/kg, 15 mg/kg, and 25 mg/kg, respectively.
   h. Mechanism of toxic action
      i.   Blocks vitamin K_1-dependent clotting factor synthesis by inhibiting vitamin K_1 epoxide
           reductase
           1. Prevents the recycling of vitamin K_1 from inactive to active form
           2. Affects clotting factors II, VII, IX, and X
           3. Intrinsic, extrinsic, and common pathways are affected.

Box 39.5. Anticoagulant rodenticides.
- Intoxication is uncommon in cats.
- Intoxication most often associated with hemorrhage into body cavities.
- Atypical clinical signs can occur if hemorrhage occurs within organs such as 4. the brain, joints, or
  pericardial sac.
- Vitamin K_1 is antidotal but takes time for active clotting factors to become available (12 to 36 hours).
- FFP +/– whole blood provides clotting factors immediately.
- Monitoring PT after cessation of vitamin K_1 therapy is important to avoid a relapse.

i. Clinical signs

    i. Onset of clinical signs is delayed for 3–5 days after ingestion due to lag time in consumption of active clotting factors.

        1. Clotting factor VII has the shortest half-life and is therefore the first factor to be affected.

    ii. Initially, clinical signs can be vague and include lethargy, weakness, and anorexia. More significant signs include dyspnea, epistaxis, hemoptysis, hematoma formation, bleeding into body cavities, melena, hematuria, and gingival bleeding. Other signs can include coughing, pallor, emesis, lameness, ecchymoses or skin bruising, acute collapse, acute upper airway obstruction, uterine bleeding, seizures, abdominal distention, and pain.

        1. Localized hemorrhage into joints, the brain, or pericardial sac many manifest as atypical signs

    iii. Radiographs may show pleural effusions or loss of abdominal detail.

        1. Thoraco- or abdominocentesis produces frank blood with a high hematocrit that does not clot.

j. Diagnosis

    i. Clotting time abnormalities

        1. One-stage prothrombin (OSPT) time is prolonged first.

        2. Often, by the time of presentation, OSPT, activated partial thromboplastin time (APTT), and activated clotting times (ACT) are all prolonged.

        3. The PIVKA (proteins induced by vitamin k antagonists) test is also abnormal.

    ii. Detection of specific anticoagulant rodenticides is widely available for serum or whole blood, although it may take several days to receive results.

k. Treatment

    i. If the animal has been exposed to a potentially toxic amount of rodenticide but is not showing clinical signs and if the animal is presented soon after ingestion, decontamination should be considered.

    ii. If decontamination is performed or if the animal is presented well after the exposure (too late for decontamination to be performed), either clotting times are monitored and vitamin K_1 therapy instituted if they become prolonged, or prophylactic vitamin K_1 is administered (1.5–5 mg/kg PO q12h for 2–4 weeks).

    iii. If the animal is showing clinical signs, the first concern is to stabilize the patient (e.g., thoracocentesis to improve respiration).

        1. Vitamin K_1 therapy should be instituted (1.5–5 mg/kg PO or SQ q12h) and consideration should be given to administering fresh frozen plasma (FFP) +/– whole blood, depending on the animal's condition.

            a. IM or IV administration of vitamin K_1 is generally not recommended (IV administration can be associated with anaphylactic reactions and IM administration can cause painful hematomas).

            b. Administration of FFP instantly provides active clotting factors, whereas following only vitamin K_1 administration, there will be a delay in formation of active clotting factors for 2–4 weeks.

        2. Once patients are stable and clotting times have returned to normal, oral vitamin K_1 can be started in lieu of continued parenteral administration.

        3. Vitamin K_1 therapy may be needed for several weeks following intoxication with second-generation rodenticides due to their prolonged half-lives.

        4. Clotting times should be monitored for up to 96 hours after cessation of vitamin K_1 treatment to avoid a relapse.

        5. If a queen is lactating, kittens should be weaned early and started on vitamin K_1.

        6. Pregnant queens should be treated as above with vitamin K_1 until queening occurs; consideration should be given to providing vitamin K_1 to neonates.

9. Boric acid/borates

a. Boric acid is used in medical, household, and industrial settings.
  i. Household products that can contain boric acid/borates include medicated powders, skin lotions, mouthwash, toothpaste, topical astringents, and eyewashes.
  ii. Boric acid is commonly used for the control of ants, roaches, and flies.
    1. Insecticide formulations can contain 90% or greater concentrations of boric acid.
    2. Formulations include powders, granules, and gels
b. Toxicity
  i. Relatively nontoxic, but concentrated formulations increase risk.
  ii. No toxicity information specific to cats; nontoxic oral doses in dogs reported to be 1 to 3 g/kg.
c. Relevant kinetics
  i. Readily absorbed across mucosal surfaces, abraded skin and from the GI tract
  ii. Relatively short (hours) half-life expected, although cat-specific data is lacking
  iii. Eliminated unchanged via kidneys
d. Mechanism of action
  i. Unknown
e. Clinical signs
  i. Blue-green emesis and diarrhea, ptyalism, abdominal pain, ataxia, hyperesthesia, seizures, coma, tremors, muscle weakness, metabolic acidosis, erythroderma, desquamation and erosion of mucosal surfaces, shock, DIC, mild hyperthermia, and renal impairment.
f. Diagnosis
  i. Measurement of serum boric acid concentrations can confirm exposure.
    1. Serum boric acid concentrations do not correlate well with severity of intoxication.
    2. Acute, fatal human pediatric intoxications had serum boric acid concentrations ranging from 2 to 160 mg/dL.
g. Treatment
  i. Decontamination
    1. Spontaneous emesis and diarrhea often preclude use of emetics or cathartics.
    2. Boric acid is not effectively adsorbed by activated charcoal.
    3. Hemodialysis or exchange transfusions have been used in human neonates.
    4. Wash skin with warm, soapy water.
    5. Efficacy of induced diuresis is unknown.
  ii. Fluid support
  iii. Diuresis may enhance clearance
  iv. Acid-base monitoring and correction of abnormalities
  v. Antiemetics
  vi. Oral gastrointestinal protectants once vomiting is controlled
10. Bromethalin (box 39.6)
  a. Neurotoxic rodenticide
    i. Formulations: grain or all-weather (paraffin) baits, bulk pellets, or concentrated solutions
  b. Toxicity
    i. Cats appear to be one of the more sensitive species; 0.54 mg/kg is an oral LD_{50} for powdered bromethalin bait.
      1. Minimum oral toxic dose is 0.3 mg/kg
  c. Relevant kinetics
    i. Rapid absorption
      1. Peak plasma concentrations reached within 4 hours
    ii. Rapid hepatic metabolism to toxic metabolite (desmethyl bromethalin)
    iii. Significant elimination via the bile with possible enterohepatic recirculation
  d. Mechanism of toxic action
    i. Uncouples oxidative phosphorylation, which reduces ATP production

> **Box 39.6.** Bromethalin.
> - Rodenticide that is used much less frequently than anticoagulants
> - Neurotoxic
> - Clinical signs are somewhat dependent on the amount ingested.
> - Treatment goal is to decrease cerebral edema.
> - Prognosis is poor in symptomatic animals.

       1. Reduced ATP-dependent sodium-potassium pumps

       2. Movement of fluid into myelinated regions of the brain and spinal cord

       3. Increased cerebral lipid peroxidation

e. Clinical signs

    i. Onset usually within 12–24 hours of ingestion, but can be as soon as 2 hours with large ingestions

       1. Can be a delayed onset of clinical signs following exposure; 0.54 mg/kg ingestion resulted in signs occurring after 2–7 days

    ii. Signs can be quite variable and are somewhat dose dependent.

    iii. Higher doses: severe muscle tremors, hyperexcitability, hyperthermia, running fits, hyperesthesia, and focal motor and/or generalized muscle tremors that may be exacerbated by light or noise

    iv. Lower doses: hind limb ataxia, paresis, patellar hyperreflexia, upper motor neuron bladder paralysis, loss of conscious proprioception leading to paralysis and loss of deep pain, and CNS depression

    v. Abdominal distention occasionally observed in cats

    vi. Decerebrate posture terminally

    vii. Increased CSF pressure manifested as papilloedema, abnormal pulsing of retinal vessels, depression, stupor or coma, and elevated blood pressure with bradycardia

    viii. EEG changes: increase spike and spike-and-wave activity associated with an irritative or seizure focus, marked voltage depression consistent with cerebral hypoxia, and abnormal high-voltage, and slow-wave activities consistent with cerebral edema.

    ix. Other signs: emesis, abnormal postures (Schiff-Sherrington syndrome) and forelimb extensor rigidity, opisthotonus, and fine muscle tremors

f. Diagnosis

    i. Detection of bromethalin in serum or plasma

g. Treatment

    i. Delay in onset of clinical signs may necessitate extended observation.

    ii. Decontamination

       1. Emesis

       2. Gastric lavage if emesis is contraindicated

       3. Activated charcoal + cathartic

          a. Multiple-dose AC indicated due to likely enterohepatic recirculation

          b. Avoid magnesium-containing cathartics.

          c. Avoid cathartics if ileus is present.

    iii. Control seizures and severe muscle tremors, keeping in mind that severe CNS depression and coma often occur at later times.

       1. Diazepam, 1–2 mg/kg IV as needed

       2. Phenobarbital, 5–15 mg/kg as needed

    iv. Control cerebral edema (see chaps. 25 and 26).

       1. Mannitol, 0.5 g/kg IV over 20 minutes; repeated doses are likely to be needed.

      2. Furosemide, 1 mg/kg IV

      3. Dexamethasone, 2 mg/kg every 6 hours IV

      4. Use colloids to avoid excessive amounts of crystalloid fluids.

    v.   Maintain hydration and electrolyte balance.

    vi. Prolonged recovery with associated anorexia will likely necessitate nutritional support.

    vii. Poor prognosis

11. Bufo toads (box 39.7)

    a. There are two species of poisonous Bufo toads: *B. marinus* (FL and HI) and *B. alvarius* (desert S.W. U.S.).

    b. Toxins are contained in parotid glands and are secreted when the toad is disturbed.

    c. Dogs are more commonly affected than cats.

    d. Relevant kinetics

      i. Toxins are readily absorbed across mucous membranes of the oral cavity.

    e. Toxicity

      i.   *B. marinus* is more toxic than *B. alvarius*.

      ii. Larger toads produce more secretions from parotid gland.

      iii. As little as 1 mL secretions per kg can cause clinical signs.

    f. Mechanism of toxic action

      i.   Secretion is a complex mixture containing dopamine, catecholamines, and a variety of bufotoxins that have digitalis-like effects.

      ii. Bufotoxins such as the bufogenins inhibit potassium-dependent ATPases, resulting in alterations of sodium and potassium transport across cell membranes.

      iii. Some bufotoxins have vasopressor and hallucinogenic effects.

    g. Clinical signs

      i.   Brick-red mucous membranes, hypersalivation, pawing at the mouth, vocalizing, restlessness, disorientation, circling, stumbling and falling, blank stares, tachypnea, opisthotonus, seizures, hyperthermia, and coma

      ii. Cardiac arrhythmias: range from bradycardia, heart block, ventricular tachycardia, and ventricular fibrillation

    h. Treatment

      i.   The mouth should be flushed copiously (2–3 times for 5–10 minutes at a time) with water as soon as possible following exposure.

      ii. Control seizures

        1. Diazepam or midazolam boluses (0.2–1 mg/kg IV) or phenobarbital (4 mg/kg IV q6–12h)

      iii. Control hyperthermia.

      iv. Monitor ECG for arrhythmias and treat accordingly (see chap. 17).

        1. Bradycardia or heart block: atropine (0.02 mg/kg IV as needed)

        2. Tachycardia: beta-blockers

Box 39.7. Bufo toads.
- Toxicity not well defined for cats
- Intoxication generally as a result of mouthing the toads
- Initial clinical signs include red mucous membranes, salivation, and pawing at the mouth; cardiac arrhythmias are the most serious clinical signs.
- Initial decontamination includes thorough flushing of the mouth.
- Treatment is symptomatic, with correction of arrhythmias and amelioration of nervous system signs most important.
- Prognosis is good.

a. Propanolol (0.5–2 mg/kg IV, followed by CRI of 0.02–0.06 mg/kg/min)

b. Esmolol (0.5 mg/kg IV, followed by CRI of 50–200 μg/kg/min)

3. Ventricular tachycardias

a. 0.25–0.5 mg/kg IV (over 1 minute); CRI at 10–20 μg/kg/min—lower dose compared to dogs because cats are sensitive to the toxic effects of lidocaine)

b. Procainaminde (1–2 mg/kg IV (over 1 minute); CRI: 10–20 μg/kg/min CRI

c. If ventricular arrhythmias are refractory, check serum Mg concentration, and if low use magnesium sulfate (0.15–0.3 mEq/kg IV given over 5–10 minutes).

v. Digoxin-specific Fab fragments might be effective, but efficacy and doses have not been established.

vi. If neurologic condition deteriorates, consider prednisolone sodium succinate or methylprednisolone (10–20 mg/kg given slowly IV).

vii. Lactated Ringer's at maintenance doses of 60 mL/kg/day

12. Calcium channel blockers

a. Examples include verapamil, diltiazem, nifedipine, and nimodipine

b. Relevant kinetics

i. Rapid absorption

c. Toxicity

i. Unknown in cats; therapeutic index in people is only 2–3.

ii. One case of verapamil intoxication of a cat reported an oral dose of 14.5 mg/kg associated with clinical signs.

d. Mechanism of toxic action

i. Prevent the opening of voltage-gated calcium channels (L-type), thus slowing calcium influx and inhibiting calcium-dependent processes in cardiac cells.

d. Clinical signs

i. Nausea, emesis, disorientation, bradycardia, hypotension, and loss of consciousness

e. Treatment

i. Decontamination protocol if deemed appropriate

1. If sustained release medication, multiple-dose AC is warranted

ii. Monitor ECG

iii. Correct hypotension

1. Fluids IV

2. Administer calcium as calcium chloride (0.1–0.3 mg/kg IV slowly of 100 mg/mL solution) or calcium gluconate (0.5–1.5 mL/mg IV slowly of 100 mg/mL solution).

3. Refractory hypotension can be treated with glucagon (recommended dose for dogs is 70 μg/kg/min IV), isoproterenol (0.01–0.2 mg/kg/min CRI), or vasopressors (e.g., dopamine 2–10 μg/kg/min IV infusion).

4. In humans, severe intoxication with calcium channel blockers has been treated effectively with hyperinsulinemia plus euglycemia therapy.

a. Insulin has positive inotropic effects.

b. In human intoxications (based upon studies in dogs), dextrose is given as an initial bolus of 0.5–1 g/kg followed by a dextrose infusion of 0.25–0.5 g/kg/h. This is followed by an initial insulin bolus of 0.1 U/kg followed by an insulin infusion at the rate of 0.5 U/kg/h, which should be increased if no hemodynamic response is noted within 1 hour.

c. Increases need to be done in a stepwise manner along with increases in the dextrose infusion rate to maintain a euglycemic state.

d. Serum glucose concentrations need to be monitored closely during therapy and for several hours after cessation of therapy.

13. Carbon monoxide (box 39.8)

a. Results from the incomplete combustion of hydrocarbons

Box 39.8. Carbon monoxide.
- Recognition of intoxication is often difficult since the gas is colorless and odorless, and bright red mucous membrane color is uncommon.
- Carboxyhemoglobin can be measured by co-oximetry, but pulse oximeters do not differentiate carboxyhemoglobin and oxyhemoglobin.
- Oxygen therapy is primary treatment.
- Fetal hemoglobin has greater affinity for CO than maternal hemoglobin.

---

    i. Automobile exhaust, propane-powered engines (e.g., forklifts, chainsaws), portable generators, kerosene heaters, gas log fireplaces, smoke inhalation, and gas furnaces or appliances
    ii. CO is clear, odorless, and nonirritating.
  b. Relevant kinetics
    i. CO is absorbed from the lungs at a rate proportional to the respiratory exchange rate.
    ii. Approximate half-life of CO in room air is 4 hours.
  c. Toxicity
    i. Lethal concentration is 1,000 ppm (0.1%) with a 1-hour exposure.
  d. Mechanism of toxic action
    i. CO combines with hemoglobin to form carboxyhemoglobin.
    ii. Reduces availability of oxygen to tissues
      1. Direct combination with hemoglobin (displacing O)
      2. Decreases release of O from remaining carboxyhemoglobin sites
    iii. Tissue hypoxia and anoxia occurs.
    iv. Binding to myoglobin may be responsible for cardiac arrhythmias, ischemia, and hypotension.
    v. Binding to cytochrome oxidase may be the initiating event that leads to CNS ischemic reperfusion injury and delayed neuronal death.
  e. Clinical signs
    i. Nausea, emesis, ataxia, tachypnea, dyspnea, tachycardia, syncope, hypotension, weakness, lactic acidosis, seizures, pulmonary edema, and coma
    ii. ECG: PVCs, atrial fibrillation, and heart block
    iii. Intoxicated animals seldom display characteristic bright red gums or blood.
  f. Diagnosis
    i. Measure arterial carboxyhemoglobin
      1. Carboxyhemoglobin absorbs light at the same wavelength as oxyhemoglobin, so pulse oximeters can give a falsely elevated or normal oxyhemoglobin saturation level.
      2. Co-oximetry on arterial blood samples directly measures oxy- and carboxyhemoglobin percent.
      3. Carboxyhemoglobin concentrations do not correlate well with severity of intoxication.
    ii. Diagnosis often relies on the history, clinical signs, and response to oxygen administration.
  g. Treatment
    i. 100% oxygen via endotracheal tube, oxygen cage, or mask
      1. Half-life of CO with 100% O_2 is approximately 1 hour compared to 4 hours with ambient air.
      2. Continue treatment until the patient is asymptomatic.
    ii. Monitor cardiac function and correct arrhythmias.
    iii. Correct hypotension.
    iv. Use of bicarbonate to treat acidemia is controversial since it can exacerbate cellular hypoxia secondary to a left shift of the oxyhemoglobin dissociation curve.
    v. Fetal hemoglobin has a greater affinity for CO than does maternal hemoglobin.

   1. Symptomatic pregnant animals should be maintained on 100% O_2 for approximately 5x the length of time it requires for maternal symptoms to resolve.
   2. CO exposure can increase the incidence of stillbirths.
   3. CO is a known teratogen, causing limb and cranial deformities.
14. Cholecalciferol (vitamin D) and analogues (box 39.9)
   a. Cholecalciferol is used as a rodenticide (0.075%) and can be found in dietary supplements; vitamin D analogs such as calcipotriene and calcipotriol are found in human medications.
   b. Relevant kinetics
      i. Following ingestion, cholecalciferol is rapidly absorbed and transported to the liver, where it is metabolized to 25-(OH)-cholecalciferol, which is further metabolized by the kidneys to 1,25-$(OH)_2$-cholecalciferol (calcitriol) and 24,25-$(OH)_2$-cholecalciferol. Calcitriol is the principal active form and is tightly regulated.
      ii. Half-lives of cholecalciferol, 25-(OH)-cholecalciferol, and calcitriol are believed to be months, days, and hours, respectively.
      iii. Elimination is primarily via bile and feces.
   c. Toxicity
      i. Cats are more sensitive with lethal doses of 5–10 mg/kg of cholecalciferol.
      ii. Calcitriol is much more toxic (toxic doses in dogs of 50 μg/kg)
   d. Mechanism of toxic action
      i. Increases calcium and phosphorus absorption from the GI tract
      ii. Increases calcium and phosphorus reabsorption from the kidneys
      iii. Mobilizes calcium from bones
      iv. Causes increases in total and ionized calcium and metastatic tissue mineralization
   e. Clinical signs
      i. Result from hypercalcemia
      ii. Signs related to effects on CNS, muscles, GI tract, cardiovascular system, and kidneys
         1. Depression, weakness, anorexia, emesis, polyuria, polydipsia, constipation, dehydration, melena, hematemesis, altered ECG (shortened QT and prolonged PR intervals), bradycardia, seizures, shock, coma, and death
         2. Increased total and ionized serum calcium concentrations, increased BUN and creatinine, hyperphosphatemia, and decreased intact PTH
         3. Radiographs may show metastatic tissue calcification of soft tissues and bronchi.
   f. Diagnosis
      i. History of ingestion, increased total and ionized calcium, increased serum concentrations of 25-(OH)-cholecalciferol, and decreased intact PTH
   g. Treatment
      i. General decontamination procedures if presented early

---

Box 39.9. Cholecalciferol and analogues.
- Vitamin D analogues used in human medicine are much more toxic than cholecalciferol rodenticide.
- Cholecalciferol has to be metabolized to active form of vitamin D to cause hypercalcemia.
- Hypercalcemia from increased absorption from GI tract, reabsorption from kidneys, and bone resorption
- Multiple treatment interventions to try to lower hypercalcemia: diuresis, furosemide, corticosteroids, and calcitonin or pamidronate
- Pamidronate preferred over calcitonin
- 25-OH cholecalciferol has a long half-life, which can result in need for prolonged treatment.

      ii. Reduce serum calcium concentrations
         1. Normal saline diuresis (4–6 mL/kg/h or above)
         2. Furosemide (2–5 mg/kg IV q8–12h)
         3. Prednisolone (0.5 mg/kg PO, SQ, IM q12h)
         4. Salmon calcitonin (4 to 6 IU/kg SQ q2–3h)
            a. Since this is a foreign protein, pre-evaluation with an intradermal skin test is recommended.
         5. Biphosphonates may be better than salmon calcitonin
            a. Pamidronate disodium (1.3–2 mg/kg in 0.9% sodium chloride slow IV over 2–4 hours. Another infusion may be needed.)
      iii. Monitor serum and ionized calcium concentrations every 24–48 hours to monitor effectiveness of therapy. Monitoring should continue for up to 6 days after cessation of therapy.
      iv. Minimize dietary calcium intake.
      v. Antiemetics such as metaclopramide (0.2–0.5 mg/kg IM or IV q4–6h)
      vi. Gastric mucosal protectants such as sucralfate (0.25 g PO q8–12h)
15. Cholinesterase-inhibiting insecticides (organophosphorus and carbamate insecticides) (box 39.10)
    a. Although commonly used in agricultural settings, their use on animals or in home or garden environments has declined significantly.
    b. Cats and younger animals more commonly affected
    c. Relevant kinetics
      i. Good absorption via all routes of exposure
      ii. Bioactivation of some organophosphorus insecticides is required for toxicity.
    d. Toxicity
      i. Quite variable—LD_{50}s from the low mg/kg range to nearly 1,000 mg/kg; most that are found in home or garden environments are moderately toxic (i.e., LD_{50}s of several hundred mg/kg).
    e. Mechanism of toxic action
      i. Inhibition of cholinesterase enzymes (specific inhibition of acetylcholinesterase) is responsible for clinical signs.
      ii. Acetylcholine is a neurotransmitter at several sites, including autonomic ganglia of both sympathetic and parasympathetic nervous systems, between postganglionic parasympathetic nerve fibers and cardiac muscle, smooth muscle and exocrine glands, at neuromuscular junctions of the somatic nervous system, and at cholinergic synapses in the CNS. Increased acetylcholine at these sites is the cause of clinical signs (see fig. 39.1).
      iii. Cholinesterase enzyme binding is irreversible with organophosphorus insecticides but reversible with carbamates. This accounts for the delayed recovery following organophosphorus insecticide exposure.

Box 39.10. Cholinesterase-inhibiting insecticides (organophosphorus and carbamate insecticides).
- Intoxications are less frequent as many have been removed from the market and have been replaced by safer insecticides.
- Acute signs are related to muscarinic and nicotinic receptor stimulation.
- An intermediate syndrome has been described in cats.
- Atropine reverses muscarinic signs, and early administration (even before decontamination) can be life-saving.
- Atropine is combined with 2-PAM for OP intoxications, whereas 2-PAM is not needed for carbamate intoxications.
- Recovery from carbamate intoxication is generally much more rapid than that following OP intoxication.

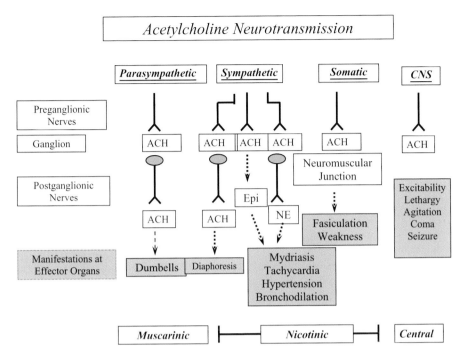

Fig. 39.1.   Acetylcholine neurotransmission.

    iv.   Death is most often due to hypoxia secondary to bronchial secretions and respiratory muscle paralysis.

f. Clinical signs

    i.   Onset is often rapid.

    ii.   Onset may be delayed in cats dermally exposed to chlorpyrifos (an OP insecticide).

    iii.   Acetylcholine receptors are classified as muscarinic or nicotinic; clinical signs can be variable due to which receptors are stimulated and to what degree.

    iv.   Signs secondary to muscarinic receptor stimulation include hypersalivation, lacrimation, urination, defecation, increased respiratory sounds, respiratory distress, bradycardia (although tachycardia can occur), and miosis.

    v.   Signs secondary to nicotinic receptor stimulation include skeletal muscle stiffness, muscle fasciculations, tremors, weakness, and paralysis.

    vi.   Clinical signs can vary depending on the degree of acetylcholine stimulation at various target sites. For example, ganglionic stimulation may predominate in some situations resulting in tachycardia or mydriasis. CNS effects may predominate, causing restlessness, anxiety, hyperactivity, seizures, or depression.

    vii.   An "intermediate syndrome" has been described with more lipophilic organophosphorus compounds.

        1. The syndrome is believed to be secondary to down-regulation of muscarinic receptors with sublethal, more prolonged exposures.

            a. Nicotinic signs predominate since nicotinic receptors are not down-regulated.

        2. Signs associated with chlorpyrifos exposure of cats are consistent with this syndrome.

            a. Generalized weakness (including ventroflexion of the neck), anorexia, muscle tremors, seizures, and depression

g. Diagnosis
   i. Cholinesterase activity can be measured in whole blood samples and compared to species-specific normal ranges. A decrease in activity of 50% or greater is strongly suggestive of exposure to a cholinesterase-inhibiting insecticide.
      1. The reversibility of cholinesterase inhibition by carbamates can sometimes make test interpretation difficult, since spontaneous reactivation can occur following sample collection.
   ii. Samples of stomach contents can be analyzed for specific compounds as well as possible sources for exposure (baits, etc.).
   iii. If administration of 0.02 mg/kg of atropine IV does not cause anticholinergic effects such as mydriasis and tachycardia, then cholinesterase inhibition is possible.
h. Treatment
   i. Decontamination should be considered if appropriate following oral or dermal exposures.
   ii. Atropine (0.1–0.2 mg/kg, ¼ dose IV and ¾ dose IM or SQ). The goal is to relieve CNS and respiratory signs. The amount and frequency of the dose is dependent on the occurrence of clinical signs amenable to atropine reversal. Atropine does not relieve signs due to nicotinic receptor stimulation.
      1. Glycopyrrolate does not cross the blood-brain barrier and therefore is not as effective as atropine for controlling CNS signs.
   iii. Nicotinic signs can be ameliorated by midazolam (0.5–1.0 mg/kg IV).
      1. The efficacy of diphenhydramine has not been determined.
   iv. For known organophosphorus insecticide exposures, pralidoxime hydrochloride or 2-PAM (10 mg/kg q12h IV) should be administered in addition to atropine.
      1. 2-PAM facilitates the regeneration of cholinesterase activity and is more effective the sooner after exposure it is administered.
      2. 2-PAM should be administered at any point following exposure to an OP to see if a clinical improvement occurs. If improvement is noted, 2-PAM administration should be continued until the patient is asymptomatic. If no improvement is seen within 24–36 hours, then 2-PAM should be discontinued.
   v. In cases of suspected cholinesterase-inhibiting insecticide intoxication in which it is unknown whether an OP or carbamate was involved, 2-PAM should be administered to see whether a clinical improvement occurs.
   vi. In cases of known carbamate intoxication, 2-PAM is not needed due to rapid enzyme regeneration.
   vii. Recovery following carbamate exposure is generally rapid while recovery following OP exposure may be prolonged.
   viii. Diazepam use in combination with atropine may be beneficial for reversing some CNS effects and bradycardia.
   ix. Atropine and 2-PAM are recommended for treating the intermediate syndrome, although atropine administration may not be needed in the absence of muscarinic signs.
16. Citrus oils
   a. Examples of citrus oil extracts include d-limonene and linalool.
   b. Products containing citrus oil or citrus oil extracts include insect sprays, pet dips, shampoos, and soaps. Solvents (degreasers), fragrances, and cleansers also contain citrus oils or citrus oil extracts.
   c. Relevant kinetics
      i. Lipid soluble; good oral and dermal absorption
      ii. Excretion via kidneys
   d. Toxicity
      i. Cats appear to be more sensitive than dogs.
      ii. Clinical signs in cats associated with the use of a pet dip containing 78.2% d-limonene used at 5x recommended rate; severe clinical signs in a cat following use of a 1% d-limonene shampoo

  e. Mechanism of toxic action
     i.   Not certain; d-limonene causes direct vasodilatation.
  f. Clinical signs
     i.   Hypersalivation (transient), ataxia, muscle tremors (shivering), and hypothermia. Other reported
          clinical signs include weakness, lethargy, vocalization, aggressive behavior, recumbency, paraly-
          sis, hypotension, mydriasis, and slow PLR.
     ii. Skin irritation or necrotizing dermatitis
  g. Diagnosis
     i.   Citrus smell may be noted
  h. Treatment
     i.   Decontamination protocol if appropriate; bathing with mild dish detergent if dermal exposure
     ii. Fluids IV if hypotensive
     iii. Skin reactions should be treated with antibiotics, corticosteroids, and pain medication if severe.
17. Cleaning agents
  a. Common household cleaning agents include hypochlorite-containing bleaches, ammonia products,
     soaps, detergents, and glass cleaners.
  b. Relevant kinetics
     i.   Not generally applicable
  c. Toxicity
     i.   Concentrated product is more likely to cause signs, compared to a product that has been diluted
          prior to exposure.
     ii. Some ingredients can cause CNS depression (e.g., glycol ethers found in glass cleaners).
  d. Mechanism of toxic action
     i.   In general, locally irritating to mucous membranes
  e. Clinical signs
     i.   Signs are generally soon after exposure and are rarely delayed.
     ii. Primarily irritants; therefore, signs generally associated with irritation to oropharyngeal or
          respiratory mucosa. Abdominal discomfort, nausea, and emesis can occur. Ocular, oral, and
          upper airway exposure can manifest as lacrimation, erythema, dyspea, tachypnea, and general
          discomfort.
  f. Diagnosis
     i.   Characteristic odors can help confirm exposures.
     ii. Laboratory analysis of limited value
  g. Treatment
     i.   Oral exposures: standard decontamination approaches (emesis, AC, etc.) are generally not
          recommended.
          1. Dilution with milk or water should be considered, although the efficacy of dilution is not
             known.
          2. Neutralization of an acidic or basic product should be avoided.
     ii. Dermal or ocular exposures: irrigation with tepid tap water or normal saline
     iii. Respiratory care includes oxygen supplementation, airway management including intubation,
          and possibly bronchodilators.
18. Cocaine
  a. A rarely recognized intoxication, possibly due to low frequency of exposure, reluctance on the part
     of owners to admit exposure, and lack of readily available testing for animals
  b. Relevant kinetics
     i.   Rapid absorption with peak plasma concentrations achieved within approximately 1 hour
          (humans)
     ii. Rapidly metabolized with a half-life of 0.5–1.5 hours (humans)
  c. Toxicity

       i. Not known
- d. Mechanism of toxic action
  - i. CNS stimulation through sympathetic discharge
- e. Clinical signs
  - i. CNS signs range from hyperactivity and seizures to depression and coma. Tachypnea, emesis, hypersalivation, tachycardia, cardiac arrhythmias, hyperthermia, and pulmonary edema are possible. Rhabdomyolysis is possible.
- f. Treatment
  - i. Rapidity of onset of clinical signs makes use of emetics problematic.
  - ii. Mainstay of treatment should focus on the ABCs.
    1. Control seizures with diazepam or midazolam (0.5–1 mg/kg IV), pentobarbital (2–30 mg/kg slowly IV to effect) or propofol (6.6 mg/kg IV slowly over 60 seconds; CRI IV infusions at 5 mg/kg slowly IV followed by 100–400 μg/kg/min IV).
    2. Correct hyperthermia
       a. May resolve once animal is sedated
    3. Monitor ECG and treat arrhythmias (see chap. 17—Management of Life-Threatening Arrhythmias)
    4. Monitor blood glucose

19. Corrosives (box 39.11)
    - a. Acids
      - i. Acetic, boric, carbolic (phenols), chromic, formic, hydrochloric, oxalic, nitric, phosphoric, and sulfuric acids
      - ii. Toxicity: injury is related to factors such as pH, concentration, volume, duration of contact with tissue, stomach contents, and titratable acid reserve.
      - iii. Mechanism of toxic action
        1. Induce tissue injury by causing protein desiccation and coagulation necrosis.
        2. Results in the formation of an eschar which generally limits deeper tissue injury
    - b. Alkalis
      - i. Sodium hydroxide, sodium hypochlorite (bleach), sodium carbonate, phosphate or silicate, ammonia, Clinitest tablets, denture cleaners, hair dyes, cement, and alkaline batteries
      - ii. Toxicity: injury related to many factors (see "Acids")
      - iii. Mechanism of toxic action.
        1. Alkalis cause tissue dissolution, collagen destruction, fat saponification, and cell membrane emulsification (liquefactive necrosis)
        2. Allow for greater penetration to deeper tissue layers.
    - c. Clinical signs
      - i. Oral burns, ptyalism, salivation, pain, vocalization, dysphagia, panting, laryngeal edema with possible airway obstruction, abdominal pain, emesis, hematemesis, refusal to swallow, coughing, and melena
      - ii. Perforation of esophoagus (Esophageal injury is much less common following acid ingestion vs. alkali ingestion.)

Box 39.11. Corrosives.
- Damage from acids is less penetrating than that associated with alkalis.
- Standard decontamination protocols are not effective; evidence for the efficacy of dilution with milk or water is lacking.
- Primary concerns relate to airway management, mucosa perforation, or later stricture formation.

      iii.   Perforation of the GI tract can lead to peritonitis, pleuritis, sepsis, circulatory shock, collapse, and death.

      iv.   Absence of clinical signs or evidence of upper GI damage (i.e., burns) does not rule out damage to esophagus or stomach.

      v.   Most common sequela is development of strictures, although esophageal motility problems have been described.

  d. Treatment

      i.   Personnel should wear protective clothes and equipment during initial examination.

      ii.   All acid or alkali ingestions should be considered life-threatening.

      iii.   Airway management and stabilization should be of immediate concern.

      iv.   Decontamination

        1. Typical decontamination procedures are not useful.

          a. Emetics re-expose the esophagus and oropharynx

          b. Cathartics may extend injury farther down the GI tract.

          c. Acids and alkalis are not effectively adsorbed by AC

      v.   Dilution is controversial

        1. Early dilution with milk or water may decrease tissue damage.

        2. Care must be taken to avoid inducing vomiting.

        3. Contraindicated if esophageal perforation is suspected

      vi.   Neutralization is not recommended

      vii.   Corticosteroid use is controversial and is not recommended

      viii. Endoscopy may be warranted to assess the extent and severity of injury.

20. Ethylene glycol (EG) (box 39.12)

  a. EG is most commonly encountered in antifreeze products.

  b. Undiluted antifreeze is 95% EG; often diluted 1:1 with water for use in vehicles.

  c. Does not appear to be a seasonally dependent intoxication

  d. Sweet taste so readily consumed

  e. Relevant kinetics

      i.   Rapid absorption and metabolism

      ii.   Metabolized to toxic products such as glycoaldehyde, glycolic acid, glyoxylic acid, and oxalic acid

      iii.   The first step in metabolism is production of glycoaldehyde by alcohol dehydrogenase in the liver (this enzyme is targeted by EG antidotes).

      iv.   Metabolism of EG to glycoaldehyde and glycolic acid to glyoxylic acid are rate-limiting steps.

  f. Toxicity

      i.   The minimum lethal dose of undiluted EG reported for cats is 1.5 mg/kg.

  g. Mechanism of toxic action

      i.   Parent EG causes CNS depression and GI irritation.

Box 39.12. Ethylene glycol.
- Cats are somewhat more sensitive than dogs to EG, although most cases occur in dogs.
- EG is not highly toxic; metabolites are responsible for most of the clinical signs.
- Rapid absorption and metabolism of EG to toxic metabolites makes early treatment essential.
- Early diagnosis often depends on occurrence of high anion and osmolar gaps and characteristic crystalluria.
- Fomepizole is an alcohol dehydrogenase inhibitor that has significant advantages over ethanol as an antidote; effective doses for cats have been established.

  ii. Glycoaldehyde is thought to contribute to CNS effects, but it is rapidly metabolized to glycolic acid.

  iii. Glycolic acid is a major contributor to the occurrence of metabolic acidosis, which stimulates respiratory compensation.

  iv. Glyoxylic acid is the most toxic metabolite; it inhibits cellular energy production.

  v. EG metabolites inhibit oxidative phosphorylation, cellular respiration, glucose metabolism, protein synthesis, and DNA replication.

  vi. The parent compound and metabolites increase serum osmolality.

  vii. Metabolites are toxic to renal tubular epithelium.

  viii. Oxalic acid complexes with calcium to form calcium oxalate crystals.

    1. The crystals contribute to renal tubular damage.

h. Clinical signs

  i. Signs are dose dependent and can be attributed to either the parent EG or metabolites.

  ii. Onset of signs can be within 30 minutes and early clinical signs can persist for up to 12 hours.

    1. Gastric irritation causes nausea and emesis.

    2. CNS signs include depression, ataxia, knuckling, and decreased withdrawal reflexes and righting ability.

    3. Muscle fasciculations, hypothermia, and an osmotic diuresis causing polyuria can occur (cats remain markedly depressed and do not develop polydipsia). Diuresis without increased water intake results in dehydration.

  iii. Metabolites of EG increase the pool of unmeasured anions causing an increased anion gap.

    1. The anion gap is increased by 3 hours and peaks at 6 hours postingestion; it remains elevated for up to 48 hours.

  iv. A metabolic acidosis occurs primarily as a result of glycolic acid accumulation (metabolism of glycolic acid to glyoxylic acid is a rate-limiting step).

    1. Evident from blood-gas analysis

  v. Oliguric renal failure becomes evident by 36–72 hours postingestion.

    1. Signs include severe lethargy or coma, seizures, anorexia, emesis, oral ulcers and salivation, oliguria with isothenuria, or anuria.

    2. Kidneys are painful.

    3. There can be apparent recovery between the onset of early signs and the occurrence of acute renal failure.

  vi. Calcium binding by oxalic acid can result in hypocalcemia.

i. Diagnosis

  i. The diagnosis is based on the history, physical exam findings, characteristic clinical pathologic abnormalities, urinalysis, and detection of ethylene glycol in serum, plasma, or urine.

  ii. Large anion and osmolar gaps are evident.

    1. Metabolites of ethylene glycol increase the pool of unmeasured anions in the serum, resulting in an increased anion gap.

    2. Hyperosmolality occurs because ethylene glycol is an osmotically active, small molecular weight substance. In intoxication, measured osmolality vs. calculated osmolality increases up to 150 mosm/kg.

      a. Multiplying the osmole gap by 5 approximates the serum ethylene glycol concentration in mg/dL.

  iii. Typical calcium oxalate crystals in large numbers are noted in urine.

    1. Crystals may be observed as soon as 3–6 hours postingestion.

    2. Calcium oxalate crystals are either in monohydrate (six-sided prisms; fig. 39.2) or dehydrate forms (envelope or Maltese cross; fig. 39.3); monohydrate crystalluria is more common.

      a. A less common form includes a "dumbbell" shape.

  iv. Ethylene glycol can be detected by bedside colorimetric tests of serum (e.g., PRN Pharmacal, Pensacola, FL or Kacey, Asheville, NC).

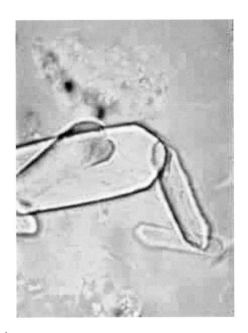

Fig. 39.2. Calcium monohydrate.

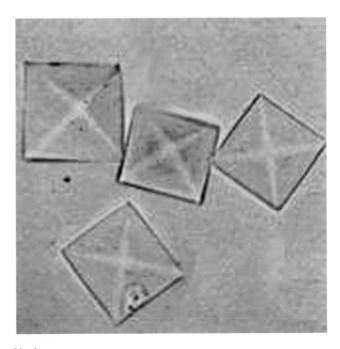

Fig. 39.3. Calcium dihydrate.

            1. Such colorimetric tests are relatively insensitive, so they are only useful if used soon after an exposure (before EG is metabolized).

                a. Colorimetric tests are not specific for EG; glycerol or propylene glycol can give false + results.

       v. Commercial or veterinary diagnostic laboratories can detect EG, but results are often not available quickly enough to guide initial treatment.

            1. Such tests are more sensitive than the bedside test.

       vi. Early after exposure, detection of fluorescence using a Wood's lamp in the oral cavity, in vomitus, or on face and paws can be helpful due to the presence of fluorescein dye in antifreeze products.

  j. Treatment

       i. The rapidity of absorption of EG or presentation after the onset of acute renal failure often precludes effective decontamination.

       ii. In addition, the rapid metabolism of EG to toxic metabolites necessitates early antidotal administration to improve survival.

       iii. Ideally, immediate hemodialysis should be provided if available.

       iv. The most critical aspect of treating EG intoxication is prevention of EG metabolism.

            1. Ethanol (5 mL of 20% ethanol/kg [hyperosmolar and has been reported to cause mild hemolysis] IV q6h for five treatments and then q8h for four additional treatments, or 1.3 mg/kg of 30% ethanol given IV as a bolus, followed by a CRI of 0.42 mg/kg/h for 48 hours)

                a. Ethanol is a competitive substrate for alcohol dehydrogenase.

                b. The CRI protocol maintains a more constant serum concentration.

                c. If the situation calls for administration of ethanol before presentation to a veterinary hospital, 1–1.5 mL/kg of an 80-proof (40% ethanol) alcoholic beverage can be used orally.

                d. Ethanol causes some undesirable side effects, including CNS and respiratory depression, impaired glucose metabolism, and exacerbation of metabolic acidosis and the osmolar gap.

            2. Fomepizole (125 mg/kg IV at 1, 2, and 3 hours postingestion followed by 31.25 mg/kg IV at 12, 24, and 36 hours) has been shown to be efficacious in cats. It is important to note the difference in doses in cats compared to dogs.

                a. Fomepizole is an alcohol dehydrogenase inhibitor (not a competitive substrate for the enzyme).

                b. It does not have appreciable side effects (in contrast to ethanol).

            3. Alcohol dehydrogenase inhibitors should be administered up to 36 hours postingestion to prevent metabolism of residual EG.

       v. Peritoneal dialysis or hemodialysis can also be utilized.

       vi. Close attention needs to be given to acid-base, electrolyte, and fluid imbalances.

            1. Calcium gluconate (10%, 0.94–1.4 mL/kg IV over 20–30 minutes or to effect) should be used to correct severe hypocalcemia.

            2. Administration of dopamine (3 µg/kg/min CRI) and furosemide (1 mg/kg/hr CRI) may help to maintain urine output.

21. Hypertonic sodium phosphate enemas

  a. Intoxication most commonly seen in cats

  b. Mechanism of toxic action

       i. High sodium and phosphate content causes hypernatremia, hyperosmolality, hyperphosphatemia, and hypocalcemia.

       ii. Rapid electrolyte changes result in CNS dehydration and dysfunction and tetany due to hypocalcemia.

  c. Clinical signs

        i. Onset of clinical signs can occur within 30–60 minutes

       ii. Depression, ataxia, emesis, diarrhea (+/– bloody), stupor, coma, miosis, and tetany

  d. Treatment

        i. Primarily supportive with low-sodium fluids. Sodium concentrations can fall quickly since hypernatremia is rapid and of short duration. Fluid diuresis can help correct hyperphosphatemia. If treatment is delayed by several hours, isotonic fluids should be used to lower sodium more slowly to avoid cerebral edema.

       ii. Extreme hypocalcemia can be treated with 10% calcium gluconate (50–100 mg/kg slow IV).

22. Lead (box 39.13)

  a. Many potential sources for lead exposure: old paints, contaminated dust and soil, vehicular batteries, linoleum, plumbing materials, grease, golf balls, caulking material, toys, lead weights, fishing gear, leaded glass, and solder

  b. Relevant kinetics

        i. Bioavailability is greater in young animals.

       ii. Lead can cross the blood-brain barrier.

      iii. Lead is excreted via the bile.

  c. Toxicity

        i. Acute and chronic toxicity not established for cats; an acutely toxic dose for dogs is 191 to 1,000 mg/kg, whereas a chronic cumulative toxic dose is 1.8–2.6 mg/kg.

  d. Mechanism of toxic action

        i. Most cellular damage due to lead is caused by the ability of lead to substitute for a variety of polyvalent cations, especially calcium and zinc, in their binding sites.

       ii. Metal transport, energy metabolism, apoptosis, ionic conduction, cell adhesion, inter- and intracellular signaling, diverse enzymatic processes, protein maturation, and genetic regulation can all be affected.

      iii. The neurotoxicity of lead is most likely due to such diverse mechanisms as lipid peroxidation; excitotoxicity (i.e., cell damage secondary to receptor overstimulation due to excitatory neurotransmitters such as glutamate); alterations in neurotransmitter synthesis, storage, and release; alterations in expression and functioning of receptors; interference with mitochondrial metabolism; interference with second messenger systems; and damage to astroglia and oligodendroglia.

      iv. The mechanism of lead-induced altered GI motility is not entirely clear, but it does not appear to be related to an effect of lead on peripheral nerves or calcium flux. Lead-induced relaxation may be due to stimulation of adenylate cyclase activity resulting in an increase in intracellular cyclic AMP.

       v. Lead causes anemia by increasing erythrocyte fragility, delaying erythrocyte maturation, and inhibiting heme synthesis.

  e. Clinical signs

        i. GI and neurologic signs are most commonly noted.

Box 39.13. Lead.
- Most intoxications result from subacute to chronic exposures.
- Clinical signs are nonspecific but most often are referable to CNS or GI dysfunction.
- Diagnosis is based on whole blood lead determination; such testing is readily available and quick.
- Treatment relies on chelation; succimer has several significant advantanges over the use of $CaNa_2EDTA$.
- Identification of the source of exposure is important.
- Lead is a significant public health concern; diagnosis in a household pet warrants assessment of the pet owners for possible exposure.

      ii.   Neurologic signs

         1. Seizures, hysteria, behavioral changes, ataxia, tremors, blindness, and jaw clamping

      iii. GI signs

         1. Anorexia, emesis, abdominal pain, and diarrhea

         2. Regurgitation, secondary to megaesophagus, can occur.

      iv. Clinical pathologic changes include mild anemia, increased nucleated red blood cells, anisocytosis, polychromasia, poikilocytosis, hypochromasia, basophilic stippling of red blood cells, and elevated ALT and ALP reported in cats.

  f. Diagnosis

      i.   Measurement of lead concentrations in whole blood (generally >0.4 ppm is diagnostic; lower concentrations may be significant but must be interpreted in conjunction with history and clinical signs)

         1. Most blood collection tubes, including those containing EDTA, can be used for blood collection; consult laboratory to verify.

      ii. Radiographs may reveal radiodense material in the GI tract.

  g. Treatment

      i.   Attempts to remove lead from GI tract are warranted.

      ii. Use of cathartics or an enema may be useful.

         1. Overuse of cathartics should be avoided.

         2. Magnesium or sodium sulfate may promote formation of lead sulfate, which is less bioavailable.

      iii. Whole bowel irrigation may be useful, but this approach has not been evaluated in cats.

      iv. Lead chelation

         1. Calcium disodium EDTA (25 mg/kg SC q4h for 2–5 days; dilute to 10 mg/mL with 5% dextrose)

           a. Total dose should not exceed 2 g/day

           b. May require multiple courses of chelation

           c. Potentially nephrotoxic—monitor renal function

           d. Can chelate essential elements such as zinc

         2. Succimer (10 mg/kg PO q8h for 5 days followed by 10 mg/kg PO q12h for 2 weeks)

           a. Not nephrotoxic

           b. Does not chelate essential elements

         3. D-penicillamine (33–55 mg/kg PO q6h for 7 days)

      v. A rest period should be employed after each course of chelation.

         1. Whole blood lead should be determined 3–5 days after cessation of chelation; continued chelation is warranted until blood lead <0.2 ppm.

      vi. Control seizures—diazepam or midazolam (0.5–1 mg/kg IV)

      vii. Lessen cerebral edema—mannitol (0.25–2 g/kg of 15–25% solution, slow IV infusion over 30–60 minutes (repeat in 6 hours if necessary); dexamethasone (2 mg/kg IV)

23. Marijuana (*Cannabis sativa*)

  a. All parts of the plant are considered to be toxic.

      i.   Hashish is more concentrated

  b. The psychoactive substance in the plant is 9-tetrahydrocannabinol (THC)

  c. Relevant kinetics

      i.   Not known in dogs or cats, but potentially has a prolonged half-life

      ii. Metabolized by the liver and eliminated via bile and feces

  d. Toxicity

      i.   Not known for cats

  e. Mechanism of toxic action

      i.   Specific cannabinoid receptors identified within the brain

        1. Primarily a CNS depressant
      ii. Stimulates sympathetic receptors and inhibits parasympathetic receptors in cardiac tissue
  f. Clinical signs
    i. Ataxia, emesis, depression, mydriasis, and disorientation
    ii. Bradycardia or tachycardia can occur.
    iii. Depression may be prolonged.
  g. Diagnosis
    i. History of exposure
    ii. Testing urine for THC
  h. Treatment
    i. Decontamination protocol should be followed where appropriate.
    ii. Monitoring and nursing care appropriate for CNS and respiratory depression

24. Melaleuca (tea tree oil)
  a. Oil derived from the Australian tea tree (*Melaleuca alternifolia*)
  b. The oil contains terpenes, sesquiterpenes, and hydrocarbons.
  c. Variety of commercial products contain the oil and the pure oil has been sold for use on animals.
  d. Relevant kinetics
    i. Little information, although likely to be well absorbed following dermal application
  e. Toxicity
    i. Not certain
  f. Mechanism of toxic action
    i. Unknown
  g. Clinical signs
    i. Hypothermia, ataxia, dehydration, nervousness, trembling, and coma
  h. Treatment
    i. Dermal decontamination using mild dishwashing detergent
        1. Possible decontamination if significant oral exposure
    ii. Treatment is symptomatic and supportive.

25. Metaldehyde (box 39.14)
  a. Used as a molluscicide (slug and snail control); present in various bait formulations (often granular) at 1.5–5%
  b. Intoxications more common in dogs
  c. Relevant kinetics
    i. Little information concerning kinetics
    ii. In stomach, may undergo some hydrolysis to acetaldehyde
    iii. Rapid metabolism is likely
  d. Toxicity
    i. An acute oral LD_{50} for cats is 207 mg/kg.
  e. Mechanism of toxic action
    i. Hypothesized to be related to decreased GABA in the CNS
  f. Clinical signs

Box 39.14.   Metaldehyde.
- Slug or snail products more commonly found in certain regions; high concentrations of active ingredient increase risk for intoxication.
- Rapidly acting neurotoxin that causes CNS stimulation
- "Shake and bake" describes the classic clinical presentation: muscle tremors and hyperthermia.
- Treatment relies on amelioration of CNS stimulation and correction of hyperthermia.

    i. Locomotor signs, dyspnea, hyperthermia, muscle spasms, mydriasis, opisthotonus, nystagmus, sensitivity to external stimuli, and seizures

  g. Diagnosis

    i. Use of products in the area

    ii. History of exposure

    iii. Detection of metaldehyde in stomach contents, serum, or urine

  h. Treatment

    i. Standard decontamination procedures if presented early

    ii. Control muscle tremors and seizures

      1. Treat tremors and seizures with either diazepam or midazolam boluses (0.2–1 mg/kg IV) or phenobarbital (4 mg/kg IV BID to QID)

      2. If refractory to anticonvulsants, induce general anesthesia.

      3. Methocarbamol (50 to 220 mg/kg slow IV; total daily dose not to exceed 330 mg/kg) for muscle tremors

    iii. Control hyperthermia

      1. Cold lactated Ringer's or 0.9% saline with dextrose 20–60 mL/kg/h IV

      2. Surface cooling from skin and hair using room temperature water; fans can enhance evaporation and result in cooling.

    iv. Correct acidosis

26. Methylxanthines

  a. Includes caffeine, theobromine, theophylline, and aminophylline. Caffeine is found in many drinks, as an OTC stimulant, in dietary supplements, and in chocolate. Theobromine is also found in chocolate and cocoa bean mulch. Theophylline and aminophylline are respiratory smooth muscle relaxants.

  b. Concentrations of theobromine and caffeine vary depending on the type of product (table 39.1).

  c. Intoxication of cats is much less frequent than that of dogs.

  d. Relevant kinetics

    i. Kinetics of methylxanthines not known with certainty in cats, with the exception of theophylline

Table 39.1. Amounts of caffeine and theobromine in various sources.

Source	Amount
Caffeine sources:	
OTC stimulants (Vivarin)	200 mg/tablet
Dexatrim diet pill	200 mg/tablet
Excedrin	65 mg/tablet
Coffee beans	1–2%
Tea	20–90 mg/5-oz cup
Chocolate products	2–40 mg/oz
Guarana seeds	3–5%
Theobromine sources:	
Cacao beans	300–1,500 mg/oz
Unsweetened baking chocolate	390–450 mg/oz
Cacao powder	400–737 mg/oz
Dark semisweet chocolate	135 mg/oz
Milk chocolate	44–60 mg/oz
White chocolate	0.25 mg/oz
Cacao bean mulch	56–900 mg/oz
Cacao bean hulls	150–255 mg/oz

1. Peak plasma concentration reached at 1.5 hours after ingestion of regular release formulations of theophylline; $T_{1/2}$ of 7.8 hours
   a. Delay of absorption with sustained-release formulations
2. Undergo rapid liver metabolism
3. Evidence for enterohepatic recirculation

e. Toxicity
   i. Cats more sensitive than dogs
      1. Oral lethal doses of caffeine range from 80–150 mg/kg.
      2. An oral LD_{50} for theobromine is 200 mg/kg.
      3. An oral LD_{50} for theophylline is 800 mg/kg.

f. Mechanism of toxic action
   i. Adenosine receptor antagonism
   ii. Inhibit cyclic nucleotide phosphodiesterases causing an increase in cAMP
   iii. Increase intracellular calcium concentrations
   iv. Stimulate catecholamine synthesis and release

g. Clinical signs
   i. Somewhat dependent on methylxanthine ingested
      1. Emesis, diarrhea, restlessness, hyperactivity, tachycardia, tachypnea, muscle tremors, muscle weakness, seizures, cyanosis, cardiac arrhythmias (premature ventricular contractions), hyperthermia, and polyuria

h. Treatment
   i. Decontamination protocols when deemed appropriate
      1. Multiple-dose AC due to likely enterohepatic recirculation
      2. Urinary catheterization may prevent reabsorption via the bladder
   ii. There is no specific antidote.
   iii. General principles of support for a critically ill patient
   iv. Monitor ECG and blood pressure.
      1. Treat ventricular tachycardia with lidocaine boluses (0.25–0.5 mg/kg IV (over 1 minute); CRI at 10–20 µg/kg/min.
      2. Supraventricular arrhythmias may be treated with a constant rate infusion of esmolol (10–100 µg/kg/min), propranolol (0.01–0.06 mg/kg IV over 1 minute; up to a maximum of 1 mg/kg), or metaprolol (0.5–1 mg/kg PO q8h).
   v. Treat tremors and seizures with either diazepam or midazolam boluses (0.2–1 mg/kg IV) or phenobarbital (4 mg/kg IV BID to QID).
   vi. Methocarbamol (50 to 220 mg/kg slow IV; total daily dose not to exceed 330 mg/kg) for muscle tremors
   vii. If refractory to anticonvulsants, induce general anesthesia.
   viii. Gastric protectants may decrease GI irritation (ranitidine or famotidine and Amphojel).

27. Mushrooms (box 39.15)
   a. There are a variety of mushrooms that can cause clinical signs following ingestion; the most toxic mushrooms contain the hepatotoxic cyclopeptide toxins called amanitins and belong to the genera *Amanita*, *Galerina*, and *Lepiota*.
   b. Relevant kinetics
      i. Amanitins probably have a relatively short half-life (hours), although kinetic data following oral exposure of animals is lacking.
      ii. A high percentage is eliminated via the kidneys (80–90%); can be detected for up to 3–4 days in urine.
      iii. May be detectable in liver and kidney tissue for many days after exposure
   c. Toxicity
      i. Not well established in cats, although an oral LD_{50} for methyl-γ- amanitin in dogs is 0.5 mg/kg.

Box 39.15. Mushrooms: hepatotoxic.
- Three genera of mushrooms contain the hepatotoxic amanitins.
- Early clinical signs are attributable to GI upset, but fulminant hepatic failure follows within 36–48 hours of ingestion.
- Recent availability of testing for amanitin can confirm exposure.
- Treatment is symptomatic and supportive, although early decontamination may be critical to prevent onset of clinical signs.

---

      ii. An average concentration of amanitin in toxic *A. phalloides* is 4 mg/g.
   d. Mechanism of toxic action
      i. Amanitins inhibit nuclear RNA polymerase II and interfere with RNA and DNA transcription. They inhibit ribosomal protein synthesis leading to cell death.
      ii. Metabolically active cells (e.g., hepatocytes) are most commonly affected.
   e. Clinical signs
      i. Early clinical signs (6–24 hours) are related to GI upset and include emesis, diarrhea, and abdominal pain; after several hours the animal may appear to recover.
      ii. Subsequent clinical signs (36–84 hours) are due to liver and kidney damage.
         1. Icterus and azotemia are noted.
         2. Tachycardia, acid-base abnormalities, hepatic encephalopathy, coagulopathy, hypoglycemia, and circulatory shock can occur.
         3. Serum liver enzyme concentrations indicative of fulminant hepatic failure are noted.
   f. Diagnosis
      i. Tests for amanitin in GI contents, serum, urine, and liver are available.
         1. The only veterinary laboratory testing for amanitin is the California Animal Health and Food Safety Laboratory at UC-Davis, (530)752-6322.
      ii. Suspicious mushrooms should be identified by a trained mycologist.
   g. Treatment
      i. Decontamination protocols should be followed if appropriate.
         1. Multiple doses of AC are recommended.
      ii. Forced diuresis may be beneficial.
      iii. Good supportive care is critical.
         1. Severe hypoglycemia significant contributor to mortality.
      iv. Coagulopathies should be treated with vitamin K_1.
      v. Penicillin G may decrease hepatic uptake of amanitins.
      vi. Silymarin (doses equivalent to 1.4–4.2 mg/kg/day PO for 4–5 days) may be hepatoprotective; available as milk thistle
28. Paraquat (box 39.16)
   a. Paraquat is a contact herbicide that is widely used in agriculture.
   b. When used according to label directions, the herbicide is safe.
   c. Has been used to intentionally poison pets
   d. Relevant kinetics
      i. Relatively low bioavailability following ingestion
      ii. Highest tissue concentrations are found in the kidneys and the lungs.
      iii. Slow release from select tissues such as the lungs accounts for prolonged elimination phase via the kidneys; prolonged elimination is also due to renal impairment.
   e. Toxicity
      i. The oral LD_{50} for cats is 40–50 mg/kg.
   f. Mechanism of toxic action

> **Box 39.16.** Paraquat.
> * Contact herbicide that is often used for malicious poisoning of pets
> * Initial clinical signs are due to its irritating properties, but significant irreversible pulmonary damage occurs within several days of ingestion.
> * There are no known antidotes and significant pulmonary involvement warrants a grave prognosis.

     i. Paraquat is selectively concentrated in type I and type II avelolar and Clara cells.

     ii. A metabolite acting as a free radical is produced in lung cells.

     iii. Oxidation of NADPH also occurs; this prevents reduction of reactive metabolite.

  g. Clinical signs

     i. Paraquat is irritating and can cause erythema, blistering, and ulceration of skin following dermal exposure.

     ii. Ocular exposure results in significant ocular irritation and corneal ulceration.

     iii. Initial clinical signs following ingestion (emesis, abdominal pain, and diarrhea) are due to the irritating properties of the chemical. Gastric ulceration and perforation with associated hemorrhage can occur.

     iv. Subsequent signs are often delayed for 2–3 days postingestion; signs are due to acute renal failure and hepatocellular necrosis.

     v. A final phase of intoxication is due to severe pulmonary edema, respiratory distress, and death. In animals that do not die from acute pulmonary damage, pulmonary fibrosis occurs with resultant hypoxemia and delayed death.

  h. Treatment

     i. Decontamination procedures should be undertaken if appropriate.

       1. Activated charcoal is the adsorbent of choice; it is better than Fuller's earth and bentonite.

     ii. Since paraquat is primarily eliminated via the kidneys, fluids should be administered at a rate to enhance urine flow; adequate fluid administration also helps to correct an underlying hypotension associated with paraquat intoxication.

     iii. Charcoal hemoperfusion increases paraquat clearance.

     iv. Supplemental oxygen is contraindicated due to exacerbation of free radical–induced lung damage.

29. Penitrem A

  a. A mycotoxin produced by *Penicillium crustosum*. The toxin has been found in moldy dairy products, bread, walnuts, and compost piles.

  b. Reported cases only in dogs; no reported cases in cats

  c. Relevant kinetics

     i. Penitrem A is readily absorbed following ingestion and undergoes enterohepatic recirculation.

     ii. The toxin is lipophilic and readily crosses the blood-brain barrier.

  d. Toxicity

     i. Specific toxicity information for cats is not available; ingestion of 0.175 mg/kg is sufficient to cause clinical signs in dogs.

  e. Mechanism of toxic action

     i. Hypothesized to alter presynaptic acetylcholine release, antagonize glycine production, or alter GABA-mediated neurotransmission

  f. Clinical signs

     i. Onset can be rapid and include irritability, weakness, muscle tremors, rigidity, hyperactivity, panting, opsithotonus, seizures, sensitivity to noise, hyperthermia, nystagmus, and recumbency with paddling.

  g. Diagnosis

      i. Ingestion of moldy food

      ii. Detection of penitrem A in moldy food, stomach contents, or urine

  h. Treatment

      i. Standard decontamination if indicated

      ii. Control muscle tremors and seizures.

         1. Diazepam or midazolam boluses (0.2–1 mg/kg IV), may repeat

         2. Phenobarbital (6 mg/kg IV)

         3. Pentobarbital (2–15 mg/kg IV mg/kg IV—give slowly as onset is delayed for 2–3 minutes).

         4. Control muscle tremors and seizures with methocarbamol (55–220 mg/kg IV; the total dose of methocarbamol should not exceed 330 mg/kg/day).

      iii. Other concerns include hyperthermia, rhabdomyolysis, metabolic acidosis.

30. Pyrethrin/pyrethroids (box 39.17)

  a. Pyrethrins are naturally occurring chemicals; pyrethroids are synthetic derivatives of pyrethrins.

  b. Exposure is primarily via use of flea- or other insect-control products.

      i. Intoxication frequently associated with the dermal application of concentrated pyrethroid products intended for use on dogs

      ii. Contact with dermally treated dogs can cause intoxication of cats

  c. Young female cats are most commonly affected, although the reason is unknown

  d. Relevant kinetics

      i. Information specific to cats is limited.

      ii. Although most exposures are dermal, grooming behavior of cats results in significant oral exposures.

  e. Toxicity

      i. Toxicity for cats is not well defined, although cats appear to be more sensitive than dogs.

  f. Mechanism of toxic action

      i. Slow the opening and closing of neural sodium channels.

      ii. Repetitive discharges occur with some pyrethroids, while membrane depolarization occurs with others.

      iii. Paresthesia may be related to direct action of pyrethroids on sensory nerve endings, causing repetitive firing.

      iv. Some pyrethroids also act on GABA-gated chloride channels.

  g. Clinical signs

      i. Signs can be limited to mild hypersalivation and paresthesia. Other signs include more severe and prolonged salivation, paw shaking, ear twitching, flicking of the tail, twitching of the skin of the back, abnormal locomotion, hiding, and reluctance to move.

      ii. Permethrin intoxication is manifested by agitation, muscle tremors, and seizures. Phenothrin exposures are associated with similar but milder clinical signs.

  h. Diagnosis

      i. History of exposure to a pyrethrin/pyrethroid-containing product

      ii. Detection of specific compounds is possible, although testing is not frequently productive.

  i. Treatment

      i. Decontamination should be considered.

Box 39.17. Pyrethrins and pyrethroids.
- Most cat intoxications are due to dermal application of concentrated pyrethroid products.
- Clinical signs are due to nervous system stimulation.
- Treatment is aimed at decontamination (dermal and GI) and controlling muscle tremors with methocarbamol.

   1. Bathing with mild dishwashing or keratolytic shampoo is warranted following dermal exposure.

   2. The possibility of enterohepatic recirculation suggests the need for multiple doses of activated charcoal (1–2 g/kg q4h).

  ii. Control muscle tremors and seizures with methocarbamol (55–220 mg/kg IV; dose is administered as a bolus not to exceed 2 mg/min). Once the cat relaxes, the remainder of the dose is given to effect. The total dose of methocarbamol should not exceed 330 mg/kg/day.

  iii. Refractory tremors or seizures may require use of diazepam or midazolam boluses (0.2–1 mg/kg IV) along with methocarbamol.

  iv. Occasionally, phenobarbital (6 mg/kg IV) or pentobarbital (4–20 g/kg IV) may be necessary to control signs.

  v. Additional concerns include hyperthermia (with possible rhabdomyolysis) or hypothermia and hypoglycemia.

31. Pennyroyal oil
 a. Essential oil derived from *Mentha pulegium* or *Hedeoma pulegoides*
 b. Has been added to a variety of products and the pure oil is available; used primarily for insect (flea) control
 c. Relevant kinetics
  i. Not certain, likely to have good bioavailability after dermal application
 d. Toxicity
  i. Unknown for cats (approximately 2 g/kg applied dermally was lethal to a dog).
 e. Mechanism of toxic action
  i. The primary constituent of the oil, pulegone, is bioactivated in the liver to a hepatotoxic metabolite; mechanism of hepatotoxicity is not known.
 f. Clinical signs
  i. Secondary to fulminant hepatic failure: lethargy, emesis, diarrhea, and coagulopathy
 g. Treatment
  i. Dermal decontamination with a mild dishwashing detergent
   1. If oral exposure, consider routine decontamination protocol.
  ii. Additional treatment involves hepatoprotective therapies and symptomatic and supportive care (see "Mushrooms").

32. Salicylates
 a. Aspirin (acetylsalicylic acid), oil of wintergreen (methylsalicylate), trolamine salicylate, keratolytics containing salicylic acid, sunscreens with homomethyl salicylate, and antidiarrheals containing bismuth subsalicylate
  i. Two types of intoxication can occur
   1. Similar to that caused by other NSAIDs: renal disease, gastric ulceration, hepatotoxicity, and inhibited platelet aggregation
   2. Acute metabolic abnormalities
 b. Toxicity
  i. Cats: 25 mg/kg or greater
 c. Relevant kinetics
  i. Rapid absorption from the stomach and proximal intestine
  ii. Delayed absorption can occur following overdoses due to formation of insoluble concretions, ingestion of coated tablets, contraction of the pylorus, or co-ingestion of drugs delaying gastric emptying.
  iii. Prolonged half-life in cats (38 hours vs. 8 hours in dogs)
   1. Due to lack of glucuronidation
  iv. Salicylic acid is the active form
   1. 70–90% protein bound

   d. Mechanism of toxic action
      i. Acute metabolic abnormalities
         1. Respiratory alkalosis
            a. Direct stimulation of respiratory center
            b. Uncoupling of mitochondrial oxidative phosphorylation resulting in $\uparrow$ O_2 consumption and CO_2 production
         2. Metabolic acidosis
            a. Renal excretion of bicarbonate, sodium, and potassium
            b. Uncoupling of oxidative phosphorylation resulting in $\uparrow$ pyruvic and lactic acid production
            c. Increased ketone formation
   e. Clinical signs
      i. Nausea, vomiting, hyperpnea (early), depressed respiration (later), metabolic acidosis, pyrexia, seizures, coma, and toxic hepatitis
   f. Diagnosis
      i. History of ingestion along with compatible clinical signs
      ii. Analysis of plasma/serum or urine
         1. Test results are unlikely to be available quickly.
   g. Treatment
      i. There is no specific treatment for salicylate intoxication.
         1. Decontamination should be considered; multiple doses of AC have been shown to increase elimination of unabsorbed salicylates over a single dose.
         2. Monitor patient's volume, glucose (hypo- or hyperglycemia), and electrolyte (hypo- or hypernatremia and hyperkalemia) status and correct as needed.
         3. Urinary alkalinization increases the renal elimination of salicylates.
            a. Administer sodium bicarbonate IV to achieve a urine pH of 7–8.
33. Selective serontonin reuptake inhibitors
   a. Examples include sertraline, fluoxetine, paroxetine, and fluvoxamine
      i. Used to treat depression, obsessive-compulsive disorders, bulimia, panic, and other behavioral problems in people; fluoxetine has been used to treat fear or anxiety disorders, acral lick dermatitis, and narcolepsy in dogs.
   b. Relevant kinetics
      i. Well absorbed orally with peak plasma concentrations within 2–8 hours
      ii. Slowly eliminated in dogs; kinetics not known in cats
   c. Toxicity
      i. Not considered to be extremely toxic; a minimum lethal dose of fluoxetine in cats is reported to be >50 mg/kg.
   d. Mechanism of toxic action
      i. Inhibit serotonin reuptake at presynaptic membranes; this results in an increase of serotonin
      ii. Selective: other neurotransmitters are not affected.
   e. Clinical signs
      i. Depression, emesis, anorexia, tremors, and cardiac arrhythmias
         1. Arrhythmias vary from drug to drug.
            a. Fluoxetine: tachycardia
            b. Fluvoxamine: bradycardia
      ii. Serotonin syndrome is described in humans and a similar clinical syndrome has been described in dogs.
         1. Seizures, tremors, emesis, diarrhea, hypersalivation, abdominal pain, and hyperthermia can occur.
   f. Treatment

     i. Decontamination protocol when deemed appropriate
     ii. Cyproheptadine is a serotonin antagonist that might be useful (1.1 mg/kg PO or per rectum q1–4h until clinical improvement
     iii. Seizure control using diazepam or midazolam boluses (0.2–1 mg/kg IV)

34. Spider bites (box 39.18; see chap. 40—Environmental Emergencies)
   a. The two primary toxic spiders in the U.S. are the black widow spiders (*Latrodectus* spp.) and the brown recluse spiders (*Loxosceles* spp.)
   b. Black widow spiders (five species) are found throughout the U.S.
   c. Brown recluse spiders (thirteen species) are found in the South, South central, and Western U.S.
   d. Venoms
     i. Black widow—several toxic components, but α-latrotoxin is the most toxic constituent.
       1. Neurotoxic—initial stimulation of nerve impulses, but later there is a neuromuscular block as a result of depletion of synaptic vesicle contents.
     ii. Brown recluse—venom consists of several constituents; primary function is to digest prey
       1. Sphingomyelinase D is a dermonecrotic factor; venom also induces rapid coagulation and occlusion of small capillaries, resulting in tissue necrosis.
       2. Immune response to venom appears to mediate the severity of the local reaction
   e. Toxicity
     i. Black widow venom: not determined for cats, but LD_{50} likely <1 mg/kg
     ii. Brown recluse: not known
   f. Clinical signs
     i. Black widow—local tissue reaction at the bite site is uncommon.
       1. Signs dependent on a number of factors, including spider and victim variables
       2. Apparent pain manifested as howling and loud vocalizations, hypersalivation, restlessness, emesis, diarrhea, muscle tremors, cramping, ataxia, inability to stand and paralysis, Cheyne-Stokes respiration pattern, and death
       3. In one experimental study, the average survival time was 115 hours.
     ii. Brown recluse
       1. Mild stinging sensation at bite site, pruritis, edema (characteristic bull's-eye appearance has been described, which consists of an area of erythema within which is a dark necrotic center)
        a. Bite sites can become ulcerated and be slow to heal.
       2. Systemic signs are uncommon.
        a. Hemolytic anemia, hemoglobinuria, fever, arthralgia, emesis, weakness, maculopapular rash, DIC, and thrombocytopenia
   g. Diagnosis
     i. Difficult since bites are rarely witnessed; there are no diagnostic tests.
   h. Treatment
     i. Black widow—antivenin available (Lyovac antivenin)
       1. Since adverse effects are infrequent when antivenin is used properly, it generally provides quick relief (within 30 minutes of administration), and it is inexpensive. Consideration should be given to its administration in the absence of a confirmed bite.

Box 39.18.   Spider bites.
- Black widow spiders and brown recluse spiders
- Black widow venom is highly neurotoxic and does not cause localized reaction.
- Brown recluse spider venom causes severe local reactions.
- Antivenin is available for black widow venom.
- Wound management is the most important component of treating brown recluse spider bites.

       2. Pretreat with diphenydramine (2–4 mg/kg SQ) or skin test
       3. Give antivenin in 100 mL saline solution over 30 minutes.
          a. One vial is generally sufficient.
          b. Monitor inner ear pinna closely for signs of hyperemia.
          c. If hyperemia noted, stop infusion and repeat diphenhydramine dose; if hyperemia resolves, infusion can be restarted.
       4. Provide pain relief when needed (see chap. 7).
       5. Fluids should be administered IV carefully since hypertension may occur as a result of envenomation.
    ii. Brown recluse—no antivenin available
       1. Wound cleaning with Burrow's solution and 3% hydrogen peroxide
       2. Some wound debridment may be necessary.
       3. Dapsone, a leukocyte inhibitor, has been recommended but efficacy is questionable.
       4. Systemic signs can be serious if they occur.
          a. Analgesics, anti-inflammatory, and antipyretics may be useful.
          b. Systemic corticosteroids early after bite

35. Smoke inhalation
  a. The most common cause of mortality involving fires
  b. Complex mixture of vapors, gases, fumes, heated air, and particulate matter
  c. Smoke can contain a large number of potentially toxic combustion products depending on the material burning.
  d. Toxicity
    i. Quite variable due to compositional differences
  e. Mechanism of toxic action
    i. Toxic combustion products are classified as simple asphyxiants, irritant toxins, or chemical asphyxiants.
       1. Simple asphyxiants cause oxygen deprivation leading to hypoxia or anoxia.
       2. Irritant toxicants are chemically reactive and cause local tissue damage.
       3. Chemical asphyxiants produce systemic tissue damage (e.g., carbon monoxide).
       4. Cyanide exposure is not unusual with smoke inhalation.
       5. Some degree of methemoglobin formation can also occur.
  f. Clinical signs
    i. Signs consistent with respiratory compromise: cough, dyspnea, tachypnea, tachycardia, and open-mouth breathing. Other signs include lacrimation, conjunctivitis, pharyngitis, and rhinitis.
    ii. Lung auscultation reveals rales, rhonchi, and wheezing (focal or diffuse in nature).
    iii. Early thoracic radiographs can be normal.
    iv. Systemic signs can include agitation, confusion, ataxia, abnormal posturing, loss of consciousness, seizures, hypotension, and cardiac arrhythmias.
    v. Upper airway burns are a complicating factor.
    vi. Skin, eyes, and other mucous membranes can be damaged.
  g. Treatment
    i. The most important component of treatment is maintenance of airway patency, adequate ventilation and oxygenation, and hemodynamic stability.
       1. Intubation may be needed.
          a. Regular suctioning is often needed.
       2. Inhalant β_2-adrenergic agonists may be useful to ameliorate bronchoconstriction.
       3. Supplemental oxygen should be humidified to prevent drying of respiratory tissue and secretions.
       4. Mechanical ventilation (continuous + airway pressure or + end-expiratory pressure) may be necessary.
       5. Tracheostomy may be necessary in cases of complete upper airway obstruction.

     ii. Corticosteroid use has not been shown to be efficacious and may result in increased risk of infection.

    iii. Antibiotics should be avoided unless there is a documented infection.

    iv. A variety of treatment interventions have been proposed (e.g., NSAIDs, antioxidants and free radical scavengers, inhaled nitric oxide, and hyperbaric oxygen treatment). However, their efficacy is unknown.

     v. Fluid administration in burn patients can contribute to upper airway edema.

    vi. Animals with ocular injury should have their eyes irrigated copiously with ophthalmic flush solution or normal saline.

36. Stinging insects (see Chap. 40—Environmental Emergencies)

   a. Examples include bites from bees, wasps, hornets, yellow jackets, and ants.

   b. Venoms are generally complex mixtures of biologically active agents.

   c. Four types of reactions are possible: local reactions, regional reactions, an anaphylactic response, or a delayed-type hypersensitivity (not as common).

     i. Anaphylactic reactions occur very quickly.

   d. Clinical signs

     i. Localized swelling, erythema, and pain at sting site; more severe reactions involve regional edema and cellulitis.

    ii. Anaphylactic signs include urticaria, pruritis, angioedema, dyspnea, and cardiovascular alterations.

    iii. Uncommon delayed responses can include serum sickness, vasculitis, glomerulonephritis, neuropathy, DIC, lymphadenopathy, low grade fever, rashes, and polyarthropathy.

   e. Treatment

     i. Localized reactions may not require treatment; possible pain management or topical corticosteroids may be needed.

    ii. Corticosteroids (prednisolone sodium succinate 10 mg/kg IV followed by 1 mg/kg PO, tapering dose over 3 to 5 days) may be indicated for more severe reactions.

      1. Fluid therapy for hypotension

      2. Monitor electrolytes.

    iii. Anaphylactic reactions require aggressive intervention.

      1. Epinephrine 1:1000 (0.1–0.5 mL SC)

      2. Fluid therapy—crystalloid fluids at shock volumes

37. Strychnine (box 39.19)

   a. Primarily used to control small mammal pests

     i. Baits generally 0.5–1% strychnine sulfate

    ii. OTC or restricted use depending on individual states

   b. Relevant kinetics

     i. Rapidly absorbed and metabolized

   c. Toxicity

     i. Oral LD_{50} in cats of 2.0 mg/kg

   d. Mechanism of toxic action

     i. Reversible, competitive inhibition of glycine at the postsynaptic receptor sites in the spinal cord and medulla. Glycine is an inhibitory neurotransmitter that opens chloride channels in postsynaptic neurons, causing hyperpolarization. Loss of glycine inhibition results in continuous muscular stimulation.

    ii. Death is due to hypoxia.

   e. Clinical signs

     i. Apprehension, anxiety, salivation, muscle spasms and stiffness (often beginning with face, neck, and limb muscles), sawhorse stance, severe extensor rigidity, tetanic seizures (often induced or exacerbated by external stimulation) apnea, and death

   f. Diagnosis

Box 39.19. Strychnine.
- Still used as a rodenticide and to maliciously poison pets, although availability varies
- Rapid onset of clinical signs
- Tonic-clonic seizures, often induced by loud noises, lead to hypoxia, anoxia, and death.
- Clinical signs can be treated with methocarbamol or barbiturates.
- Relatively rapid metabolism and elimination of strychnine results in rapid recovery.

---

    i. Detection of strychnine in baits, stomach contents, serum, or urine is widely available from veterinary diagnostic laboratories.
  g. Treatment
    i. Early decontamination
    ii. Control muscle spasms and seizures.
      1. Methocarbamol (50–220 mg/kg slow IV; total daily dose not to exceed 330 mg/kg)
      2. Pentobarbital (3–15 mg/kg slow IV or to effect)
    iii. Mechanical ventilation if needed
    iv. Fluid and electrolyte therapy as needed
      1. Correct metabolic acidosis.
      2. Maintain urine flow to prevent myoglobinuria and renal damage secondary to rhabdomyolysis.
    v. Minimize sensory stimulation.
38. Tricyclic antidepressants (TCAs)
  a. Examples include amitriptyline, amoxapine, clomipramine, despiramine, doxepin, imipramine, maprotiline, nortriptyline, protriptyline, and trimipramine.
  b. TCAs vary in their ability to block neurotransmitter reuptake and in their anticholinergic, antihistaminic, and sedative properties.
  c. Relevant kinetics
    i. Good bioavailability and rapidly absorbed
    ii. Liver metabolism is the primary mechanism for elimination; some metabolites contribute to toxicity.
  d. Toxicity
    i. Therapeutic index is low; toxicity information for specific TCAs is unknown for cats
  e. Mechanism of toxic action
    i. Extension of pharmacologic effects: neurotransmitter reuptake inhibition (dopamine, norepinephrine, and serotonin) and anticholinergic effects
  f. Clinical signs
    i. Ataxia, lethargy, hypotension, disorientation, hyperactivity, emesis, tachycardia, mydriasis, dyspnea, urinary retention, ileus, cardiac arrhythmias, acidosis, hyperthermia, coma, seizures, myoclonus, pulmonary edema, and death
  g. Treatment
    i. Follow decontamination protocol if appropriate.
    ii. Fluid support to maintain blood pressure (1.5–2x maintenance)
    iii. Tachycardia often resolves with fluid therapy.
    iv. If bradycardia is present, avoid atropine due to anticholinergic effects of TCAs.
    v. Seizures or myoclonus generally respond to diazepam or midazolam boluses (0.2–1 mg/kg IV).
    vi. Monitor blood gases due to frequency of acidosis. Maintaining blood pH between 7.5 and 7.55 can reduce cardiotoxicity (in dogs), and hypertonic sodium bicarbonate has been recommended for treating human TCA intoxication.

  vii. Patients should be monitored for at least 24 hours after cessation of clinical signs for potential complications including pulmonary edema, coagulopathy, or pancreatitis.

39. Zinc phosphide
 a. Used to control small mammalian pests
 b. Available in OTC products (2–5% zinc phosphide) or via certified pest control operators
 c. Unlike anticoagulant rodenticides, secondary intoxication from ingestion of poisoned animals is unlikely.
 d. Relevant kinetics
  i. Rapidly forms phosphine gas in the acidic stomach
  ii. Production of phosphine gas is delayed if the stomach is empty due to higher pH.
 e. Toxicity
  i. An oral lethal dose for cats is 40 mg/kg.
  ii. Phosphine gas is responsible for toxicity.
 f. Mechanism of toxic action
  i. Not certain; phosphine gas blocks cytochrome oxidase and can increase reactive oxygen species.
 g. Clinical signs
  i. Onset of clinical signs can be rapid and can include anorexia, depression, dyspnea, emesis, hypotension, shock, and cardiac arrhythmias (due to myocardial damage).
 h. Diagnosis
  i. Phosphine gas has a characteristic odor: rotten fish or acetylene.
  ii. Phosphine can be detected in stomach contents or vomitus.
 i. Treatment
  i. Decontamination if early after ingestion
  ii. Gastric lavage with 5% sodium bicarbonate may help slow phosphine gas production in the stomach.
  iii. Monitor acid-base status and correct as needed.
  iv. Provide supplemental oxygen if dyspneic.
  v. Provide other standard supportive care.

40
ENVIRONMENTAL EMERGENCIES

Lori S. Waddell and Elise Mittleman Boller

Unique Features
- Heatstroke from exertion occurs infrequently in cats, and environmental causes are also rare with the exception of cats being trapped in a clothes dryer.
- Although cats' small sizes can predispose them to more severe hypothermia and frostbite, they usually exhibit more successful behavioral responses to cold, which prevents prolonged exposure.
- Because cats have a natural dislike of water, they rarely experience drowning or near-drowning; most drowning cases are due to intentional submersion.
- Due to their smaller size, cats that are bitten by rattlesnakes tend to get more venom per kilogram of body weight than dogs and may be more sensitive to it, which makes their prognosis more guarded.
- Cats are much more sensitive to black widow spider venom than dogs. Signs are severe and often include muscle spasms, abdominal and hind limb rigidity, pain, and vomiting. The spider may be seen in the vomitus.
- Electrical injury is not uncommon in cats who are playful and have an inherent curiosity about linear materials.

A. Heatstroke—hyperthermia
   a. Definition/general points
      i. Heat cramps—characterized by dehydration, muscle cramps, and electrolyte depletion; not recognized in cats because they do not lose excessive salts from sweating; most common heat illness in humans
      ii. Heat exhaustion—inability to perform work due to heat-induced illness, including headache, nausea, vomiting, tachycardia, weakness, excessive panting
      iii. Heat stroke—includes the signs of heat exhaustion but also CNS signs such as depression, blindness, ataxia, collapse, stupor, coma, and seizures
   b. Pathophysiology—nonpyrogenic hyperthermia occurs when heat-dissipating mechanisms are overcome by heat-producing mechanisms (environmental or exercise induced), leading to increased body temperature.
      i. Environmental—confinement to an area that is exceptionally hot, such as a car. This occurs less frequently in cats than in dogs, as cats are less likely to be passengers in cars and are more tolerant of heat. Even in homes or apartments without air-conditioning, cats will usually find the coolest part of the house and remain inactive. Cats or kittens can get into dryers if left open. If they get closed in the dryer and it is turned on, they may present with heatstroke, thermal injuries, and blunt trauma. Dryer-induced hyperthermia is probably the most common cause of environmental hyperthermia in cats.
      ii. Exertional—usually not a problem in cats, but there are anecdotal reports of cats chasing a bird or other small animal in a closed, hot apartment or home becoming hyperthermic from the activity. Very rare.

      iii.   Predisposing causes can include lack of acclimatization to increased temperature, confinement, poor ventilation, high humidity, water deprivation, restriction of airway (e.g., brachycephalic breeds, obesity, or laryngeal dysfunction), cardiac disease, pediatric or geriatric status, toxicities such as amphetamines, pyrethrin toxicity, hyperthyroidism, seizures, and eclampsia.

   c. History/presenting complaint

      i.   History of exposure to high environmental temperature

      ii.   Cat may be found recumbent, open-mouth breathing/panting, tachypneic, and/or neurologically inappropriate.

   d. Clinical signs/PE findings

      i.   Cardiovascular

         1.   Tachycardia, vasodilation, initially increased cardiac output, decreased intravascular volume as fluid loss increases

         2.   Cardiac dysfunction secondary to hyperthermia, decreased perfusion of myocytes, electrolyte and acid-base disturbances, and thromboembolism leading to poor perfusion from hypotension and arrhythmias

      ii.   Respiratory

         1.   Direct thermal injury to pulmonary endothelium

         2.   Noncardiogenic pulmonary edema and/or acute respiratory distress syndrome (ARDS)

         3.   Leads to increased respiratory rate, effort, respiratory distress

         4.   Auscultation—harsh lung sound to crackles depending on severity. May develop serous to serosanguineous nasal discharge

      iii.   Nervous system

         1.   Cerebral edema, hemorrhage, infarction, and neuronal death may be seen.

         2.   Disorientation, blindness, coma, and seizures

         3.   Thermoregulatory center (in hypothalamus) may become damaged and predispose to future episodes of heatstroke.

      iv.   Hematologic

         1.   Dehydration and hemoconcentration

         2.   Hemolysis of red blood cells and blood loss into GI tract can result in anemia in some patients.

         3.   Disseminated intravascular coagulation (DIC) secondary to stasis of blood in capillaries, endothelial damage from direct thermal injury, hyperthermia-induced platelet activation, and decreased synthesis of coagulation factors by the liver

         4.   Megakaryocyte damage from hyperthermia and consumption of platelets can cause thrombocytopenia, which persists for several days after the hyperthermic event.

         5.   Clinical signs may include petechia, ecchymoses, excessive bleeding from venipuncture sites, hemolyzed serum, and weakness.

      v.   Gastrointestinal

         1.   Decreased perfusion to GI tract causes ischemia, loss of GI wall integrity, and bacterial translocation.

         2.   Leads to bacteremia, endotoxemia, and sepsis—important cause of death in heatstroke patients

         3.   Vomiting, diarrhea with pieces of mucosa, melena, and hemotachezia may be seen.

         4.   Hepatic damage results from decreased perfusion and direct thermal injury.

         5.   Increased values for alanine transaminase, alkaline phosphatase, and total bilirubin are common.

      vi.   Renal

         1.   Acute renal failure caused by tubular necrosis from direct thermal injury, hypoxia, and decreased perfusion.

         2.   Prerenal azotemia is common.

      3. Renal azotemia may develop, including oliguria.

      4. Myoglobinuria may contribute to renal failure.

e. Diagnosis/laboratory testing

  i. History of heat exposure with/without exertion

  ii. PE findings

      1. Hyperventilation/panting

      2. Tachycardia, poor pulse quality, tacky dark red mucous membranes, rapid CRT

      3. Diarrhea—melena, mucosal sloughing, hematochezia

      4. Petechia, ecchymosis

      5. Neurologic signs—ataxia, disorientation, cortical blindness, coma, seizures

  iii. CBC/CS/ UA

      1. CBC—hemoconcentration or anemia, leukopenia, thrombocytopenia, increased numbers of nucleated red blood cells

      2. Chemistry screen—hypoglycemia, increased alanine transaminase, aspartate aminotransferase, alkaline phosphatase, total bilirubin, blood urea nitrogen and creatinine, decreased albumin and cholesterol

      3. UA—hematuria, pigmenturia, inappropriate glucosuria, and granular casts

  iv. Acid-base—metabolic acidosis from lactate, respiratory alkalosis from hyperventilation

  v. Coagulation screening—thrombocytopenia, prolonged PT, PTT, ACT

f. Treatment

  i. Cooling—should be started by owners!

      1. Move to a cool environment (air-conditioned).

      2. Wet down with water.

      3. Place fan blowing on cat to increase convective heat loss.

      4. Shave if cat has a heavy coat.

      5. Do not place ice bags on patient—will vasoconstrict skin vessels and decrease heat loss.

  ii. IV fluids

      1. Room-temperature fluids will aid in cooling.

      2. Shock bolus of crystalloids (up to 45–60 mL/kg) is indicated if cardiovascular compromise is present, then matching ins and outs (see chap. 8—Fluid Therapy).

      3. Colloids (hydroxyethyl starch) may also be needed if significant hypoalbuminemia occurs (3–5 mL/kg as a bolus over 30 minutes, 1–2 mL/kg/hr as CRI).

      4. Measurement of CVP can guide fluid therapy if central catheter placement is not contraindicated because of coagulopathy (OSPT and aPTT are no more than 25–30% prolonged, and platelets ≥50,000/uL).

  iii. Oxygen—supplemental O_2 if hypoxemic based on pulse oximetry or arterial blood gas analysis: SPO_2 <93–94%, or PaO_2 <80–90 mm Hg.

  iv. GI protectants—H_2 blocker (famotidine 0.5 mg/kg IV q12–24h), proton pump inhibitor (omeprazole 0.7 mg/kg PO q24h, esomeprazole 0.5–0.7 mg/kg IV q24h), or sucralfate (250 mg PO q8h if patient is able to swallow oral medications)

  v. Correction of hypoglycemia (0.5 g/kg of 25% dextrose IV), then monitor blood glucose concentrations closely and supplement 2.5%–5% dextrose in fluids depending on patient's needs. Avoid hyperglycemia if possible.

  vi. Address acid base and electrolyte abnormalities.

  vii. Mannitol to reduce cerebral edema if patient is showing significant neuorologic impairment (blindness, disorientation, seizures, or coma) and to increase UOP if oliguric or anuric (oliguria: UOP 1.0 mL/kg/hr) after reestablishing euvolemia—0.5 g/kg over 20–30 minutes. Crystalloid fluid therapy should be increased if a diuresis occurs to prevent dehydrating the patient.

  viii. FFP if coagulopathy is present, 10 mL/kg

  ix. Pressors if refractory hypotension (systolic <90 mm Hg)

      1. Dopamine 5–15 μg/kg/min

         2. Norepinephrine 0.05–0.3 μg/kg/min
- x. Antibiotic therapy for translocation of bacteria across GI wall
  1. Not indicated in all patients
  2. If severe GI signs are present, broad-spectrum coverage for gram negative, gram positive, and anaerobes should be considered. Protocols that can be used include clindamycin 10 mg/kg IV q12h and cefoxitin 20 mg/kg IV q6h or timentin 50 mg/kg IV q6h and metronidazole 10 mg/kg IV q12h.
- xi. Corticosteroids and NSAIDS are not indicated and may be contraindicated due to increased risk of sepsis from bacterial translocation, and risk of hyperglycemia secondary to antagonism of insulin. Hyperglycemia may worsen neurologic injury.
- g. Monitoring
  - i. Temperature—active cooling should only be performed until temperature <103.5°F. Continued cooling will occur, and prevention of hypothermia is indicated.
  - ii. PCV/TS/glucose/Azo—can help assess hydration status, need for glucose supplementation, colloid, and blood product administration.
  - iii. Venous blood gas/electrolytes—monitor for metabolic acidosis (usually secondary to lacate), hypernatremia, hyper- or hypokalemia.
  - iv. Blood pressure
  - v. ECG for arrhythmias
  - vi. Urine output—monitor for oliguria or anuria. If oliguria (<1–2 mL/kg/hr) occurs after the cat's hydration status, intravascular volume, and blood pressure are normalized, treat for ARF with furosemide and mannitol.
  - vii. Neurologic function, especially mentation and cranial nerve function
- h. Prognosis—associated with the severity and duration of hyperthermia, at least in other species. No information available specifically on cats. Potential for life-threatening complications including renal failure, liver failure, DIC.

B. Frostbite—hypothermia
- a. Definitions/general points
  - i. Primary hypothermia—the body possesses normal compensatory responses (thermoregulation) to decreased environmental temperatures, but the exposure to cold is overwhelming.
  - ii. Secondary hypothermia—mild to moderate exposure to cold results in hypothermia because of an alteration in the body's normal thermoregulatory responses.
  - iii. Frostbite results in tissue necrosis and generally occurs in the distal extremities and ears; the final area of tissue necrosis can take weeks to become apparent.
- b. Pathophysiology
  - i. Thermoregulation involves a dynamic balance between heat production and heat loss, the overall goal of which is to maintain the core temperature within a narrow range called the "set point." The central control of thermoregulation is in the preoptic region of the anterior hypothalamus.
  - ii. Mechanisms of heat loss from the body include convection, conduction, radiation, and evaporation. Mechanisms of heat conservation include vasoconstriction, shivering, piloerection, chemical thermogenesis, and behavioral responses.
  - iii. Primary hypothermia occurs when a conscious animal with normal thermoregulation is exposed to extreme low environmental temperatures.
  - iv. Secondary hypothermia occurs with alterations in the body's normal thermoregulatory mechanisms (e.g., certain disease processes, as a consequence of drug therapy, anesthesia, or surgery).
  - v. Physiologic consequences and severity of hypothermia have been better described in the human literature and seem based on severity of cardiovascular compromise. There is less known about the physiologic significance of varying degrees of hypothermia in veterinary patients, especially in cats. The following proposals have been made:
    1. Mild: 32–37°C (90–99°F)

   2. Moderate: 28–32°C (82–90°F)
   3. Severe: <28°C (<82°F)
  vi. Frostbite injury is due to prolonged exposure to low environmental temperatures or prolonged contact with frozen metal objects. It starts as an initial freeze injury followed by vascular impairment due to inflammatory mediators and thrombosis.
c. History, presenting complaint, predisposing factors
  i. The patient may present with a history of exposure to cold temperatures (in primary hypothermia) or with signs attributable to, or a history of, the underlying disease process that led to the hypothermia (in secondary hypothermia).
  ii. Predisposing factors include small size, immobility, very young and very old age, anesthesia, surgery, hypothyroidism, uremia, hypoadrenocorticism, shock, hypopituitarism, cachexia, malnutrition, hypoglycemia, burns, trauma, and central nervous system disorders.
d. Clinical signs/PE findings
  i. Cardiovascular—vasoconstriction (early), vasodilation (late), decreased cardiac output, hypotension, arrhythmias (see below)
  ii. Respiratory—bronchospasm (acute), bronchorrhea (excessive bronchial mucus production), pulmonary congestion and edema, depression of the medullary respiratory center (decreased respiratory rate, minute ventilation, tidal volume), respiratory arrest
  iii. Nervous system—decreased cerebral blood flow causing mentation changes, hyperreflexia, pupillary dilation, coma
  iv. Hematologic—coagulopathy, thrombocytopathia, platelet sequestration, decreased inhibition of fibrinolysis, increased blood viscosity
  v. GI—decreased motility, mucosal ulceration, hemorrhagic pancreatitis
  vi. Renal—"cold diuresis" (due to increased central blood volume and GFR, suppression of ADH, decreased activity in renal tubular concentrating segments), acute tubular necrosis
  vii. Metabolic—catecholamine release, insulin resistance, suppression of ADH release
  viii. Frostbite generally involves the distal extremities, tail tip, scrotum, and ear tips. The affected areas are pale and cool to the touch. The ears may droop when frostbitten. In addition to locally affected areas, the patient may also suffer systemic consequences of hypothermia as described above.
e. Diagnosis/laboratory testing
  i. History of exposure to low environmental temperatures, disappearance from home, trauma, or a disease process that may predispose to secondary hypothermia.
  ii. PE findings
    1. Low measured temperature
      a. Note that some thermometers have a temperature below which they will not measure, and other methods such as esophageal or rectal probes should be employed (fig. 40.1).
    2. Mental depression or lethargy
    3. Shivering
    4. Muscle stiffness
    5. Profoundly hypothermic animals may appear dead, as respiratory efforts and heart sounds are difficult to detect. An adage that seems to describe a shared experience in emergency medicine says, "A hypothermic animal should not be considered dead until it is warm and dead." This simply states that detection of vital signs should be attempted after a patient is warmed prior to pronouncing a severely hypothermic animal dead (e.g., ECG and end-tidal CO_2).
  iii. CBC/chemistry/UA
    1. CBC—hemoconcentration, thrombocytopenia, leukopenia
    2. Chemistry—hyper/hypoglycemia, hypo/hyperkalemia, hyponatremia, evidence of organ insult (azotemia, increased hepatic transaminases)
    3. UA—decreased urine specific gravity

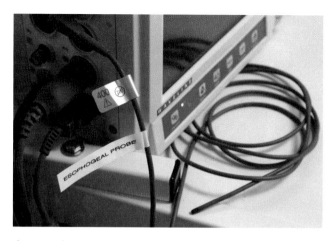

Fig. 40.1. Esophageal (or rectal) temperature probe.

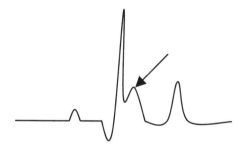

Fig. 40.2. J wave, also called Osborne deflection, as seen in hypothermia.

    iv. Acid-base—metabolic acidosis, respiratory acidosis

    v. Coagulation screening—PT and PTT prolongation, changes consistent with DIC. The enzymes of the coagulation cascade are temperature dependent and hypothermia is associated with prolongation of coagulation times. Note that coagulation tests are routinely performed at 37°C and therefore will not reflect activity of the coagulation cascade at the hypothermic patient's temperature (i.e., coagulation in vivo may be more abnormal than in vitro).

    vi. ECG abnormalities include:

        1. Sinus bradycardia

        2. T-wave inversion

        3. Prolonged PR, QRS and QT intervals

        4. Osborn (J) waves—positive deflection following the S wave in the early part of the ST segment (fig. 40.2).

        5. Ventricular fibrillation

        6. Asystole

  f. Treatment

    i. For the previously healthy patient with mild hypothermia (32–37°C [90–99°F]), institute passive rewarming by heating the patient's environment and wrapping the patient in dry blankets.

    ii. Active rewarming should be instituted for severely hypothermic patients (less than 32°C [90°F]) with cardiovascular instability, loss of thermoregulation, risk factors predisposing the patient to hypothermia or when previous attempts with passive rewarming have failed.

        1. Active external rewarming of the thorax

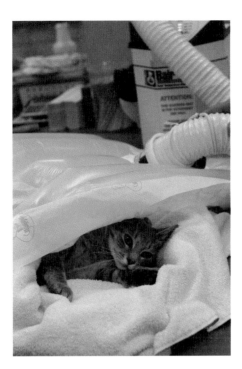

Fig. 40.3.   Forced air warming blanket.

      a. Conductive rewarming—direct application of an exogenous heat source to the patient's body. The heat source should not be directly applied to the patient's skin but rather on top of a layer of dry blankets; patients may be predisposed to burns because of the inability to vasodilate and conduct heat away from the heat source. Heat should be applied to the trunk only.

        i.   Forced warm air blankets (fig. 40.3)

        ii. Recirculating water blankets

        iii. Hot water bottles

      b. Radiant rewarming

        i.   Heat lamps

  2. Active core rewarming

      a. Administration of warmed IV fluids—up to 65°C (18°F). Relatively inefficient due to large difference between administered fluids and patient's body mass. Most useful when large volumes of fluids are being given rapidly. Note that fluid bags cool very quickly at room temperature.

      b. Administration of warmed and humidified air either by oxygen mask or intubation. Airway rewarming achieves a 1–2°C per hour increase in temperature. Newer commercial ventilators and nebulizers have the capacity to heat inhaled air. One can also cover the patient's head and blow warm air into and under the blanket in order to force breathing of warmed air.

      c. Body cavity lavage

        i.   Peritoneal lavage using 10–20 mL/kg heated (40–45°C; 104–113°F) crystalloids via an abdominal catheter. The fluid should be allowed to flow in rapidly by gravity flow and should be removed immediately. Adequate rewarming is generally achieved with 6–8 exchanges. It should be noted that active rewarming should be discontinued prior to reaching normal body temperature (at 37°C [98.5°F]) to avoid rebound hyperthermia.

    ii. Pleural lavage with active suction via a second catheter may also be employed. No more than 10–20 mL/kg should be in the chest at any given time.

    iii. Bladder, colonic, and gastric lavage has been reported but may not be as practical and may be complicated by electrolyte disturbances. Colonic lavage will interfere with monitoring rectal temperature; therefore, temperature should be monitored by other methods when using colonic lavage for rewarming.

3. Complications of rewarming

    a. Rewarming shock—with active external rewarming, there are increased peripheral metabolic demands that may exceed the ability of the cardiovascular system to meet them. The term *rewarming shock* describes the overwhelming effects of rewarming on the patient's metabolism and cardiovascular system, which may lead to sudden death. It is therefore suggested that core rewarming be combined with active external rewarming in moderately to severely hypothermic patients. Rewarming shock is also a part of the reasoning behind rewarming the thorax prior to the extremities so that the heart has a chance to rewarm and is more able to perfuse the extremities.

    b. Afterdrop—further decline in temperature after removal from the cold environment due to countercurrent cooling of the blood until the gradient between the periphery and the core is eliminated.

    c. Movement of the patient may lead to cardiac arrhythmias, including fibrillation.

4. It may take up to 2 weeks before frostbitten areas that are irreversibly damaged become evident. Frostbitten areas should be thawed by application of warm water. Necrotic tissue will require resection (in some cases amputation). Experimental studies suggest that pentoxifylline and topical aloe vera cream may be helpful in treating frostbitten ears.

g. Monitoring

    i. Temperature—rectal or core (esophageal, rectal probe). With active core warming techniques, rewarming efforts should be stopped prior to reaching normal body temperature (at 37°C [98.5°F]), as the patient temperature will continue to rise after active core rewarming has stopped.

    ii. PCV/TS/blood glucose/azo—can help assess hydration status, need for glucose supplementation, need for colloid vs. crystalloid fluid therapy

    iii. Venous blood gas and electrolytes—pH should be interpreted at 37°C and should not be corrected to patient temperature.

    iv. Blood pressure

    v. ECG

    vi. Urine output—monitor for cold diuresis (which may lead to hypovolemia) or oligo/anuria.

    vii. Neurologic function—monitor serial mental status and cranial nerve function.

    viii. PT, PTT, d-dimers, and CBC—monitor for abnormalities in primary and secondary hemostasis.

h. Prognosis

    i. Prognosis for hypothermia is difficult to predict and may depend to some extent on the presence of underlying predisposing disease processes. In humans, some predictors of outcome include prehospital cardiac arrest, low or absent blood pressure, azotemia, the need for endotracheal intubation, severe hyperkalemia, and evidence of thromboembolism.

    ii. Prognosis for viability of frostbitten tissue should be delayed until a distinction between viable and nonviable tissue can be made.

C. Fresh and salt water drowning

a. Definitions/general points

    i. Near-drowning refers to submersion under water followed by some period of survival. Drowning refers to death caused by water submersion.

    ii. Fresh or salt water aspiration may result in laryngospasm, neurogenic pulmonary edema, and acute respiratory distress syndrome (ARDS).

iii. There is little available information in the veterinary literature on drowning or near-drowning in dogs, and there is even less on drowning or near-drowning in cats.

b. Predisposing causes—because cats have a natural dislike of water, they rarely experience drowning or near-drowning; most cases are due to intentional submersion; however, curious kittens can fall into toilets, tubs, and so forth. In dogs and cats, near-drowning may be associated with falling into water, swimming mis-events, seizures, and breaking through ice.

c. Pathophysiology

   i. Fresh water near-drowning

      1. Aspirated fresh water dilutes surfactant and contributes to alveolar collapse and low ventilation perfusion (V/Q) mismatch. The hypotonic aspirated water is relatively quickly absorbed and only contributes to electrolyte disturbances or hemolysis if the volume is large (via dilution).

   ii. Salt water near-drowning

      1. Aspirated salt water is hypertonic to plasma and is therefore not readily absorbed. Alveolar flooding with hypertonic salt water causes fluid transudation from the intravascular space into the alveoli, leading to hypoxemia, hypovolemia, hypotension, and hemoconcentration. Electrolyte disturbances may occur if the aspirated volume is large (via fluid shifts and added sodium).

   iii. "Dry drowning" refers to intense laryngospasm that may occur resulting in upper airway obstruction. Intense efforts at breathing in this situation result in negative pressure pulmonary edema. Additionally, severe drops in intrapleural pressure cause increased intrathoracic blood volume, increased pulmonary artery pressure, and decreased pulmonary interstitial pressure. The combination of these changes results in edema formation due to fluid movement into the interstitial space.

   iv. Near-drowning resulting in hypoxemia is generally characterized as acute lung injury (ALI) or ARDS.

   v. The associated hypoxemia and hypotension may precipitate multiple organ dysfunction.

d. History/presenting complaint

   i. Diagnosis is generally made based on the history of finding the patient submerged in or found near a body of water.

e. Clinical signs/PE findings

   i. Cardiovascular—cardiovascular disturbances may occur secondary to hypoxemia, brain insult, massive sympathetic discharge, and fluid fluxes. Tachycardia, arrhythmias, and hypotension may be present.

   ii. Respiratory—varying degrees of dyspnea, tachypnea, pulmonary crackles, cyanosis

   iii. Nervous system—depressed mentation, obtundation, coma

   iv. The patient may be significantly hypothermic if cold water near-drowning occurred.

f. Diagnosis/laboratory testing

   i. History—history is often diagnostic (the owner may find the patient in or near the water either unconscious or struggling).

   ii. PE findings—the patient may be in shock from hypoxemia +/− hypovolemia. Dyspnea, tachypnea, and cyanosis may be present. The patient may be mentally inappropriate, obtunded, or comatose. The Small Animal Coma Scale may be employed during initial evaluation and for serial monitoring, but use of this scale has not yet been reported (see chap. 25—General Approach and Overview of the Neurologic Cat).

   iii. CBC/chemistry/UA—changes reflective of shock (increased hepatic transaminases, stress leukogram, hyperglycemia). Hemolysis can occur with fresh water aspiration due to swelling and rupture of of red blood cells secondary to rapid decrease in plasma osmolality.

   iv. Acid-base—respiratory acidosis or alkalosis, metabolic acidosis

   v. Electrolyte disturbances may be present when aspirated fluid volumes are large (e.g., hyponatremia due to dilution or hypernatremia due to hemoconcentration and added sodium).

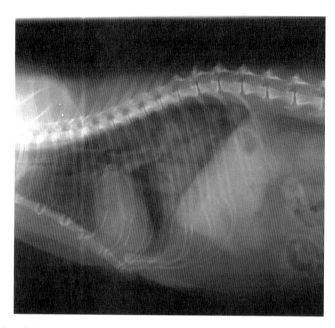

Fig. 40.4. Caudodorsal distribution of alveolar infiltrates in a patient with noncardiogenic pulmonary edema (courtesy of the University of Pennsylvania Department of Radiology archives).

    vi. Thoracic radiographs—pulmonary alveolar infiltrates (can be diffuse or caudodorsally distributed in cases with intense laryngospasm; fig. 40.4).

g. Treatment

    i. Supplemental oxygen is mandatory and positive pressure ventilation (PPV) would be indicated in most cases. As a general rule of thumb, PPV is indicated in patients that are unable to maintain normal blood pH due to inadequate ventilation and/or are unable to maintain adequate tissue oxygen delivery and/or are clearly severely dyspneic. Many clinicians use the 50:50 or 60:60 rule (PPV when PaO_2 <50 or 60 mmHg, or $PaCO_2$ >50 or 60 mmHg) as a starting point in the decision to initiate PPV. Positive end–expiratory pressure (PEEP) would enable alveolar units to stay open throughout the respiratory cycle, optimizing gas exchange and minimizing shear injury.

    ii. Optimizing cerebral perfusion by maintaining normotension and normoxemia and recognizing and treating increased intracranial pressure is mandatory.

    iii. Antibiotics should be administered, as inhaled water can be contaminated with bacteria, algae, and debris. Additionally, animals that are ventilated may be especially prone to secondary pneumonia. Broad spectrum antibiotics should be considered. Protocols that can be used include clindamycin 10 mg/kg IV q12h and cefoxitin 20 mg/kg IV q6h or timentin 50 mg/kg IV q6h and metronidazole 10 mg/kg IV q12h.

    iv. Balanced electrolyte crystalloid solutions +/– synthetic colloids should be administered. Note that ALI and ARDS patients may have increased pulmonary capillary endothelial permeability and excessive fluid rates may cause further alveolar flooding. Serial body weights, urine output and specific gravity, measurement of albumin, total solids by refractometry, colloid osmotic pressure, and central venous pressure may aid in choosing fluid rates and types (see chap. 8— Fluid Therapy).

    v. Diuretics may help by decreasing intravascular hydrostatic pressure, thereby aiding in fluid movement from the alveoli to the intravascular space; however, hypovolemia and hypotension should be avoided. There is no evidence to say that diuretics hasten the resolution of the disease. 0.5–1.0 mg/kg furosemide IV may be administered once, but it should be acknowledged that near-drowning is not a primary problem of increased hydrostatic pressure.

    vi. Passive or active rewarming should be commenced in hypothermic patients (see "Frostbite–hypothermia").

  h. Monitoring as for any critically ill patient with special attention to:

    i. Arterial blood gases, pulse oximetry, capnography

    ii. Blood pressure, ECG, and cardiovascular function

    iii. Central venous pressure, urine output, and urine specific gravity

    iv. Neurologic function

    v. Thoracic radiographs

    vi. Serial acid-base measurements

    vii. Serial electrolyte monitoring

    viii. Temperature

    ix. Venous blood gas and electrolytes

    x. ECG

    xi. Consider advanced imaging if head trauma or organic brain disease is suspected.

  i. Prognosis

    i. Prognosis for cats that suffer near drowning is unknown. In humans, prognosis is related to level of mentation at presentation. Positive pressure ventilation will optimize the chance of a successful outcome.

D. Snakebite

  a. Pit vipers (Viperidae) include rattlesnakes (*Crotalus* spp.), copperheads, cottonmouths, water moccasins (*Agkistrodon* spp.), and massasaugas (*Sisturus* spp.) and are found throughout North America.

    i. General points

      1. These snakes strike and release prey, then find it after it dies.

      2. Dry bites (no release of venom) occur in 20–25% of bites from North American pit vipers.

      3. Eastern diamondback rattlesnake is one of the most dangerous snakes in United States (long fangs, high yield of venom, and large size and strength).

      4. Most snakebites in cats occur on forelimbs, head, or neck.

      5. Bites on the head and neck can become life threatening because of edema resulting in airway obstruction.

      6. Bites on the thorax often are more prone to complications and may be more common in cats than in dogs due to their defensive posture, which exposes the lateral aspects of the thorax.

      7. Agonal bites often contain the highest amount of venom.

      8. Bites from larger snakes and bites that occur when snakes first come out of hibernation often have higher amounts of venom.

    ii. Pathophysiology

      1. Venom contains phospholipase A, hyaluronidase, collagenase, L-amino-oxidase, and other enzymes, proteins, and peptides.

      2. Phospholipase A causes echinocytosis, spherocytosis, hemolysis, and endothelial damage.

      3. Hyaluronidase and collagenase enhance tissue penetration.

    iii. History/presenting complaint

      1. Exposure to snake

      2. Swelling and pain at site of bite—most cats get bitten on front limbs.

    iv. Clinical signs/PE findings

      1. Usually can see two fang marks

      2. Pain and swelling at site

      3. May see color change of tissue around bite—becomes dark red to black

          4. May present with shock (tachycardia, poor pulses), fever, dyspnea, vomiting, hematuria, pigmenturia, ataxia, mental dullness

    v. Laboratory testing

          1. CBC—echinocytes are common finding after rattlesnake bites, appear soon after envenomation and are evident for at least 24–48 hours. Thrombocytopenia, leukocytosis, and increased nucleated red blood cells may be seen.

          2. Chemistry screen—hypoalbuminemia, azotemia, and increased liver enzymes may be present.

          3. Coagulation tests—thrombocytopenia, prolonged PT/aPTT, ACT

          4. Urinalysis—hematuria, pigmenturia

    vi. Treatment

          1. Treatment for cardiovascular and respiratory compromise

             a. IV fluid therapy—may require shock boluses initially (crystalloids 45–60 mL/kg/hr, colloids 10–15 mL/kg/hr)

             b. Supplemental oxygen

          2. Antivenin—produced by Wyeth Laboratories, Marietta, PA

             a. Equine origin so can cause allergic/anaphylactic reaction

             b. If used, 1 vial per cat is given slowly IV over 1–2 hours.

             c. Intradermal testing does not accurately predict anaphylaxis.

             d. Pretreatment with diphenhydramine, 1–2 mg/kg IM or IV, and close monitoring of respiratory (respiratory rate and effort, ausculatation) and cardiovascular parameters (heart rate, rhythm, blood pressure) during infusion is recommended.

             e. Use of antivenin may result in serum sickness (a type III hypersensitivity reaction) 5–25 days after administration (reported in humans and one dog). Signs in humans may include fever, urticaria, lymphadenopathy, edema, vomiting, and peripheral neuritis.

          3. Corticosteroids—not currently recommended

          4. Antibiotics—broad-spectrum antibiotics pending culture and sensitivity results. Protocols could include clindamycin 10 mg/kg IV q12h and cefoxitin 20 mg/kg IV q6h, or timentin 50 mg/kg IV q6h and metronidazole 10 mg/kg IV q12h.

          5. Pain management is essential; snakebites can be very painful (see chap. 7—Pain Management in Critically Ill Feline Patients).

          6. Surgical debridement if tissue necrosis occurs.

    vii. Monitoring as for any critical cat. Especially consider:

          1. Cardiovascular parameters—heart rate, ECG, blood pressure

          2. Respiratory status—RR, RE, pulse oximetry

          3. Urine output

          4. Degree of swelling and any respiratory compromise secondary to swelling

    viii. Prognosis—unknown for cats. Cats tend to get more venom/kg body weight than dogs (smaller size resulting in higher venom dose/kg), and they may be more sensitive to it. Fair to poor prognosis depending on severity of signs.

  b. Coral snakes, cobras, mambas, kraits, and tiger snakes (Elapidae)

    i. General points

          1. Eastern (*Micrurus fulvius*) and Western (*Micruroides euryxanthus*) coral snakes are the only two species present in North America.

          2. Eastern coral snake responsible for envenomations, *Micrurus fulvius fulvius* found in area from eastern North Carolina through tip of Florida and in the Gulf coastal plain to the Mississippi River, and *Micrurus fulvius tenere* found west of the Mississippi River in Louisiana, Arkansas, and Texas; western coral snake *Micruroides euryxanthus* found in southeastern Arizona and southwestern New Mexico but not medically important.

          3. Adult coral snake is usually 20–44 inches long, with a black nose and alternating yellow, black, and red bands around the body. Albino, all black, and partially pigmented forms may be seen.

          4. Dry bite rate of 25%–40%

      5. Coloration of coral snakes is very similar to nonvenomous kingsnake—use the rhyme "red next to yellow, kill a fellow; red next to black, venom lack" to differentiate

      6. Coral snakes usually strike and hold on, using a chewing motion to introduce more venom.

      7. Coral snakes are nonaggressive and bites are rare—only approximately 20 bites/year in humans.

      8. Clinical signs usually begin within a few hours but may be delayed for up to 18 hours after the bite (at least in humans).

  ii. Pathophysiology

      1. Neurotoxic venom causes postsynaptic nondepolarizing blockade of the neuromuscular junction, resulting in flaccid paralysis.

      2. May also cause intravascular hemolysis (reported in dogs and humans but not cats)

  iii. History/presenting complaint

      1. Exposure to coral snake

      2. May only have history of acute flaccid paralysis

  iv. Clinical signs/PE findings

      1. May see scratch marks or puncture wounds, mild to moderate edema, erythema, and pain at the bite site

      2. Systemic signs can include lethargy, weakness, vomiting, hypersalivation, dyspnea, seizures, and paralysis (in humans and dogs).

      3. Paralysis and death from respiratory failure can occur within a few hours.

      4. Cats most often present with acute flaccid quadriplegia to paralysis.

  v. Diagnosis/laboratory testing

      1. Identification of snake

      2. Clinical signs

      3. Laboratory testing is not helpful in making diagnosis. Mild hypokalemia, hyperglycemia, increased creatinine kinase and aspartate aminotransferase, and a stress leukogram may be present.

      4. Electromyogram will be consistent with neuromuscular junction blockade.

  vi. Treatment

      1. Supportive care

      2. Antivenin—produced by Wyeth Laboratories, Marietta, PA. Can administer one vial/cat slowly IV over 1–2 hours. Monitor for allergic or anaphylactic reactions (equine origin), including edema, urticaria, tachycardia, hypotension, arrhythmias, and increased respiratory rate and/or respiratory distress.

  vii. Monitoring

      1. Monitor ability to ventilate as paralysis can be ascending and affect muscles of respiration. This can be accomplished by observing the patient during respiration watching for signs of paradoxical breathing as well as arterial or venous blood gases. An arterial CO_2 of >45 mm Hg or a venous CO_2 of >50–55 mmHg indicates hypoventilation.

      2. ECG for arrhythmias (appears rare in cats, common in dogs)

      3. PCV for evidence of hemolysis (appears rare in cats, common in dogs)

      4. Recovery may take 7–10 days.

  viii. Prognosis—unknown as many cases may go undiagnosed. In case report of three cats, all three survived. Same publication mentions two other cats that died either just after presentation or en route to hospital.

E. Insect bites/stings

  a. Bee and wasp stings, ant bites (*Hymenoptera* order—includes bees, wasps, hornets, and ants)

    i. General points

      1. Includes bees (Apidae); yellow jackets, wasps, and hornets (Vespidae); and fire ants (Formicidae)

       2. Venom contains histamine, hyaluronidase, phospholipase, polyamines, melittin, and kinins

       3. Severity of signs depends on number and location of stings, hypersensitivity, age (kittens and older cats are more susceptible), and preexisting disease processes.

       4. Yellow jackets are more aggressive in late August/September when new colonies are being formed ("yellow jacket delirium").

       5. Yellow jackets form colonies in the ground, making them more of a risk to cats than wasps and hornets, which form nests along rooflines and in trees.

       6. Africanized honey bees are more aggressive than other honey bees and more likely to swarm and result in many stings. These are primarily present only in the southern portion of the U.S.

  ii. Three categories of reaction

       1. Local reaction

         a. Includes pain, pruritis, erythema, angioedema, and urticaria

         b. Often affects paws or head (playing with or trying to eat insect)

         c. Can result in airway obstruction due to swelling if tongue or oral cavity is affected

       2. Systemic toxicosis (massive envenomation)

         a. Requires large dose of venom from many stings or bites

         b. Severe depression, fever, neurologic signs (ataxia, seizures), vomiting, anorexia, petechiation

         c. Can result in hepatic dysfunction, hemoglobinuria, myoglobinuria, acute renal failure, DIC, cerebral and pulmonary edema, and myocardial damage

         d. CBC abnormalities may include thrombocytopenia, leukopenia or leukocytosis, and anemia

         e. Chemistry screen abnormalities may include increased BUN, creatinine, liver enzymes, and hypoalbuminemia

         f. Coagulation abnormalities may include thrombocytopenia, prolongation of the PT and aPTT, and increased FDPs and D-dimers

       3. Anaphylaxis

         a. A single sting or bite can cause anaphylactic reaction in a hypersensitized patient.

         b. Clinical signs of anaphylaxis in cats include shock (tachycardia, hypotension), laryngeal edema, salivation, dyspnea, bronchial constriction, pruritis, vomiting, diarrhea, salivation, ataxia, collapse, seizures, and death.

         c. Signs usually occur within 15 minutes but can be delayed for a few hours.

         d. Anaphylaxis to insect bites and stings appear to be very rare in cats.

  iii. Treatment

       1. Localized—often self-limiting and do not require treatment

         a. If more severe swelling occurs, treat with diphenhydramine, 1–2 mg/kg SQ or IM. Can continue with oral diphenhydramine at 1 mg/kg q12h if needed.

         b. Dexamethasone sodium phosphate 0.1–0.2 mg/kg can be used IV or IM, followed by oral prednisone at 0.5–1.0 mg/kg/day tapered over 5–7 days if severe swelling.

         c. Usually treated as outpatients, unless swelling is severe or compromising airway. Emergency tracheostomy may be needed rarely.

       2. Systemic toxicosis (massive envenomation)

         a. Supplemental oxygen if respiratory signs are present.

         b. IV fluids—may require shock bolus of crystalloids (up to 45–60 mL/kg). Given in incremental doses, as needed, based on cardiovascular parameters of patient.

         c. Colloids may also be required if hypoproteinemia and increased leakiness of vessels are present (tissue edema). 3–5 mL/kg of hetastarch or Dextran-70 IV over 20–30 minutes can be given or a CRI of 1–2 mL/kg/hr. This will reduce volume of fluids needed for resuscitation and hopefully reduce edema formation.

         d. Diphenhydramine 1–2 mg/kg IM. May need to be repeated every 8 hours.

         e. Dexamethasone sodium phosphate 0.1–0.2 mg/kg IV

f. Blood products such as FFP, whole blood, and/or pRBC if coagulopathic or anemic

g. Monitoring and treatment for cardiac arrhythmias

3. Anaphylaxis—see chap. 3—Shock.

iv. Prognosis—depends on number of stings/bites and severity of reaction. Excellent for localized reactions. Cats with systemic toxicosis or anaphylactic reactions are very critical and a guarded prognosis should be given.

b. Brown recluse spider bites (*Loxosceles* spp.)

i. General points

1. This species is generally limited to central Midwestern U.S. southward to the Gulf of Mexico.

2. Has characteristic violin-shaped marking on the cephalothorax (fused head and thorax of spider)—also called fiddleback spiders or violin spiders

a. Also has six eyes arranged in pairs—most spiders have eight eyes—and has fine hairs, not spines, covering legs

ii. Pathophysiology

1. Venom causes a characteristic dermonecrotic lesion from the hyaluronidase, sphingomyelinase D, and other proteases in the venom.

iii. History/presenting complaint

1. May have history of playing with a spider

iv. Clinical signs/PE findings

1. Lesion on skin that is often a bull's-eye pattern with black center surrounded by white areas from ischemia, and finally a ring of erythema

2. Lesions are often located on extremity or face

3. Most severe cases are those that involve adipose tissue due to poor blood supply and ischemic effects of venom

4. Development of abscess is uncommon.

5. Fever, lameness, seizures, renal failure, hemolytic anemia, thrombocytopenia, and DIC may develop, but these complications are all rare.

v. Diagnosis/laboratory testing

1. Presumptive diagnosis unless spider can be located and identified

2. Rarely, hemolytic anemia, thrombocytopenia, or DIC can be seen

vi. Treatment

1. Small lesions may heal without treatment but take a prolonged time to heal, often weeks to months.

2. Larger wounds may require surgical debridement but this is rare.

3. Reconstructive surgery involving flaps or grafts may be required for severe cases.

4. Broad-spectrum antibiotics are indicated for large open lesions. Cultures should be taken and antibiotics chosen based on culture and sensitivity.

5. Dapsone (leukocyte inhibitor) has been suggested as a therapy to decrease inflammation early in the course of treatment in humans, although some studies have not shown a benefit. Dose: 1 mg/kg/day PO for 10 days. There are no published clinical reports of its use in cats with brown recluse spider bites. Cats may be more prone to side effects, including hemolysis, methemoglobinemia, and peripheral neuropathy.

6. Hyperbaric oxygen therapy and/or oxyglobin (to increase oxygen delivery to the tissues) have been recommended for severe cases, since oxygen inactivates some of the necrotizing enzymes. Oxyglobin should be used with caution in cats due to potential for volume overload and pulmonary edema. Dose of oxyglobin is 5–10 mL/kg IV given over 2–3 hours, with close monitoring of cardiovascular and respiratory parameters.

7. Corticosteroids and IV fluids are indicated if hemolytic anemia or severe thrombocytopenia (platelet count <30,000/uL, consistent with an immune-mediated destruction of platelets) develop.

    vii. Monitoring
        1. Monitor for signs of secondary bacterial infection in wound.
        2. Temperature, heart rate, respiratory rate, mucous membrane color, capillary refill time, blood pressure should be monitored for signs of secondary sepsis or SIRS
   viii. Prognosis—most cases respond well to supportive care and surgical treatment of wound, if needed.
  c. Black widow spider bites (*Lactodectus* spp.)
      i. General points
        1. Found throughout the temperate and tropical regions of the world, including most of the U.S.
        2. Only the females have fangs long enough to envenomate animals and humans.
        3. Female has orange to red hourglass shape on the ventral, black abdomen.
        4. Venom is more potent and bites are more common in late summer to early fall.
        5. Cats are much more sensitive to black widow spider venom than dogs.
     ii. Pathophysiology
        1. The venom contains alpha-latrotoxin, which binds to sympathetic, parasympathetic, and motor nerve terminals.
        2. Membrane channels open, allowing calcium to move intracellularly and releasing neurotransmitters (acetylcholine and norepineprhine).
        3. This causes muscle spasm and pain, followed by flaccid paralysis. It also causes salivation, lacrimation, tachycardia, bradycardia, and hypertension.
    iii. History/presenting complaint
        1. Owner may have seen black widow spider.
        2. Agitation, anorexia, ataxia, pain, skeletal muscle spasms and rigidity, followed by weakness and recumbency due to flaccid paralysis
     iv. Clinical signs/PE findings
        1. Signs are severe in cats, often fatal.
        2. May have a small erythematous lesion at site of bite
        3. Vocalization, hypersalivation, and severe abdominal pain are most common.
        4. Muscle spasms, with abdominal and hind limb rigidity and pain
        5. Tachypnea secondary to pain; may develop respiratory failure as muscles of respiration are affected
        6. Vomiting may occur, and spider may be present in vomitus.
      v. Diagnosis/laboratory testing
        1. Often a presumptive diagnosis
        2. Increased creatinine kinase and AST
        3. Myoglobinuria
        4. Hypocalcemia due to influx of calcium into nerve terminals
        5. Hypokalemia
        6. Azotemia
     vi. Treatment
        1. Muscle relaxants (methocarbamol 50–100 mg/kg IV q6–8h, do not exceed 330 mg/kg/day) during the early phase of muscle rigidity and pain control with opioids or other pain management drugs (see chap. 7—Pain Management in Critically Ill Feline Patients).
        2. Fluid therapy
        3. Calcium supplementation
          a. Calcium gluconate 10% solution: 0.5–1.5 mL/kg slowly IV over 10–15 minutes if patient has ionized hypocalcemia (<0.8 mmol/L). Administration of calcium may help relieve muscle pain and is thought to antagonize the release of synaptic vesicles by the toxin while potentiating normal neurotransmitter release.
        4. Antivenin—black widow spider antivenin (Merck & Co., Inc. West Point, PA) of equine origin

        a. Single vial is given after reconstitution in 50 mL 0.9% NaCl IV over 15 minutes.

        b. Prior to administration, test dose of 0.1 mL is given intradermally. The cat should be monitored for signs of anaphylaxis including tachypnea, increased respiratory effort, tachycardia, hypotension, erythema, and edema. If noted, antivenin should not be administered. Intradermal test may not be very reliable in cats.

        c. Clinical response is usually seen within 1–2 hours of administration and is characterized by a return of muscle strength and function, initially including an improvement in respiratory function and ability to lay sternally.

   vii. Monitoring

      1. Electrolyte and acid-base monitoring

      2. Blood pressure monitoring (may become hypertensive due to the autonomic effects of the toxin)

  viii. Prognosis

      1. Incidence and mortality not known in cats, but thought to be often fatal if untreated

      2. Early recognition and appropriate therapy improve prognosis

F. Electrical injury/electrocution

  a. Definitions/general points

    i. Electrical injury is not uncommon in cats that are playful and have an inherent curiosity about linear materials.

    ii. Electrical injury causes a form of neurogenic pulmonary edema that is secondary to severe brain insult and involves massive sympathetic discharge.

    iii. Electrocution technically refers to death caused by exposure to electrical current; however, the term is often used interchangeably with "electrical injury."

  b. Pathophysiology

    i. Predisposing causes—kittens and cats who are playful and curious may be predisposed.

    ii. The amount of tissue injury caused by electrocution depends upon the amount of current, duration of exposure, and tissues traversed. Generally, low-voltage exposure (e.g., household sources) causes less injury than high-voltage exposure (e.g., lightning strikes).

    iii. Electrical injury can cause acute dyspnea. The dyspnea is thought to be caused by massive release of catecholamines resulting in intense peripheral vasoconstriction and redistribution of blood to the pulmonary circulation. There may also be increased pulmonary capillary endothelial permeability.

    iv. Injury and/or death may be caused by depolarization of muscles and nerves, launching of abnormal electrical rhythms in the heart and brain, and production of burns.

    v. Alternating current (AC) may produce ventricular fibrillation if the path of the current traverses the chest.

    vi. Protracted exposure to electrical current may interfere with respiratory muscle movement and can cause rhabdomyolysis, myoglobinemia, and myoglobinuria.

  c. History/presenting complaint

    i. In unwitnessed electrical injury, the owner may present the patient for signs of respiratory distress, collapse, or neurologic abnormalities but without a known cause. The owner may find the cat with the electrical cord in its mouth.

  d. Clinical signs/PE findings

    i. Tissue injury is generally the worst at the point of contact, where it causes deep focal burns that appear pale and bloodless on examination. Cutaneous burns involving the commissures of the lips, tongue, and hard palate may be present.

    ii. Cardiovascular—tachycardia, poor pulses, and arrhythmias may be present. The patient may also suffer cardiac (or respiratory) arrest.

    iii. Respiratory—varying degrees of dyspnea, tachypnea, crackles, and coughing may be present.

    iv. Nervous system—seizures, mental obtundation, unconsciousness

    v. GI—vomiting and diarrhea

      vi. Renal—pigmenturia
  e. Diagnosis/laboratory testing
      i. History—known exposure to an electrical source
      ii. PE findings—cutaneous burns (especially in and around the mouth), dyspnea. Note that lack of oral or mucocutaneous burns does not rule out electrocution
      iii. Thoracic radiographs—caudodorsal pulmonary alveolar infiltrates consistent with neurogenic pulmonary edema initially but can progress to diffuse changes rapidly (fig. 40.4)
      iv. CBC/chem/UA—increased CK, azotemia, myoglobinemia, myoglobinuria, stress leukogram
      v. Acid-base—metabolic acidosis, respiratory alkalosis or acidosis
      vi. ECG—ventricular arrhythmias
  f. Treatment
      i. Witnessed electrical injury must initially be treated by removal of the patient from the electrical source once the power supply has been interrupted.
      ii. Initial triage and stabilization as with any critical case with possible pulmonary parenchymal disease (supplemental oxygen and fluid resuscitation) and is mainly supportive. Judicious IV fluid therapy should be employed when the patient has pulmonary manifestations. Guiding fluid therapy with central venous pressure monitoring, urine output, urine specific gravity, and serial body weights may be helpful.
      iii. Local burn injury should be treated by clipping and cleaning the lesion(s). If larger areas of necrosis develop, treatment with surgical debridement may be indicated. Oronasal fistulas may need surgical intervention.
      iv. Patients with large surface area burns will have excessive fluid losses and will require more aggressive and tailored fluid therapy (e.g., they may require colloidal support in the form of synthetic colloids or fresh frozen plasma if coagulopathic).
      v. In patients with signs of increasing intracranial pressure (deteriorating mentation, hypertension, bradycardia), mannitol or hypertonic saline solution may be indicated. Mannitol at 0.5 g/kg can be administered over 15–20 minutes. Mannitol should be avoided in hypovolemic patients, as it will cause volume loss via osmotic diuresis. Hypertonic saline at 3 mL/kg can be administered over 15 minutes and is a better choice for hypovolemic patients. Dehydration is a relative contraindication to administration of hypertonic saline solution, and serum sodium should be monitored.
      vi. Diuresis with IV fluids, mannitol (0.5–1.5 g/kg) or furosemide (0.5–1.5 mg/kg) may be warranted in patients with rhabdomyolsis-associated myoglobinuria (suggested by presence of red-brown pigmenturia that is positive for blood on a dipstick but is devoid of RBCs on sediment exam). Care should be taken to strictly avoid hypovolemia and electrolyte disturbances with use of diuretics.
  g. Monitoring
      i. Arterial blood gasses, pulse oximetry, capnography
      ii. Blood pressure, ECG and cardiovascular function
      iii. Central venous pressure, urine output, and urine specific gravity
      iv. Neurologic function
      v. Thoracic radiographs
      vi. Serial acid-base measurements
      vii. Serial electrolyte monitoring
      viii. Temperature
      ix. Venous blood gas and electrolytes
      x. ECG
      xi. Temperature
  h. Prognosis
      i. There is little veterinary literature to describe prognoses of cats with electrical injury. In humans without burns, prognosis depends on CNS function. If it promptly returns, prognosis can be excellent, even with arrest.

Index

Page references followed by b denote boxes; those followed by f denote figures; those followed by t denote tables.